American Academy of Orthopaedic Su

D0851878

OKU

Orthopaedic Knowledge Update:

Hip and Knee Reconstruction

3

American Academy of Orthopaedic Surgeons

OKU

Orthopaedic Knowledge Update:

Hip and Knee Reconstruction

3

Edited by
Robert L. Barrack, MD
Robert E. Booth, Jr, MD
Jess H. Lonner, MD
Joseph C. McCarthy, MD
Michael A. Mont, MD
Harry E. Rubash, MD

Developed by

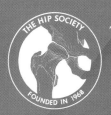 The Hip Society

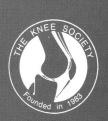 The Knee Society

Published 2006
by the American Academy of Orthopaedic Surgeons
6300 North River Road
Rosemont, IL 60018
1-800-626-6726

The material presented in the *Orthopaedic Knowledge Update Hip and Knee Reconstruction 3* has been made available by the American Academy of Orthopaedic Surgeons for educational purposes only. This material is not intended to present the only, or necessarily best, methods or procedures for the medical situations discussed, but rather is intended to represent an approach, view, statement, or opinion of the author(s) or producer(s), which may be helpful to others who face similar situations.

Some drugs or medical devices demonstrated in Academy courses or described in Academy print or electronic publications have not been cleared by the Food and Drug Administration (FDA) or have been cleared for specific uses only. The FDA has stated that it is the responsibility of the physician to determine the FDA clearance status of each drug or device he or she wishes to use in clinical practice.

The FDA has expressed concern about potential serious patient care issues involved with the use of polymethlymethacrylate (PMMA) bone cement in the spine. A physician might insert the PMMA bone cement into vertebrae by various procedures, including vertebroplasty and kyphoplasty. Orthopaedic surgeons should be alert to possible complications.

PMMA bone cement is considered a device for FDA purposes. In October 1999, the FDA reclassified PMMA bone cement as a Class II device for its intended use "in arthroplastic procedures of the hip, knee and other joints for the fixation of polymer or metallic prosthetic implants to living bone." Some bone cements have recently received marketing clearance for the fixation of pathological fractures of the vertebral body using vertebroplasty or kyphoplasty procedures. Orthopaedic surgeons should contact their manufacturer for the FDA-clearance status. The use of a device for other than its FDA-cleared indication is an off-label use. Physicians may use a device off-label if they believe, in their best medical judgment, that its use is appropriate for a particular patient (eg, tumors).

The use of PMMA bone cement in the spine is described in Academy educational courses, videotapes and publications for educational purposes only. As is the Academy's policy regarding all of its educational offerings, the fact that the use of PMMA bone cement in the spine is discussed does not constitute an Academy endorsement of this use.

Furthermore, any statements about commercial products are solely the opinion(s) of the author(s) and do not represent an Academy endorsement or evaluation of these products. These statements may not be used in advertising or for any commercial purpose.

Some of the authors or the departments with which they are affiliated have received something of value from a commercial or other party related directly or indirectly to the subject of their chapter.

Third Edition
Copyright ©2006 by the
American Academy of Orthopaedic Surgeons

ISBN 0-89203-348-7

Printed in the USA

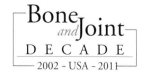

Acknowledgments

Editorial Board,
OKU: Hip and Knee Reconstruction 3

Robert L. Barrack, MD
Department of Orthopaedics
Washington University School of Medicine
Saint Louis, Missouri

Robert E. Booth, Jr, MD
Chief, Department of Orthopaedic Surgery
Pennsylvania Hospital
Booth Bartolozzi Balderston Orthopaedics
Philadelphia, Pennsylvania

Jess H. Lonner, MD
Director of Knee Arthroplasty Service
Booth Bartolozzi Balderston Orthopaedics
Pennsylvania Hospital
Philadelphia, Pennsylvania

Joseph C. McCarthy, MD
Clinical Professor of Orthopedic Surgery
New England Baptist Hospital
Boston, Massachusetts

Michael A. Mont, MD
Director, Center for Joint Preservation and Reconstruction
  Orthopedics
Sinai Hospital of Baltimore
Rubin Institute for Advanced Orthopedics
Baltimore, Maryland

Harry E. Rubash, MD
Chairman
Department of Orthopedic Surgery
Massachusetts General Hospital
Boston, Massachusetts

The Hip Society

Board of Directors, 2005

James D'Antonio, MD
  President
John Callaghan, MD
  First Vice-President
Lawrence Dorr, MD
  Second Vice-President
William Maloney, MD
  Secretary-Treasurer

Paul Lachiewicz, MD
  Member at Large
William Maloney, MD
  Chairman Education Committee
Richard White, MD
  Immediate Past President
Richard Johnston, MD
  Historian
Kevin Garvin, MD
  Membership Committee Chairman
Richard White, MD
  Committee on Hip Fellowships Chairman
Karen V. Andersen
  Executive Director

The Knee Society

Executive Board, 2005-2006

Russell E. Windsor, MD
  President
Gerard A. Engh, MD
  First Vice President
Michael A. Kelly, MD
  Second Vice President
Douglas A. Dennis, MD
  Third Vice President
Thomas P. Sculco, MD
  Treasurer (2005-2008)
Arlen D. Hanssen, MD
  Secretary (2004-2007)
Steven B. Haas, MD
  Membership Committee Chair
Ray Wasielewski, MD
  Membership Committee Chair-Elect
John J. Callaghan, MD
  Education Committee Chair
Daniel J. Berry, MD
  Education Committee Chair-Elect
Paul F. Lachiewicz, MD
  Member at Large (2004-2006)
William L. Healy, MD
  Member at Large (2005-2007)
Merrill A. Ritter, MD
  Past President
Cecil H. Rorabeck, MD
  Past President
Priscilla Majewski
  Executive Director

Contributors

Robert L. Barrack, MD
Department of Orthopaedics
Washington University School of
  Medicine
Saint Louis, Missouri

Richard A. Berger, MD
Department of Orthopaedics
Rush-Presbyterian St. Luke's
  Medical Center
Chicago, Illinois

Daniel J. Berry, MD
Professor of Orthopedics
Mayo Clinic College of Medicine
Consultant in Orthopedic Surgery
Mayo Clinic
Rochester, Minnesota

Anil Bhave, PT
Division Head, Rehabilitation
Rubin Institute of Advanced
  Orthopedics
Sinai Hospital
Baltimore, Maryland

Michael P. Bolognesi, MD
Assistant Professor
Division of Orthopaedic Surgery
Duke University Medical Center
Durham, North Carolina

Peter M. Bonutti, MD, FACS
Associate Clinical Professor
University of Arkansas
Little Rock, Arkansas
Director, Bonutti Clinic
Effingham, Illinois

Robert E. Booth, Jr, MD
Chief, Department of Orthopaedic
  Surgery
Pennsylvania Hospital
Booth Bartolozzi Balderston
  Orthopaedics
Philadelphia, Pennsylvania

Thomas D. Brown, PhD
Richard and Janice Johnston Chair
  of Orthopaedic Biomechanics
University of Iowa
Orthopaedic Biomechanics
  Laboratory
Iowa City, Iowa

Joseph A. Buckwalter, MD
Professor and Chair of Orthopaedics
Orthopaedics and Rehabilitation
University of Iowa
Iowa City, Iowa

John J. Callaghan, MD
Lawrence and Marilyn Dorr Chair
  and Professor
Orthopaedics and Rehabilitation
University of Iowa
Iowa City, Iowa

Charles R. Clark, MD
Dr. Michael Bonfilio Professor of
  Orthopaedic Surgery
Orthopaedic Surgery
University of Iowa
Iowa City, Iowa

Henry D. Clarke, MD
Attending Orthopaedic Surgeon
Insall Scott Kelly Institute for
  Orthopaedics and Sports Medicine
Beth Israel Medical Center-Singer
  Division
New York, New York

Clifford W. Colwell, Jr, MD
Director, Shiley Center for Orthopaedic
  Research and Education at Scripps
  Clinic
Orthopaedic Surgery of the Lower
  Extremity
Scripps Clinic
La Jolla, California

Francis W. Cooke, PhD
Director of Orthopaedic Research
Orthopaedic Research Institute
Via Christi Regional Medical
  Center
Wichita, Kansas

Darin Davidson, MD
Department of Orthopaedics,
  Faculty of Medicine
University of British Columbia
Vancouver, British Columbia, Canada

Craig J. Della Valle, MD
Assistant Professor
Department of Orthopaedic Surgery
Rush University Medical Center
Chicago, Illinois

Douglas A. Dennis, MD
Professor
Biomedical Engineering
Mechanical, Aerospace and Biomedical
  Engineering
University of Tennessee
Knoxville, Tennessee

Rahul V. Deshmukh, MD
Department of Orthopedic Surgery
New England Baptist Hospital
Boston, Massachusetts

Anthony M. DiGioia III, MD
Director
Institute for Computer Assisted
  Orthopaedic Surgery (ICAOS)
The Western Pennsylvania Hospital
Pittsburgh, Pennsylvania

Lawrence D. Dorr, MD
Medical Director
Arthritis Institute
Centinela Hospital
Inglewood, California

John Dumbleton, PhD, DSc
Consultant
Consultancy in Medical Devices, Bio-
  materials, and Technology Assessment
Ridgewood, New Jersey

Clive P. Duncan, MD, FRCSC
Professor and Chairman
Department of Orthopaedics
Faculty of Medicine
University of British Columbia
Vancouver, British Columbia, Canada

Charles A. Engh, Sr, MD
Anderson Orthopaedic Clinic
Alexandria, Virginia

Gracia Etienne, MD, PhD
Attending Physician
Department of Orthopedics
Rubin Institute for Advanced Orthopedics
Sinai Hospital of Baltimore
Baltimore, Maryland

Jorge O. Galante, MD, DMSc
Professor of Orthopedic Surgery
Orthopedic Surgery
Rush University
Chicago, Illinois

Victor M. Goldberg, MD
Professor
Orthopaedic Surgery
University Hospitals of Cleveland
Cleveland, Ohio

Stuart B. Goodman, MD, PhD, FRCSC, FACS
Professor, Orthopaedic Surgery
Stanford University
Stanford, California

Andrew Grose, MD
New York Medical College
Valhalla, New York

Thomas A. Gruen, MS
Consultant
Zonal Concepts
Wesley Chapel, Florida

Thomas R. Hackett, MD
Steadman Hawkins Clinic
Vail, Colorado

William G. Hamilton, MD
Clinical Instructor
Anderson Orthopaedic Research
    Institute
Alexandria, Virginia

Arlen D. Hanssen, MD
Professor of Orthopedics
Mayo Clinic
Rochester, Minnesota

Mary E. Hardwick, MSN, RN
Manager, Research Publications
Shiley Center for Orthopaedic
    Research and Education
Scripps Clinic
La Jolla, California

Sanaz Hariri, MD
Department of Orthopedic Surgery
Harvard Combined Orthopedic Surgery
    Program
Boston, Massachusetts

Aaron A. Hofmann, MD
Professor
Department of Orthopaedics
University of Utah School of Medicine
Salt Lake City, Utah

David S. Hungerford, MD
Johns Hopkins Orthopaedics at
    Good Samaritan Hospital
Baltimore, Maryland

Marc W. Hungerford, MD
Assistant Professor
Orthopaedics
Johns Hopkins University
Baltimore, Maryland

David J. Jacofsky, MD
Instructor
Department of Orthopedics
Mayo Clinic School of Medicine
Rochester, Minnesota

Branislav Jaramaz, PhD
Associate Director
Scientific Director
Institute for Computer Assisted
    Orthopaedic Surgery (ICAOS)
The Western Pennsylvania Hospital
Pittsburgh, Pennsylvania

Julie M. Keller, MD
Department of Orthopaedic Surgery
Center for Hip & Knee Replacement
Columbia University
New York, New York

Ira H. Kirschenbaum, MD
Adjunct Attending
Orthopaedic Surgery
Hospital for Joint Disease/Orthopaedic
    Institute
New York, New York

Richard D. Komistek, PhD
Professor
Biomedical Engineering
Mechanical, Aerospace and Biomedical
    Engineering
University of Tennessee
Knoxville Tennessee

Kenneth A. Krackow, MD
Professor and Vice Chairman
Department of Orthopaedic Surgery
State University of New York at Buffalo
Clinical Director
Department of Orthopaedic Surgery
Kaleida Health-Buffalo General Hospital
Buffalo, New York

Richard S. Laskin, MD
Hospital for Special Surgery
New York, New York

Wayne B. Leadbetter, MD
Attending Orthopedic Surgeon
Center for Joint Preservation and
    Replacement
Rubin Institute for Advanced
    Orthopedics
Sinai Hospital
Baltimore, Maryland

Jo-ann Lee, MS
New England Baptist Hospital
Boston, Massachusetts

David G. Lewallen, MD
Professor of Orthopedic Surgery
Mayo Medical School
Chair, Division of Adult
    Reconstruction
Department of Orthopedic Surgery
Mayo Clinic
Rochester, Minnesota

Jess H. Lonner, MD
Director of Knee Arthroplasty
    Service
Booth Bartolozzi Balderston
    Orthopaedics
Pennsylvania Hospital
Philadelphia, Pennsylvania

William Macaulay, MD
Director, Center for Hip and Knee
    Replacement
Department of Orthopaedic Surgery
Columbia University
New York, New York

Mohamed R. Mahfouz, PhD
Associate Professor
Biomedical Engineering
Mechanical, Aerospace and
    Biomedical Engineering
University of Tennessee
Knoxville, Tennessee

William J. Maloney, MD
Elsbach-Richard Professor and Chairman
Department of Orthopaedic Surgery
Stanford University Medical Center
Stanford, California

Michael T. Manley, FRSA, PhD
Consultant Bioengineer
Ridgewood, New Jersey

Bassam A. Masri, MD, FRCSC
Associate Professor and Head of
    Reconstructive Orthopaedics
Department of Orthopaedics
University of British Columbia
Vancouver, British Columbia, Canada

Joseph C. McCarthy, MD
Clinical Professor of Orthopedic
    Surgery
New England Baptist Hospital
Boston, Massachusetts

William A. McGann, MD
Associate Director
San Francisco Orthopaedic Residency
    Program
Chief, Department of Orthopaedics
St. Mary's Medical Center
San Francisco, California

David A. McQueen, MD
Program Director, Department of
    Surgery
University of Kansas School of
    Medicine-Wichita
Medical Director, Orthopaedic
    Research Institute
Kansas Joint & Spine Institute
Wichita, Kansas

William M. Mihalko, MD, PhD
Associate Professor
Department of Orthopaedic Surgery
University of Virginia
Charlottesville, Virginia

Michael A. Mont, MD
Director, Center for Joint Preservation
    and Reconstruction Orthopedics
Sinai Hospital of Baltimore
Rubin Institute for Advanced
    Orthopedics
Baltimore, Maryland

Andrew B. Mor, PhD
Research Scientist
Institute for Computer Assisted
    Orthopaedic Surgery (ICAOS)
The Western Pennsylvania Hospital
Pittsburgh, Pennsylvania

Kevin J. Mulhall, MD, MCh, FRCSI
    (Tr & Orth)
Department of Orthopaedic Surgery
Mater Misericordiae University Hospital
Dublin, Ireland

Orhun K. Muratoglu, PhD
Co-Director, Orthopaedic Biomechan-
    ics & Biomaterials Laboratory
Massachusetts General Hospital
Boston, Massachusetts

Nicholas O. Noiseux, MD, FRCSC
Adult Reconstruction
Department of Orthopedic Surgery
Mayo Clinic
Rochester, Minnesota

Mark W. Pagnano, MD
Associate Professor of Orthopedic
    Surgery
Mayo College of Medicine
Mayo Clinic
Rochester, Minnesota

Wayne G. Paprosky, MD, FACS
Associate Professor
Department of Adult Joint
    Reconstruction
Rush University Medical Center
Chicago, Illinois

Phillip S. Ragland, MD
Physician
Orthopaedics
Sinai Hospital of Baltimore
Baltimore, Maryland

Chitranjan S. Ranawat, MD
Chairman, Department of Orthopaedic
    Surgery
Chairman, Ranawat Orthopaedic Center
Lenox Hill Hospital
New York, New York

Vijay J. Rasquinha, MD
Attending Orthopaedic Surgeon
Lenox Hill Hospital
New York, New York

Aaron G. Rosenberg, MD
Professor
Department of Orthopaedic Surgery
Rush University Medical Center
Chicago, Illinois

Harry E. Rubash, MD
Chairman
Department of Orthopedic Surgery
Massachusetts General Hospital
Boston, Massachusetts

Khaled J. Saleh, MD, MSc (Epid),
    FRCSC, FACS
Associate Professor, Department of
    Orthopaedic Surgery, School of
    Medicine
Adjunct Associate Professor,
    Health Services Research &
    Policy, School of Public Health
Director of Orthopaedic Research,
    Veterans Affairs Medical Centre
University of Minnesota
Minneapolis, Minnesota

Carlton G. Savory, MD
Hughston Orthopaedics and Sports
    Medicine
Columbus, Georgia

Thomas P. Schmalzreid, MD
Orthopaedics
University of California–Los Angeles
Los Angeles, California

John R. Schurman II, MD
Assistant Professor
University of Kansas School of
    Medicine-Wichita
Kansas Joint & Spine Institute
Wichita, Kansas

Richard D. Scott, MD
Professor of Orthopaedic Surgery
Harvard Medical School
Boston, Massachusetts

W. Norman Scott, MD
Professor and Chairman of
  Orthopaedic Surgery
Orthopaedic Surgery at Beth Israel
  Insall Scott Kelly Institute
New York, New York

Giles R. Scuderi, MD
Director
Insall Scott Kelly Institute
New York, New York

Nigel E. Sharrock, MB, ChB
Attending Anesthesiologist
Senior Scientist
Anesthesiology
Hospital for Special Surgery
New York, New York

Scott M. Sporer, MD, MS
Assistant Professor Orthopaedic
  Surgery
Rush University Medical Center
Chicago, Illinois

Steven H. Stern, MD
Clinical Associate Professor of
  Orthopaedics
Northwestern University
Chicago, Illinois

James B. Stiehl, MD
Clinical Associate Professor of
  Orthopaedic Surgery
Department of Orthopaedic Surgery
Medical College of Wisconsin
Milwaukee, Wisconsin

Steven A. Stuchin, MD
Associate Professor of Orthopedics
New York University School of Medicine
Director of Orthopedic Surgery
New York University Hospital for
  Joint Diseases
New York, New York

Issada Thongtrangan, MD
Adult Reconstructive Surgery
Department of Orthopaedic Surgery
University of Minnesota
Minneapolis, Minnesota

Robert T. Trousdale, MD
Professor of Orthopaedic Surgery
Mayo Clinic
Rochester, Minnesota

John H. Velyvis, MD
Desert Orthopaedic Center
Rancho Mirage, California

Peter S. Walker, PhD
Professor, Department of Surgery
New York University School of
  Medicine
Hospital for Joint Diseases
Veterans Administration Medical Center
New York, New York

Jean F. Welter, MD, PhD
Assistant Professor
Orthopaedics
Case Western Reserve University
Cleveland, Ohio

Steven T. Woolson, MD
Adjunct Clinical Professor
Orthopaedic Surgery
Stanford University Medical School
Stanford, California

Steven B. Zelicof, MD, PhD
Associate Professor of Clinical
  Orthopaedic Surgery
Department of Orthopaedic Surgery
New York Medical Center
Valhalla, New York

Preface

*O*rthopaedic Knowledge Update: Hip and Knee Reconstruction 3 complements and expands information that was published in the two previous editions. The first edition was published in 1995 and the second in 2000, with the current edition encompassing knowledge current through the first 10 months of 2005. The previous updates can be used as information resources, but the current editors have tried to use the third edition as an update that can stand on its own.

This edition should provide residents, fellows, and practicing orthopaedists with a clear understanding of the state-of-the-art knowledge relevant to adult hip and knee reconstruction. As in the previous publications, it can be used as a resource for both general orthopaedic surgeons as well as hip and knee specialists.

The third edition has been expanded from the previous volumes. There are at least ten unique chapters that we believe are relevant to practicing orthopaedists. Some of the exciting new chapters include minimally invasive approaches to the hip and knee, computerized navigation methods, hip arthroscopy, as well as metal-on-metal resurfacing hip arthroplasty. All of the chapters have been written by experts in each field, with an attempt made to reflect the current state of hip and knee reconstruction knowledge by being as objective as possible.

We, the editors, would like to thank all of the authors for their efforts and timely completion of their chapters. We also gratefully acknowledge the invaluable assistance of Keith Huff, Lisa Claxton Moore, Kathleen Anderson, Sophie Tosta, and Marilyn Fox, PhD, in the Publications Department at the American Academy of Orthopaedic Surgeons. They did tremendous work to make this book of the highest quality.

Robert L. Barrack, MD
Robert E. Booth, Jr, MD
Jess H. Lonner, MD
Joseph C. McCarthy, MD
Michael A. Mont, MD
Harry E. Rubash, MD
Editors

Table of Contents

Section 1: The Knee

Section Editors: Robert L. Barrack, MD
Robert E. Booth, Jr, MD
Jess H. Lonner, MD

Section 2: Basic Science and General Knowledge
Section Editors: Michael A. Mont, MD
Harry E. Rubash, MD

Section 3: The Hip

Section Editors: Joseph C. McCarthy, MD
Harry E. Rubash, MD

Section 1

The Knee

Section Editors:
Robert L. Barrack, MD
Robert E. Booth, Jr, MD
Jess H. Lonner, MD

Chapter 1

Surgical Exposure in Total Knee Arthroplasty

Steven H. Stern, MD

Introduction

As with any surgery, adequate surgical exposure is required in knee arthroplasty to optimize the surgical outcome. Visualization of the relevant anatomy allows surgeons to optimize alignment and fixation, both of which are required to achieve a successful result. The basic anterior surgical approach allows for dissection through a region that minimizes risk to neurovascular structures. However, there are several unique aspects of knee arthroplasty that place extra emphasis on surgical exposure and handling of the soft tissues. The knee is a relatively superficial joint; although this allows for a relatively straightforward dissection down to the knee capsule, it also means that the soft-tissue envelope protecting the knee and prosthesis is not extensive. In addition, surgeons who perform knee arthroplasty are faced with the twin goals of obtaining soft-tissue healing and maximizing knee motion. These two goals are often difficult to achieve without one compromising the other. In certain patients, excessive early motion may put the soft-tissue envelope at risk, whereas extensive immobilization to enhance wound healing may result in an unacceptable risk of stiffness and fibrosis. Thus, adequate exposure needs to be achieved and excessive skin and soft-tissue tension needs to be minimized.

Historically, exposure in knee arthroplasty has followed some of the basic tenets of surgical dissection in general. An extensile approach is commonly used. Thus, dissection can be extended either proximally or distally if needed. One long incision is preferred to several shorter incisions. However, it is widely accepted that prior transverse incisions can be successfully crossed at right angles by newer longitudinal incisions. If possible, previous vertical incisions should be incorporated into current skin incisions, and parallel incisions should be avoided. However, old vertical incisions are occasionally in areas that make their inclusion in a current longitudinal approach impractical and undesirable. In such instances, it may be necessary to make a second vertical incision, leaving as wide a soft-tissue bridge between the two wounds as possible. Finally, the possible need for future surgical procedures should always be considered at the time of any skin incision.

Primary Procedures

A standard anterior midline incision with a medial parapatellar arthrotomy remains the most common method of exposure for knee arthroplasty procedures. However, there are certain circumstances that require (and certain surgeons who prefer) alternative surgical approaches. Alternate methods include a lateral arthrotomy and variation in the location, length, and soft-tissue interval used with the medial arthrotomy. The medial arthrotomy options tend to vary the amount of dissection through the extensor mechanism. The standard anterior approach with a midline or medial parapatellar arthrotomy dissects directly through the extensor mechanism. Because of this disruption, some authors advocate either a midvastus or subvastus approach for total knee replacements. In addition, for certain revision procedures and/or for knees that have undergone ankylosis, it is often necessary to perform either proximal soft-tissue releases or distal bone osteotomies to enhance visualization.

Anterior Approach for Knee Arthroplasty

The anterior approach is extensile, allowing access to both the distal femur and proximal tibia. Patellar eversion permits excellent visualization of all knee compartments. An anterior knee approach can be used for fracture, arthroplasty, and extensor mechanism procedures. Multiple procedures can be performed through the same incision with excellent visualization of medial and lateral structures and minimal risk of neurovascular injury. Although the basic philosophy behind all anterior exposures is similar, there are slight variations in technique. Skin incisions can be made directly midline or with slight medial or lateral curves (Figure 1). Some surgeons believe there is a theoretic benefit to wound healing with a curved medial parapatellar skin incision. A medial parapatellar skin incision is preferred by a small number of surgeons, but most favor a straight midline

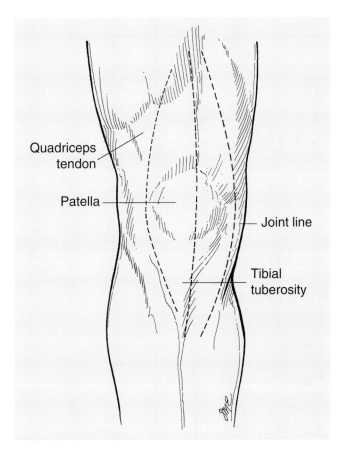

Figure 1 Schematic representation of skin incisions for an anterior knee approach (*dashed lines*). *(Reproduced with permission from Stern SH: Surgical exposure in total knee arthroplasty, in Harner CD, Vince KG, Fu FH (eds): Knee Surgery. Baltimore, MD, Williams & Wilkins, 1994, pp 1289-1302.)*

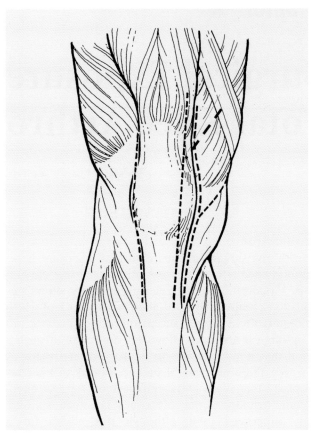

Figure 2 Schematic representation of possible retinacular capsular incisions in total knee arthroplasty (*dashed lines*): lateral parapatellar, straight medial, medial parapatellar, midvastus, and subvastus approaches. *(Reproduced with permission from Stern SH: Surgical exposure in total knee arthroplasty, in Harner CD, Vince KG, Fu FH (eds): Knee Surgery. Baltimore, MD, Williams & Wilkins, 1994, pp 1289-1302.)*

incision. Others favor a compromise with a straight or very gently curved incision made slightly medial to midline. Lateral skin incisions associated with medial arthrotomies are normally not encouraged because of the extensive skin flaps they require.

After the skin is incised, dissection is carried down directly through the subcutaneous tissue. This method allows for exposure of the extensor mechanism, including the quadriceps and patellar tendons. After adequate visualization of the extensor mechanism, most surgeons perform a medial retinacular arthrotomy. A medial arthrotomy allows for eversion of the patella laterally and exposure of the knee joint proper. The medial retinacular incision can be either curved or straight (Figure 2). Insall advocated a straight medial retinacular exposure and suggested starting the medial arthrotomy incision along the medial aspect of the quadriceps tendon, continuing over the medial aspect of the patellar, and finishing distally on the anterior tibial cortex. In this technique, the quadriceps expansion, including periosteum, is sharply dissected from the medial patella. Theoretically, this results in less damage to the distal insertion of the vastus medialis. Insall preferred this technique to a

curved parapatellar retinacular incision because the curved retinacular incision transected the insertion of the vastus medialis into the patella.

Others advocate a medial parapatellar retinacular incision in which the retinacular incision is medial to the patella. The incision starts through the medial portion of the quadriceps tendon. With this method, however, dissection proceeds distally through the anteromedial knee capsule, not directly over the patellar bone. The incision then curves back to the medial aspect of the patellar tendon and extends distally onto the proximal tibia. This method allows for a thicker cuff of soft tissue for closure at the level of the patellar bone.

After the arthrotomy is performed, the knee is flexed and the patellar tendon everted. Care should be taken to avoid placing excessive tension on the patellar tendon. In revision surgery or with obese patients, it may be necessary to extend the dissection further proximally to help facilitate patellar eversion. In certain patients, patellar eversion may not be possible and/or desirable. In these circumstances, the knee arthroplasty may be performed by retracting the extensor mechanism and patella laterally. At this point, exposure should

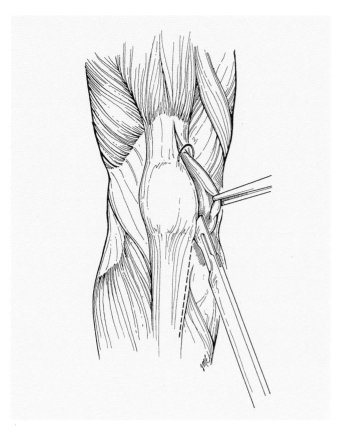

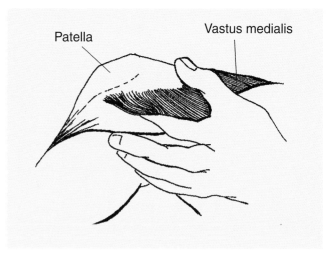

Figure 4 Schematic representation showing blunt dissection allowing the vastus medialis to be released from the intermuscular septum. *(Reproduced with permission from Roysam GS, Oakley MJ: Subvastus approach for TKA: A prospective, randomized, and observer-blinded trial.* J Arthroplasty *2001;16:454-457.)*

Figure 3 Schematic representation of the placement of an initial retinacular suture during closure to minimize patella baja complications. *(Reproduced with permission from Stern SH: Surgical exposure in total knee arthroplasty, in Harner CD, Vince KG, Fu FH (eds):* Knee Surgery. *Baltimore, MD, Williams & Wilkins, 1994, pp 1289-1302.)*

be adequate to perform a knee arthroplasty. The exact order of cuts and instruments used depends on the knee alignment and prosthesis to be implanted.

During closure, care should be taken when positioning the initial sutures to appropriately realign the previously incised extensor mechanism. Specifically, care should be taken to minimize patella baja, which is associated with prior knee procedures, by placing the initial suture in a specific oblique manner (Figure 3). The arthrotomy and subcutaneous tissue can be approximated in a variety of ways depending on surgeon preference.

Subvastus Approach

The subvastus approach was first described in 1929, but it fell out of favor over the next several decades. One advantage of the subvastus technique is that it preserves an intact extensor mechanism. Thus, advocates of the subvastus approach believe it results in less postoperative pain and a stronger extensor mechanism. The procedure also preserves patellar vascularity, thereby theoretically minimizing patellar fractures, patellar prosthesis loosening, and anterior knee pain. Additionally, preservation of the extensor mechanism allows surgeons to more accu-

rately judge patellar tracking in knee arthroplasty and minimizes the need for lateral retinacular releases.

However, advocates of this approach also stress its limitations. Specific relative contraindications include revision total knee arthroplasty, previous arthrotomy, or previous high tibial osteotomy. In addition, obese patients represent a relative contraindication to this method because of the difficulty in everting the patella in this patient population.

Technique

The patient is positioned in a standard supine fashion on the surgical table. The subvastus approach begins with the knee flexed to at least 90°. A straight longitudinal anterior skin incision is made. The superior portion of the incision extends approximately 4 cm superior to the patella. The distal portion of the incision is carried to a point that is 1 cm distal and slightly medial to the tibial tubercle. A slightly longer incision than is used with the standard midline approach is made to minimize skin tension. Dissection is carried through deeper levels until the first fascial layer is identified proximally. This layer is incised in line with the skin incision down to the level of the patella. In the patella region, dissection is carried slightly medially. After incising the fascial layer, blunt dissection raises this layer off the underlying vastus medialis. Dissection is meticulously carried down the fascial layer of the vastus medialis to its insertion site. This dissection continues until the inferior edge of the vastus medialis is clearly identified. After identification of the inferior edge of the vastus medialis obliquus, the muscle belly is bluntly dissected free of the periosteum and intramuscular septum (Figure 4). Dissection is carried superior for approximately 10 cm proximal to the adductor tubercle. During this approach, blunt dissec-

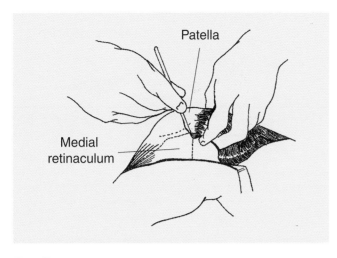

Figure 5 Schematic representation of a transverse incision made at the level of the midpatella through the medial capsule. Dissection is carried down onto the proximal tibia in a manner similar to that used in a standard medial parapatellar approach. *(Reproduced with permission from Roysam GS, Oakley MJ: Subvastus approach for TKA: A prospective, randomized, and observer-blinded trial. J Arthroplasty 2001;16: 454-457.)*

tion minimizes risk of injury to the underlying neurovascular structures.

The vastus medialis muscle is continually retracted anteriorly to clearly identify its musculotendinous insertion onto the medial capsule. When dissection allows clear visualization, the medial capsule is transversely incised at the level of the midportion of the patella (Figure 5). The arthrotomy is continued distally in a curvilinear manner. The distal limb of the incision continues along the medial aspect of the patella and patellar tendon to the region of the tibial tubercle. This method is similar to the dissection used in a standard anterior approach. The patella is then everted and dislocated laterally. The knee is slowly flexed with continued blunt dissection of the vastus medialis muscle belly off the intermuscular septum. A theoretic advantage of this approach is that the bulk of the vastus medialis remains attached to the patella and quadriceps tendon.

At this point, the prosthetic knee component can be placed in a standard fashion. Patellar tracking is assessed through the arthrotomy. If the patella does not track in an acceptable manner, a lateral retinacular release can be performed in an outside to inside fashion with the knee in full flexion. In an attempt to minimize injury to the anterior tibia and the lateral geniculate vessels, the release is made at least 1.5 cm lateral to the patella.

After the components are implanted, the wound is closed in a routine manner. The vertical limb of the incision and the proximal horizontal limb are closed with interrupted sutures. The distal arthrotomy is also closed with interrupted sutures. No reattachment of the vastus muscle belly to the intermuscular septum is needed.

Results

In a recent prospective, randomized, blinded trial of 89 consecutive knees undergoing total knee arthroplasty, a standard medial parapatellar approach was used in 43 knees, and a subvastus approach was used in the remaining 46 knees. All knees were implanted with the identical posterior-substituting knee prosthesis. After 1 week, the patients in the subvastus approach group had significantly earlier return of straight-leg raise, less consumption of narcotic analgesics in the first postoperative week, less blood loss, and greater knee flexion. No significant difference was noted between the groups in regard to length of hospital stay, knee motion at 4 weeks, or knee motion at 3 months. The authors advised wider use of the subvastus approach in knee arthroplasty.

Another recent study compared the results of two consecutive patient groups undergoing total knee arthroplasty; 169 medial parapatellar arthroplasties were performed in the first group from 1988 to 1992 and 167 were performed in the second group using a subvastus approach from 1992 through 1996. At 6-month follow-up, no significant differences were found between the two groups in terms of knee motion, stair climbing ability, and Knee Society knee and function scores. However, the patella tracked centrally in significantly more knees in the subvastus approach group, and there was a significantly lower rate of lateral retinacular releases in the subvastus approach group. Although the authors concluded that the subvastus approach led to improved patellar tracking and stability, they acknowledged that their results may have been affected by changing circumstances over the 9-year period of the study.

An earlier study compared the results achieved with a subvastus approach to those achieved with a standard midline exposure. Although the authors concluded that no correlation was found between postsurgical recovery and morbidity related to the surgical approach, they thought the vastus medialis sparing method was more technically demanding than the standard medial arthrotomy.

Midvastus Approach

The midvastus approach gained popularity in the 1990s. Advocates of this technique believe it offers some of the benefits of both the anterior and subvastus approaches. In the midvastus technique, the vastus medialis muscle fibers are divided in their midsubstance along the line and directions of the fibers. Thus, dissection is carried through an interval in the midsubstance of the vastus medialis muscle beginning at the superior medial border of the patella. The main advantage of this approach over the standard anterior exposure is that the vastus medialis insertion onto the medial border of the quadriceps tendon is not disrupted. Theoretically, this helps maintain the stabilizing contribution of the intact extensor mechanism, allows for a rapid restoration of postoperative extensor mechanism function, and minimizes the need for a lateral retinacular release. Compared with the subvastus approach, however, complete eversion and lateral displacement of the patella are less difficult to achieve because a portion of the vastus medialis attached to the medial side of the patella is released.

The midvastus approach is commonly recommended for patients with at least 80° of knee flexion. Obesity, hypertrophic arthritis, and previous high tibial osteotomies are believed to be relative contraindications to the midvastus approach.

Technique

The midvastus approach commences with a standard anterior medial skin incision. It has been recommended that the incision be made with the knee in flexion to provide tension to the skin and help retract the skin margins. Dissection is carried directly down through the subcutaneous tissue. The superior medial corner of the patella is identified with the knee in flexion, and a parallel interval between the vastus medialis muscle fibers is created. This interval starts at the superior medial corner of the patella and extends obliquely in a superomedial direction approximately 4 cm through the full thickness of the muscle (Figure 6). The quadriceps tendon is not incised. Releasing the capsular folds of the suprapatellar pouch proximal to the patella has been recommended to allow full patellar eversion. Distal dissection is carried along the medial side of the patella onto the proximal tibia just medial to the tibial tubercle. This portion of the exposure is identical to the standard medial arthrotomy performed with a basic anterior approach. A cuff of soft tissue attached to the patella is normally preserved to aid in capsular repair at the conclusion of the procedure. Surgical exposure is completed by inverting the patella and releasing the patellofemoral ligament.

Knee closure is done with the knee held in about 60° of flexion, which tenses the extensor mechanism and thereby helps in aligning the tissues for repair. Closure normally commences by placing a suture at the intersection of the capsular and muscular segments of the incision. It is not usually necessary to suture the split muscle at the superior portion of the approach because the muscle fibers approximate well once the capsular segment is repaired. With this technique, most of the vastus medialis, including the entire portion of the muscle inserting into the quadriceps tendon, remains intact.

Results

Initial results with a midvastus exposure were reported in 1997, at which time the midvastus muscle-splitting approach was found to be an effective alternative to the medial parapatellar approach for primary total knee procedures.

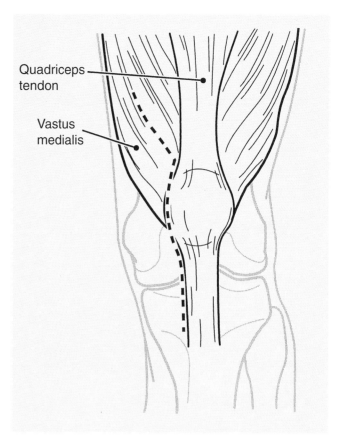

Figure 6 Schematic representation of the incisions for a midvastus approach (*dashed line*). Note that dissection is carried between the fibers of the vastus medialis. The quadriceps muscle is not incised. (*Reproduced with permission from Engh GA, Holt BT, Parks NL: A midvastus muscle splitting approach for total knee arthroplasty. J Arthroplasty 1997;12:322-331.*)

More recently, the results of a medial parapatellar approach and a midvastus approach in 109 patients undergoing bilateral primary total knee arthroplasties were compared and statistically significant differences in several parameters were noted, all of which favored the midvastus approach. The patients with knees exposed using the midvastus approach required fewer lateral retinacular releases, had less pain and a higher incidence of ability to straight-leg raise at 8-day follow-up, and had less pain at 6-week follow-up.

Another study reported the results of 100 patients undergoing bilateral total knee replacements who were randomized to undergo either a midvastus muscle-splitting approach or a medial parapatellar approach. In this series, there was no difference in range of motion at 2-day follow-up, discharge straight-leg raise ability, terminal knee extension, or extensor lag. There were two postoperative hematomas and one manipulation, all in the muscle-splitting approach group. It was concluded that the midvastus muscle-splitting approach could not be recommended as superior to the median parapatellar approach.

Another study prospectively evaluated 51 knees undergoing knee arthroplasty with either a midvastus or a median parapatellar approach, and no significant differences in postoperative strength, range of motion, knee scores, tourniquet time, proprioception, or patellar replacement were noted in the two groups. There were significantly more lateral releases performed and greater blood loss in the knees exposed with the medial parapatellar exposure. All postoperative electromyograms were normal in the medial parapatellar approach group; however, 43% of the electromyograms obtained for patients in the vastus splitting approach were abnormal. The postoperative electromyographic results were believed to reveal neurologic injuries in the vastus medial muscle that were present only after the vastus splitting approach. The clinical significance of the denervation of the vastus medial muscle was believed to be undetermined at that time.

Lateral Approach for Knee Arthroplasty

Some authors advocate a lateral approach for knee arthroplasty, especially when operating on knees with a fixed preoperative valgus deformity. It is believed that the standard medial approach can result in an increased incidence of patellar maltracking and extensor mechanism problems because the medial exposure requires lateral displacement and eversion of the extensor mechanism, which is accomplished with external tibial rotation. Therefore, in a valgus knee, the standard medial arthrotomy and the external tibial rotation retract the most severely involved lateral pathologic anatomy of the posterolateral corner farther away from the surgical field. Additionally, in valgus knees, the medial exposure usually requires an extensive lateral release, thereby violating the blood supply to the extensor mechanism on both the medial and lateral sides.

The lateral approach was developed in an attempt to address these issues, and it has been used when performing a total knee arthroplasty in patients with knees with a valgus deformity. One advantage of this technique is that it allows a more direct approach to the pathologic lateral anatomy. A lateral retinacular release is routinely performed as an integral part of the exposure; this is in contrast to a medial exposure in which it represents an additional step. The lateral approach allows for medial displacement of the extensor mechanism and internal rotation of the tibia, further exposing the posterolateral corner. Vascularity is preserved because the medial blood supply of the extensor mechanism is not violated. Finally, optimal tracking of the patella is accomplished with the inherent self-centering tendency of the retained extensor mechanism.

There are some limitations to a lateral knee exposure. Advocates of this technique concede that it is technically more demanding than the traditional medial approach. The anatomy is less familiar to most surgeons and orientation is reversed. Medial eversion and displacement of the extensor mechanisms is more difficult than traditional lateral eversion.

Technique
The lateral approach to the knee begins with a long longitudinal incision made just lateral to the midline. The incision is carried distally to a point 1 to 2 cm lateral to the lateral aspect of the tibial tubercle. As with other knee approaches, prior longitudinal incisions should be incorporated into the current incision whenever possible.

The lateral retinacular arthrotomy originates proximally along the lateral border of the quadriceps tendon. The arthrotomy line extends distally 1 to 2 cm lateral to the lateral patellar border and then proceeds along the medial border of Gerdy's tubercle. Dissection is carried distally in the anterior compartment fascia to a point approximately 2 cm lateral to the lateral patellar tendon border (Figure 2). Care should be taken during the exposure to minimize trauma to the fat pad because preservation of its blood supply is necessary for soft-tissue closure.

After the arthrotomy is performed, testing for any iliotibial band contracture has been recommended. This test is done by applying a varus stress to the extremity with the knee held in full extension. If the knee cannot be brought to an acceptable anatomic alignment, the proximal iliotibial band is released approximately 10 cm proximal to the joint line. If it is necessary to release the iliotibial band, it is exposed with blunt finger dissection. The dissection is carried from proximal to distal. The peroneal nerve should be palpated and protected. Although there are several methods for releasing the iliotibial band, making multiple small punctures in the iliotibial band has been recommended. These punctures are made while an assistant maintains a constant varus stress on the extremity. This technique is thought to allow the release to be titrated to the extent necessary to achieve acceptable limb alignment. If acceptable alignment cannot be achieved with this method, then further posterior lateral release is required.

As opposed to the proximal release noted previously, some surgeons favor a distal iliotibial band release in patients with knees with severe fixed valgus deformities. Advocates of distal releases normally perform this step after medial displacement of the extensor mechanism with the knee flexed. The distal release can include elevation of Gerdy's tubercle with a sleeve of anterolateral fascia. In addition, fibular head resection can be added to minimize stress on the peroneal nerve.

The next step is mobilization of the fat pad and capsule. Soft-tissue mobilization is necessary to provide an adequate envelope to close the lateral retinacular gap that is created with correction of a valgus knee. Soft-tissue mobilization can be achieved by sharply dissecting the area along the underside of the patellar tendon. Dissection is carried to the medial extent of the intermeniscal ligament, which is then incised to bone. This technique allows the fat pad, capsule, intermeniscal ligament, and rim of lateral meniscus to be mobilized laterally. Care is taken not to dissect through the lateral fat pad, which is the region for its blood supply.

The extensor mechanism is then translocated medially by creating an osteoperiosteal sleeve off the lateral tibial tubercle with a sharp osteotome. This technique is done with great care to allow for a gradual peel of the lateral 50% of the patellar tendon. Patellar eversion and medial patellar displacement can then be achieved. Medial eversion is slightly more difficult than the traditional lateral displacement technique, but it has been reported that it can be performed safely. The patella is everted medially while a varus moment is applied to the flexed knee. The patellar tendon attachment is observed at all times during this maneuver. Occasionally, adhesions or large patellar osteophytes must be resected to achieve patellar eversion. In addition, patellar resection, which is part of prosthetic resurfacing, can be performed at this point to further aid in eversion. After medial patellar displacement has been achieved, it has been reported that the tibia will rotate internally, thereby enabling direct visualization and a more accurate analysis of the posterolateral corner and arcuate complex.

If necessary, a posterior lateral release can be carried out at this time. This osteoperiosteal release is carried out along the femur after all osteophytes are excised. The release can be carefully titrated so that only the minimum amount of soft-tissue stripping necessary to achieve an anatomic valgus limb alignment is performed.

In general, the posteromedial compartment is the most difficult area of the knee to visualize with this lateral exposure technique. Curved retractors can be placed over the posteromedial corner to aid visualization. In addition, rotating the tibia back to a neutral position also helps improve visualization. At this point, exposure should be adequate to perform the bone cuts and proceed with component implantation.

Patellar tracking is evaluated after the components are inserted. It has been reported that the lateral approach allows the extensor mechanism to more naturally adjust to the midline. Thus, this technique minimizes the tendency for lateral patellar subluxation commonly seen with the traditional medial exposure. In addition, a lateral retinacular release has already been performed as part of the initial approach. Arthrotomy closure uses the previously developed lateral soft-tissue composite (lateral meniscus, capsule, and fat pad) to fill any gap in the lateral retinaculum. If needed, significant expansion of the fat pad can be achieved while preserving vascularity by making a transverse relaxing incision

in line with the retained lateral meniscal rim. This soft-tissue composite can then be sutured to the proximal capsular flap, thereby helping to restore the soft-tissue retinacular envelope. The knee is held in a flexed position while final closure of this composite to the border of the lateral extensor mechanism is completed. Skin closure and postoperative rehabilitation are done in a standard manner.

Results

In a study of 53 knees in which the lateral approach was used, it was reported that knee motion improved from an average of 85° preoperatively to 115° postoperatively. Complications included five nonfatal pulmonary embolisms, two subcutaneous hematomas that healed uneventfully, and one wound dehiscence that required débridement and secondary closure. Intraoperative complications included three minor split type fractures, and one failure of an uncemented patellar component that required revision to a cemented component. In one patient with a complex deformity, a meniscal-bearing tibial component was malpositioned and required reoperation 1 week after surgery. One transient sensory and one transient motor peroneal nerve palsy resolved uneventfully after 6 months. No patellofemoral maltracking problems were reported.

Exposure in Revision or Difficult Knees

It is not always possible to evert the patella and achieve adequate knee exposure with routine exposure techniques. This can be especially problematic in knees that have undergone prior surgical procedures, knees with severe flexion contractures, malaligned knees, or the knees of obese patients. In these instances, it is often necessary to improve visualization with some additional exposure techniques, which include extending the quadriceps incision proximally, performing a lateral retinacular release, and externally rotating the tibia. External tibial rotation enhances medial subperiosteal dissection of the proximal tibia. If patellar eversion and adequate exposure cannot be achieved with these methods, the surgeon must consider using additional exposure enhancement techniques.

Exposure enhancement normally falls into one of two categories. Some surgeons advocate proximal soft-tissue techniques to allow additional retraction of the extensor mechanism laterally and distally. Other surgeons advocate a distal tibial tubercle osteotomy, thereby letting the extensor mechanism and tibial tubercle retract laterally and superiorly. A proximal soft-tissue release minimizes the risk of major mechanical complications that have been reported with tubercle osteotomy. However, this technique theoretically jeopardizes the blood supply to the extensor mechanism, but advocates of proximal soft-tissue release believe that this has not been a clinical problem. Distal tibertcle osteotomy allows for excellent visualization and permits bone-to-bone healing, which is believed to be superior to soft-tissue healing. However, the osteotomy carries a risk of bone fracture, even though advocates of tibial tubercle osteotomy believe an appropriately sized osteotomy will minimize complications.

Basic Techniques

Windsor and Insall first documented the basic principles of surgical exposure in revision knee arthroplasty in 1988. In general, the prior skin incision is used for exposure in revision knee procedures. If needed, prior midline longitudinal incisions can be lengthened proximally and distally to aid in visualization. If more than one longitudinal incision is present, the more lateral incision should be selected if it affords adequate access to the joint because the medial knee theoretically has a better blood supply. Medial and lateral skin flaps can be created, but only to the extent necessary to expose the extensor mechanism. Excessive undermining of the skin flaps should be avoided. Blunt dissection techniques with minimal skin flap retraction and soft-tissue undermining have been recommended.

After adequate exposure of the extensor mechanism is achieved, a medial retinacular incision can be made. Depending on surgeon preference and soft-tissue anatomy, either a straight longitudinal or a medial parapatellar retinacular incision can be used. Care should be taken to ensure that the proximal extension of the quadriceps tendon is not transversely cut at this time. Distal dissection continues with a careful subperiosteal elevation of soft tissue from the medial tibial cortex. Subperiosteal dissection is extended medially and posteriorly until the soft tissue is stripped to the posterior margin of the tibial plateau. The need for a full posterior medial exposure has been recommended, which includes sharply dissecting the insertion of the semimembranosus muscle off of the proximal medial tibia. This should leave an intact sleeve of medial soft tissue, including the medial collateral ligament. Scar tissue should then be removed from the medial and lateral gutters. These adhesions are normally dissected and released with a combination of sharp and blunt techniques.

After adequate soft-tissue release and exposure, patellar eversion can be attempted. This is normally best performed with the knee flexed to 90°. Certain maneuvers can help facilitate patellar eversion and minimize the risk of patellar tendon disruption. First, a combination of anterior tibial translation and external rotation helps move the extensor mechanism laterally. In addition, a bent Hohmann type retractor may facilitate further lateral retraction of the extensor mechanism. These maneuvers aid in achieving adequate knee exposure and patellar eversion. Finally, a lateral retinacular release

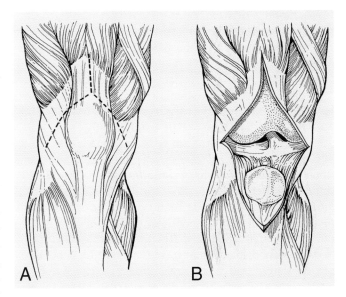

Figure 7 **A** and **B,** Schematic representations of the original Coonse-Adams V-Y turn-down technique. *(Reproduced with permission from Stern SH: Surgical exposure in total knee arthroplasty, in Harner CD, Vince KG, Fu FH (eds): Knee Surgery. Baltimore, MD, Williams & Wilkins, 1994, pp 1289-1302.)*

can also increase knee exposure and aid in patellar eversion. However, if adequate exposure is not achieved with these techniques, either proximal soft-tissue techniques or distal tubercle osteotomy may be required.

If further dissection is required after the tibia and femur are adequately exposed, surgeons can proceed with what has been described as a femoral peel, in which the posterior capsule and scar are released from the distal femur with a large curet, the femoral periosteum is incised supramedially and supralaterally, and the scar is then peeled off of the femur subperiosteally in a single soft-tissue layer, effectively skeletonizing the bone. Care is taken to preserve the medial and lateral collateral ligaments. Knees with severe flexion deformities may require further posterior capsular dissection and release.

Proximal Soft-Tissue Releases
V-Y Turndown (Coonse-Adams Approach)
A patellar turndown approach as an alternative method for knee exposure that involved making an inverted Y incision through the extensor mechanism was first described by Coonse and Adams in 1943. Starting at the proximal pole of the quadriceps tendon, an incision was carried distally through the middle of the tendon. The incision was carried to a point 0.25 to 0.50 inches superior to the patella. Two oblique limbs arising from the distal end of the midline incision were then created, both traveling medially and laterally to the patella (Figure 7). The patella and patellar tendon were then reflected distally to obtain adequate knee exposure. This method minimized the need for soft-tissue retraction, thereby reducing trauma to the surrounding knee structures. Although

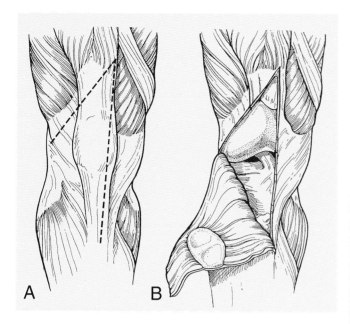

Figure 8 **A** and **B,** Schematic representations of the modified Coonse-Adams turndown as described by Insall. This technique incorporates a routine longitudinal medial arthrotomy. The second incision is inclined approximately 45° inferiorly. It can be performed at any point in the procedure. *(Reproduced with permission from Stern SH: Surgical exposure in total knee arthroplasty, in Harner CD, Vince KG, Fu FH (eds): Knee Surgery. Baltimore, MD, Williams & Wilkins, 1994, pp 1289-1302.)*

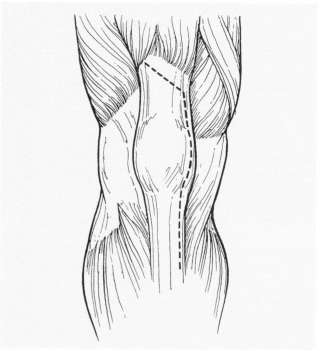

Figure 9 Schematic representation of the quadriceps (rectus) snip. As with the modified Coonse-Adams turndown, this approach uses a routine medial retinacular incision. In this exposure, the additional incision extends superiorly and laterally across the proximal portion of the quadriceps tendon. As with the modified Coonse-Adams turndown, this technique can be performed at any point in the procedure. *(Reproduced with permission from Stern SH: Surgical exposure in total knee arthroplasty, in Harner CD, Vince KG, Fu FH (eds): Knee Surgery. Baltimore, MD, Williams & Wilkins, 1994, pp 1289-1302.)*

it was first thought that this technique would be applicable to fractures, synovectomies, and internal derangements of the knee joint, it was not widely used because of the extensive dissection intrinsic to this technique.

There were specific difficulties with the original technique with regard to its applicability in knee arthroplasty. The original method, like most proximal soft-tissue releases, required a broad-based distal flap to maintain an adequate blood supply for the extensor mechanism. In addition, a routine knee exposure could not be converted to the Coonse-Adams approach. Thus, the surgeon was forced to choose whether to use this technique at the commencement of the retinacular exposure. In part because of these limitations, the technique was modified to a more accommodating patellar turndown technique.

Patellar Turndown (Modified Coonse-Adams Approach)
The patellar turndown approach (modified Coonse-Adams approach) offers several advantages over the original technique. Importantly, this technique may be used at any stage of the procedure and can easily be added to a routine knee exposure if required. A standard medial arthrotomy is used (Figure 8). Intraoperatively, if quadriceps tightness is excessive or adequate exposure is unobtainable, a second quadriceps incision is made. This second incision extends distally at a 45° angle from the superior pole of the initial incision. The dissection is carried distally and laterally through the

vastus lateralis and upper portions of the iliotibial tract, and this second incision should be ended short of the inferior lateral geniculate artery. During wound closure, the medial vertical incision is always repaired. However, the oblique lateral incision can be left open, if needed, to enhance patellar tracking.

Quadriceps Snip (Rectus Snip)
The patellar turndown approach was later modified to the currently popular quadriceps snip. This technique was designed to achieve adequate exposure while reducing trauma to the proximal soft-tissue envelope. As with the modified Coonse-Adams exposure, a standard medial arthrotomy is used. If intraoperative visualization is not adequate (Figure 9), the apex of the quadriceps retinacular incision is extended superiorly and laterally. The release extends across the superior portion of the quadriceps tendon into the distal aspect of the vastus lateralis. Lateral mobilization of the entire extensor mechanism can then be achieved. Arthrotomy closure is performed in a standard manner.

Results With Proximal Soft-Tissue Techniques
Early results of using the modified V-Y turndown for primary knee arthroplasties in ankylosed knees revealed

that the average range of motion increased from 15° preoperatively to 67° postoperatively. The mean postoperative flexion contracture was 8°. The authors of another early study reported that this technique was safer than tibial tubercle osteotomy for total knee arthroplasty and recommended using it in patients who required extraordinary exposure methods because of the satisfactory knee motion, strength, and low complication rate. Yet another early study reported that arthroplasty results were not compromised by using this technique.

Initial results with using the quadriceps snip revealed that this surgical technique was safe and simple and did not require special equipment nor changes in postoperative rehabilitation.

A recent study reported the results of comparing a standard medial parapatellar exposure (57 knees) and a rectus snip (50 knees) for revision knee arthroplasty. No difference in terms of function, pain, stiffness, and satisfaction was noted between the two groups, and the authors concluded that the rectus snip had no effect on surgical outcome.

An earlier study reported on the results of 123 revision total knee replacements performed at multiple centers with 2- to 4-year follow-up. A quadriceps turndown was used in 14 knees, and a tibial tubercle osteotomy was used in 15 knees. The remaining 94 knees were exposed with a standard medial parapatellar capsular incision, 31 of which required a quadriceps snip to aid in exposure. Postoperatively, the patients who had a quadriceps snip were equivalent in every parameter measured with the patients who underwent a standard approach. The patients in the quadriceps turndown group and the tibial tubercle osteotomy group had equivalent scores postoperatively; however, both of these groups had significantly lower scores than the standard group. The patients who had a quadriceps turndown had a significantly greater increase in knee motion compared with the tibial tubercle osteotomy group. Although the tibial tubercle osteotomy group had less extension lag, a higher percentage of patients in this group had difficulty with kneeling and stooping and a higher percentage believed the surgery was unsuccessful in relieving pain and in returning them to normal daily activities.

Tibial Tubercle Osteotomy

Tibial tubercle osteotomy is an alternative method for optimizing exposure. This technique is especially useful when previous scarring makes patellar eversion difficult. The distal osteotomy technique can be technically difficul, however, and complications are associated with this method. Tibial tubercle osteotomy advantages include bone-to-bone healing and superior exposure compared with proximal soft-tissue techniques. In addition, this technique theoretically does not jeopardize the patellar blood supply.

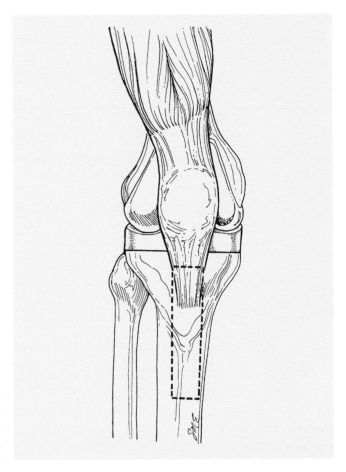

Figure 10 Schematic representation of the area of exposure needed for a tibial tubercle osteotomy. *(Reproduced with permission from Stern SH: Surgical exposure in total knee arthroplasty, in Harner CD, Vince KG, Fu FH (eds): Knee Surgery. Baltimore, MD, Williams & Wilkins, 1994, pp 1289-1302.)*

Technique

Tibial tubercle osteotomy commences with a standard skin and subcutaneous tissue exposure. Both sides of the tubercle are exposed (Figure 10). The medial periosteum is incised approximately 6 to 7 cm distal to the tubercle. It is generally believed that a larger tubercle fragment is beneficial. The actual osteotomy can be created with either oscillating saws or osteotomes. The osteotomy is created medial to lateral, with the goal of creating a bone wedge approximately 2 cm wide and 6 cm long. The wedge is tapered so it is thicker proximally (approximately 1 cm) and tapers to a few millimeters distally. A step-cut proximally can aid in minimizing proximal migration of the fragment. When performing the osteotomy, an attempt is made to retain an adequate lateral periosteal hinge. The osteotomized bone is then reflected laterally (Figure 11). At closure, the multiple wires can be used to repair the bone. The wires are commonly passed through the lateral aspect of the tibial tubercle and then distally and medially through the tibial crest. Tightening the wires helps pull and hold the osteotomy distally (Figure 12). If a tibial tubercle osteot-

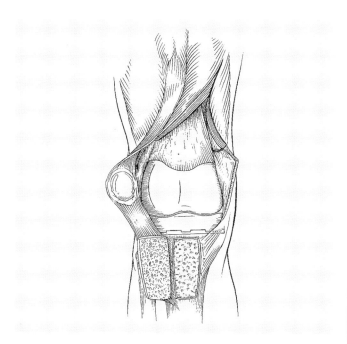

Figure 11 Schematic representation of knee exposure with a tibial tubercle osteotomy. Note the tubercle is retracted laterally to aid in knee exposure. *(Reproduced from Whiteside LA: Surgical exposure in revision total knee arthroplasty.* Instr Course Lect *1997;46:221-225.)*

omy is performed, use of a stemmed tibial component should be considered to bypass the cortical defect.

Results

Early results with the use of this technique varied. One study reported that tibial tubercle osteotomy allowed for initiation of an early physical therapy protocol and that all patients could move the knee and bear weight in the first week after surgery. No fixation failures or nonunions were reported. Another study found that complications occurred in 35% of the knees for which tibial tubercle osteotomy was used to perform knee arthroplasty (N = 26). Major nonmechanical complications, ranging from superficial skin necrosis to deep infections or deep wound necrosis requiring a gastrocnemius flap, occurred in 23% of knees. Major mechanical complications (one knee had both mechanical and nonmechanical complications), ranging from displacement of the osteotomized segment to patellar tendon rupture, occurred in 15% of knees. The complication rate was higher in patients with rheumatoid arthritis. The authors found higher rates of osteotomy union when two cortical lag screws were used. They recommended long osteotomy segment to minimize stress concentrations in the osteotomized bone.

A later study reported the results of 136 total knee arthroplasties in which a tibial tubercle osteotomy was performed. Two or three wires were used to reattach the bone fragment and patellar tendon. Mean range of motion at 2-year follow-up was 94°. Although quadriceps

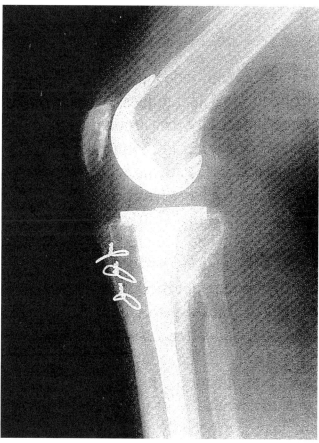

Figure 12 Lateral radiograph showing multiple wire fixation of repaired tibial tubercle osteotomy. *(Reproduced with permission from Kelly MA, Clarke HD: Stiffness and ankylosis in primary total knee arthroplasty.* Clin Orthop Relat Res *2003;416:68-73.)*

function was not compromised in any of the patients, the authors urged caution with this technique in knees with Charcot arthropathy or after manipulation.

A recent study reported on the results of 67 tibial tubercle osteotomies in knees undergoing revision arthroplasty. Mean follow-up was 30 months. Knee Society scores showed 87% good or excellent results. No patellofemoral complications, no component malalignment, and no patellar tendon avulsions occurred. However, serious complications directly related to the osteotomy occurred in 7% of patients.

Summary

There are multiple methods of surgical exposure that can be successfully used when performing total knee arthroplasty. During exposure, surgeons should attempt to achieve adequate exposure to visualize the relevant anatomy and allow for appropriate component alignment. In revision procedures or in difficult cases, the basic principles of exposure still should be followed, although it may be necessary to use the additional techniques previously discussed. In general, surgeons should remember that appropriate and sufficient anatomic exposure will aid in the performance of total knee arthroplasty; therefore, surgical exposure is the first, integral step toward achieving an optimal surgical outcome.

Annotated Bibliography

Primary Procedures

Matsueda M, Gustilo RB: Subvastus and medial parapatellar approaches in total knee arthroplasty. *Clin Orthop* 2000;371:161-168.

In this retrospective comparison of two consecutive groups of patients who underwent primary total knee arthroplasty, 169 arthroplasties were performed using a medial parapatellar approach, and 167 arthroplasties were performed using a subvastus approach. No significant differences were found between the two groups for range of motion, Knee Society knee and function scores, and stair-climbing ability. In the subvastus approach group, the patella tracked centrally in significantly more knees, and significantly fewer knees required a lateral retinacular release. The authors cautioned that the results may have been affected by changing circumstances during the 9-year period of the study.

Roysam GS, Oakley MJ: Subvastus approach for total knee arthroplasty: A prospective, randomized, and observer-blinded trial. *J Arthroplasty* 2001;16:454-457.

This prospective, randomized, and blinded trial of 89 consecutive primary knee arthroplasties compared a standard medial parapatellar arthrotomy (43 knees) with a subvastus approach (46 knees). The subvastus approach group had significantly earlier return of straight-leg raise, lower consumption of narcotic analgesics in the first postoperative week, less blood loss, and greater knee flexion at 1-week follow-up. The authors concluded that the subvastus approach offered early advantages over the standard medial parapatellar arthrotomy because it preserves the integrity of the vastus medialis and peripatellar plexus of vessels.

Exposure in Revision or Difficult Knees

Kelly MA, Clarke HD: Stiffness and ankylosis in primary total knee arthroplasty. *Clin Orthop* 2003;416:68-73.

The authors discuss the techniques for handling exposure in stiff or ankylosed knees. A systematic review of these techniques, including indications and results, based on published reports and experience, is presented.

Meek RM, Greidanus NV, McGraw RW, Masri BA: The extensile rectus snip exposure in revision of total knee arthroplasty. *J Bone Joint Surg Br* 2003;85:1120-1122.

In this study, 107 patients who underwent revision of total knee arthroplasty were followed for a minimum of 2 years. A standard medial parapatellar approach was used in 57 patients and the rectus snip was used in 50 patients. The two groups had equivalent age, sex, and comorbidity scores. The Western Ontario and McMaster Universities Osteoarthritis Index function, pain, stiffness, and satisfaction scores demonstrated no statistically significant difference between the two groups. The

authors concluded that the use of a rectus snip as an extensile procedure had no significant effect on outcome.

Mendes MW, Caldwell P, Jiranek WA: The results of tibial tubercle osteotomy for revision total knee arthroplasty. *J Arthroplasty* 2004;19:167-174.

Tibial tubercle osteotomy was used for patients undergoing revision total knee arthroplasty (67 knees). Knee Society scores confirmed good or excellent results in 87% of the knees, and the mean Knee Society score was 86. The authors found that the procedure was particularly effective in two-stage exchanges for patients with infected total knee arthroplasty. In this series, no patellofemoral complications, no component malalignments, and no avulsions of the patellar tendon occurred. Serious complications directly related to the tibial tubercle osteotomy occurred in five patients (7%).

Classic Bibliography

Barrack RL, Smith P, Munn B, Engh G, Rorabeck C: The Ranawat Award: Comparison of surgical approaches in total knee arthroplasty. *Clin Orthop Relat Res* 1998;356:16-21.

Buechel FF: A sequential three-step lateral release for correcting fixed valgus knee deformities during total knee arthroplasty. *Clin Orthop Relat Res* 1990;260:170-175.

Coonse K, Adams JD: A new operative approach to the knee joint. *Surg Gynecol Obstet* 1943;77:344.

Dolin MG: Osteotomy of the tibial tubercle in total knee replacement: A technical note. *J Bone Joint Surg Am* 1983;65:704-706.

Engh GA, Holt BT, Parks NL: A midvastus muscle-splitting approach for total knee arthroplasty. *J Arthroplasty* 1997;12:322-331.

Engh GA, Parks NL: Surgical technique of the midvastus arthrotomy. *Clin Orthop* 1998;351:270-274.

Erkes F: Weitere Erfahrungen mit physiologischer Schnittfuhrung zur Eroffnung des Kniegelenks. *Bruns Beitr zur Klin Chir* 1929;147:221.

Garvin KL, Scuderi G, Insall JN: Evolution of the quadriceps snip. *Clin Orthop Relat Res* 1995;321:131-137.

Hofmann AA, Plaster RL, Murdock LE: Subvastus (Southern) approach for primary total knee arthroplasty. *Clin Orthop* 1991;269:70-77.

Insall JN: Surgical approaches to the knee, in Insall JN, Scott WN (eds): *Surgery of the Knee*. New York, NY, Churchill Livingstone, 1984, pp 41-54.

Johnson DP, Houghton TA, Radford P: Anterior midline or medial parapatellar incision for arthroplasty of the knee: A comparative study. *J Bone Joint Surg Br* 1986; 68:812-814.

Keating EM, Faris PM, Meding JB, Ritter MA: Comparison of the midvastus muscle-splitting approach with the median parapatellar approach in total knee arthroplasty. *J Arthroplasty* 1999;14:29-32.

Keblish PA: The lateral approach to the valgus knee: Surgical technique and analysis of 53 cases with over two-year follow-up evaluation. *Clin Orthop Relat Res* 1991;271:52-62.

Miller DV, Urs WK, Windsor RE, Insall JN: Quadricepsplasty in total knee arthroplasty. *Orthop Trans* 1988;12:706.

Parentis MA, Rumi MN, Deol GS, Kothari M, Parrish WM, Pellegrini VD Jr: A comparison of the vastus splitting and median parapatellar approaches in total knee arthroplasty. *Clin Orthop* 1999;367:107-116.

Ritter MA, Keating EM, Faris PM: Comparison of two anterior medial approaches to total knee arthroplasty. *Am J Knee Surg* 1990;3:168-171.

Scott RD, Siliski JM: The use of a modified V-V Quadricepsplasty during total knee replacement to gain exposure and improve flexion in the ankylosed knee. *Orthopedics* 1985;8:45-48.

Stern SH: Surgical exposure in total knee arthroplasty, in Harner CD, Vince KG, Fu FH (eds): *Knee Surgery*. Baltimore, MD, Williams & Wilkins, 1994, pp 1289-1302.

Trousdale RT, Hanssen AD, Rand JA, Cahalan TD: V-Y quadricepsplasty in total knee arthroplasty. *Clin Orthop* 1993;286:48-55.

White RE Jr, Allman JK, Trauger JA, Dales BH: Clinical comparison of the midvastus and medial parapatellar surgical approaches. *Clin Orthop* 1999;367:117-122.

Whiteside LA: Exposure in difficult total knee arthroplasty using tibial tubercle osteotomy. *Clin Orthop* 1995; 321:32-35.

Whiteside LA: Surgical exposure in revision total knee arthroplasty. *Instr Course Lect* 1997;46:221-225.

Windsor RE, Insall JN: Exposure in revision total knee arthroplasty: The femoral peel. *Tech Orthop* 1988;3:1-4.

Wolff AM, Hungerford DS, Krackow KA, Jacobs MA: Osteotomy of the tibial tubercle during total knee replacement: A report of twenty-six cases. *J Bone Joint Surg Am* 1989;71:848-852.

Chapter 2

Biomechanics of the Knee

Richard D. Komistek, PhD

Mohamed R. Mahfouz, PhD

Douglas A. Dennis, MD

Introduction

Mechanics traditionally includes two main concepts: kinematics and kinetics. The understanding of knee biomechanics should therefore involve the determination and explanation of knee kinematics (motion) and knee kinetics (forces and torques). Orthopaedic surgeons should also have an understanding of in vivo knee kinematics, for both the implanted and nonimplanted knee, and the prediction of knee kinetics through mathematical modeling techniques.

Kinematics includes both translational and rotational motions. Translational motion involves changes in the position of a point fixed on a rigid body when this body moves relative to another body or in a reference frame (a newtonian reference frame). In contrast to translation, rotational motion occurs when changes take place in the relative orientation of two bodies or reference frames. Rotational motions and associated angular velocities cannot be defined with respect to a point.

Kinematics were historically determined using in vitro cadaveric analyses, in vivo roentgen stereophotogrammetric analyses (RSA), or in vivo motion analysis techniques. Unfortunately, cadaveric studies often do not simulate in vivo conditions because the actuators used to apply joint loads are unable to accurately reproduce in vivo motions. RSA analyses have often been performed under non–weight-bearing conditions and are quasidynamic. Error analyses of gait laboratory evaluations have suggested that these systems can induce significant out-of-plane rotational and translational error because of motion between skin markers and underlying osseous structures. It has been determined that the out-of-plane rotational error could be as high as 18° for internal/external knee rotation, which is unacceptable for analyses of total knee arthroplasty (TKA) rotation because it is often less than 5° during certain activities.

As an alternative to these other techniques, video fluoroscopy has been used to assess kinematics of TKA. Although most fluoroscopic analyses have focused on single surgeon series, two recent studies report the results of multicenter analyses of 811 knees to assess in vivo anteroposterior kinematics and 1,027 knees to assess in vivo axial rotation patterns. The kinematic findings from these fluoroscopic studies have enhanced the understanding of how the knee functions under in vivo weight-bearing conditions.

In contrast to kinematics, the understanding of forces and torques are more vague and more easily misused when referring to mechanics. First, there are only two types of forces: contact forces and distance forces (gravitational forces). Second, when describing human body mechanics, contact forces can be bearing surface forces (for example, when bones contact each other) or they can be muscle or ligament forces arising at points where a ligament is in contact with a bone or muscle.

The term most easily misused in biomechanics is torque. In mechanics, moments and torques are not the same and do not have the same definition. All torques are moments, but not all moments are torques. Torque is defined as the sum of the moments, about any point whatsoever, of a set of forces whose resultant is zero (and such a set of forces is called a couple). In the context of knee mechanics, it often is best to work with a single force and a single torque, which is possible because it is known that any set of forces can be replaced with a couple together with a single force. A helpful way to think of torque at the knee joint is to imagine the muscles being replaced by a motor that creates the motion of the femur relative to the tibia.

The two main techniques that have been used to determine in vivo kinetics are telemetry, which is a direct experimental approach, and mathematical modeling, which predicts in vivo contact loads on the basis of a theoretic evaluation. Although telemetry has been used successfully to determine in vivo forces and moments at the human hip joint, researchers have been less successful in their attempts to use this technique to determine the in vivo loads of the human knee. Mathematical modeling is an alternative theoretic methodology that relies on the derivation of mathematical equations to predict the in vivo loading of the human knee. Mathematical modeling approaches can be categorized two

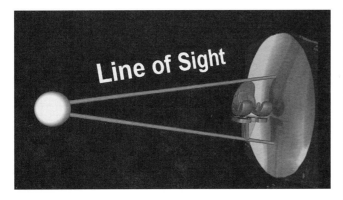

Figure 1 Illustration of the computer model fitting of a three-dimensional computer-aided design model onto a two-dimensional fluoroscopic image.

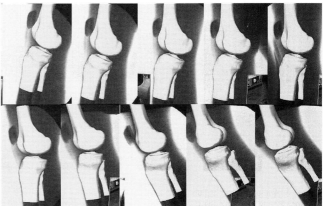

Figure 2 Illustration of the computer model-fitting process as used to extract femorotibial motion under in vivo conditions.

ways: those that use optimization techniques to solve an indeterminate muscle force system and those that use a reduction method that minimizes the number of muscle force unknowns, keeping the system solvable as the number of equations of motion are equal to the number of unknown quantities. Recently, a new, fully in vivo approach has been developed that models the human body as a system, rather than modeling each rigid body independently, and uses input data specific to each test subject. Also, all of the input data entered into the model are derived from fluoroscopy, MRI, and a new approach for extracting rigid body orientation from only two external markers on each bone segment. In light of this, mathematical modeling techniques can be used to explain the in vivo kinematics of implanted and nonimplanted knees and predict the bearing surface forces acting at the knee.

Kinematics

Multicenter kinematic analyses have determined the in vivo anteroposterior contact positions and axial rotations for implanted and nonimplanted knees. In these studies, patients either performed normal gait or a deep knee bend while under fluoroscopic surveillance. Three-dimensional kinematics for each knee are recovered from the two-dimensional fluoroscopic images using a previously described model-fitting technique that determined the in vivo orientation of the femoral component relative to the tibial component (Figure 1).

The images are projected onto the image plane, and the corresponding computer-aided design implant models are added to the scene. The operator manipulates the models into an initial position and then allows the computer to iteratively determine an accurate fit. The correct fit is achieved when the silhouettes of the femoral and tibial implant components perfectly match the corresponding components in the fluoroscopic image. The pose of each component is then recorded and each measurement of interest is digitized using a computer-aided design modeling program. Femorotibial contact anterior to the mid-

coronal plane of the tibial articular surface is denoted as positive, and posterior contact is denoted as negative. Extensive error analyses of the three-dimensional model fitting technique have demonstrated a translational three-dimensional error of less than 0.5 mm.

To determine normal knee kinematics, computer-generated three-dimensional models of each subject's femur, tibia, and fibula are precisely registered to the two-dimensional fluoroscopic images using an optimization algorithm that automatically adjusts the pose of the model at various knee flexion angles. For each activity, femorotibial contact paths are determined for the medial and lateral condyles and plotted with respect to knee flexion angle (Figure 2). For the purposes of this chapter, only the relative change in contact position between the femur and the tibia and the axial rotation of the femur with respect to the tibia will be discussed. This change in contact position and axial rotation is plotted with respect to femorotibial flexion/extension.

Kinetics

The only alternative to direct measurement of joint forces using telemetry is to theoretically predict interactive contact forces and the torques acting across each joint by developing a mathematical model. In real life, the interactive forces and torques are represented by muscle, ligament, and contact forces, and these contact forces are, in fact, contact surfaces with distributed pressure across them. Using mathematical modeling techniques, the joint is modeled using three interactive forces and torques after the joints are idealized and replaced with a single force and a torque. Additionally, the human knee joint is composed of three rigid bodies: the femur, tibia, and patella. Therefore, this joint can be defined by six interactive forces and six active torques. Fluoroscopic analysis has determined that the patella remains in contact with the femur, but rotates and translates with respect to the tibia. Therefore, modeling the

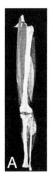
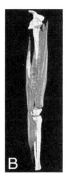
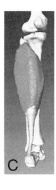
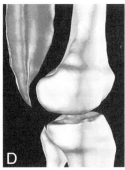
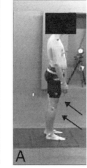

Figure 3 Computer modeling of muscle attachment sites derived from MRI data for the front view of the whole leg **(A)** and the sagittal view **(B)**, posterior view **(C)**, and close-up sagittal view **(D)** of the knee joint.

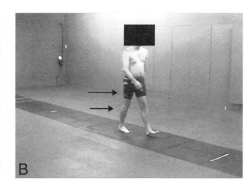

Figure 4 **A** and **B,** Photographs showing two markers (*arrows*) attached to each rigid body; the markers are representative of joint rotation points.

human knee joint is quite difficult because it involves three bodies, which are assumed to be rigid, that experience motion patterns unlike those of any other joint in the human body. The human leg is composed of numerous muscles and interactive forces, represented by resultant forces and torques. Hence, the lower leg system is indeterminate because only 30 equations of motion can be derived. Although other researchers use optimization criteria to solve for the unknowns in the indeterminate system, a reduction technique that limits the number of unknowns to the number of equations is recommended.

Most prior models have used either in vitro data or a combination of in vivo and in vitro data. More recently, a mathematical modeling protocol has been developed that uses only in vivo data from MRI and fluoroscopy. Initially, this approach was used to create a two-dimensional sagittal plane model, which was then extended to create a three-dimensional one. Each model was created with the aid of the Autolev (Kane Dynamics, Stanford, CA) software package, which is a symbolic manipulator that facilitates the implementation of a method reported by Kane in 1985.

This three-dimensional mathematical model was created to study intrabody forces (forces exerted on each other by anatomic structures forming parts of the subject's body, such as the femur, tibia, patella, cruciate ligaments, pelvis, hamstring, and quadriceps) that come into play when a human subject is engaged in activities such as walking, running, jumping, and squatting. Although such forces only rarely can be determined by purely experimental means, use of fundamental laws of physics, particularly those of mechanics, can allow force information to be deduced from motion data together with measurements of extrabody forces (forces exerted on the subject's body by objects that are not parts of the body, such as the ground on which the subject walks and a handrail the subject grips). Gravitational forces are exerted on all parts of the body by the earth and are therefore extrabody forces.

As in connection with the two-dimensional model, patients are asked to perform normal gait and deep knee bends under fluoroscopic surveillance. A relative transformation is then created by defining three points on each body and determining the translation and rotations of the femur relative to the tibia. Also, variable expressions are created for the distance from each contact position to a fixed point on each body. Then MRI is used to determine the in vivo contact positions of the muscle and ligament attachment sites with respect to each subsequent body (Figure 3). With respect to a fixed point on each rigid body, constant expressions are derived for each muscle from the attachment sites to this fixed position. A unique difference between this model and the model that was previously discussed is the use of only two markers on each rigid body to define the gross motion of each bone with respect to the newtonian reference frame (Figure 4). External markers are attached at locations representing rotation points between pairs of bodies.

Gross motions derived from the external markers are defined as temporal functions and entered into the mathematical model of the system. The three-dimensional model is composed of two components: use of external marker data to determine resultant forces and torques and use of internal fluoroscopic and MRI data to distribute the resultant forces and torques to muscle and interaction forces.

In the three-dimensional model, instead of inputting force-plate data, force-plate data can be used to validate the values of the foot/ground forces predicted by the model. Eighteen auxiliary generalized speeds are introduced to solve for the resultant forces and torques in the system. Determination of forces using Kane's methodology, when motion is input to the model, requires the introduction of auxiliary generalized speeds. These auxiliary generalized speeds are defined as imaginary motion that is introduced into the system so that the partial angular velocity and partial velocity equations do not equate to zero. After the system resultant forces and

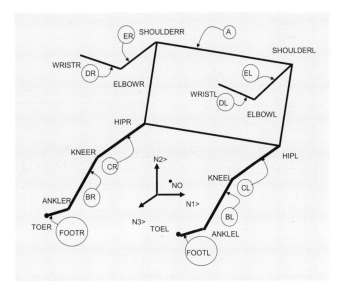

Figure 5 Free-body diagram in which each point is referenced using the name of the joint followed by either the letter R (right side) or L (left side).

torques are determined, they are distributed to muscle forces acting across the joint and interactive forces at the bearing interfaces. The knee resultant forces and torques are distributed using the reduction method technique to the bearing interactive forces between the medial condyle and tibial plateau, the lateral condyle and tibial plateau, the patellar ligament force, hamstring force, and muscles representing the abductor/adductor muscles. The shear forces exerted on the tibial plateau by the medial and lateral condyles are found by using a friction coefficient multiplied by the normal forces. Once the patellar ligament force is known, the patellofemoral interactive force and quadriceps muscle forces can be determined because the patella represents a three-force system.

In the three-dimensional model, the human subject is treated as a set of eleven rigid components to which specific names are assigned. When dealing with the mass distribution properties of these components, the human head and the pelvis form parts of TRUNK, the toes are parts of FOOT, the fibula and all soft tissue between an ankle and a knee are parts of TIBIA, and all soft tissue between a knee and a pelvis are a part of FEMUR. A schematic representation of these components is shown in Figure 5. Each of these points corresponds to a skin marker in connection with gait-lab measurements.

A dynamic analysis involving this system represented serves to provide input information for a second dynamic analysis that deals directly with certain intrabody forces, such as the forces exerted on a tibia by a patellar ligament, hamstring, cruciate ligaments, and femur (via the femoral condyles).

For purposes of the first dynamic analysis, it is assumed that the motion of each of the 14 labeled points shown in Figure 5 is known throughout some time interval. More specifically, it is presumed that gait-lab data provide three Cartesian coordinates of each point for a large number of instants of time. This information is used to determine, as a function of time, the velocity and the acceleration of each of the points. Additionally, the position information is used to establish a set of mutually perpendicular unit vectors in each of the 14 components of the model (for example, FOOTR and TIBIAR).

Once the unit vectors fixed in a given component have been established, the direction cosine matrix relating these unit vectors to the unit vectors fixed in the laboratory are known, and they can be used to determine the angular velocity and the angular acceleration of the component. For example, if C_{ij} (i = 1, 2, 3) are the direction cosine elements for TIBIAR, and C_{ij}' (i = 1, 2, 3) are their first time-derivatives, then the angular velocity of TIBIAR in the newtonian reference frame in which $\underline{N}_1$, $\underline{N}_2$, and $\underline{N}_3$ are fixed is given by:

$$^{TIBIAR}\underline{\omega}^N = (C_{13} \cdot C_{12}' + C_{23} \cdot C_{22}' + C_{33} \cdot C_{32}') \cdot \underline{TIBIAR}_1 + (C_{11} \cdot C_{13}' + C_{21} \cdot C_{23}' + C_{31} \cdot C_{33}') \cdot \underline{TIBIAR}_2 + (C_{12} \cdot C_{11}' + C_{22} \cdot C_{21}' + C_{32} \cdot C_{31}') \cdot \underline{TIBIAR}_3$$

and the angular acceleration of TIBIAR in the newtonian reference frame is then obtained by differentiation of $^{TIBIAR}\underline{\omega}^N$ with respect to time in the newtonian reference frame.

The velocity of each of the 14 points labeled in Figure 5 is found as the first time-derivative in the newtonian reference frame of the position vector from a point fixed in the newtonian reference frame to the point under consideration; the velocity of the mass center of each component can be determined similarly; and all mass center accelerations are then available as the first time-derivatives of corresponding velocities. The accelerations and angular accelerations mentioned previously are used to determine the inertia force and the inertia torque for each component.

Although each of the 14 components forming the system under consideration can undergo full three-dimensional rotational and translational motions, all such motions are completely determined by the motions of the 14 points labeled in Figure 5 and, as has been stated, the latter motions are presumed to be known a priori. Thus, in the sense in which the phrase number of degrees of freedom is generally used in analytic mechanics, this number is equal to zero for the present system; concomitantly, the number of independent generalized speeds required to characterize the instantaneous motion of the system is equal to zero. However, because certain forces and torques associated with these motions are to be determined, 18 auxiliary generalized speeds are introduced. As an illustrative example, consider the right

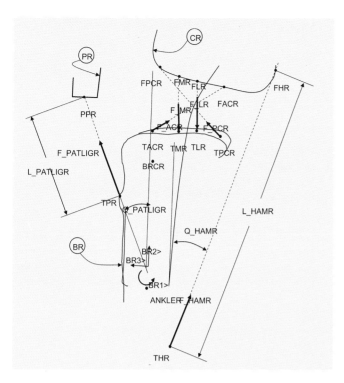

Figure 6 Free-body diagram of the knee joint depicting relevant points and angles. PR, BR, and CR refer to different bones at the right knee. Q_HAMR and Q_PATLIGR refer to the angles of the hamstring muscle and the patellar ligaments with respect to the tibial bone. L_HAMR and L_PATLIGR refer to the length of the hamstring muscle and patellar ligament muscle. All other terms refer to points on each of the bones for reference purposes.

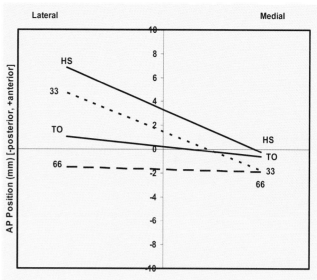

Figure 7 Graph comparing the average medial and lateral condyle contact positions for the normal knee from heel strike to toe-off.

mitted to the tibia by the femur is equivalent to a couple of torque $T_{FEMRTIBR}$ together with the force $F_{FEMRTIBR}$ applied at point KNEER. Analogous steps allow determination of forces and torques relevant to the interaction of FOOTR with the ground and with TIBIAR as well as the interaction of FEMURR with TRUNK.

Mathematical Modeling Techniques
Predicting Knee Kinematics

During gait, no statistically significant difference between the normal knee and any of the TKA groups was noted in the magnitudes of femorotibial translation from heel strike to toe-off ($P > 0.1$). However, kinematic patterns occurring during individual interval segments of stance phase (heel strike to 33% of stance phase, 33% to 66% of stance phase, and 66% of stance phase to toe-off) were often visibly different. Additionally, although the magnitude of anteroposterior translation during gait was similar among groups, the contact location for normal knees was typically centrally located on the tibia, whereas the contact for most of the patients in the TKA groups was posterior, particularly in patients with posterior cruciate ligament–retaining TKA (Figure 7). The only TKA groups to experience more centrally located contact points were the posterior cruciate ligament–sacrificing (Figure 8) and posterior-stabilized (Figure 9) mobile-bearing rotating platform TKAs. The other TKA groups experienced incidences of femorotibial sliding that were often opposite in motion compared with the normal knee. It was hypothesized that the larger sagittal radii of the mobile-bearing TKA, especially the posterior cruciate ligament–sacrificing rotating platform TKA, leads to greater constraint in the

knee. In Figure 6, this is represented by the point KNEER. Two more points are introduced: one a point of TIBIAR, called TIBRFEMR, the other a point of FEMURR, called FEMRTIBR, and both instantaneously coincident with KNEER; with $^{TIBRFEMR}V^N$ as the velocity of TIBRFEMR in the newtonian reference frame, and $^{FEMRTIBR}V^N$ as the velocity of FEMRTIBR in the newtonian reference frame, the latter is expressed as

$$^{FEMRTIBR}V^N = {}^{FEMRTIBR}V^N + U_{11} \cdot N_1 + U_{12} \cdot N_2 + U_{13} \cdot N_3$$

where U_{11}, U_{12}, and U_{13} are three of the aforementioned auxiliary generalized speeds. Three more, U_7, U_8, and U_9, enter the analysis when $^{TIBIAR}\omega^N$ is expressed, the angular velocity of TIBIAR in the Newtonian reference frame, as

$$^{TIBIAR}\omega^N = {}^{FEMURR}\omega^{TRUNK} + {}^{TRUNK}\omega^N + U_7 \cdot N_1 + U_8 \cdot N_2 + U_9 \cdot N_3$$

The introduction of these auxiliary generalized speeds subsequently allows a force ($F_{FEMRTIBR}$) and a torque ($T_{FEMRTIBR}$) to be determined that together represent the set of all forces of interaction between the tibia and femur. Specifically, the set of all forces trans-

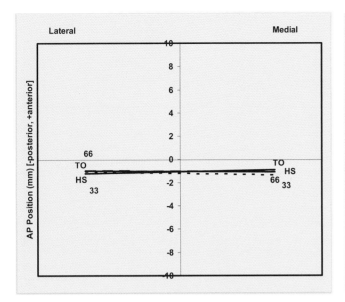

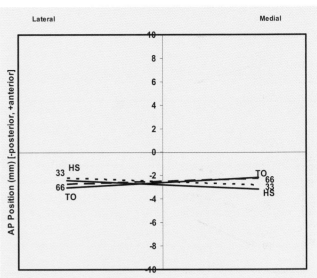

Figure 8 Graph comparing the average medial and lateral condyle contact positions for the mobile-bearing posterior cruciate ligament–sacrificing TKA from heel strike to toe-off.

Figure 9 Graph comparing the average medial and lateral condyle contact positions for the mobile-bearing posterior-stabilized TKA from heel strike to toe-off.

anteroposterior direction and also more reproducible kinematic patterns.

A summary comparison of each study group revealed some interesting findings during the stance phase of gait. Patients with a normal knee experienced the highest incidence (90%) and magnitude (–5.8 mm) of posterior motion of the lateral femoral condyle. On average, the kinematic patterns for patients in the fixed- and mobile-bearing posterior-stabilized TKA groups were similar, as were the kinematic patterns for those in the various mobile-bearing designs (posterior cruciate ligament–retaining mobile-bearing, posterior-stabilized mobile-bearing, and posterior cruciate ligament–sacrificing mobile-bearing TKA groups). On average, for all TKA groups during the stance phase of gait, only 125 of 236 patients (53.0%) had posterior motion of the lateral condyle, and 102 of 236 patients (43.4%) experienced posterior motion of the medial condyle. The lateral condyle translated posteriorly an average of –0.5 mm (SD, 3.3), and the medial condyle translated anteriorly an average of 0.2 mm (SD, 3.1). Although it was expected that those patients with intact anterior and posterior cruciate ligaments (patients with normal knees and those in the anterior cruciate ligament–retaining TKA group) would demonstrate less variability in kinematic data, the opposite was observed. Also, the pivot location for the normal and implanted knees was similar.

A summary comparison of each study group, for axial rotation, revealed some interesting findings during the stance phase of gait. Patients with a normal knee experienced the highest incidence (80%) and magnitude (average = 5.7°; average maximum = 24.0°) of axial rotation. The axial rotation patterns for patients in the

fixed- and mobile-bearing posterior-stabilized TKA groups were similar, as were the axial rotation patterns for those in the fixed- and mobile-bearing posterior cruciate ligament–retaining TKA groups. Patients having a fixed-bearing posterior cruciate ligament–retaining (2.1°) and mobile-bearing posterior-stabilized (2.2°) TKA achieved the largest average axial rotation from heel strike to toe-off. Although most patients with a posterior cruciate ligament–sacrificing mobile bearing TKA experienced axial rotation, the average rotation for this group was 0°. On average, for all TKA groups during the stance phase of gait, only 146 of 252 knees (58%) experienced a normal axial rotational pattern; normal knees experienced 80% normal rotation, but this difference was not statistically significant ($P = 0.15$). In addition, only 86 of 252 patients (34%) experienced greater than 5.0° of axial rotation at any increment, which was a significant decrease from that observed in normal knees (90%; $P = 0.01$). This trend continued for knees experiencing greater than 10.0° of axial rotation. Only 15 of 252 patients (6%) experienced greater than 10.0° of axial rotation compared with 50% of those in the normal knee group ($P = 0.01$).

As with gait activity, overall comparison of each group revealed some interesting phenomena for anteroposterior translation. The normal knee and anterior cruciate ligament–retaining fixed-bearing TKA groups experienced similar results and had the highest variability (widest SDs) of any knee group. Patients in the normal and anterior cruciate ligament–retaining TKA groups showed the highest magnitudes of posterior femoral rollback of both the medial and lateral femoral condyles when compared with those in any of the other TKA

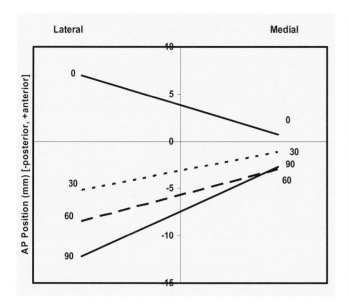

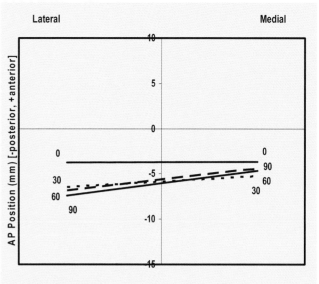

Figure 10 Graph comparing the average medial and lateral condyle contact positions during a deep knee bend for the normal knee from full extension to 90° of knee flexion.

Figure 11 Graph comparing the average medial and lateral condyle contact positions during a deep knee bend for a fixed-bearing posterior cruciate ligament-retaining TKA from full extension to 90° of knee flexion.

groups ($P < 0.01$) (Figure 10). Patients with fixed-bearing posterior-stabilized TKAs demonstrated greater posterior femoral rollback of the medial and lateral condyles than those with fixed- or mobile-bearing posterior cruciate ligament–retaining and posterior cruciate ligament–sacrificing mobile-bearing TKAs ($P < 0.01$), but this was statistically comparable to that of patients with posterior-stabilized mobile-bearing TKAs ($P > 0.5$). No statistically significant differences were observed among patients with fixed- and mobile-bearing posterior cruciate ligament–retaining TKAs or those with posterior cruciate ligament–sacrificing mobile-bearing TKAs ($P > 0.2$) When investigating the effects of surgeon variability on anteroposterior motion patterns of patients with the same TKA design, no differences were observed ($P > 0.2$) when analyzing the mobile-bearing TKA groups. In contrast, statistically significant differences among differing surgeons were observed in patients with fixed-bearing TKAs ($P < 0.05$) (Figure 11). Overall, only 55% of all knee groups demonstrated a medial pivot pattern during a deep knee bend, whereas 37% showed a lateral pivot pattern, and 8% did not exhibit a pivot motion pattern.

A summary comparison of each study group revealed some interesting findings for axial rotation during knee flexion from full extension to 90° of knee flexion. Patients with a normal knee experienced the highest incidence (100%) and magnitude (average = 16.5°, maximum = 27.7°) of axial rotation. The axial rotation patterns for the fixed- and mobile-bearing posterior-stabilized TKA groups were similar, as were the axial rotation patterns for the fixed- and mobile-bearing posterior cruciate ligament–retaining TKA

groups. Patients with a mobile bearing posterior cruciate ligament–retaining (3.9°) and mobile-bearing posterior-stabilized (3.9°) TKA achieved the highest average axial rotation during a deep knee bend. Substantial variability of average and maximum axial rotation values were observed within each implant group. For example, the range of average axial rotation was –1.1° to 7.6° for the posterior cruciate ligament–retaining mobile-bearing TKA group and 1.0° to 7.2° for the posterior-stabilized mobile-bearing TKA group. Similarly, the maximum amount of normal rotation ranged from 7.0° to 35.9° and 9.5° to 22.4° for patients with posterior cruciate ligament–retaining and posterior-stabilized mobile-bearing TKAs, respectively. On average, for all TKAs, only 551 of 745 knees (74%) had a normal axial rotational pattern during deep knee bending, a significant decrease from the normal knee group in which 100% (10 of 10) demonstrated a normal axial rotational pattern ($P = 0.001$). Additionally, only 425 of 745 patients with a TKA (57%) experienced greater than 5.0° of axial rotation at any increment, which was a significant decrease compared with normal knee group (100%, 10 of 10; $P = 0.001$). This trend continued for the number of knees experiencing greater than 10.0° of axial rotation. Only 127 of 745 (17%) patients with a TKA experienced greater than 10.0° of axial rotation compared with 90% (9 of 10) of the normal knees ($P = 0.001$).

Predicting Knee Kinetics
The initial results from this analysis revealed good correlation between the predicted foot/ground forces compared with the experimentally derived forces from the

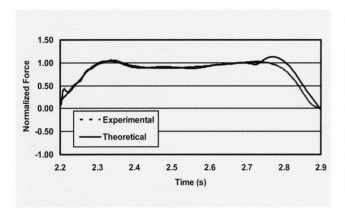

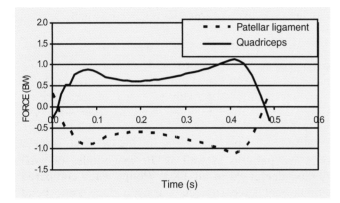

Figure 12 Graph comparing the predicted and experimental vertical forces at the ground/foot interface.

Figure 14 Graph comparing the forces acting in the quadriceps and patellar ligament during normal, slow walking.

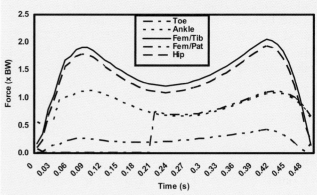

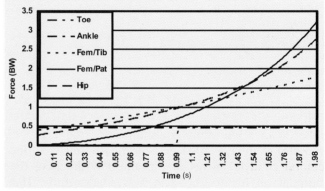

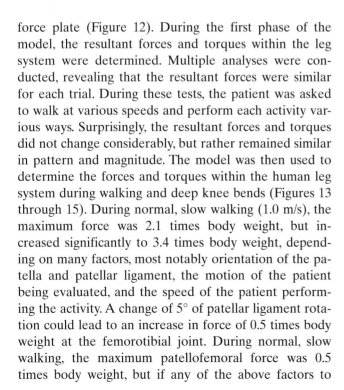

Figure 13 Graph comparing the interactive contact forces occurring at various bearing interfaces within the leg.

Figure 15 Graph comparing the joint reaction forces at the hip, knee, ankle, and patella during normal gait.

force plate (Figure 12). During the first phase of the model, the resultant forces and torques within the leg system were determined. Multiple analyses were conducted, revealing that the resultant forces were similar for each trial. During these tests, the patient was asked to walk at various speeds and perform each activity various ways. Surprisingly, the resultant forces and torques did not change considerably, but rather remained similar in pattern and magnitude. The model was then used to determine the forces and torques within the human leg system during walking and deep knee bends (Figures 13 through 15). During normal, slow walking (1.0 m/s), the maximum force was 2.1 times body weight, but increased significantly to 3.4 times body weight, depending on many factors, most notably orientation of the patella and patellar ligament, the motion of the patient being evaluated, and the speed of the patient performing the activity. A change of 5° of patellar ligament rotation could lead to an increase in force of 0.5 times body weight at the femorotibial joint. During normal, slow walking, the maximum patellofemoral force was 0.5 times body weight, but if any of the above factors to

which the model is sensitive is altered, this force could increase to 1.0 times body weight (Figure 13). Also, the quadriceps and patellar ligament forces remain similar in magnitude but opposite in direction during normal walking. The maximum amount of force for both was 1.25 times body weight (Figure 14).

During a deep knee bend, the maximum amount of force acting between the femur and the tibia was 1.8 to 3.0 times body weight, but the patellofemoral bearing interactive force became more significant (Figure 15). The maximum amount of force during a deep knee bend between the femur and the patella increased to 3.2 to 4.5 times body weight. During this activity, the maximum amount of force in the quadriceps muscle increased to 2.4 to 3.5 times body weight.

In a recent multicenter study to determine anteroposterior translation, patients with either a fixed- or mobile-bearing posterior cruciate ligament–retaining TKA experienced the highest incidence and magnitude of paradoxical anterior femoral translation of either femoral condyle. During a deep knee bend, 72% of patients having a posterior cruciate ligament–retaining fixed-bearing TKA and 60% of patients with a posterior cruciate ligament–retaining mobile-bearing TKA experienced greater than 3 mm of paradoxical femoral translation during knee flexion. At cam-post engagement, the medial condyle typically experiences the greatest shear forces and translates anteriorly as the lateral femoral condyle levers posteriorly. This finding was determined by analyzing the data in flexion increments greater than 60°. Once a patient achieves 60° flexion, the medial femoral condyle typically shifts anteriorly a similar amount as the lateral condyle translates posteriorly.

Contact position of the medial and lateral femoral condyles usually remains near the midline of the tibial component during gait with minimal anteroposterior motion in patients with mobile-bearing TKAs. These patients also usually have less paradoxical anterior femoral sliding during the stance phase of gait. This results in reduced polyethylene shear stresses and may account, at least in part, for the low polyethylene wear rates reported with clinical use of mobile-bearing TKAs. These phenomena may be secondary to the higher sagittal femorotibial conformity typically present in most mobile-bearing TKA designs. Condylar motion in rotating platform mobile-bearing TKA designs predominantly occurs because of polyethylene bearing rotation rather than femorotibial translation on the articular (topside) of the polyethylene bearing. Routinely, as one femoral condyle moves in the anterior direction, the contralateral femoral condyle moves posteriorly. This occurrence was supported by data from a recent study in which tantalum beads were implanted into mobile-bearing polyethylene tibial inserts before implantation in nine patients. The metallic beads were then tracked using the same fluoroscopic method described previously. All nine patients achieved polyethylene bearing rotation, whereas minimal motion occurred between the femoral component and polyethylene insert, which also may contribute to the low polyethylene wear rates observed in clinical reports of mobile-bearing TKAs.

Additionally, it is clear that surgeon variability can play a significant role in eventual knee kinematic patterns. In surgeon-to-surgeon comparisons of patients implanted with the same fixed-bearing TKA implant, a statistically significant difference in anteroposterior motion patterns was observed ($P < 0.05$). For example, three different studies were done by three different surgeons, all of whom implanted the same type of fixed-bearing posterior-stabilized TKA prosthesis. In two of these studies, 95% and 100% of patients experienced posterior rollback of the lateral femoral condyle during deep flexion. In the third evaluation, only 65% of patients had posterior motion of the lateral condyle. This statistically significant variance among surgeons was not observed in subjects implanted with mobile-bearing TKA designs. This occurrence may be attributed, at least in part, to the increased sagittal plane conformity typically

found in mobile-bearing TKA designs, which provides enhanced control of kinematic patterns and therefore lessens the effect of differences in surgical technique among surgeons.

There also was great variability among TKA types within each group (those with posterior-stabilized fixed-bearing TKAs or posterior cruciate ligament–retaining fixed-bearing TKAs, etc). For example, one recent study reported that patients having a posterior cruciate ligament–retaining fixed-bearing TKA with asymmetric femoral condyles experienced more than twice the amount of posterior femoral motion and substantially less paradoxical anterior femoral translation compared with patients having a posterior cruciate ligament–retaining fixed-bearing TKA with symmetric femoral condyles. Although it often has been assumed that all posterior-stabilized fixed-bearing TKA designs have similar kinematic patterns, the opposite actually is true. Differing incidences and magnitudes of posterior femoral rollback were typically seen when comparing differing fixed-bearing posterior-stabilized TKA designs. One fixed-bearing posterior-stabilized TKA design, for example, showed an excessively posterior contact position throughout the flexion range, thereby never achieving cam-post engagement.

The percentage of subjects experiencing normal rotational patterns as well as the magnitudes of axial rotation decreased in all TKA groups when compared with normal knee subjects during a deep knee bend ($P < 0.01$). More axial rotation occurred during deep flexion than in gait in all study groups. Average axial rotational magnitudes in both gait and a deep knee bend were similar among major implant categories (fixed-verus mobile-bearing TKA and posterior cruciate ligament–retaining versus posterior-stabilized TKA). The maximum magnitudes of axial rotation occurring during extreme flexion in posterior-stabilized TKA designs may be underestimated when analysis is performed only to a maximum of 90° of flexion (as was the case in a previously discussed recent study). Many posterior-stabilized implants are designed to have late (> 70° of knee flexion) cam-post engagement, which may result in additional axial rotation at flexion increments greater than 90°. Increased axial rotation has been reported to be present in deep flexion if the anterior cruciate ligament is intact. Average values in normal knees and those with anterior cruciate ligament–retaining TKAs (16.5° and 8.1°, respectively) were significantly higher than in TKA study groups in which the anterior cruciate ligament was absent ($< 4.0°$; $P < 0.01$).

Reverse axial rotational patterns during individual increments of gait or a deep knee bend were common in all study groups but were more frequently observed in patients with TKA. It was uncommon for patients in any TKA group to demonstrate a progressive normal rotational pattern throughout all increments of deep flexion.

Alternating patterns of internal and external tibial rotation were typically observed as flexion increased. Reverse axial rotation is undesirable because it poses a risk of patellofemoral instability resulting from lateralization of the tibial tubercle during deep flexion as well as lessening maximum knee flexion because of reduced posterior femoral rollback of the lateral femoral condyle.

High variability in axial rotation patterns and magnitudes have been reported among differing TKA categories, among differing implant designs within the same implant category, and among identical implant designs implanted by differing surgeons. This suggests axial rotation is determined by many factors, including implant design, individual patient anatomic variances, and the surgical technique of TKA.

Both telemetry and mathematical modeling approaches have been used to determine the in vivo forces of the human hip joint, but these approaches have not yet provided verifiable in vivo loads. Attempts to determine in vivo loads of the human knee joint using telemetry has not yet produced a prosthesis that can be implanted, and mathematical modeling approaches have not verified the predicted results using an error analyses. The best possible solution for determining in vivo loads of the human knee should use both approaches. If a telemetric knee could be implanted successfully in one patient, the loads predicted using mathematical models could be validated. A protocol for this analysis should include determination of in vivo kinematics simultaneously as the telemetric mechanics are determined. Then the in vivo kinematics could be entered into the mathematical model, and the results for both the predicted (mathematical model) and experimentally (telemetry) derived analyses could be sent to an independent researcher for verification. This independent researcher could then compare the predicted and experimentally derived results and conduct a statistical analysis to determine the accuracy of the predicted results from a mathematical model. Therefore, if the predicted values are within an acceptable range of the experimentally derived values, it could be independently concluded that the mathematical model is accurate. Once a model has been determined to be accurate, parametric analyses and sensitivity analyses could then be conducted to determine more meaningful information.

The mathematical model discussed at length in this chapter and the model developed by Wimmer and Andriacchi highlight the importance of patellofemoral kinematics. Both demonstrate that if patellofemoral kinematics are altered, femorotibial forces tend to increase. This is a reasonable determination because altering the patellofemoral kinematics directly affects the forces within the quadriceps muscle, possibly leading to increased tension and directly leading to greater compression at the femorotibial bearing interface. These results suggest that the loading at the femorotibial joint may also be sensitive to loading at other joints.

Although effective, there are limitations and challenges associated with these new methods. For example, each patient must undergo an evaluation using MRI and fluoroscopy, which is time consuming, costly, and requires radiation exposure. Moreover, the muscles in the systems are modeled using a reduction technique, whereas they must be grouped together to create a determinate system. Nonetheless, the benefits for this approach outweigh the liabilities. Because this approach uses a reduction technique, there is no issue with choosing the correct cost function, and there is no need to determine specific parameters to model each muscle-tendon actuator (optimal muscle fiber length, peak isometric force, tendon slack length, and maximum shortening velocity). The MRI analysis ensures that only accurate moment arms are modeled in terms of patient-specific muscle-related parameters. More importantly, all collected input data are for the same subject, rather than approximating soft-tissue parameters and contact positions from a cadaver and determining the in vivo motions using an ex vivo approach.

When only in vivo data from MRI and fluoroscopy was used as input data to the mathematical model, the forces at the knee joint seemed to be less than those previously reported. By altering parameters associated with the knee joint, the resultant bearing surface force between the femur and tibia ranges from 2.1 to 3.4 times body weight. The most important parameter seems to be the rotation between the patellar ligament and the tibia and between the patella and the patellar ligament because both structures influence the quadriceps muscle, the key determining factor that increases the femorotibial forces. As the quadriceps force increases, the bearing surface force between the femur and the tibia increases at a proportional rate.

Summary

The biomechanics of the knee involve the determination and explanation of knee kinematics (motion) and knee kinetics (forces and torques). An understanding of in vivo knee kinematics and the ability to predict knee kinetics through mathematical modeling techniques, imaging techniques, and Kane's multibody dynamics can help orthopaedic surgeons formulate treatment plans and optimize outcomes for patients undergoing knee implantation. Knee biomechanics can be assessed using MRI, CT, and fluoroscopy to exact in vivo soft-tissue locations, bone geometry, and kinematics, respectively.

Annotated Bibliography
Kinematics/Kinetics

Bertin KC, Komistek RD, Dennis DA, Hoff WA, Anderson WA, Langer T: In vivo determination of posterior femoral rollback for subjects having a NexGen posterior cruciate-retaining total knee arthroplasty. *J Arthroplasty* 2002;17:1040-1048.

Patients who underwent posterior cruciate ligament–retaining TKA with asymmetrical condylar geometry were analyzed during a deep knee bend. All of the subjects routinely experienced posterior femoral rollback of the lateral condyle with increasing knee flexion. These findings differed from those of previous studies that found that patients who underwent posterior cruciate ligament–retaining TKA have symmetrical condylar geometry as they experienced an anterior sliding motion with increasing flexion.

Dennis DA, Komistek RD, Cheal EJ, Walker SA, Stiehl JB: In vivo femoral condylar lift-off in total knee arthroplasty. *J Bone Joint Surg Br* 2001;83:33-39.

Fluoroscopy was performed on 40 patients who underwent TKA to determine the presence and magnitude of femoral condylar lift-off. Femoral lift-off was observed at some increment of knee flexion in 75% of patients (posterior cruciate ligament–retaining TKA, 70%; posterior cruciate ligament–substituting TKA, 80%). The mean values for lift-off were 1.2 mm for patients who underwent posterior cruciate ligament–retaining TKA and 1.4 mm for patients who underwent posterior cruciate ligament–substituting TKA. Lift-off occurred mostly laterally for patients who underwent posterior cruciate ligament–retaining TKA and both medially and laterally for patients who underwent posterior cruciate ligament–substituting TKA. Separation between the femoral condyles and the articular surface of the tibia was recorded at 0°, 30°, 60°, and 90° of flexion.

Dennis DA, Komistek RD, Mahfouz MR, Haas BD, Stiehl JB: Multicenter determination of in vivo kinematics after total knee arthroplasty. *Clin Orthop Relat Res* 2003;416:37-57.

A summation analysis of more than 70 individual kinematic studies involving normal knees and patients who underwent TKA with 33 different implant designs was done with the objective of analyzing implant design variables that affect knee kinematics. Eight hundred eleven knees (733 patients) were analyzed either during the stance phase of gait or a deep knee bend while under fluoroscopic surveillance. The highest magnitude of translation was found in the normal and anterior cruciate ligament–retaining TKA groups. Substantial variability in kinematic patterns was observed in all groups. The least amount of variability during gait was observed in patients with mobile-bearing TKA implants, whereas those with posterior-stabilized TKA implants (fixed or mobile-bearing) showed the least variability during a deep knee bend. A medial pivot kinematic pattern was observed in only 55% of patients during deep knee flexion.

Dennis DA, Komistek RD, Mahfouz MR, Walker SA, Tucker A: A multicenter analysis of axial femorotibial rotation after total knee arthroplasty. *Clin Orthop Relat Res* 2004;428:180-189.

A multicenter analysis was done to determine in vivo femorotibial axial rotation magnitudes and patterns in 1,027 knees (normal knees, nonimplanted anterior cruciate ligament–deficient knees, and multiple designs of TKA implants). Normal knees showed 16.5° and 5.7° of internal tibial rotation during a deep knee bend and gait, respectively. Average axial rotational magnitudes in gait and a deep knee bend were similar among major implant categories (fixed-bearing implant versus mobile-bearing implant, etc). Average values in normal knees and patients who underwent TKA with anterior cruciate ligament–retaining implants (16.5° and 8.1°, respectively) were higher than in groups in which the anterior cruciate ligament was absent (< 4.0°). All TKA groups had at least 19% of patients with a reverse axial rotational pattern during a deep knee bend and at least 31% during gait.

Dennis DA, Komistek RD, Mahfouz M: In vivo fluoroscopic analysis of fixed-bearing total knee replacements. *Clin Orthop Relat Res* 2003;410:114-130.

Subjects who underwent TKA with either a fixed posterior cruciate ligament–retaining or posterior-stabilized implant were analyzed using fluoroscopy during the stance phase of gait and a deep knee bend. During gait, kinematics were similar for the two groups, but during a deep knee bend, patients with posterior-stabilized implants experienced greater posterior femoral rollback.

Komistek RD, Dennis DA, Mabe JA, Walker SA: An in vivo determination of patellofemoral contact positions. *Clin Biomech (Bristol, Avon)* 2000;15(1):29-36.

The objective of this study was to determine patellofemoral contact patterns in two dimensions for normal subjects and patients who have undergone TKA. The patellofemoral kinematics of the TKA group analyzed in the study were statistically different than those of the normal subjects and patients with anterior cruciate ligament–deficient knees. The kinematic variations observed between normal subjects and patients with implanted knees may be related to disturbed femorotibial kinematics that have been observed to occur after TKA.

Komistek RD, Dennis DA, Mahfouz MR: In vivo fluoroscopic analysis of the normal human knee. *Clin Orthop* 2003;410:69-81.

Using CT, three-dimensional bone geometry was recovered for subjects having a normal knee and fluoroscopy was used to determine their in vivo kinematic patterns. During both gait and a deep knee bend, 80% of the subjects experienced more motion for the lateral condyle than the medial condyle. The other 20% of the subjects experienced a more variable kinematic pattern.

Komistek RD, Dennis DA, Mahfouz MR, Walker S, Outten J: In vivo polyethylene bearing mobility is maintained in posterior stabilized total knee arthroplasty. *Clin Orthop Relat Res* 2004;428:207-213.

Nine patients who underwent TKA with a posterior-stabilized mobile-bearing implant were analyzed using fluoroscopy to determine the amount of bearing rotation during a deep knee bend. All patients experienced bearing rotation, but most experienced less than 2.0° of polyethylene bearing rotation.

Mahfouz MR, Hoff WA, Komistek RD, Dennis DA: A robust method for registration of three-dimensional knee implant models to two-dimensional fluoroscopy images. *IEEE Trans Med Imaging* 2003;22(12):1561-1574.

An error analysis was conducted using a fresh cadaver to determine the relative and absolute errors for a robust method used for registering three-dimensional knee implant models to two-dimensional fluoroscopic images. The relative error for this process is less than 0.5 mm in translation and 0.5° in rotation.

Mathematical Modeling Techniques

Anderson FC, Pandy MG: Dynamic optimization of human walking. *J Biomech Eng* 2001;123:381-390.

A three-dimensional, neuromusculoskeletal human model was combined with dynamic optimization theory to simulate normal walking on level ground. Quantitative comparisons of the model predictions with patterns of body-segmental displacements, ground-reaction forces, and muscle activations demonstrated that the simulation reproduces the salient features of normal gait, suggesting that minimum metabolic energy per unit distance traveled is a valid measure of walking performance.

Buechel FF Sr, Buechel FF Jr, Pappas MJ, Dalessio J: Twenty-year evaluation of the New Jersey LCS rotating platform knee replacement. *J Knee Surg* 2002;15:84-89.

The clinical results of the initial cemented and cementless series of 233 New Jersey Low Contact Stress Rotating Platform Knee Replacements in 184 patients surviving at least 10 years were analyzed using a strict knee scoring scale. Survivorship of the patients who underwent primary cemented rotating platform knee replacements with end points of revision for any mechanical reason or a poor clinical knee score was 97.7% at 10- and 20-year follow-up. Survivorship of the patients who underwent cementless rotating platform knee replacements with end points of revision for any mechanical reason or a poor clinical knee score was 98.3% at 10- and 18-year follow-up.

Burny F, Donkerwolcke M, Moulart F, et al: Concept, design and fabrication of smart orthopedic implants. *Med Eng Phys* 2000;22:469-479.

The authors discuss the concept, design, and fabrication of orthopaedic implants instrumented with strain gauges connected to a Wheatstone bridge by means of percutaneous leads, particularly two fully implantable wireless designs that are powered from the outside by magnetic induction.

Komistek RD, Kane TR, Mahfouz M, Ochoa JA, Dennis DA: Knee mechanics: A review of past and present

techniques to determine in vivo loads. *J Biomech* 2005;38(2):215-228.

The authors of this article evaluated various techniques that were used to determine in vivo loads in the human knee, particularly telemetry, which is an experimental approach, and mathematical modeling, which is a theoretical approach. The authors also discuss another approach that relies on the use of in vivo data obtained from fluoroscopy, CT, MRI, and a revised motion analysis technique. A review of all techniques revealed a wide range of forces at the human knee, ranging from 1.9 to 7.2 times body weight during level walking.

Morris BA, D'Lima DD, Slamin J, et al: e-Knee: Evolution of the electronic knee prosthesis: Telemetry technology development. *J Bone Joint Surg Am* 2001;83-A (suppl 2):62-66.

The authors describe the development of the first telemetric tibia prosthesis. After conducting experimental tests on this device, modifications are being implemented before implantation.

Piazza SJ, Delp SL: Three-dimensional dynamic simulation of total knee replacement motion during a step-up task. *J Biomech Eng* 2001;123:599-606.

The authors developed a three-dimensional dynamic model of the tibiofemoral and patellofemoral articulations to predict the motions of knee implants during a step-up activity. The simulation reproduced an experimentally measured flexion-extension angle of the knee (within 1 SD), but translations at the tibiofemoral articulations were larger during the simulated step-up task than those reported for patients with total knee replacements.

Classic Bibliography

Andriacchi TP: Functional analysis of pre- and post-knee surgery: Total knee arthroplasty and ACL reconstruction. *J Biomech Eng* 1993;115:575-581.

Brand RA, Crowninshield RD, Wittstock CE, Pedersen DR, Clark CR, van Krieken FM: A model of lower extremity muscular anatomy. *J Biomech Eng* 1982;104(4): 304-310.

Draganich LF, Andriacchi T, Anderson GBJ: Interaction between intrinsic knee mechanics and the knee extensor mechanism. *J Orthop Res* 1987;5:539-547.

Kane TR, Levinson D: *Dynamics: Theory and Applications.* New York, NY, McGraw-Hill Publishing Company, 1985.

Karrholm J, Jonsson H, Nilsson KG, Soderqvisy I: Kinematics of successful knee prosthesis during weight-bearing: Three dimensional movements and positions of screw axes in the Tricon-M and Miller-Galante designs. *Knee Surg Sports Traumatol Arthrosc* 1994;2:50-59.

Komistek RD, Stiehl JB, Dennis DA: Mathematical model of the lower extremity joint reaction forces using Kane's method of dynamics. *J Biomech* 1998;31:185-189.

Lu TW, O'Connor JJ, Taylor SJG, Walker PS: Validation of a lower limb model with in vivo femoral forces telemetered from two subjects. *J Biomech* 1998;31:63-69.

Morrison JB: The mechanics of the knee joint in relation to normal walking. *J Biomech* 1970;3:51-61.

Murphy M: Geometry and the kinematics of the normal human knee. PhD thesis. Cambridge, MA, Department of Mechanical Engineering Massachusetts Institute of Technology 1990.

Murray DW, Goodfellow JW, O'Connor JJ: The Oxford medial unicompartmental arthroplasty: A ten year survival study. *J Bone Joint Surg Br* 1998;80:983-989.

Nilsson KG, Karrholm J, Gadegaard P: Abnormal kinematics of the artificial knee: Roentgen stereophotogrammetric analysis of 10 Miller-Galante and five New Jersey LCS knees. *Acta Orthop Scand* 1991;62:440-446.

Paul JP: Force actions transmitted by joints in the human body. *Proc R Soc Lond B Biol Sci* 1976;192(1107): 163-172.

Seireg A, Avikar RJ: A mathematical model for evaluation of forces in lower extremities of the musculoskeletal system. *J Biomech* 1973;6:313-326.

Wimmer MA, Andriacchi TP: Tractive forces during rolling motion of the knee: Implications for wear in total knee replacement. *J Biomech* 1997;30:131-137.

Chapter 3

Total Knee Implant Design

Peter S. Walker, PhD

Introduction

Most of the features of total knee implants used in current designs were first introduced in the 1970s, notwithstanding the numerous refinements in design and technique that have occurred since that time. Subsequent biomechanical studies and clinical experience have identified the features that provided satisfactory function, durability, and absence of problems over the long term. From the beginning, there were two types of condylar replacements: those that were more anatomic, characterized by less constraint and a reliance on at least the posterior cruciate ligament for stability; and those that adopted a more mechanical approach by sacrificing the cruciate ligaments and relying on the constraint of the bearing surfaces or intercondylar guiding surfaces for stability. In general, both of these design types have had a similar clinical performance based on criteria such as survivorship and clinical evaluation schemes.

At the opposite extremes of the condylar replacements have been the unicompartmental knee implants and the linked or constrained implants. Unicompartmental knee implants have had limited indications, mainly the requirements for an intact anterior cruciate ligament and reasonably normal lateral and patellar components, but successful long-term results of some designs and minimally invasive techniques have led to a recent upsurge of application. Linked or constrained implants have had an important place in revision and salvage, with an intercondylar mechanism requiring less bone resection, and the incorporation of tibial rotation features, adding benefit to these otherwise nonconservative approaches.

The numerous augmentations such as stem extensions, wedges, and blocks have played an important role in expanding and optimizing the use of condylar replacements and constrained designs to otherwise difficult reconstructive procedures. Until a few years ago, the availability of this range of implants seemed to be sufficient and seemed to have solved the problem of restoring the arthritic knee to an acceptable functional level, with the expectation of at least a 95% success rate at 10-year follow-up and longer. However, based on studies in which patients have been categorized by expectations and capabilities, it has recently been noted that the designs and techniques can be further developed to enhance performance and rehabilitation. In addition, the introduction of new technology has led to the development of innovative surgical techniques. As a result, new total knee implant design goals have emerged (Table 1).

Although until recently it appeared that the field of total knee replacement had reached a plateau, the field is experiencing an increase in new developments as a result of the new design goals. The principles of design and technique that have evolved and succeeded in the past few decades provide the platform for these new total knee implant design goals, which are likely to result in substantial benefits in the years ahead.

Table 1 | New Total Knee Implant Design Goals

Extended durability	This has resulted in the identification of net-shape molded polyethylene and highly cross-linked polyethylene for tibial and patellar bearing surfaces; ceramic surfaces can also reduce wear. New cementless modalities are emerging.
Extended range of flexion	Modifications have been made to the implant designs and to the surgical techniques to make this possible.
Improved functional ability	This is being addressed by new design concepts and by improvements in rehabilitation.
Greater consistency of clinical results with a minimization of problems	One of the major areas of development is computer-assisted surgery using navigation.
Reduced trauma and shorter recovery times	Smaller incisions (minimally invasive surgery), possibly augmented by navigation, will reduce trauma and recovery time.

Geometry of the Bearing Surfaces

A dimensional description of condylar replacements is necessary for component definition and for manufacturing purposes (Figure 1). However, the parameters can be used for a range of evaluations. The shape of the components can be compared with that of the natural knee for determining the closeness of fit and for sizing schemes. In computer models, the kinematics as well as the muscle and joint forces can be predicted. Calculations can be made of the contact stresses on the plastic surface as an indicator of the wear and deformation. In Figure 1, the major radii are shown in both the sagittal and frontal planes.

In the sagittal plane of the femur, symmetric total knee implants take an average contour between the anatomic lateral and medial profiles. However, some designs preserve a lateral and medial difference to obtain a differential rollback in early flexion, assuming that rolling does occur in this range. For example, if the distal radii of the lateral and medial femoral radii are 70 mm and 40 mm, respectively, for a 10° flexion arc, the lateral condyle would roll posteriorly by 5 mm more than the medial condyle, producing an internal rotation of about 6°. The sagittal radii at the posterior of the femoral condyles will influence the range of flexion because of the effect of the tensions in the posterior cruciate and medial collateral ligaments. Reducing the radius at high flexion angles may reduce the possibility of high ligament tensions, but it will increase the likelihood of bony impingement on the posterior of the tibia.

An important parameter in the sagittal plane is the transition angle between the large distal radius and the smaller posterior radius. If the transition angle is 20° or more, the large distal radius will contact the tibia during the entire stance phase of gait, reducing the contact stresses on the plastic. This scheme has been used on the Low Contact Stress (LCS) Rotating Platform (DePuy, Warsaw, IN) design and in many other condylar designs. However, there are two possible consequences to this scheme. First, because of geometric design constraints, the distal anterior trochlea can be abnormal in shape, which can require higher forces in the quadriceps and patellar ligament. Second, there can be a kinematic abnormality such that, in moving from extension to mid-flexion, the femur will displace anteriorly, which is opposite to the behavior in the natural knee. This is because, in the presence of axial compressive forces and relatively low shear forces, the femur locates close to the dwell point on the tibia. This phenomenon has been observed in fluoroscopy studies of deep knee bends or step ascending and descending, where the femur is found to slide anteriorly with flexion and posteriorly with extension, so-called paradoxical motion. The anterior femoral sagittal radii determine the tracking of the patella. It is important that the sagittal profile closely

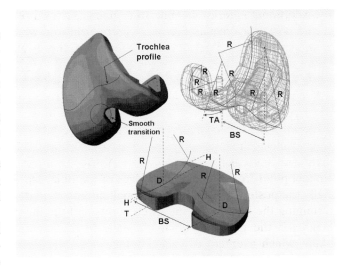

Figure 1 Schematic representation of the parameters describing the geometry of the bearing surfaces of a total knee implant. R = radius, H = jump height, T = thickness, TA = transition angle, BS = bearing spacing, D = dwell point (bottom of the dish).

replicates the anatomic profile to preserve the correct lever arm of the quadriceps. The largest patellar femoral forces occur at the higher flexion angles when the patella traverses the intercondylar notch. Hence, there should be a smooth transition region between the trochlea bearing surfaces and the distal femoral surfaces that articulate with the tibia.

Although the sagittal femora radii are determined largely by the requirement of closely replicating the anatomic profile, the sagittal tibial radius can range from infinite (a flat surface) to a value equal to the largest distal sagittal femoral radius. The former, which is analogous to the lateral tibial compartment, would produce no inherent constraint, whereas the latter, resembling the medial tibial compartment, would provide the maximum constraint. Most current designs use a value between the two. Using round numbers for an average-sized knee, a sagittal tibial radius of 80, 70, and 60 mm will provide low, moderate, and high constraint, respectively, to anteroposterior shear forces and torques. The larger radii will result in higher contact stresses. An interesting alternative to symmetric tibial surfaces is the medial pivot concept, which includes low constraint on the lateral side and maximum constraint on the medial. This scheme more closely replicates the anatomic motion, in which the contact location on the lateral side moves progressively posterior with flexion, while the contact on the medial side remains in the same location. In high flexion, the lateral contact is at the very posterior edge of the tibia, and the medial side displaces posteriorly by a few millimeters and levers upward on the posterior horn of the meniscus.

The sagittal tibial radii and the location of the dwell point determine the anterior and posterior jump heights, which is one measure of anteroposterior stability. Additional anterior stability to compensate for a resected posterior cruciate ligament can be achieved with a smaller anterior tibial radius. Anatomically, the dwell point is located about 40% from the posterior edge. When axial compression forces are applied, the femur will contact at the dwell point. When a shear force is superimposed, the contact will displace along an anteroposterior line. The smaller the tibial radius, the less the displacement; the larger the tibial radius, the more ligament and muscular control is required to prevent the contact point from reaching the edges of the tibia, especially the posterior edge. An additional parameter in determining the location of the dwell points and the jump heights is the posterior tibial tilt angle in the sagittal plane, which averages 8° (SD, 3°). For each total knee implant design, the angle needs to be defined for the particular geometry and technique. The dwell point moves approximately 1 mm posteriorly for every 1° of posterior tibial tilt.

In regard to the frontal radii, the femur and tibia need to be considered in combination. The frontal profile is usually constant around the femoral condyles and from the anterior to posterior of the tibia. The femorotibial conformity is preferably close to maintain the maximum contact area. However, the values of the frontal radii make a major difference to the constraint in internal-external rotation. This is important because a rotation of approximately ± 10° in extension and ± 20° in flexion is required for normal function. For a given relative femorotibial conformity, as the radius increases, the rotational constraint decreases. Eventually, a point is reached where the mediolateral jump height becomes so small that stability in this direction is inadequate. A further limiting consideration is the stability to varus-valgus movements. If lift-off occurs, a stable pivot point is an advantage. For a constant frontal radius, a value of approximately 40 to 50 mm is seen as optimal, although different inner and outer radii can be an alternative option. The bearing spacing is an important parameter in the frontal plane. The larger the bearing spacing, the greater the varus-valgus stability; a high bearing spacing will increase rotational constraint. A suitable value for average bearing space size is approximately 46 mm.

With these bearing geometries, the contact areas on each condyle will be elliptical, with the major axis being mediolateral. It is important that the contact area does not diminish for different relative displacement and rotational positions of the femur and tibia. Any digging in that occurs can lead to excessive damage of the plastic. Achieving high contact areas and smooth boundaries also applies to the patellofemoral joint. Because there is now strong evidence that replacing or retaining the patella are equally viable clinical options, the femoral trochlea should be anatomic in profile and blend smoothly around the intercondylar notch.

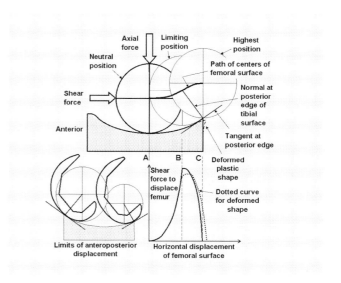

Figure 2 Schematic representation of an anteroposterior constraint test in which the femur is loaded and a shear force is applied. In a cyclic test, the shear force is reversed from anterior to posterior. A, B, and C line up with the center of the femoral surface in the neutral, limiting, and highest positions, respectively.

Constraint and Laxity

Constraint and laxity are frequently used to describe a total knee implant, whereas a test to quantify these properties is a US Food and Drug Administration requirement for a new total knee implant design. Constraint is the resistance provided to anteroposterior displacement and internal-external rotation (mediolateral and varus-valgus can also be included) because of the shape of the bearing surfaces or other mechanical features. Laxity refers to the measured displacement and rotation values in a constraint test. To measure kinematics in fluoroscopy studies, the displacements and rotations that have occurred in various test activities have been related to the constraint; the higher the constraint, the lower the measured laxity. Variation between patients, however, is considerable. Regarding the significance of constraint, using standard clinical evaluations or survivorship analysis, the results of total knee implants with high or low constraint, with posterior cruciate ligament preservation or substitution, have been similar. However, tests on specific groups of patients, especially those who are more active, may demonstrate differences in the function, wear, satisfaction level, and feel of the implant.

The characteristics of constraint are shown in Figure 2. If there is a compressive force between the femur and tibia and then a shear force is applied, there will be a displacement until equilibrium is reached. For an implanted total knee replacement, the restraints are the ligaments, muscle forces, curvature of the tibial bearing surfaces, and friction of the metal-plastic interface. For a test with the total knee implant in isolation, the curvatures and friction only are involved, and the test becomes reproducible and can be used to compare one total knee im-

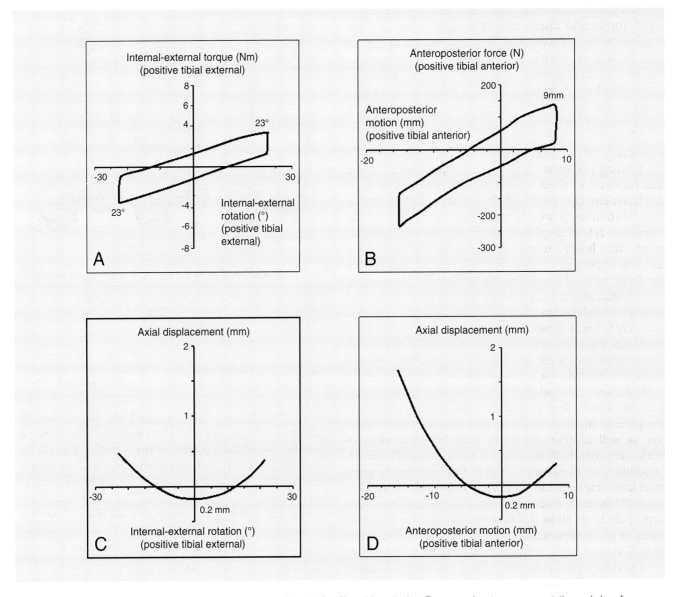

Figure 3 **A** and **B,** Schematic representation of the constraint curves for a NexGen CR total knee implant. The curves show torque versus rotation, and shear force versus displacement. The stiffness is the slope of the curves. **C** and **D,** Schematic representation of the axial displacement of the femoral component during the tests. Test conditions included NexGen CR total knee implant, 155° of flexion, axial force of 712 N (one times the body weight), and posterior tibial tilt of 3°.

plant with another. The limits of the contact point extend from the tangent points at the anterior and the posterior edges of the implant. In general, evidence indicates that this range is not used in normal function because it would represent extreme instability. However, results from retrieval studies show that damage at the anterior or posterior edges of the implant has frequently been observed, typical of failure caused by instability. Most contemporary total knee implant designs provide dishing of the tibial surfaces with radii between 60 and 80 mm to compensate for the absence of one or both cruciate ligaments; in such designs, instability is relatively infrequent.

In the test, the assumption is that the femur is in the neutral position at the dwell point on the tibial surface, and an axial compressive force is applied. If a shear force is now applied, the femur displaces. The shear force increases with the displacement until an equilibrium position is reached. The shear force can be increased so that the femur reaches the limiting position at the common tangent point at the very edge of the component, the posterior edge in the example provided in Figure 2. Further displacement will result in the femur pivoting over the edge of the plastic, whereas the shear force that can be carried diminishes, resulting in an unstable situation. Such contact at the edge results in deformation of the plastic, produces further instability and if repeated, severe damage to the plastic.

Figure 3 provides examples of constraint curves for a posterior cruciate ligament–retaining design with low-moderate constraint (NexGen Cruciate Retaining [CR],

Zimmer). The tests were performed in a special rig in which forces and displacements in all degrees of freedom could be controlled and monitored. In the shear test, the limiting position of the femur displacing posterior was 9 mm at a shear force of little over 100 N. The femur could displace anteriorly by more than 20 mm, at which point the shear force was greater than 300 N, which is an unlikely scenario; hence, the test was limited to 16 mm of displacement. A cyclic torque was applied to produce internal and external rotation; the angles to the limiting positions were 23°. A torque of only 3 Nm was required to reach the limits. The amounts of axial displacement that occurred during the anteroposterior and rotation tests were surprisingly small. Except for when the femur displaced anteriorly, all the displacements were limited to approximately 0.5 mm, indicating the low constraint of this type of geometry (primarily the large radii of the curvature of the tibial surface in the sagittal and frontal planes). The amount of actual penetration of the femoral surface into the tibial surface was only 0.2 mm. Based on the radii of curvature of the particular knee being tested, even this small amount of penetration indicated an area of contact of approximately 70 mm^2 on each condyle as measured by contact area studies, even when the tests were performed at 155° of flexion. This particular total knee implant was designed to maintain full contact at that degree of flexion, as well as allow for more than 20° of rotation in both directions, both of which were achieved. However, in addition to allowing rotation in flexion, fixed-bearing total knee implants ideally require rotational laxity of at least 10° in each direction when the knee is in extension. This is to allow for nonoptimal rotational placement of the components and to avoid the transmission of high torques.

The rotating platform or mobile-bearing knee implant is a type of total knee prosthesis that is specifically designed to provide rotational freedom at all angles of flexion. The theoretic advantages of this design are that component placement at surgery is not critical, freedom of motion for any activity is provided, and the femorotibial bearing surfaces can be made with high conformity, which minimizes contact stresses and wear. The latter has been confirmed with the Oxford Unicompartmental Knee System (Biomet, Warsaw, IN), for which wear rates of only 0.02 mm/year with molded polyethylene have been measured in vivo. Although some rotating platform knees have been successful clinically, no particular advantage has yet been demonstrated clinically with total knee implant designs. However, as noted previously, it may be that mechanical features such as freedom of rotation or high flexion capability are only an advantage for patients who are capable of performing specific activities.

For a mobile-bearing knee implant with a fixed axis of internal-external rotation, the location of the axis affects the mechanics (Figure 4). When the axis is central, the

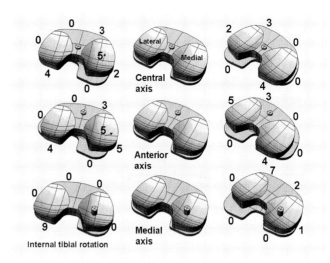

Figure 4 Schematic representation of the effects (in mm) on the overhang and the movements of the lateral and medial sides for different centers of rotation in a rotating platform knee implant. The rotation is 15° in each direction. Top row = central axis, middle row = anterior axis, bottom row = medial axis.

movements on the medial and lateral sides are equal and opposite. If the femoral component is seated in the dwell points, in high flexion, when the lateral condyle tends to displace posteriorly, there will be an anteromedial displacement. However, in the normal knee, the medial contact remains in the same location with little deviation, in part because of the tightness of the medial collateral ligament. Furthermore, anterior displacement of the medial femoral condyle is likely to cause posterior impingements that will limit the maximum flexion. This disadvantage can be avoided; however, in a posterior stabilized knee implant design in which the intercondylar cam causes femoral rollback in high flexion and the displacement behavior is therefore similar to that of the normal knee. In this instance, the femoral condyles do have to ride up the posterior ramp of the plastic surfaces, which will tend to tighten soft tissues and possibly limit flexion.

If the axis of rotation is central in the mediolateral direction but anterior, the kinematics still have the disadvantage of anteromedial displacement as well as another disadvantage of sideways motion. In the example shown in Figure 4, the overhang on the medial or lateral sides for 15° of rotation is 5 mm. The plastic could then impinge on the medial collateral ligament.

A medial pivot point provides the closest replication of normal motion, in which instance the medial femoral condyle remains in a constant location for both internal and external rotation, but the displacements of the lateral side are increased. For 15° of internal tibial rotation, there is 9 mm of posterior overhang in the example shown in Figure 4. For the lateral femoral condyle seated in the dwell point, this overhang would reproduce normal knee motion in high flexion where the lateral femoral condyle actually locates at the very posterior of the tibial bearing surface. The plastic, therefore, may be subject to excessive stresses because of the overhang. This is certainly possible because it has been calculated that joint compressive forces of greater than two times body weight are likely to occur when rising from a deep squat. If such a force occurred at the very posterior of an overhung plastic component, high stresses would occur on the upper surface as well as along the line where the plastic overhangs the metal tray. A possible compromise is to place the medial pivot point on the medial side but only halfway to the bearing spacing (Figure 1). For example, if the bearing spacing was 48 mm (as in an average normal knee), a pivot point at 12 mm from the midline would only result in about 2 mm of anterior displacement of the medial condyle for 15° of internal rotation.

How much rotation occurs between the plastic and the metal plate in a mobile-bearing knee implant? Both laboratory and clinical studies have shown that the amounts of rotation are limited, and no more than on the femorotibial bearing surfaces of fixed-bearing knee implants. One of the likely reasons for this is that the rotation occurs preferentially on the femoral-tibial surface when this is partially conforming (this applies to the LCS implant design after 20° of flexion). The reason for this relates to the friction. The friction coefficient (friction force/axial compressive force) of polyethylene on metal is not constant but varies with the contact pressure: the lower the pressure, the higher the friction coefficient. Hence, if there is a compressive force and a torque simultaneously applied to the knee, the lowest frictional resistance occurs at the upper bearing surfaces and not between the plastic and the plate. Figure 5 shows the substantial frictional torque that is required to initiate rotation when an axial force of two times the body weight is applied. In this test, the plastic was oscillated in internal and then external rotation, and the frictional torque was measured. With bovine serum as the lubricant, the breakaway torque was almost 30% higher than the dynamic torque once motion had been initiated. The magnitude of the torque (greater than 3 Nm) is considerable and indicates that in many activities the applied torque would be insufficient to cause rotation at that bearing. Conversely, both sliding and rolling could occur at the femoral-plastic interface.

Overall, specifying the ideal constraint for a total knee implant is a complex problem. Because designs with a wide range of constraints seem to function similarly based on traditional evaluation methods, it can be assumed that the knee adapts to the implant during the months following implantation. However, if restoration of normal constraint is a goal of total knee implant design, then in a laboratory test in which a total knee prosthesis is implanted in a cadaveric knee, the constraint characteristics in response to several tests should be indistinguishable from those of the knee in its intact state. For the patient with a normal knee on one side and a total knee implant on the

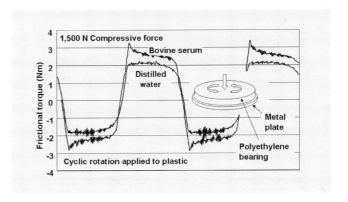

Figure 5 Graphic representation of the frictional torque between a polished metal plate and polyethylene bearing in a rotating platform implant model that was axially loaded and then a cyclic torque applied. The curve shows the magnitude of the torque to cause rotational movement.

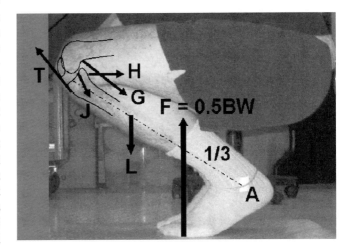

Figure 6 Photograph illustrating a method for calculating forces in squatting. The forces acting on the tibia are the ground reaction force (F) (one half of body weight [BW]), patellar tendon force (T), hamstring force (H), gastrocnemius force (G), weight of the leg (L), and joint force (J). The ground reaction force intersects the tibia approximately one third the distance from the center of rotation of the ankle joint (A) to the top of the tibia.

other, the constraints should be similar, and the total knee implant ought to feel like a normal knee.

Requirements for High Flexion

The average ranges of flexion achieved by total knee implants have generally been from 100° to 110°. The postoperative range is usually close to the preoperative range, which implies that soft-tissue effects such as capsular thickening and muscle adhesions are limiting factors. Nevertheless, in recent years efforts to modify both the surgical technique and the implant design have been undertaken to achieve high flexion activities such as kneeling, crouching, and squatting.

Deep flexion activities can be characterized as those requiring relatively low muscle forces such as kneeling and those requiring high forces such as squatting and ris-

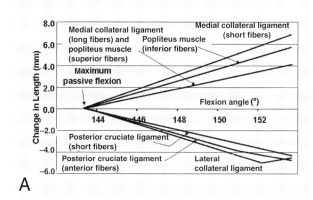
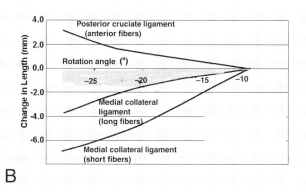

Figure 7 Graphic representation of the changes in the lengths of ligaments when a specimen with a total knee implant was forcibly hyperflexed **(A)** and forcibly rotated **(B)** at the natural maximum flexion angle. The posterior tibial slope was 3°. Shaded area (in B) indicates popliteus muscle (superior and inferior fibers), posterior cruciate ligament (posterior fibers), and lateral collateral ligament.

ing. These activities involve flexion angles in the range of 135° to 155° or more. The most common method of achieving these angles in squatting with comfort is to place the foot flat on the ground and externally rotate the foot or to elevate the foot as shown in Figure 6. In such a position, the ground reaction force (half of the body weight in symmetric squatting) intersects the tibia approximately one third the distance from the center of rotation of the ankle joint to the top of the tibia. Elevation from that position is achieved by tension in the quadriceps, with gastrocnemius and hamstring forces acting as antagonists. With only the quadriceps active, both the muscle force and the resultant joint force are two to three times the body weight. The joint force can be resolved into a compressive component acting down the tibial axis and a shear force in a direction such that it would tense the posterior cruciate ligament. The compressive force component is of similar magnitude, but there is a shear force component acting on the tibia of approximately one time the body weight. A force in the gastrocnemius, acting closely parallel to the tibia, would increase the patellar tendon force and the joint force in an equal amount. The hamstrings force exerts a posterior force on the tibia, and its effect on the magnitude of the resultant force is small. However, it slightly reduces the compressive component but increases the shear component, a value of one and one half times body weight being possible. In this analysis, the additional inertia forces that are present during rising quickly, for instance, have not been accounted for nor has the weight of the shank.

Because this activity requires delicate balance and high quadriceps forces in a fully elongated muscle, it is not easy even for normal individuals to perform. The compressive forces on the implant are more than for level walking or stair climbing and descending. However, unless there is a full area of contact between the posterosuperior femoral condyles and the tibial plateau, digging in will occur, which would eventually lead to serious

damage of the plastic. There is also the possibility of impingement of the posterior femur just above the component and the posterior edge of the plastic. The effect of the high shear force (one to one and one half times the body weight) needs to be considered. In a posterior stabilized knee implant, this force will act on the posterior of the plastic post. In a posterior cruciate ligament–retaining design, the posterior cruciate ligament will be tensed and the femorotibial contact point will tend to move anteriorly when rising from a squat, a phenomenon that has been observed in fluoroscopic studies.

In achieving the higher flexion angles, either actively or passively, the limitations to motion can be a combination of the tightness of soft tissues, including the anterior muscles and retinacula, impingements of bone against the implant components, and the pressing together of the thigh and shank. However, impingements will always be reacted by soft tissues within the joint itself. Studies have been performed to investigate this, both in the intact knee and after total knee replacement. In one study, the knee was loaded to 5 kg and passive maximum flexion was achieved. Using a three-dimensional space tracker to digitize the attachment points of soft tissues in a starting reference position and to track the three-dimensional motion continuously, the lengths of the soft tissues could be computed using vector analysis. When the knee was at maximum flexion, a moment was applied to forcibly hyperflex the knee (Figure 7). In this example, knee flexion was from 143° to 153°, as if a person were kneeling with body weight applying the final flexion range. The structures that elongated were the short and long fibers of the medial collateral ligament and the popliteus muscle. These structures were already elongated at 143° of flexion, so it is likely that they were among the limiting factors to high flexion. Conversely, even though the anterior fibers of the posterior cruciate ligament elongated up to approximately 135° of flexion, beyond that both the anterior and posterior fibers reduced in length in hyperflexion. Hence, the anterior and posterior fibers of the posterior cruciate ligament and the lateral collateral ligament were not limiting hyperflexion.

High flexion was shown to be accompanied by internal tibial rotation (external femoral rotation) in some situations. At the limit of flexion (143°), the knee was forcibly rotated and the soft-tissue lengths were determined. The only structures that elongated were the anterior fibers of the posterior cruciate ligament. Significantly, both bands of the medial collateral ligament shortened considerably; therefore, although the medial collateral ligament limited hyperflexion, it would not have limited the motion if accompanied by internal tibial rotation. Regarding the anterior fibers of the posterior cruciate ligament, hyperflexion accompanied by internal tibial rotation would have resulted in little change of length. Clearly, there are many factors that determine the limitations to high flexion, including surgical technique, implant design, and the prevailing condition of the knee joint. However, these study results indicate that particular attention should be given at the time of surgery to the tensions in the medial collateral ligament (especially the short fibers), the anterior fibers of the posterior cruciate, and the popliteus muscle.

As to the design of the total knee replacement components themselves, several modifications can be made to standard designs to facilitate high flexion (Figure 8). Preservation of a full area of contact is necessary to avoid digging in of the posterior-superior edge of the femoral condyles into the plastic. This can be achieved by increasing the posterior cut on the bone and thickening the posterior condyle itself, which allows the posterior condylar radius to continue farther. In the example shown, the tangent at the tip is 20°, allowing up to 155° of flexion with full contact. Along with this feature, however, any bone remaining about the superior corner must be removed to avoid impingement and plastic damage, which is a difficult procedure. In individuals whose lifestyle has included frequent kneeling, this area of the femur is typically more recessed. The provision of a minus (in-between) size recognizes the difficulty in matching exactly the correct tensions of the medial collateral ligament, posterior cruciate ligament, and other soft tissues throughout flexion and especially in high flexion. This minus size, which can be used to loosen a tight knee or tighten a loose knee (from the size below), allows for such fine tuning but requires extra inventory. When high flexion is accompanied by internal tibial rotation, as in a kneeling position (Figure 8), the interior of the posterior lateral femoral condyle can impinge on the posterior cruciate ligament. To relieve this, the femoral condyle can be chamfered. This also prevents the condyle from contacting the edge of the notch in the plastic. There is a small but acceptable reduction in contact area with this adjustment. On the plastic compo-

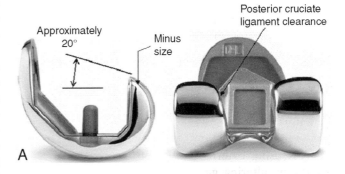

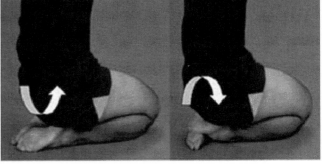

Figure 8 **A,** Photographs showing the features of a total knee implant that have been especially adapted for high flexion. The minus size, between the standard size and the size below, allows for fine tuning of the soft-tissue balancing. **B,** Photographs showing that kneeling and squatting can involve tibial rotation.

nent, the posterior edges should be chamfered to reduce the possibility of deformation from posterior contacts under load. The anterior edge of the plastic needs to be rounded and recessed to allow for the passage of the patellar tendon to avoid problems when there is high flexion and high tendon forces. On the question of whether a rotating platform implant will result in higher flexion angles than a fixed-bearing design, this is probably a topic for controlled clinical studies. However, biomechanical studies in the laboratory using special high-flexion test rigs can provide insight about forces, contact point locations, and impingements that is not readily determined from clinical studies. For example, in a fixed-bearing design, if the posterior of the plastic is shallow and relieved and there is a mechanism for achieving femoral rollback (from the posterior cruciate ligament or from a cam), high flexion is possible. In a mobile-bearing design, if there is relatively high femorotibial conformity, the plastic shape at the posterior of the implant must be such as to avoid bony impingements. Other schemes are possible to facilitate high flexion. In the Bisurface knee prosthesis (Kyocera, Kyoto, Japan), an intercondylar spherical bearing is used to provide both posterior femoral displacement and freedom of rotation in high flexion. In fact, freedom of rotation is just as important as a bias toward internal tibial rotation, which is the natural way the knee moves. However, squatting positions and even kneeling (Figure 8) can involve external tibial rotation, which is imposed by each patient's choice of position.

Summary

Total knee implant design, technique, and materials are going through a period of rapid development. More attention will likely be given to addressing arthritis in its early stages, including the potential for arresting the progress using external orthotic devices such as shoe wedges, by altering gait patterns, or by pharmacologic means. Smaller components such as local resurfacing and unicompartmental devices will play an increasing role. Tissue-engineered solutions involving osteochondral grafts are even possible. However, total knee replacement is likely to remain the primary treatment for generalized arthritis of the knee, the incidence of which has been predicted to steadily increase over the coming years. Total knee implant designs will be modified to allow for high flexion and will include materials that will reduce wear and damage. Other modifications such as reduction in the length of the tibial post and modular tibial posts and even modular femoral components will be developed to facilitate the insertion of total knee implants through small incisions. There is evidence that along with smaller incisions, use of computer-assisted surgery will become more widespread, especially when it allows not only for improved accuracy but for reduced surgical time. The possibility of making curved bone cuts will in turn allow for implants that are more anatomic and that preserve much more of the bone. These features may result in a general improvement in patient function, especially for those who are potentially more active.

Annotated Bibliography

General

Insall JH, Clarke HD: Historical development, classification and characteristics of knee prosthesis, in Insall JH, Scott WN (eds): *Surgery of the Knee*, ed 3. New York, NY, Churchill Livingstone, 2001, pp 1516-1552.

The authors discuss the basic design concepts of knee prostheses that were developed in the 1970s, including condylar replacement with and without preservation of cruciate ligaments, posterior-stabilized designs, and constrained condyles for instability.

Walker PS, Sathasivam S: Controlling the motion of total knee replacement using intercondylar guide surfaces. *J Orthop Res* 2000;18(1):48-55.

The authors devised a computerized method for generating and analyzing intercondylar cams such as those used in posterior-stabilized devices. Optimized cams were derived depending on the type of stability required.

Walker PS, Wang CJ, Masse Y: Joint laxity as a criterion for the design of condylar knee prostheses. *Clin Orthop* 2003;410:5-12.

In this study, a theoretic analysis provided the basis of condylar bearing surfaces that were partially conforming in both frontal and sagittal planes, providing a combination of stability and laxity according to which cruciate ligaments were preserved or resected.

Weiss JM, Noble PC, Conditt MA, et al: What functional activities are important in patients with knee replacements? *Clin Orthop* 2002;404:172-188.

A wide range of everyday activities were analyzed in patients who underwent knee replacement. Some activities, those of high biomechanical demand, were found to be still beyond the capability of many patients.

Geometry of the Bearing Surfaces

Dennis DA, Komistek RD, Mahfouz MR, Haas BD, Stiehl JB: Multicenter determination of in vivo kinematics after total knee arthroplasty. *Clin Orthop* 2003;416:37-57.

The authors analyzed the kinematic patterns of 811 knee replacements with a range of implant designs. There was a wide range of patterns for each type of knee implant, and factors such as paradoxical motion were identified when there was insufficient dishing of the surfaces.

Iwaki H, Pinskerova V, Freeman MA: Tibiofemoral movement 1: The shapes and relative movements of the femur and tibia in the unloaded cadaver knee. *J Bone Joint Surg Br* 2000;82(8):1189-1195.

The authors produced a model for the distal femur based on sagittal radii of different centers and described motion in flexion based on axes through the arc centers. The motion consisted primarily of a twisting about the medial condyle, with the lateral femoral condyle displacing posteriorly.

Nakagawa S, Kadoya Y, Todo S, et al: Tibiofemoral movement 3: Full flexion in the living knee studied by MRI. *J Bone Joint Surg Br* 2000;82(8):1199-1200.

The authors used MRI to assess active flexion from 90° to 133° and passive flexion to 162° in 20 unloaded knees. They found that flexion over this arc was accompanied by backward movement of the medial femoral condyle of 4.0 mm and by backward movement laterally of 15 mm.

Silva M, Shepherd EF, Jackson WO, Pratt JA, McClung CD, Schmalzried TP: Knee strength after total knee arthroplasty. *J Arthroplasty* 2003;18:605-611.

The authors of this study report that the peak torque generated by the quadriceps in knee extension was reduced by up to 30% in patients who underwent total knee arthroplasty, whereas flexion torque was reduced by 32%. The authors suggested that improved rehabilitation would increase muscle strength and enhance function in this patient population.

Yu CH, Walker PS, Dewar ME: The effect of design variables of condylar total knees on the joint forces in step climbing based on a computer model. *J Biomech* 2001;34:1011-1021.

A computer model was used to analyze the quadriceps force required to extend the knee for different total knee implant design variables. Although an implant design with a smaller distal radius reduced the forces by 12%, other variables had smaller effects.

Constraint and Laxity

Forster MC: Survival analysis of primary cemented total knee arthroplasty. *J Arthroplasty* 2003;18:265-270.

The author of this study combined survival analysis data from 16 articles (5,950 knees) to compare design features. No difference was found in survival rates when comparing posterior-stabilized implants and implants that were not stabilized or when comparing metal-backed and all-polyethylene tibial components. All-polyethylene tibial components that were not stabilized had significantly better survival rates than metal-backed, nonstabilized tibial components and posterior-stabilized, metal-backed components ($P < 0.05$).

Haider H, Walker PS: Measurements of constraint of total knee replacement. *J Biomech* 2005;38:341-348.

The laxity of different total knee replacement designs were measured in anterior-posterior and rotation with a load across the joint. The different designs had a wide range of laxity. The method was recommended as a standard to characterize the constraint of a total knee replacement and estimate its reliance on ligaments and its functional capabilities.

Misra AN, Hussain MRA, Fiddian NJ, Newton G: The role of the posterior cruciate ligament in total knee replacement. *J Bone Joint Surg Br* 2003;85:389-392.

In this study, two groups of patients (129 knees) were randomized to undergo total knee replacement using a standard posterior cruciate ligament–retaining cemented implant; in one group, the posterior cruciate ligament was retained, and in the other group it was resected. On average there were no differences in clinical results. The authors suggested that the posterior cruciate ligament was not functional in many patients, and based on satisfactory results of this study, they also questioned the need for a posterior-stabilized implant.

Ranawat AS, Rossi R, Loreti I, Rasquinha VJ, Rodriguez JA, Ranawat CS: Comparison of the PFC sigma fixed-bearing and rotating-platform total knee arthroplasty in the same patient. *J Arthroplasty* 2004;19:35-39.

The authors found that there were no significant differences in knee score, patient preference, range of flexion, and knee pain when comparing two types of implants that were inserted bilaterally in the same patients. The study period, however, was quite short (46 months for the fixed-bearing implants and 16 months for the rotating-platform implants.)

Straw R, Kulkarni S, Attfield S, Wilton TJ: Posterior cruciate ligament at total knee replacement. *J Bone Joint Surg Br* 2003;85:671-674.

Three cohorts of patients undergoing total knee replacement were compared and randomized to have either the posterior cruciate ligament retained, excised, or substituted with a posterior-stabilized implant. There were no differences between the groups for the knee score, function score, and range of flexion; however, patients who had partial posterior cruciate ligament release had poorer function scores.

Walker P, Haider H: Characterizing the motion of total knee replacement in laboratory tests. *Clin Orthop* 2003;410:54-68.

The authors review the methods used for testing the laxity and motion characteristics of total knee replacement implants, and conclusions were made regarding the most suitable tests to perform to assess different implant characteristics.

Weiss JM, Noble PC, Conditt MA, et al: What functional activities are important in patients with knee replacements? *Clin Orthop* 2002;404:172-188.

This was also a review of the methods used for testing the laxity and motion characteristics of total knees; in this article the authors also made conclusions regarding the most suitable tests to perform to assess different characteristics.

Requirements for High Flexion

Banks S, Bellemans J, Nozaki H, Whiteside LA, Harman M, Hodge WA: Knee motions during maximum flexion in fixed and mobile-bearing arthroplasties. *Clin Orthop* 2003;410:131-138.

The authors of this study reported a relationship between the maximum flexion achieved by patients who underwent total knee replacement and the anterior-posterior position of the femur on the tibia as measured by fluoroscopy. Posterior impingement was cited as a major reason for this finding.

Hung CT, Lima EG, Mauck RL, et al: Anatomically shaped osteochondral constructs for articular cartilage repair. *J Biomech* 2003;36:1853-1864.

The authors analyzed grafts consisting of bovine chondrocytes that were seeded into an agarose scaffold on a bony substrate and cultured for different times. They concluded that this may be a feasible method for replacing large areas of cartilage defects.

Miner AL, Lingard EA, Wright EA, Sledge CB, Katz JN: Knee range of motion after total knee arthroplasty. *J Arthroplasty* 2003;18:286-294.

In 684 patients who underwent total knee replacement, measures of patient satisfaction, including the Western Ontario and McMaster Universities Osteoarthritis Index pain and function questionnaire scores, patient satisfaction, and perceived improvement in quality of life, were compared with the range of flexion achieved. Only weak correlations were found, and the Western Ontario and McMaster Universities Osteoarthritis Index was suggested as a more useful overall measure.

Nagura T, Dyrby CO, Alexander EJ, Andriacchi TP: Mechanical loads at the knee joint during deep flexion. *J Orthop Res* 2002;20:881-886.

The authors conducted a biomechanical analysis of the external forces at the knee in deep squatting using radiographs and a knee model. High loads were predicted, including a high anterior shear force on the tibia.

Said RM, Walker PS, Kim DE, Ieaka K, Wei C-S: Factors influencing flexion in total knee replacement, in Proceedings of the *Transactions of the Annual Meeting of the Orthopaedic Research Society*, 2004. Available at: http://www.ors.org/Transactions/ TransactionsSearchResult.asp. Accessed June 6, 2005.

The authors of this study reported that the most influential factors in limiting deep flexion were the deep fibers of the medial collateral ligament; however, after 120° of flexion, the posterior cruciate ligament had little influence. Experiments were also conducted to assess internal and external rotation.

Sultan PG, Most E, Schule S, Li G, Rubash HE: Optimizing flexion after total knee arthroplasty. *Clin Orthop* 2003;416:167-173.

This preliminary study developed the technique of using a robot to investigate the mechanics of high flexion in a total knee replacement. Factors such as posterior impingement, tibial dishing and slope, and femoral component design were assessed.

Zalzal P, Papini M, Petruccelli D, deBeer J, Winemaker MJ: An in vivo biomechanical analysis of the soft-tissue envelope of osteoarthritic knees. *J Arthroplasty* 2004;19: 217-223.

A tensioning device was used in this study to quantify soft tissue tensions at the time of total knee replacement surgery. The tensions were significantly higher with retention of the posterior cruciate ligament. The authors concluded that these data can improve surgical technique and possibly patient function.

Classic Bibliography

Sathasivam S, Walker PS: The conflicting requirements of laxity and conformity in total knee replacement. *J Biomech* 1999;32:239-247.

Walker PS, Sathasivam S: The design of guide surfaces for fixed-bearing and mobile-bearing knee replacements. *J Biomech* 1999;32:27-34.

Chapter 4

Osteotomy

Mark W. Pagnano, MD

Introduction

Osteotomy for the treatment of unicompartmental knee arthrosis associated with malalignment of the lower limb has a well documented record of success. High tibial osteotomy for patients with varus knee deformity and medial compartment disease and distal femoral osteotomy for patients with valgus knee deformity and lateral compartment disease remain appropriate treatment options for a subgroup of patients with unicompartmental osteoarthritis. An evolving role exists for osteotomy in association with cartilage restoration procedures in those knees with concomitant varus or valgus malalignment.

The current role for periarticular osteotomies around the knee is strongly influenced by three trends in the treatment of knee problems. First, there is an increased willingness among some surgeons to bypass osteotomy and instead proceed directly to knee arthroplasty for patients in their 50s. Second, there has been a reemergence of unicompartmental knee replacement, in part because of the introduction of so-called minimally invasive techniques and in part because of encouraging midterm survivorship data. Third, there is an interest in intervening early in the treatment of some full-thickness articular cartilage defects of the knee, a trend that has been led by the introduction of osteochondral grafting techniques and cell-based therapies such as autologous chondrocyte implantation. Although many surgeons now use osteotomy for young or active patients and unicompartmental or total knee replacement for older, more sedentary patients, the exact role of each treatment option remains a source of debate.

The biomechanical rationale for osteotomy and the pathogenesis of degenerative arthrosis accompanying malalignment have been delineated well in the literature. Malalignment of the limb results in added stress on damaged articular cartilage and causes further loss of articular cartilage that subsequently exacerbates limb malalignment. This results in a downward spiral of progressive deformity and additional loss of articular cartilage over time. Osteotomy can be used to realign the limb, reduce stress on the articular cartilage at risk, and share the load with the opposite compartment of the knee. In appropriately selected patients, osteotomy is a reliable procedure to improve pain and function. Over the past two decades, osteotomy has been viewed largely as a temporizing measure to buy time for patients before they ultimately have a total knee arthroplasty. In this role, osteotomy has largely been accepted as successful. Substantial improvements in pain and function have been documented and seem to hold up well over a 7- to 10-year period after the osteotomy. The introduction of meniscal and articular cartilage restoration techniques has led to considerable interest in applying the favorable biomechanical effects of osteotomy to the younger patient who has a full-thickness chondral lesion or an absent meniscus. Osteotomy alone or in conjunction with techniques to restore articular or meniscal cartilage appears to be a reasonable treatment option for the symptomatic patient with substantial chondral injury and associated malalignment. Similarly, osteotomy in conjunction with either simultaneous or staged cruciate ligament reconstruction appears to be reliable in decreasing pain and improving function for patients with the combination of instability and pain from limb malalignment. Relatively few clinical data are available at this time on these combined osteotomy and cartilage restoration procedures; thus, definitive statements about their reliability or durability are not currently possible.

Assessment of Malalignment

Full-length hip to ankle radiographs are required to assess the mechanical axis and the tibiofemoral angle of the lower extremity (Figure 1). The normal anatomic axis or tibiofemoral angle measures 5° to 6° of valgus and is obtained by finding the intersection of the lines drawn along the anatomic axes of the tibia and femur. Most often the mechanical axis is used to determine the extent of limb malalignment. The mechanical axis, or weight-bearing line, is defined as that line from the center of the femoral head to the center of the tibiotalar joint; it typically measures 1.2° of varus. This is consistent with the fact that in normal knees approximately 60% of weight bearing is

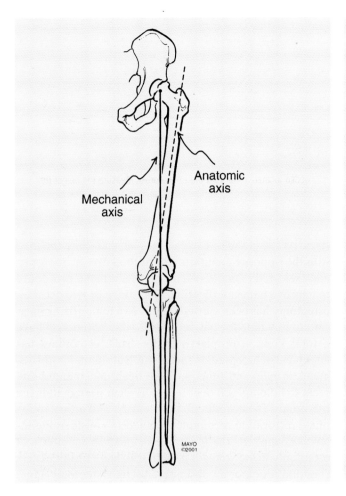

Figure 1 Schematic representation of the mechanical and anatomic axes. The mechanical axis *(solid line)* represents a line drawn from the center of the femoral head to the center of the talus and averages 1.2° of varus in the normal knee. The anatomic axis *(dashed line)* represents the difference between the longitudinal axis of the femur and tibia and averages 6° of valgus in the normal knee. *(Reproduced with permission from the Mayo Foundation, Rochester, MN.)*

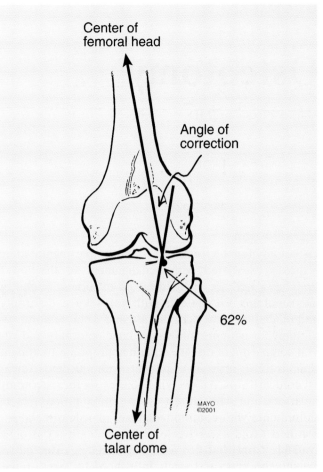

Figure 2 Schematic representation of the weight-bearing line method of preoperative planning. The 62% coordinate is measured from medial to lateral and typically lies just lateral to the lateral tibial spine. The angle that is subtended by the lines drawn from the femoral head center and the tibiotalar joint center to the 62% coordinate is the proposed angle of correction. *(Reproduced with permission from the Mayo Foundation, Rochester, MN.)*

done through the medial side of the knee. Varus malalignment with medial compartment disease is usually treated with a valgus-producing high tibial osteotomy, and valgus malalignment with lateral compartment disease is treated with a varus-producing distal femoral osteotomy. The desired postoperative alignment after a valgus-producing high tibial osteotomy and a varus-producing distal femoral osteotomy is slightly different. Most surgeons seek to correct the mechanical axis to pass through the 62% coordinate of the knee as measured from medial to lateral for valgus-producing high tibial osteotomy and to correct the mechanical axis to pass directly through the middle of the knee for a varus-producing distal femoral osteotomy (Figure 2).

High Tibial Osteotomy

The full-length weight-bearing radiograph facilitates measurement of overall limb alignment, joint line obliquity, and excess collateral ligament laxity. Ligamentous

laxity is represented by the amount of tibiofemoral joint space separation on the weight-bearing radiograph compared with the separation on a supine non–weight-bearing radiograph. Each millimeter of extra joint space opening has traditionally been thought to increase the apparent deformity by 1°; however, simple trigonometry reveals the flaw in this often-quoted rule of thumb and demonstrates that it is valid only for tibias that are 56 mm wide (Figure 3). Thus, it is best to directly measure the number of millimeters of separation and subtract that amount from the calculated size of the wedge needed to correct the deformity.

Preoperative planning should be done to facilitate an accurate and efficient surgical procedure. The weight-bearing line method of planning is appropriate for most straightforward osteotomies. This technique requires the four steps listed in Table 1.

In more complicated situations where there is associated extra-articular deformity or marked joint line

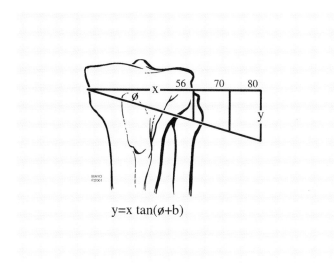

$$y = x \tan(\phi + b)$$

Figure 3 Schematic representation of the amount of correction as calculated using trigonometric methods. With this mathematical formula, it is clear that the old rule of thumb that the degree of correction would equal the size of the wedge in millimeters only applies to tibias that happen to be 56 mm wide. *(Reproduced with permission from the Mayo Foundation, Rochester, MN.)*

Table 1 | The Four Steps of the Weight-Bearing Line Method of Preoperative Planning for Osteotomy

Divide the tibial plateau from 0 to 100% from medial to lateral.

Determine the angle of correction: On a full-length hip to ankle radiograph, trace a line from the center of the femoral head to the 62% coordinate from medial to lateral and a second line from the tibiotalar center to the 62% coordinate. The angle subtended by those lines is the angle of correction.

Draw the angle of correction on the radiograph with the apex of the wedge located 1 cm from the tibial cortex. Measure the height (in millimeters) of the wedge at its base and then subtract the amount (in millimeters) of tibiofemoral separation. That calculated height is the size of the opening or closing wedge to correct the mechanical axis appropriately.

Be aware of any errors introduced by radiographic magnification.

obliquity, computerized analysis of the deformity may be used to predict the appropriate correction. In such situations, a combined high tibial and distal femoral osteotomy may be required to obtain appropriate correction and avoid excessive joint line obliquity. The data available from these computerized analyses can guide the surgeon as to the location, magnitude, and type of knee osteotomy for an individual patient and provide options among opening wedge versus closing wedge osteotomy, tibial versus femoral osteotomy, or combined osteotomies.

Surgical Technique

Lateral closing wedge osteotomy is performed with the patient supine and the knee either extended or flexed to 90° (Figure 4). The incision can be based laterally or a slightly longer midline incision may be used. Subperiosteal dissection of the anterior compartment musculature exposes the proximal tibia and the tibiofibular joint. To allow proper closure of the osteotomy, the tibiofibular joint is disrupted by removing the inner one third of the fibular head with its overlying cartilage. Subperiosteal dissection is performed along the posterior tibia, and a retractor is placed to protect the neurovascular structures. Similarly, the patellar tendon is protected anteriorly. A guide pin is placed 2 cm distal to the joint and parallel to the articular surface. A second guide pin is then placed at the distance calculated from pin one based on preoperative planning. Pin two is angled to intersect pin one at least 1 cm from the medial tibial cortex to leave a sufficient hinge for the osteotomy. Pin position and degree of correction should be confirmed fluoroscopically.

The proximal cut is made on the undersurface of pin one and care is taken to angle the saw slightly to match the patient's posterior slope. The distal cut is done on top of pin two. The most lateral wedge of bone can be removed easily, whereas the inner portion of the wedge, particularly the posteromedial corner of bone, often requires removal with a combination of osteotomes and curets. The medial cortex is left intact, but can be perforated with a narrow osteotome to facilitate closure of the osteotomy while leaving an intact osteoperiosteal sleeve. The osteotomy is closed with the gradual application of valgus stress to the tibia. Confirmation of appropriate correction is done by running a cautery cord or alignment rod from the center of the femoral head to the center of the talus and ensuring under fluoroscopy that the mechanical axis passes through the 62% coordinate of the knee. Fixation can be done with step-staples or a plate and screws per surgeon choice. If staples are used, the distal tine should be inserted after predrilling the lateral cortex in a way that promotes compression of the osteotomy site. Care must be taken not to disrupt the medial hinge when inserting the fixation device. Bone graft from the wedge can be placed around the osteotomy, and the wound is closed in layers. Postoperative care is dictated by the stability of the osteotomy. In most patients, full gentle motion and partial weight bearing is allowed with the use of a hinged knee brace or cast brace for the first 6 to 8 weeks and then progression to full weight bearing is allowed when there is radiographic evidence of healing. Patients for whom a closing wedge osteotomy is fixed rigidly with a plate and screws can safely increase range-of-motion exercises and weight bearing more quickly than those treated with staple fixation alone.

Medial opening wedge osteotomy has recently gained popularity in the United States after a long period of use in Europe. Potential advantages of the medial opening wedge technique include providing the

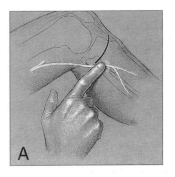
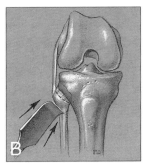
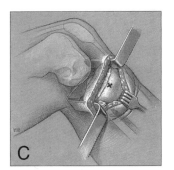
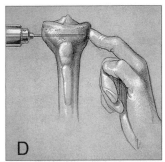

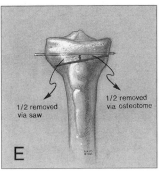
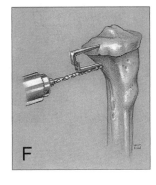
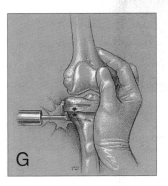

Figure 4 Illustration of the closing wedge high tibial osteotomy technique. **A,** Skin incision (*black line*). **B,** Resection of the inner one third of fibular head (*dashed line*). **C,** Retractors are placed anteriorly and posteriorly. **D,** Pin one is placed parallel to the joint and 2.0 cm distal to the joint line. **E,** The wedge is cut proximally and then distally, traversing 80% of the tibial width. **F,** A step staple is applied with the drill hole just distal to the inferior tine to promote compression of the osteotomy site. **G,** Firm counterpressure is applied during staple insertion to avoid disrupting the medial osteoperiosteal hinge. *(Reproduced with permission from the Mayo Foundation, Rochester, MN.)*

ability to easily adjust the degree of correction intraoperatively, providing the ability to correct deformities in the sagittal plane as well as the coronal plane, requiring only one bone cut, and avoiding the tibiofibular joint. The medial opening wedge technique is also less likely to introduce iatrogenic patella baja or introduce lateral collateral ligament laxity. The disadvantages of the opening wedge technique include the need for bone graft to fill the created defect, a potentially higher rate of nonunion or delayed union, and a longer period of restricted weight bearing after the procedure.

The procedure is done with the patient supine on a radiolucent table. The incision is centered between the medial border of the tibial tubercle and the posteromedial corner of the knee and is made starting just below the joint line and extending 5 to 8 cm distally. The pes tendons and superficial medial collateral ligament are elevated subperiosteally and protected. Subperiosteal dissection is done around the back of the tibia as far laterally as the tibiofibular joint, and a blunt retractor is placed to protect the neurovascular bundle. Anteriorly, the patellar tendon is identified and protected. A guide pin is placed under fluoroscopic guidance; the angle of this guide pin is along the line that connects the head of the fibula with the superomedial corner of the tibial tubercle. When the osteotomy is performed along this line, it ensures that the patellar tendon insertion is not violated and yet sufficient proximolateral tibial bone re-

mains intact to limit the chance of a fracture that would extend into the lateral compartment of the knee. The osteotomy is performed along the distal surface of the guide pin such that the guide pin limits proximal excursion of the saw blade. Appropriate depth of the cut is confirmed under fluoroscopy. The osteotomy is then gently opened with a tapered, calibrated wedge or other distraction device. Slowly opening the wedge (5 mm per minute) limits the chance of fracture through the lateral hinge or into the lateral compartment of the knee. Alignment can be progressively checked under fluoroscopy until the desired correction is obtained.

In most patients, the 62% coordinate of the knee also corresponds to the lateral margin of the lateral tibial spine. Sagittal alignment also should be assessed before fixing the osteotomy. Because of the triangular cross-section of the tibia, the wedge should be slightly wider posteromedially than it is anteriorly to maintain the normal posterior slope of the tibia. If the anterior and posteromedial portions are opened similar amounts, then the posterior slope will be increased. In patients with cruciate ligament deficiency, there may be a role for deliberately altering the tibial slope to decrease anterior or posterior tibial translation. Once the final wedge size and location has been selected, the osteotomy is fixed with a plate and screws. Special step plates that maintain the opening wedge gap are useful (Figure 5). The created defect is then grafted using autograft or

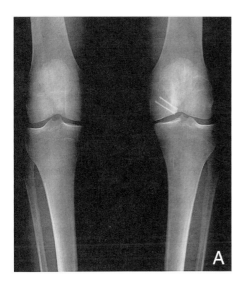
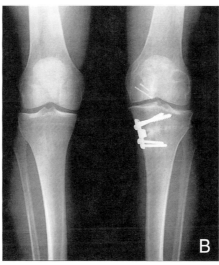
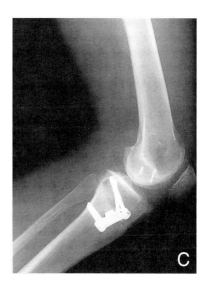

Figure 5 **A,** Preoperative AP radiograph reveals medial compartment narrowing and varus deformity in a young active patient with a history of medial sided knee pain. Screw fixation of an old osteochondral defect of the medial femoral condyle is visible. Postoperative AP **(B)** and lateral **(C)** radiographs were obtained 1 year after opening wedge high tibial osteotomy with step plate and screw fixation.

allograft bone. For wedges larger than 10 mm, some surgeons prefer to use structural graft, either tricortical iliac crest or allograft of various types, to support the osteotomy. Postoperatively, theses patients are protected in a hinged knee brace and allowed full motion but restricted to toe-touch weight bearing for the first 6 to 8 weeks. Thereafter, weight bearing is progressed gradually as indicated by a combination of clinical and radiographic findings. Typically, patients return to full activities at 4 to 6 months after surgery.

Medial opening wedge osteotomy can also be performed with an external fixator using a gradual distraction method. External fixators allow gradual correction of the deformity, and the alignment can be fine-tuned over time. Multiplanar corrections and very large corrections are possible with fixators that would be technically difficult to use with other techniques. Those advantages must be weighed against the disadvantages associated with pin site infection, possible deeper seeding of the bone, and the potential for later infection to ultimately compromise a total knee arthroplasty in the same limb. Furthermore, the patient must be willing to accept the fixator and the fact that it is bulky and requires daily care until bone healing has occurred. Both unilateral fixators and circular frame techniques have been described. In general, the circular frame is best suited to treat patients with multiplanar complex deformities. It is important with any external fixator technique to keep all pins at least 1 cm from the articular surface to minimize the risk of seeding the joint if the pin becomes infected.

Clinical Results

The results of closing wedge valgus-producing high tibial osteotomy have been well described in the literature and can be summarized as satisfactory in most appropriately selected patients at 7- to 10-year follow-up. Clinical success may be improved by avoiding undercorrection or marked overcorrection of the deformity, excluding substantially obese patients, and limiting the surgery to those patients with minimal lateral compartment disease. The results of medial opening wedge osteotomy can be summarized as encouraging. One study of 245 medial opening wedge osteotomies demonstrated satisfactory postoperative alignment in 93% of patients and survivorship rates of 94% at 5-year, 85% at 10-year, and 68% at 15-year follow-up, with conversion to total knee arthroplasty as the end point. Another study of 17 young active patients with the difficult combination of varus deformity and hyperextension with a varus thrust found all but one patient to be improved after medial opening wedge high tibial osteotomy. At a mean 5-year follow-up, nine patients remained markedly improved and seven patients remained somewhat improved than they were preoperatively. Another study of 21 patients with a mean age of 66 years found that appropriate correction was obtained reliably and that varus deformity did not recur at a mean 6-year follow-up. Those patients had a marked improvement in Knee Society score, and there were no instances of collapse or subsidence at the osteotomy site.

Complications after high tibial osteotomy are not uncommon and can be devastating. Meticulous surgical technique and care to protect the neurovascular structures about the knee are required. Peroneal nerve palsy, nonunion, malunion, patella baja, popliteal artery laceration, and deep venous thrombosis have all been reported with some frequency. Undercorrection of the deformity can result in poor results because of inadequate pain relief, whereas marked overcorrection of the defor-

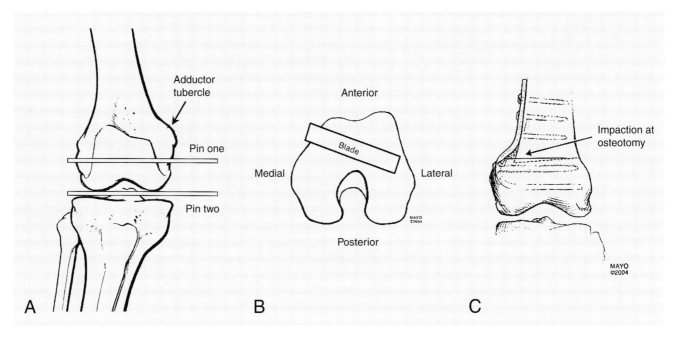

Figure 6 Illustration of the distal femoral closing wedge technique **A,** Pin one is placed across the joint, and pin two is placed in parallel 2.5 cm from the joint line. **B,** Pin two and the chisel blade are directed from anteromedial to posterolateral to accommodate the anatomy of the distal femur. **C,** A small wedge of bone (5 mm) is removed medially to accommodate the 90° blade plate; then the proximal fragment is impacted into the distal cancellous bone until the blade plate is flush against the femur. *(Reproduced with permission from the Mayo Foundation, Rochester, MN.)*

mity is a frequent cause of patient dissatisfaction because of cosmetic disfigurement.

Distal Femoral Osteotomy

For the symptomatic patient with valgus malalignment, it is possible to consider a varus-producing upper tibial osteotomy. For practical purposes, however, most varus-producing osteotomies are performed on the femoral side. For active patients with isolated lateral compartment disease, a varus-producing distal femoral osteotomy may be indicated for valgus deformities provided that the patient has adequate range of motion (≥ 90° and flexion contracture < 15°) and has not had a prior medial meniscectomy. In most patients, the mechanical axis should be corrected to zero in a valgus knee. That alignment results in a varus mechanical load with most of the load then transmitted through the intact medial compartment of the knee. The postoperative mechanical axis should pass just medial to the medial tibial spine.

Surgical Technique

Several surgical techniques exist for varus-producing distal femoral osteotomy, with the most common method being that described by the AO group as a medial closing wedge osteotomy fixed with a blade plate (Figure 6). The patient is placed supine on a radiolucent table, a 12- to 15-cm midline or medial skin incision is made, and the vastus medialis muscle is elevated to expose the distal femur. Guide pin one is placed across the knee joint parallel to the joint surface. Guide pin two is placed 2.5 cm proximal to the joint and directed from anteromedial to posterolateral to accommodate the differing geometries of the medial and lateral femoral condyles. The blade plate chisel is guided by pin two and three 4.5-mm drill holes are made in the medial cortex of the femur, after which the chisel is inserted parallel to the guide pin. The chisel is removed, and the medial aspect of the femoral shaft is marked to avoid rotational malalignment after the osteotomy. The osteotomy itself is done with a saw just proximal to the adductor tubercle. The lateral femoral cortex is not cut, but instead is perforated multiple times with a narrow osteotome to allow the osteoperiosteal hinge to remain intact. A small wedge of bone can be removed medially, but it is seldom more than 5 mm thick; instead, the proximal fragment is impacted into the distal fragment to obtain the correction. A 90° blade plate is inserted into the distal fragment, and the osteotomy is closed with gradual varus stress until the blade plate sits flat against the femoral shaft. When a 90° blade plate is inserted parallel to the joint surface and then reduced to the shaft of the femur, a neutral mechanical axis is ensured, provided the tibia itself is free of deformity. Intraoperative fluoroscopy can be used to confirm appropriate correction of overall limb alignment. Postoperatively, knee range-of-motion exercises are encouraged but toe-touch weight bearing typically is recommended for 6 to 8 weeks and progressive weight bearing thereafter.

Clinical Results

The clinical results of distal femoral varus-producing osteotomy have been good in selected patients. Substantial improvements in pain and function can be expected in approximately 90% of patients. One series of 49 patients demonstrated a 7-year survivorship rate of 87%, with conversion to total knee arthroplasty as the end point. Complications after distal femoral osteotomy include undercorrection of the deformity, nonunion, and malunion. Historically, the prevalence of complications such as nonunion and malunion was high when the method of fixation was staples. The prevalence of such complications is markedly lower when a blade plate is used for fixation.

Total Knee Arthroplasty After Osteotomy

The effect of osteotomy on the reliability and durability of subsequent total knee arthroplasty remains a focus of considerable attention. The conversion of a knee with a prior osteotomy to total knee arthroplasty often presents several surgical technical difficulties. The prior skin incision, presence of patella infera, offset of the tibial shaft from the tibial plateau, and rotational malalignment of the tibial tubercle relative to the proximal tibial plateau are factors that can complicate the total knee surgery. In those patients with prior high tibial osteotomy, longer surgical times, greater difficulty mobilizing the patella, and a greater need for lateral retinacular release during the total knee surgery should be anticipated. Some studies have suggested that the degree of pain relief is less reliable when a prior high tibial osteotomy has been done and that poor outcomes are more frequent in patients who are laborers and those receiving workers' compensation as well as those with poor pain relief after the osteotomy and multiple prior knee operations. After accounting for differences in patient age, it appears that the durability of total knee arthroplasty is not affected by the presence or absence of prior high tibial osteotomy because a 10-year survival rate of 90% or greater has been reported in several studies.

Summary

Osteotomy for the treatment of unicompartmental knee arthrosis has a well-documented record of success and continues to have a role in the surgical treatment of young and high-activity patients. In addition, an expanding role exists for osteotomy combined with cartilage, meniscal, and ligament restoration procedures for patients with full-thickness articular cartilage defects in knees with concomitant varus or valgus malalignment.

Annotated Bibliography

Assessment of Malalignment

Agneskirchner JD, Hurschler C, Stukenborg-Colsman C, Imhoff AB, Lobenhoffer P: Effect of high tibial osteotomy on cartilage pressure and joint kinematics: A biomechanical study in human cadaveric knees. *Arch Orthop Trauma Surg* 2004;124:575-584.

This study demonstrated in a cadaver model that decreasing posterior tibial slope, by adding flexion to a high tibial osteotomy, substantially decreased posterior tibial contact pressure and substantially limited posterior tibial translation. This suggests that adding a flexion component to a high tibial osteotomy may be beneficial in some patients with complex knee problems and combined degenerative arthritis and posterior or posterolateral corner instability.

Amendola A: Unicompartmental osteoarthritis in the active patient: The role of high tibial osteotomy. *Arthroscopy* 2003;19:109-116.

The author discusses the special considerations that are part of the decision making process when treating young active patients with isolated degenerative arthritis of the knee.

Brouwer RW, Jakma TS, Bierma-Zeinstra SM, Berhagen AP, Verhaar J: Osteotomy for treating knee arthritis. *Cochrane Database Syst Rev* 2005;1:CD004019.

Based on 11 studies, of which 6 were high quality, these authors concluded that there was good evidence that valgus high tibial osteotomy improves knee function and reduces pain. There is no scientific evidence whether osteotomy is more effective than conservative treatment and no conclusions can be made about the effectiveness of specific surgical techniques.

High Tibial Osteotomy

Billings A, Scott DF, Camargo MP, Hofmann AA: High tibial osteotomy with a calibrated osteotomy guide, rigid internal fixation and early motion: Long term followup. *J Bone Joint Surg Am* 2000;82:70-79.

This study of 64 high tibial osteotomies demonstrated that a calibrated osteotomy guide and rigid internal fixation with a plate and screws facilitated accurate correction of limb alignment and allowed early motion after closing wedge osteotomy. There were no instances of patella baja postoperatively, and one patient had delayed union. With conversion to total knee arthroplasty as the end point, the survivorship rate was 85% at 5-year follow-up and 53% at 10-year follow-up.

Hernigou P, Ma W: Open wedge tibial osteotomy with acrylic bone cement as bone substitute. *Knee* 2001;8:103-110.

In this study of 245 medial opening wedge osteotomies, the bone defect was held apart by a wedge of bone cement placed posteromedially, and the tibia was fixed with a plate and screws. Survivorship rate was estimated at 94% at 5-year, 85% at 10-year, and 68% at 15-year follow-up, with conversion to total knee arthroplasty as the end point.

Koshino T, Murase T, Saito T: Medial opening-wedge high tibial osteotomy with use of porous hydroxyapatite to treat medial compartment osteoarthritis of the knee. *J Bone Joint Surg Am* 2003;85-A:78-85.

Twenty-one osteotomies in 18 knees were done with the medial opening wedge technique using a structural wedge of hydroxyapatite to fill the defect. At a mean follow-up of approximately 7 years in this series of older patients (mean age, 66 years), there were no failures. Limb alignment was adequately corrected, and there were no instances of recurrence of the deformity. Mean Knee Society scores improved from 60 points preoperatively to 94 points at the time of last follow-up.

Naudie DD, Amendola A, Fowler PJ: Opening wedge high tibial osteotomy for symptomatic hyperextension varus thrust. *Am J Sports Med* 2004;32:60-70.

In this study, 17 high tibial osteotomies were done in young, active patients with symptomatic hyperextension and varus thrust. At a mean 56-month follow-up, all patients had improved their Tegner and Lysholm activity scores, with nine patients rating their improvement as significantly better and the remainder rating their improvement as somewhat better. One patient was dissatisfied with the surgical outcome.

Noyes FR, Barber-Westin SD, Hewett TE: High tibial osteotomy and ligament reconstruction for varus angulated anterior cruciate ligament deficient knees. *Am J Sports Med* 2000;28:282-296.

In this study, 41 young active patients who had anterior cruciate ligament deficiency and varus limb alignment were treated with high tibial osteotomy. In 34 patients, the anterior cruciate ligament was also reconstructed, and in 18 patients the posterolateral corner was also reconstructed. Follow-up at a mean of 4.5 years revealed an improvement in Cincinnati knee rating scores from 63 to 82 points, with 71% of patients rating their knees as good or excellent.

Sterett WI, Steadman JR: Chondral resurfacing and high tibial osteotomy in the varus knee. *Am J Sports Med* 2004;32:1243-1249.

This study of 38 patients with a mean age of 51 years demonstrated good early (2-year follow-up) outcomes after a combined medial opening wedge osteotomy and microfracture procedure for combined medial compartment degenerative arthritis and varus malalignment.

Warden SJ, Morris HG, Crossley KM, Brukner PD, Bennell KL: Delayed- and non-union following opening wedge high tibial osteotomy: Surgeons' results from 182 completed cases. *Knee Surg Sports Traumatol Arthrosc* 2005;13:34-37.

This series included 182 medial opening wedge osteotomies done by 21 different surgeons, all members of the Australian Knee Society. The prevalence of delayed union was 6.6% (12 patients), and the prevalence of nonunion was 1.6% (3 patients).

Weale AE, Lee AS, MacEachern AG: High tibial osteotomy using a dynamic axial external fixator. *Clin Orthop* 2001;382:154-167.

To determine whether opening wedge osteotomy using hemicallotasis techniques is safer than and outcomes comparable with conventional techniques, the authors performed 76 high tibial osteotomies (65 patients; mean age, 54.8 years) to treat primary osteoarthritis. At a mean 6-year follow-up, the only complication reported occurred in one patient (chronic osteomyelitis 2 years postoperatively). The authors concluded that this technique was safer than conventional techniques. With survivorship at 5 and 10 years of 89% and 63%, respectively, they also concluded that outcomes were comparable with or better than those of conventional osteotomy techniques.

Distal Femoral Osteotomy

Wang JW, Hsu CC: Distal femoral varus osteotomy for osteoarthritis of the knee. *J Bone Joint Surg Am* 2005; 87:127-133.

In this study, 30 patients underwent distal femoral varus osteotomy to treat noninflammatory lateral compartment knee arthritis; 18 patients also had demonstrable arthritic changes in the patellofemoral joint. The 10-year survival rate (determined by a patient being free of conversion to total knee arthroplasty) was 87%. The result was not affected by the presence of patellofemoral arthritis.

Total Knee Arthroplasty After Osteotomy

Karabatsos B, Mahomed NN, Maistrelli GL: Functional outcome of total knee arthroplasty after high tibial osteotomy. *Can J Surg* 2002;45:116-119.

This retrospective matched cohort study evaluated the functional outcome for patients who underwent total knee arthroplasty after high tibial osteotomy and included 20 patients who underwent total knee arthroplasty after high tibial osteotomy and 20 matched patients who underwent primary total knee arthroplasty. The authors found that functional outcomes at a mean 5-year follow-up after total knee arthroplasty in patients who underwent a prior high tibial osteotomy tended to be inferior compared with the matched cohort, but the differences were not statistically significant.

Parvizi J, Hanssen AD, Spangehl M: Total knee arthroplasty following proximal tibial osteotomy: Risk factors for failure. *J Bone Joint Surg Am* 2004;86:474-479.

In this study, 166 cemented condylar total knee arthroplasties were done at a mean of 8.6 years after a previous proximal tibial osteotomy in 118 patients (mean age, 69 years). These patients were followed for a mean of 15 years clinically and 9 years radiographically, and 8% had required total knee revision. This failure rate is comparable to that observed at the authors' institution for age-matched patients who had primary total knee arthroplasty without previous high tibial osteotomy.

Classic Bibliography

Coventry MB: Osteotomy of the upper portion of the tibia for degenerative arthritis of the knee: A preliminary report. *J Bone Joint Surg Am* 1965;47:984-990.

Coventry MB, Ilstrup DM, Wallrichs SL: Proximal tibial osteotomy: A critical long-term study of eighty-seven cases. *J Bone Joint Surg Am* 1993;75:196-201.

Geiger F, Schneider U, Lukoschek M, Ewerbeck V: External fixation in proximal tibial osteotomy: A comparison of three methods. *Int Orthop* 1999;23:160-163.

Chapter 5

Alternatives in the Treatment of Knee Arthritis: Arthroscopy and Cartilage Restoration

Henry D. Clarke, MD

W. Norman Scott, MD

Introduction

Surgical options for the treatment of the arthritic knee include arthroscopic débridement and arthroscopically assisted cartilage restoration procedures. Numerous studies have been published describing these techniques, yet their role is still controversial. Although several different techniques have been described, they can be broadly classified into three distinct groups: (1) arthroscopic lavage and débridement, (2) cartilage transplantation procedures, and (3) marrow stimulating techniques.

Arthroscopic Lavage and Débridement

Arthroscopic treatment of the arthritic knee was first reported in 1934. However, the early instrumentation essentially allowed only simple joint lavage. Since the development of improved instrumentation in the 1970s, the role of arthroscopic lavage and débridement in the treatment of gonarthrosis has been vigorously debated. Although the results of published studies have been inconsistent, independent centers have reported satisfactory outcomes in approximately two thirds of patients. Explanations for the perceived benefits include removal of mechanical irritants such as unstable meniscal and chondral fragments, removal of painful debris, and lavage of inflammatory enzymes. Factors that have been identified as favorable prognostic indicators are listed in Table 1. When these criteria are used, statistically significant improvements in objective criteria such as knee swelling and walking ability have been noted.

Table 1 | Favorable Prognostic Indicators for Arthroscopic Lavage and Débridement

Short duration of mechanical symptoms

Minimal mechanical axis malalignment of the extremity

Absence of flexion contractures

Less severe radiographic changes of osteoarthritis

Realistic patient expectations

In a study of 36 patients treated for symptomatic knee arthritis that was refractory to nonsurgical modalities, 25 patients were satisfied with the results of arthroscopic débridement at 5-year follow-up. Poor results were correlated with flexion contractures greater than 10° and lower preoperative Hospital for Special Surgery Knee Scores. In another retrospective review of 204 patients, favorable factors included smaller axial angulation of less than 5° if varus or valgus malalignment was present and absence of prior surgery.

Arthroscopic débridement has also been selectively applied as a temporizing procedure in patients with osteoarthritis of the knee who are apprehensive about the magnitude of the total knee replacement procedure. In these patients, the goal is symptomatic improvement rather than complete pain relief. For successful outcomes to be achieved, patient expectations and patient education are critical factors. Patients need to understand the importance of lifestyle changes, including activity modification. In a group of 77 patients with knee pain and radiographic changes consistent with significant osteoarthritis (Ahlbach radiographic evaluation scale grade 2 or 3) who were considered to be candidates for total knee arthroplasty but elected to undergo arthroscopic débridement as a temporizing procedure, 67% did not proceed to knee replacement at a mean of 13.2 years postoperatively. Furthermore, the mean postoperative patient satisfaction score regarding the success of the procedure was 8.6 (range, 0 to 10).

Despite many published studies that have supported the use of arthroscopic débridement in the arthritic knee, recent studies have stimulated the debate. A recent retrospective review of 126 patients questioned the accuracy of physicians in predicting which patients would benefit from this procedure. Only three variables were significantly associated with postoperative improvement: the presence of medial joint line tenderness, a positive Steinmann test, and the presence of an unstable meniscal tear at arthroscopy. Further questions have been raised by another recent blinded, prospective, randomized study that did not demonstrate any therapeutic benefit compared with the placebo effect seen in the control group. One hundred eighty patients were randomized into three treatment groups: arthroscopic lavage; arthroscopic débridement; and a sham procedure in which patients were anesthetized and received skin incisions and simulated débridement, but did not actually undergo any intra-articular intervention. The results of this study suggested that the perceived benefits of arthroscopic débridement were simply the result of the placebo effect alone because there was no difference in knee pain among the placebo group and either the lavage group or débridement group at 1 or 2 years postoperatively. These results challenged the continuing use of arthroscopic débridement for the treatment of the osteoarthritic knee.

Although this prospective, randomized study provided seemingly definitive results, the debate is still very much alive because the study methods have been widely criticized for selection bias and failure to apply the previously identified favorable prognostic indicators. Rather than applying specific selection criteria, any patient younger than 75 years with osteoarthritis of the knee and knee pain who had undergone nonsurgical treatment for 6 months but had not undergone arthroscopy of the knee in the prior 2 years was considered a candidate. Additionally, the radiologic assessment of the extent of the osteoarthritis was criticized because it was based on limited views. Other selection bias concerns were also introduced because almost all of the patients were male and were treated at a Veterans Administration facility. Furthermore, 44% of the patients who met the selection criteria refused to participate. Therefore, it is unclear whether these results can be extrapolated to the general population because the motives and expectations of the patients who did consent were not clear.

Although definitive studies have yet to be performed and results are inconsistent, a select group of patients appears most likely to achieve short-term benefits from arthroscopic débridement. These include patients with short duration of mechanical symptoms, good range of motion, less deformity, less radiographic evidence of osteoarthritis, and reasonable expectations. Essential elements of the procedure include joint lavage, excision of torn meniscal fragments, removal of loose bodies, and débridement of fibrillated or loose articular cartilage fragments, while avoiding creation of full-thickness articular cartilage defects. If these selection criteria and technical principles are followed, short-term beneficial outcomes can be expected in about two thirds of the patients undergoing arthroscopic débridement.

Cartilage Repair Techniques

Optimal management of cartilage defects is not yet known and is hindered by a lack of complete understanding of normal articular cartilage biology, as well as the natural history of focal injuries. However, it is clear that hyaline cartilage lacks both a blood and nerve supply; as a result, partial- and full-thickness injuries have very limited healing abilities in adult humans. Some in situ repair processes occur, but they generally require that the subchondral bone be penetrated. This allows mesenchymal cells from the marrow to populate the articular defect and produce a fibrocartilage substitute. However, it is also clear that the mechanical properties of this fibrocartilage substitute, which is primarily type I collagen, are inferior to the original hyaline cartilage, principally type II collagen. Based on this information, it seems reasonable to assume that patients with focal lesions are at greater risk of developing symptomatic osteoarthritis. However, the use of procedures to prophylactically repair cartilage defects in asymptomatic individuals is limited. Additionally, application of the techniques designed to stimulate the limited in vivo healing that can occur, as well as techniques to transplant either autologous or allogeneic hyaline cartilage into areas of damaged cartilage, have been primarily limited to the treatment of traumatic focal lesions on one articular surface in young patients rather than older patients with osteoarthritis in whom coexisting knee pathology exists, such as mechanical malalignment or bipolar lesions (kissing lesions) in one or more compartment.

Marrow Stimulating Techniques

Various techniques have been used to promote the limited fibrocartilage reparative process that can occur in vivo. These include mechanical abrasion, drilling, and picking or microfracture of the subchondral bone. Each of these techniques is best suited to treat small, focal lesions smaller than 1 to 2 cm^2.

Abrasion Chondroplasty

Abrasion chondroplasty was one of the first marrow stimulating techniques described during the 1980s. This technique is limited to areas of exposed bone rather than degenerative cartilage and is best performed with a mechanical burr. The superficial layer of subchondral bone is removed, allowing the mesenchymal marrow cells to be released into the lesion that stimulates the fibrocartilage repair process. Analysis of biopsy samples, obtained during second-look arthroscopy, has confirmed that the reparative material is fibrocartilage rather than the original hyaline cartilage. Long-term follow-up of these patients has documented that abrasion arthroplasty does not seem to offer any advantage to débridement alone and may in fact lead to a higher failure rate.

Subchondral Drilling

A second technique for promoting fibrocartilage formation involves drilling through the denuded articular areas into the subchondral bone. The repair process again is the result of stimulation of the native fibrocartilage repair process. Despite limited published reports, the results fail to demonstrate significant benefits compared with arthroscopic débridement alone.

Microfracture

The microfracture technique is a third method that stimulates the in vivo fibrocartilage repair process. In this technique, the exposed subchondral bone is first denuded of any remaining cartilage with a shaver or curet. Next, an arthroscopic awl is used to create multiple small puncture holes that are a few millimeters in diameter and located 3 to 4 mm apart, which penetrate 2 to 4 mm into the subchondral bone. Theoretic advantages of this technique compared with drilling include the generation of less heat and therefore less bone necrosis damage. Moreover, the awls may be contoured, which allows easier access to the entire joint. Although the use of contoured awls may indeed provide practical benefits, it is important to note the results are essentially the same as with drilling. Again, the regenerated surface seems to be composed of fibrocartilage rather than true hyaline cartilage.

The original pioneers of these three similar techniques emphasized the importance of prolonged periods of modified weight bearing postoperatively, typically with the use of crutches for 6 to 8 weeks, and avoidance of pivoting impact sports for 6 months or more. Little evidence exists to support the routine use of these procedures in the arthritic knee when compared with arthroscopic lavage and chondroplasty of unstable chondral surfaces, especially considering the significant requisite postoperative restrictions and disability.

Autologous and Allogeneic Cartilage Transplantation

A variety of techniques have been developed that aim to restore the hyaline cartilage articular surface, including the transplantation of autologous and allogeneic cartilage in the form of autologous cells cultured in vivo, the transplantation of autologous osteochondral plugs of different sizes from one area to another, and the use of allogeneic osteochondral plugs or bulk osteochondral grafts. As with the marrow stimulating techniques, most of these techniques have been developed for use in patients with focal, well defined traumatic defects or osteochondritis dissecans rather than in patients with diffuse degenerative changes with mechanical malalignment. Furthermore, evidence of reduced healing potential in older patients has generally limited the use of these techniques to patients age 50 to 60 years and younger. Again, this limits the applicability of these procedures in most patients with osteoarthritis. Furthermore, the procedures are associated with prolonged periods of activity modification and disability, generally requiring limited weight bearing for 6 to 12 weeks, followed by avoidance of impact activities for 6 months or more.

Autologous Osteochondral Plug Transfer

Mosaicplasty is performed either arthroscopically or in a limited open manner. In this technique, multiple small plugs of autologous cartilage with their subchondral bone base and measuring between 2.7 and 10 mm in diameter are harvested from non–weight-bearing areas of the knee, such as areas that are adjacent to the intercondylar notch or those located at the lateral femoral condyle superior to the sulcus terminalis. These autologous osteochondral plugs are then transplanted to the area of chondral damage. These multiple small plugs when implanted in a mosaic pattern can be used to fill lesions up to 4 cm^2, but the technique is probably best suited for lesions between 1 and 2 cm^2. Lesions of this size can usually be managed arthroscopically, but may require a limited, open arthrotomy. The treatment of larger lesions is generally limited by the availability of donor sites, and in patients with larger lesions, open arthrotomy is required. The small voids between the transplanted plugs become filled with a fibrocartilage grout. Using this technique, the resulting composite articular surface has been shown to be composed of approximately 80% transplanted hyaline cartilage and 20% fibrocartilage. The donor sites heal with a fibrocartilage cap within approximately 6 to 8 weeks. Favorable postoperative outcomes based on standardized clinical rating systems, including the modified Hospital for Special Surgery Knee Scores, Lysholm scores, and Modified Cincinnati scores have been reported, with 92% good to excellent results reported in patients with femoral lesions and 88% good to excellent results reported in those with tibial lesions. However, once again, this technique should be considered for treating only focal cartilage defects rather than diffuse arthritic changes.

Autologous Chondrocyte Transplantation

Autologous chondrocyte transplantation is best suited to treat larger lesions, typically those that are greater than 2 cm^2 and involve a single condyle of the knee. In this technique, chondrocytes from the patient's knee are harvested arthroscopically and then cultured in vitro to produce 20 to 50 times the original number of cells. During the culture process, the cells dedifferentiate, and the resulting chondrocytes are similar to mesenchymal cells. These cells are implanted weeks to months later through a second open procedure at which time they are inserted under a watertight periosteal graft patch over the cartilage defect, and cartilage is produced. Analysis of cartilage obtained through second-look arthroscopies has demonstrated hyaline-like cartilage. Favorable results at mid- to long-term follow-up have now been reported using this technique. The best results have been obtained in patients with unipolar femoral condyle lesions, 90% of whom had excellent or good results using the Modified Cincinnati score at 2- to 10-year follow-up. In a recent study, 71 salvage procedures were performed in patients with knees with multiple lesions and early arthritic changes or in those with knees with bipolar lesions. In this group, in which the mean resurfaced area was 11.66 cm^2 per knee, statistically significant improvements in Medical Outcomes Study Short Form 36-Item Health Survey quality of life scores and Knee Society scores at 24-month follow-up were reported. Eighty percent of patients reported good or excellent results and 87% were satisfied with their outcomes. Ninety-three percent of these patients thought they were better than before the procedure. Despite these results, however, this technique should be considered experimental for the treatment of diffuse cartilage damage that is encountered in the osteoarthritic knee. Furthermore, the role of this technique in conjunction with simultaneous or staged osteotomy has not been clearly defined.

Allogeneic Osteochondral Transplantation

The transplantation of large allografts of bone and overlying hyaline cartilage using a variety of techniques has been performed in patients with traumatic articular cartilage injuries and osteochondritis dissecans lesions. These techniques are best suited for large areas of cartilage damage that are larger than 3 to 4 cm in diameter, uncontained defects, or lesions with osseous defects greater than 1 cm deep that preclude the use of either autologous osteochondral plug transfer or autologous chondrocyte transplantation. Although the potential for donor site morbidity is eliminated using these allogeneic grafts, concerns exist about the risks of disease transmission because of viral and submicroscopic vector transmission as well as bacterial contamination resulting from improper graft harvest and storage techniques. Again, few published data are available about the use of these techniques either with or without supplemental procedures such as osteotomy in patients with diffuse or bipolar cartilage damage. Furthermore, the supply of graft material can limit the use of this technique. Cell viability decreases by 14 days and is significantly reduced by 28 days with fresh grafts. Therefore, scheduling requires complex logistic procedures.

In one series, fresh osteochondral allografts were used in 72 patients with posttraumatic cartilage lesions that were larger than 3 cm in diameter and 1 cm deep of the distal femur. Kaplan-Meier survivorship rates of 85% at 10 years and 74% at 15 years were reported in this series, with 12 failures among 60 grafts that were available for long-term follow-up at a mean of 10 years.

Sixty-eight percent of the patients underwent simultaneous realignment osteotomy because more than physiologic loading was demonstrated on preoperative full-length, weight-bearing radiographs. Among the 48 surviving grafts at mean 10-year follow-up, 40 patients (84%) had good or excellent Hospital for Special Surgery knee scores.

Future Trends: Growth Factors and Biologic and Synthetic Matrices

Significant research is currently underway to identify both biologic and synthetic scaffolds that can be used to fill osteochondral defects. These scaffolds may act as simple patches or stimulate extrinsic repair processes through the incorporation of growth factors and even autologous cells. Both preformed and injectable materials are currently under development. Desirable features of these scaffolds include the ability to provide good initial fixation to the host site, biodegradable substrates that are biocompatible, and the ability to encourage cell attachment and growth. The goal of this research is to produce a substitute for the native hyaline cartilage that can be implanted with minimal morbidity, yet restore articular congruity, eliminate pain, improve function, and slow or eliminate the potential for progressive degenerative cartilage damage. The durability and long-term clinical benefits of recent advances in tissue engineering are yet to be demonstrated, but they remain the focus of intensive research efforts.

Annotated Bibliography

Arthroscopic Lavage and Débridement

Dervin GF, Stiell IG, Rody K, Grabowski J: Effect of arthroscopic debridement for osteoarthritis of the knee on health-related quality of life. *J Bone Joint Surg Am* 2003; 85-A:10-19.

In this study, 126 patients (mean age, 61 years) with symptomatic knee osteoarthritis underwent arthroscopic débridement. At 2-year follow-up, 44% were rated as having had a clinically meaningful reduction in pain as determined by Western Ontario and McMaster Universities Osteoarthritis Index pain scale. Clinical variables were only partially helpful for predicting success.

Fond J, Rodin D, Ahmad S, Nirschl RP: Arthroscopic debridement for the treatment of osteoarthritis of the knee: 2- and 5-year results. *Arthroscopy* 2002;18:829-834.

In this study, 36 patients with symptomatic knee osteoarthritis underwent arthroscopic débridement. At 5-year follow-up, 25 of 36 patients were satisfied with the results. Poor results were associated with flexion contractures greater than 10° and lower preoperative Hospital for Special Surgery Knee Scores.

Moseley JB, O'Malley K, Petersen NJ, et al: A controlled trial of arthroscopic surgery for osteoarthritis of the knee. *N Engl J Med* 2002;347:81-88.

In this study, 180 patients were prospectively randomized to one of three treatment groups: arthroscopic lavage alone, arthroscopic débridement, or a sham procedure group with skin incisions but no intra-articular intervention. Results at 2-year follow-up were not statistically different. Forty-four percent of the patients who met selection criteria refused to participate.

Marrow Stimulating Techniques

Johnson LL: Arthroscopic abrasion arthroplasty: A review. *Clin Orthop Relat Res* 2001;(391 suppl):S306-S317.

The rationale and technique for abrasion arthroplasty is described. One hundred five patients who underwent the procedure to avoid total knee replacement were evaluated at 2-year and 5-year follow-up. At 2 years, 74% of patients said they were improved. At 5 years, 78% of patients had not required additional surgery.

Steadman JR, Briggs KK, Rodrigo JJ, Kocher MS, Gill TJ, Rodkey WG: Outcomes of microfracture for traumatic chondral defects of the knee: Average 11-year follow-up. *Arthroscopy* 2003;19:477-484.

In this study, 72 patients younger than 45 years (75 knees) with traumatic full-thickness chondral defects underwent microfracture treatment. Significant improvement was recorded for both Lysholm (scale 1 to 100; preoperative, 59; final follow-up, 89) and Tegner (1 to 10; preoperative, 3; final follow-up, 6) scores. At 7-year follow-up, 80% of the patients rated themselves as improved.

Autologous and Allogeneic Cartilage Transplantation

Aubin PP, Cheah HK, Davis AM, Gross AE: Long-term followup of fresh femoral osteochondral allografts for posttraumatic knee defects. *Clin Orthop Relat Res* 2001;(391 suppl):S318-S327.

In this study, 72 fresh osteochondral allografts were transplanted in patients with distal femoral chondral lesions greater than 3 cm in diameter and 1 cm deep. Kaplan-Meier survivorship rates were calculated to be 85% at 10-year follow-up and 74% at 15-year follow-up. Twelve failures occurred among 60 grafts that were available for long-term follow-up (mean, 10 years). Sixty-eight percent of the patients required simultaneous realignment osteotomy.

Hangody L, Feczko P, Bartha L, et al: Mosaicplasty for the treatment of articular defects of the knee and ankle. *Clin Orthop Relat Res* 2001;(391 suppl):S328-S336.

The technique, indications, and experience with 652 mosaicplasties for the treatment of osteochondral lesions are described. Good to excellent results were reported in 92% of pa-

tients with femoral lesions, 88% of those with tibial lesions, and 81% of those with patellar or trochlear lesions.

Minas T: Autologous chondrocyte implantation for focal chondral defects of the knee. *Clin Orthop Relat Res* 2001;(391 suppl):S349-S361.

In this study, 71 knees with early arthritis and large salvage cartilage lesions were treated with autologous chondrocyte transplantation using chondrocytes harvested from the patient's knee that were cultured in vitro and then implanted under a periosteal patch. At 24-month follow-up, 80% of patients had good or excellent results and 93% reported they were better than they were preoperatively.

Classic Bibliography

Baumgaertner MR, Cannon WD Jr, Vittori JM, Schmidt ES, Maurer RC: Arthroscopic debridement of the arthritic knee. *Clin Orthop* 1990;253:197-202.

Bert JM, Maschka K: The arthroscopic treatment of unicompartmental gonarthrosis: A five-year follow-up study of abrasion arthroplasty plus arthroscopic debridement and arthroscopic debridement alone. *Arthroscopy* 1989;5:25-32.

Burman MS, Finkelstein H, Mayer L: Arthroscopy of the knee joint. *J Bone Joint Surg Am* 1934;16A:255-268.

Brittberg M, Lindahl A, Nilsson A, et al: Treatment of deep cartilage defects in the knee with autologous chondrocyte transplantation. *N Engl J Med* 1994;331:889-895.

Hangody L, Kish G, Karpati Z, Udvarhelyi I, Szigeti I, Bely M: Mosaicplasty for the treatment of articular cartilage defects: Application in clinical practice. *Orthopedics* 1998;21:751-756.

Harwin SF: Arthroscopic debridement for osteoarthritis of the knee: Predictors of patient satisfaction. *Arthroscopy* 1999;15:142-146.

Livesley PJ, Doherty M, Needoff M, Moulton A: Arthroscopic lavage of osteoarthritic knees. *J Bone Joint Surg Br* 1991;73:922-926.

McGinley BJ, Cushner FD, Scott WN: Debridement arthroscopy: 10-year follow-up. *Clin Orthop* 1999;367:190-194.

Rand JA: Role of arthroscopy in osteoarthritis of the knee. *Arthroscopy* 1991;7:358-363.

Sprague NF III: Arthroscopic debridement for degenerative knee joint disease. *Clin Orthop* 1981;160:118-123.

Yang SS, Nisonson B: Arthroscopic surgery of the knee in the geriatric patient. *Clin Orthop* 1995;316:50-58.

Chapter 6

Unicompartmental Knee Arthroplasty: Long-Term Results

Rahul V. Deshmukh, MD

Richard D. Scott, MD

Introduction

Unicompartmental knee arthroplasty (UKA) has been controversial since its introduction approximately 30 years ago. Although lateral compartment replacement seemed to be promising, initial results suggested that medial compartment replacement did not yield early results that were satisfactory for this treatment modality to be a viable long-term option. By the early 1980s, however, good initial results were reported for medial and lateral compartment replacement and enthusiasm for the procedure began to increase. Refinements were made in patient selection, surgical technique, and prosthetic design. Ten-year follow-up studies were reported showing survivorship that although slightly lower than that reported for total knee arthroplasty was nonetheless acceptable, considering the theoretically conservative nature of unicompartmental surgery. Some reports refuted this conservative argument, whereas later reports supported it provided conservative designs and techniques were used.

Eight- to 10-year outcome data are now available for UKA in properly selected patients with osteoarthritis using skillfully implanted, proper prosthetic device design. As a result, UKA is now considered an attractive alternative to osteotomy or total knee arthroplasty, especially in selected middle-aged female patients. Patients with bilateral disease can undergo bilateral UKA procedures during the same anesthetic with full recovery expected within 3 months.

Comparison With Alternative Procedures

Compared with high tibial osteotomy, UKA has been shown to yield a higher initial success rate and fewer complications. In a 12- to 17-year follow-up study, the survival rates for these two procedures varies with time, with a 90% and 76% survival rate for UKA high tibial osteotomy, respectively, at 10-year follow-up; and an 88% and 65% survival rate for UKA and high tibial osteotomy, respectively, at 15-year follow-up. An early randomized, prospective trial provided comparable data, showing superior outcome in UKA over high tibial os-teotomy with regard to range of motion, rapid rehabilitation, and perioperative morbidity. The published results of revision total knee arthroplasty after UKA or high tibial osteotomy are somewhat equivocal. Although one study reported 50% bone loss with revisions of UKA and no major wound complications, revisions of high tibial osteotomy had a 30% major wound complication rate. Another study reported significantly higher knee scores after revision from high tibial osteotomy compared with revision from UKA. This study also reported increased osseous reconstructions in the revisions of UKAs.

Compared with tricompartmental replacement, there is general consensus that UKA is less invasive, often requires no blood transfusion, more closely approximates normal kinematics, and allows more rapid recovery, better postoperative range of motion, and better postoperative physiologic function. Recent in vivo fluoroscopic studies demonstrated nearly normal kinematics for patients who underwent UKA, noting that on average, medial UKAs remained relatively stationary in the antero-posterior plane and had normal 3° of axial rotation. Lateral UKAs had posterior femoral rollback. In contrast, a paradoxical anterior slide occurs during deep flexion and gait with cruciate-retaining total knee arthroplasty and during gait with posterior-stabilized designs. Moreover, bone stock is preserved in the unresurfaced compartments, which facilitates revision surgery as long as conservative surgical techniques and components were used. Early published results of revision surgery with UKA reported technical problems and the frequent need for bone graft, complex revision, or even custom total knee arthroplasty implants. Two more recent studies have described revision surgery of UKAs with newer prosthetic design and much better results. In both series, standard primary femoral implants were used and only autograft was required for bony deficiencies; however, half of the patients required stemmed tibial components.

To help define the current role of UKA in the orthopaedic surgeon's armamentarium, it is important to assess both short- and long-term results. Experience has shown that initial excellent early results can be achieved in more than 95% of patients provided patients are selected properly for the procedure and important surgical goals have been achieved.

Indications

The indications for UKA have varied widely. When UKA still was considered experimental, one study reserved UKA as the last option before arthrodesis in the treatment of patients with severe arthritis. One early study included patients with patellectomy and incompetent anterior cruciate ligaments or other ligamentous structures. Other studies have applied strict criteria such as patients with limited unicompartmental osteoarthritis and no patellofemoral or opposite compartment disease. Early guidelines that were published to assist surgeons in patient selection suggested that the ideal candidate for UKA has noninflammatory osteoarthritis with a mechanical axis that deviates no more than 10° from neutral for a varus knee and no more than 5° for a valgus knee, and the anterior cruciate ligament should be intact without signs of mediolateral subluxation of the femur on the tibia. These guidelines also noted that flexion contractures greater than 15° may be difficult to correct and that the patellofemoral compartment of candidates may have grade II or even grade III changes as long as patellofemoral symptoms are not present. More recently, it has been suggested that patellofemoral and opposite compartment evaluation should be evaluated using MRI or bone scanning because concurrent arthroscopy places the patient at high risk of infection. These guidelines were the accepted criteria for patient selection for many years and are still used in many centers today. Surveying a patient population of arthroplasty candidates, one study reported that only 6% of patients fulfilled these criteria if they were applied rigidly. Until recently in the United States, UKAs have consistently been performed in only 5% of patients for whom knee arthroplasty is indicated.

The UKA selection criteria for patient age and weight are controversial. Many authors believe that UKA should not be performed in young, very active, or obese patients in whom the loads placed on the joint will be too great. In a review of 67 UKAs at an average 9.7-year follow-up, an improvement was noted in the survival rates of patients older than 60 years at 5- and 10-year follow-up; a decrease in the survival rate was noted at 15-year follow-up, but this was not statistically significant. Obesity was also assessed as a selection criterion, and no significant difference was reported. One study reported a 98% 10-year survival rate without using obesity as an exclusion criterion for UKA, whereas another study reported excluding patients with significant obesity. A multicenter trial of 294 UKAs that was conducted to evaluate predictors of survival found that

the average weight of a patient with a successful UKA was 67 kg and that of a patient requiring revision for UKA was 90.4 kg. Establishing an arbitrary cutoff of 81 kg proved to be statistically significant ($P = 0.0001$). This study also reported that men had a lower rate of revision than women ($P = 0.02$) and that the rate of revision increased with polyethylene thickness of ≤ 6 mm ($P = 0.01$). In a review of 63 Compartment II knee replacements (Zimmer, Warsaw, IN), it was reported that although weight did not correlate with revision surgery, it was a statistically significant indicator of functional pain. Despite the association of weight greater than 90 kg with a higher incidence of component wear, loosening, or subsidence, experienced surgeons believe that patients who weigh as much as 80 kg are acceptable candidates for UKA, but are wary of performing this procedure on patients who weigh more than 90 kg.

Technique

Certain technical considerations must be fulfilled at the time of implantation. Overcorrection of the deformity should be avoided. Many experienced surgeons have advocated undercorrection of the mechanical axis by 2° to 3°. Overcorrection can result in mediolateral subluxation of the femorotibial articulation or result in excessive force on the unresurfaced compartment with early secondary degeneration. Peripheral and notch osteophytes should be removed, and care should be taken to resect as little bone as possible to facilitate any future revision procedure. In general, medial and lateral soft-tissue releases should be avoided because knees requiring these releases probably have too much preoperative deformity for UKA. Angular correction usually is obtained by removing peripheral osteophytes that tent-up the capsule and collateral ligaments. The components must exhibit good congruency in extension (mediolaterally and rotationally). If a flat-on-flat articulation is used, edge loading must be avoided. The leading edge of the femoral component must be recessed into the trochlear cartilage to prevent patellar impingement. Improper mediolateral placement must be avoided to prevent problems of tibial spine impingement. Varus placement of the tibial component may lead to early loosening and should also be avoided. Additionally, the surgeon should use caution in placement of proximal tibial guide pins because there have been independent case reports of these cortical perforations leading to tibial plateau stress fracture after UKA and requiring subsequent revision to TKA.

Minimally Invasive Surgical Technique

The minimally invasive surgical technique is often performed in the United States with a modified Marmor prosthesis using a freehand, inset technique. In 2002, an 8- to 9-year survival rate of 93% in 136 medial mini-

Table 1 | Long-Term Results of UKA Outcome Studies

Author	Year	Prosthesis	No. of Knees	Survivorship* 10 Year	15 Year	20 Year
Marmor	1988	Marmor	228	70%		
Scott et al	1991	Unicondylar	100	85%		
Capra and Fehring	1992	Marmor, Compartmental II	52	94%		
Heck et al	1993	Marmor, Zimmer I and II	294	91%		
Munk and Frokjaer	1994	Marmor	68	92%		
Weale and Newman	1994	St. Georg	42	90%	88%	
Cartier et al	1996	Marmor	60	93%		
Ansari et al	1997	St. Georg	461	96%		
Tabor and Tabor	1998	Marmor	67	84%	79%	
Murray et al	1998	Oxford	144	98%		
Squire et al	1999	Marmor	140	–	90%	84%
Svard and Price	2001	Oxford	94	95%		
Gioe et al	2003	Nine different designs (community-based)	516	89%		
Pennington et al	2003	Miller-Galante (patients younger than 60 years)	46	92%		
Berger et al	2005	Miller-Galante	49	98%	95.7%[†]	

*Based on revision for any reason
[†] 13-year survivorship reported

mally invasive UKAs was reported, many of which were performed on an outpatient basis if the patient's health permitted. A 6.5-mm minimum thickness all-polyethylene tibial component medially or a metal-backed tibial component can be used for the lateral compartment. The incision extends from the superior medial pole of the patella to just distal to the joint line. The deeper capsular dissection is in the same line and incorporates a subvastus extension proximally. In another recent series, a minimally invasive approach for implantation of the Oxford unicompartmental prosthesis (Biomet, Warsaw, IN) was described that involves a short incision from the medial pole of the patella to the tibial tuberosity. This causes minimal damage to the extensor mechanism because the patella is not dislocated and the suprapatellar synovial pouch remains intact. Follow-up data on these patients support the possible use of this technique on an outpatient basis, with recovery of function (measured by straight-leg raising, knee flexion, and stair climbing) reported to occur twice as fast as with open UKA and three times faster than in patients undergoing total knee replacement.

Enthusiasm for minimally invasive UKA has been met with some caution, however. One recent series demonstrated that on retrospective radiographic analysis, UKA was less accurate than total knee arthroplasty in implant placement and limb alignment. Furthermore,

when using a minimally invasive technique without eversion or dislocation of the patella, neither anteroposterior tibial placement nor postoperative limb alignment were as accurate as open UKA done through a standard median parapatellar arthrotomy. The advent of minimally invasive surgery and decreased visibility may be an appropriate indication for the increased use of surgical navigation. One study reported that UKA position was significantly improved with navigation systems when compared with standard instrumentation.

Survival Data

Table 1 presents an analysis of studies that provided a minimum of 10 years of follow-up data for patients with UKA. Several issues come to light. First, regarding the definition of survival and what constitutes UKA failure, most authors define failure as revision for any reason, whereas others include revision, recommendation for revision, or severe pain as indicators of UKA failure. Second, revision procedures are undertaken much more readily with UKA than total knee arthroplasty because the conversion of UKA to total knee arthroplasty is not as involved a procedure. It has been reported that survival of medial UKA is as good as that of total knee arthroplasty at 10-year follow-up, 74% and 75%, respectively, when pain is included in the end-point criteria. Another study assessed the causes of early failure of the porous-coated anatomic cemented UKA at 5- to 9-year follow-up and documented a 42% revision rate, with failures caused by femoral loosening, polyethylene wear, and fracture-dislocation of the femoral prosthesis. The main causes of failure were reported to be poor quality heat-pressed polyethylene with significant delamination, inadequate thickness of polyethylene, and a polycentric design with reduced contact area and high-contact stresses. In a retrieval study of Oxford UKA inserts, it was reported that a significant number of patients who had revision surgery for pain without obvious etiology continued to have pain after revision surgery; therefore, the authors recommended that revision of UKA not be undertaken without a clear cause of pain. Furthermore, although most UKAs are performed to treat patients with varus disease, one series proposed that lateral compartment arthroplasty is a reliable and successful option in the treatment of patients with a low level of physical activity, although the results demonstrated only an 89% survival rate at a minimum 5-year follow-up. The authors of this study suggested that lateral UKAs are not as susceptible to loosening because the weight is shared by both compartments and the stress on the lateral prosthesis is therefore decreased compared with medially. Lateral UKA, however, is not without unique problems. One study reported a statistically significant increase in patellar impingement with lateral over medial UKA. Overall, examination of these studies reveals that the field of UKA is evolving and that survival rates improve with advances in prosthetic design and patient selection.

First-Decade Results

Two early series documented a 70% survival rate at 10-year follow-up in 228 knees using the Marmor UKA prosthesis. Of the 21 failures in the series, 9 occurred because of the use of 6-mm polyethylene that actually provided only 4 mm of polyethylene at minimum thickness. Furthermore, six failures were attributed to inclusion of patients who now would be considered to have disease too severe for UKA.

Most series published in the late 1980s to early 1990s demonstrated improved survival rates, ranging from 87.4% to 96% at 10-year follow-up. Most of these studies defined failure as the occurrence of revision procedure. In 1991, an 85% 10-year survivorship was reported with the unicondylar prosthesis. In 1992, a 94% 10-year survivorship was reported with the Marmor and Compartmental II components. In three other reports (1993 to 1996), a 91%, 92%, and 93% 10-year survivorship was reported using the Marmor components. These later findings suggest that surgeons took advantage of lessons learned regarding patient selection and surgical technique and set the standard for a failure rate in the first decade at 1% per year of follow-up. More recent study

data regarding the Oxford UKA revealed a 98% 10-year survivorship in a series of 144 medial compartment UKAs. These findings support those from an independent recent series that reported a 95% 10-year survivorship in 94 medial Oxford UKAs implanted by three surgeons in a nonteaching hospital. Another series of 38 patients (49 knees) documented a 98% 10-year survivorship using the fixed-bearing, metal-backed Miller-Galante prosthesis. Survival data reflect revision and radiographic loosening as end points, and patients had 98% good to excellent results during the same period. Progression of arthritis in the opposite compartment (18%) and patellofemoral compartment (14%) was the leading cause of late failure. With aseptic loosening as a criterion for failure, survivorship was 100%. Including progression of arthritis leading to revision or loosening of the components, survivorship was 98% at 10-year follow-up and 95.7% at 13-year follow-up. Recently, a series was published presenting survival data for UKA performed in a community hospital setting. Using nine different designs, 23 surgeons implanted 516 UKAs and a 92.6% 5-year survivorship and an 88.6% 10-year survivorship was reported compared with a 94.8% 10-year survivorship for TKA. The authors reported that the most common reasons for revision were opposite compartment progression (50%), aseptic loosening (25%), and polyethylene wear (20%).

Second-Decade Results

Second-decade results are less promising, with studies often reflecting a rapid decline in survivorship. This decline in survivorship may be the result of a smaller patient population; in this older population, patients often die of natural causes within the first decade. Only three series have reported 15-year survivorship rates (88%, 79%, and 90%, respectively). The first of these used the St. Georg prosthesis, whereas the other two used the Marmor design. One of these studies reports the only 20-year survivorship as 84%. In light of these results, second-decade survivorship appears to be somewhat inferior to that reported for tricompartmental knee arthroplasty, with the Oxford mobile-bearing and Miller-Galante prostheses being possible exceptions.

Causes of Failure in the Second Decade

The causes of late failure in UKA include opposite compartment degeneration, component loosening, and polyethylene wear. Opposite compartment degeneration remains a point of controversy. Early series that attempted to fully restore alignment reported increased amounts of degeneration and presentation of degenerative joint disease within 5 years. With time, the trend has been to undercorrect alignment or restore alignment to neutral with favorable results. In the series of 52 arthroplasties with 94% survivorship at 10-year follow-up, five of six failures were attributable to progressive degenerative joint disease; however, two failures were overcorrected and two failures were attributable to improper patient selection (those with patellectomy or prior high tibial osteotomy). In a later series assessing 56 Oxford meniscal-bearing knee prostheses, no evidence of deterioration of knee function was found 10 years postoperatively. In addition, no radiographic evidence of degenerative joint disease was found, relief of pain remained stable, and the presence of radiolucent lines under the cemented tibial component was determined to be the rule rather than the exception (occurring in 21 of 26 knees) and was not indicative of impending failure. Regarding the patellofemoral joint, the authors of this study did not exclude patients based on patellofemoral disease because they believed that it was secondary to deformity rather than primary disease. These authors showed that with correction of alignment, no patient in the original series of 144 patients underwent revision surgery for patellofemoral disease. In the series evaluating 62 fixed-bearing metal-backed Miller-Galante prostheses, the only reported failure in the series was attributable to opposite compartment disease. These low failure rates are believed to be associated with the surgical principle of undercorrection of deformity and to the strict criteria applied in patient selection. Because the most significant factor that predisposes the postoperative knee to further degeneration was believed to be the extent of preoperative degeneration, the authors of this study allowed patients with no greater than grade II chondrosis in the other compartments to be included in their study.

Improvements in UKA Implant Design

Problems related to component loosening and polyethylene wear have changed significantly with time. From the initial implants used in the 1970s to the current designs, tibial aseptic loosening and polyethylene wear remain the most common causes of failed UKA. These two areas are linked because increased wear leads to increased deformity and therefore increased load. Additionally, wear can produce osteolysis, which plays a role in component loosening. From the initial design of a cemented femoral component with cemented tibial polyethylene, several advances have been made. Because the use of 6 mm or less of polyethylene was found to be a significant risk factor for wear, loosening, and subsequent revision, the US Food and Drug Administration now requires 6 mm of polyethylene as the absolute minimum. Another surgical advancement involved a move from inset to onlay placement of the tibial component to increase surface coverage and decrease component subsidence. As mentioned previously, improvements were made in femoral component placement and with emphasis placed on recessing the leading edge of the

femoral component into the trochlear cartilage to prevent patellar impingement. A brief trial was made of press-fit components, but these were determined to have a higher failure rate, which was attributable to component loosening.

Other changes in design to address these problems remain somewhat controversial. In an attempt to address the issue of polyethylene wear and subsidence, the concept of metal-backed tibial components was introduced. Metal backing, however, decreases the thickness of the polyethylene available for any given composite thickness of the prosthesis, ranging from just greater than 2 mm to as much as 4 mm, depending on whether the metal backing is titanium or cobalt-chromium. A projected 98% 10-year survivorship was reported in a series of fixed-bearing, minimally constrained UKAs. The authors of this study maintained that the composite tibial component thickness should be at least 8 mm (the minimum used in this series) to avoid complications of accelerated wear, deformity, and subsequent loosening. Although the authors acknowledged that this led to increased bone removal, they observed that new implant design, bone-sparing cuts, and minimal penetration of cement allow for easier revision. The one revision performed in this study was revised to a posterior cruciate ligament–retaining total knee arthroplasty without the need for blocks or wedges. Some experienced surgeons believe that use of an all-polyethylene tibial component remains an attractive option because it allows maximum polyethylene thickness with the most conservative tibial resection. With regard to polyethylene inserts in UKA, shelf age is an important consideration. A recent study of 61 knees found a 96% survivorship and improved function at 6-year follow-up when the shelf age of the insert was less than the median age of 1.7 years, compared with a 71% survivorship and poorer functional results when the shelf age of the insert was greater than 1.7 years. Because the success rate of UKA has not exceeded that of total knee arthroplasty, a UKA still must be implanted with the awareness that a revision procedure may need to be performed, which makes preservation of bone stock and polyethylene integrity an important consideration.

Another significant area of advancement has been the decreased constraint seen in more recent UKA prostheses, most notably the Oxford UKA, which has a reported 10-year survivorship of 98%. The Oxford UKA prosthesis is a meniscal-bearing design that allows increased conformity and contact area without prosthetic constraint. If prosthetic wear debris is an important inciting factor for component loosening or opposite compartment degeneration, and prosthetic constraint promotes loosening, a reasonable argument can be made for recommending a mobile-bearing UKA design. A retrieval study of liners showed that although meniscal bearings introduced the difficulty of two articulation surfaces and thinner polyethylene at the center, this was more than compensated for by the impressive 5.7 cm^2 fully congruous contact in all joint positions. The authors of this study proposed that if the problem of impingement was eliminated by improved surgical technique, then thin components (3.5 mm) would wear at the same rate as thicker ones and the wear rate would decrease to 0.01 mm per year (requiring 100 years to produce deformity of 1° if the rate of wear remains linear). As advocates of meniscal bearing components, and working outside of US Food and Drug Administration restrictions on polyethylene thickness, these authors have been able to resect minimal bone and still implant metal-backed tibial components. However, mobile-bearing knee prostheses can be technically demanding to implant, bearings can dislocate, and as long as government regulations require a minimum bearing thickness of 6 mm, significantly more bone stock must be sacrificed from the tibial side than is necessary for all-polyethylene fixed bearings. In a recent matched comparison series assessing the average 7-year outcomes of 51 fixed-bearing UKAs and 50 mobile-bearing Oxford UKAs, a 99% survivorship for the meniscal-bearing implant was reported compared with a 93% survivorship for the fixed-bearing design. Causes of failure were different for each type of implant; fixed-bearing designs failed most often because of tibial component failure, whereas mobile-bearing designs failed most often because of opposite compartment failure. The authors attributed this scenario to the significantly increased valgus alignment observed postoperatively and cautioned against the tendency to overstuff the joint as a means of preventing bearing dislocation.

Controversies in UKA
Age Criteria
Initially, UKA was thought to be appropriate for elderly, sedentary patients. With the advent of minimally invasive techniques, indications have expanded to include its use in younger patients (especially women) as an alternative to osteotomy or tricompartmental knee arthroplasty. Advantages over osteotomy include higher initial success, greater longevity, and fewer early complications. If done conservatively, salvage is not difficult. Although the extent of safe postoperative activity levels has yet to be established, failure rates seem to be higher in heavy, active males.

The results of long-term follow-up studies have caused some surgeons to reevaluate the classic selection criteria for UKA. In terms of survivorship, UKA seems to be comparable to total knee arthroplasty for the first 10 years after surgery. Within the past 2 years, two separate centers, one using a fixed-bearing design and the other using a mobile-bearing design, each reported a 98% 10-year survivorship. Second-decade survivorship,

however, except for rare reports, seems to be inferior to that of total knee arthroplasty, which undermines the advisability of doing UKA in age groups with 15 to 20 years of life expectancy. Patients in their early 70s, for example, may likely require revision of UKAs in their middle to late 80s, whereas a total knee arthroplasty is more likely to last a lifetime.

As a result, UKA candidates are typically stratified into two separate categories. The first group includes middle-aged patients, especially women, in whom UKA is used as an alternative to osteotomy. Advantages include a higher initial success rate, fewer early complications, a more acceptable cosmetic appearance, a longer-lasting result, and an easier conversion to total knee arthroplasty. The second group may include octogenarians with a level of demands and life expectancy that allow the UKA to outlive the patient. Advantages in this group include a faster recovery, less blood loss, less medical morbidity, and a less expensive procedure. In effect, UKA becomes the first arthroplasty in the middle-aged patient and the last arthroplasty in the elderly patient.

UKA in Younger Patients
There are only three known reports concerning UKA in younger patients in the English-language literature. One such report presented a 7-year follow-up of 49 patients who received a metal-backed UKA. Patient age ranged from 40 to 60 years. Survivorship, based on revision as an end point, was poor; 28% of patients had revision surgery at 7 years, many as the result of wear-through of thin polyethylene in a metal-backed design. Because failure was largely attributable to early implant design, it is impossible to reliably assess the concept of UKA in younger, high-demand patients except to say that they may be more vulnerable to prosthetic wear problems compared with older patients with similar follow-up who received the same type of implant. Nevertheless, the 7.1-year 86% survivorship reported in this study is clearly inferior to most other reported survival rates for UKA.

One study reported the 2- to 6-year follow-up of 28 UKAs in patients younger than 60 years (average age, 52 years). Ninety percent of the patients were rated as having good to excellent results, but two revisions were necessary in heavy, active males because of femoral component loosening at the prosthesis-cement interface. Again, because these failures may have been related to prosthetic design issues, conclusions cannot be made from these results regarding this patient category.

A more recent study reported the average 11-year follow-up of 46 UKAs performed in 41 patients younger than 60 years. The authors cited an 11-year 92% survivorship using the Miller-Galante prosthesis and a combination of all-polyethylene (5 knees) and metal-backed

(41 knees) tibial components and documented 93% good to excellent results. Of the three revisions, two were done for progressive polyethylene wear and one for persistent knee pain and tibial radiolucency. Of note, nine knees had progression of arthritis in the opposite compartment, but none went on to require revision surgery.

Because of renewed enthusiasm for UKA, several series of UKAs in younger, active patients are being generated at numerous centers. With the advent of minimally invasive UKA, more UKAs are being performed, and the indications are being expanded to include younger patients. This technique uses a smaller incision with minimal disturbance of the quadriceps mechanism, requires a shorter hospital stay (overnight or even on an outpatient basis), and allows a faster recovery time. Although no early or midterm results have been reported using this technique in younger patients, it is generally considered to be a temporizing procedure for delaying an eventual total knee arthroplasty, and it is mandatory that early results are documented and reported to assist surgeons with decision making in young or middle-aged patients with unicompartmental osteoarthritis.

Metallic Interposition Hemiarthroplasty

In addition to metal-to-plastic UKA, a second conservative type of arthroplasty is being revisited: metallic interposition hemiarthroplasty. Metallic interposition hemiarthroplasty was introduced in the 1950s (MacIntosh and McKeever prostheses, Howmedica, Rutherford, NJ) with limited popularity. This alternative was all but forgotten until recently when the concept was reintroduced with a prosthetic device called the UniSpacer (Centerpulse, Austin, TX). Good initial results were reported in 72 of 103 knees with a minimum 6-month follow-up. In another study, a slightly different prosthesis was used and good initial results were reported in 39 of 40 knees. A later study of patients with osteoarthritis who had either a McKeever or MacIntosh prosthesis for an average of 3 years (range, 1 to 9 years) reported good to excellent results in 17 of 19 knees.

Another study reported on 40 patients with 44 unicompartmental McKeever prostheses at an average 8-year follow-up (range, 5 to 13 years). At final follow-up, 70% of the knees were rated as good or excellent. Another study reported that at an average 5-year follow-up, 72% of 61 unicompartmental McKeever prostheses were rated as good or excellent. Despite these results, metallic hemiarthroplasty never became popular, possibly because of the advent of cemented metal-to-plastic total knee arthroplasty, which had significantly better initial and long-term results.

Certain patients, however, may still qualify for metallic interposition hemiarthroplasty as an alternative to high tibial osteotomy, metal-to-plastic UKA, or total knee arthroplasty. Indications include a young patient with osteoarthritis who has unicompartmental arthritis of either the medial or lateral side, in whom an osteotomy is contraindicated by early opposite compartment disease or poor range of motion, and who is considered too young, heavy, or active for total knee arthroplasty. It is estimated that approximately 1% of patients with osteoarthritis would be candidates. Because of the minimally invasive nature of metallic interposition hemiarthroplasty, another relative indication would be a past history of sepsis at the knee joint.

The UniSpacer implant can be thought of as a mobile McKeever or MacIntosh hemiarthroplasty implant. Rather than attempting fixation to the tibial plateau via a keel or roughened undersurface, it is designed to translate freely on the tibial plateau as determined by the conforming articulation of its top surface with the femoral condyle. This mobility makes it inappropriate for use in the lateral compartment where the femoral rollback could cause prosthetic dislocation and/or soft-tissue impingement.

In the only recently published report on this device, 71 knees in 67 patients were assessed with a minimum 1-year follow-up. Five knees (7%) were revised to a total knee arthroplasty and an additional 10 knees (14%) had the UniSpacer exchanged because of dislocation (6 knees) or pain (4 knees). The overall 1-year revision rate, therefore, was 21%. Among the 66 knees that retained a UniSpacer, the average flexion was 117°, with an average Knee Society knee score of 78 and function score of 72. Additionally, 17 patients (24%) had arthrofibrosis requiring manipulation under anesthesia for flexion ranging from 60° to 100°.

These results appear to be inferior to those previously published for McKeever hemiarthroplasty, except for a slighter higher flexion arc of 117° versus 110°. The revision rate was 50% higher for the UniSpacer implant compared with the McKeever implant at 1-year follow-up. The UniSpacer device, however, has the advantage of possible insertion through a minimally invasive approach, whereas the McKeever arthroplasty device requires a larger exposure for contouring the femur and tibia and for insertion of the prosthesis.

The role of the UniSpacer device is uncertain at this time. Indications for its use should be similar to those for the McKeever arthroplasty device. A patient with unicompartmental osteoarthritis in whom an osteotomy is contraindicated but is considered too young, heavy, or active for metal-to-plastic arthroplasty is an ideal candidate. Because fewer than 1% of patients with osteoarthritis may be appropriate candidates and the procedure is technically demanding and sensitive, its widespread success is unlikely.

Summary

UKA remains an attractive surgical option for selected patients with osteoarthritis. Ten-year survivorship is comparable to that for tricompartmental arthroplasty when the procedure is well executed using properly designed components. Second-decade survivorship series have been affected adversely by problems with prosthetic wear, loosening, and degeneration of the opposite compartment. Although initial concerns were raised about early opposite compartment degeneration, the advances described previously have significantly decreased the incidence of this problem in the first decade. Additional advances in prosthetic design have significantly reduced problems with prosthetic wear and aseptic component loosening. Mobile-bearing designs address these issues and could play a significant role in the future of UKA. Improvements in the wear characteristics of polyethylene may enhance the performance of fixed-bearing implants, and 10-year survivorship rates with fixed- and mobile-bearing designs are encouraging. Continued long-term follow-up of these series will provide important data regarding second-decade survivorship and the overall role of UKA in the treatment of osteoarthritis. Additionally, newer technology in the preparation of polyethylene bearings may enhance long-term survivorship. Until the late 1990s, many unicompartmental designs used polyethylene gamma-sterilized in air. If oxidation occurs, both surface and subsurface deterioration can lead to polyethylene failure. Polyethylene prepared with alternative techniques could have higher second-decade survivorship. The highly cross-linked polyethylene that now is available for hip arthroplasty articulation could also be beneficial in some UKA designs, whether fixed or mobile.

Annotated Bibliography

Comparison With Alternative Procedures

McAuley JP, Engh GA, Ammeen DJ: Revision of failed unicompartmental knee arthroplasty. *Clin Orthop* 2001; 392:279-282.

The authors of this study evaluated 30 patients (32 knees) at a mean of 53 months. Revision procedures were performed 9 to 204 months after UKA. Although the predominant mechanism of failure was polyethylene wear, nine prostheses failed because of loosening. Although this study assessed a small series of patients, the authors concluded that the simplicity of UKA and the complications encountered compared favorably with those of total knee revision.

Minimally Invasive Surgical Technique

Berger RA, Meneghini RM, Jacobs JJ, et al: Results of unicompartmental knee arthroplasty at a minimum of ten years of follow-up. *J Bone Joint Surg Am* 2005;87(5): 999-1006.

The authors of this study clinically and radiographically assessed 38 patients with cemented modular Miller-Galante implants (49 knees) at a minimum 10-year follow-up. Two patients (two knees) with well-fixed components required revision to total knee arthroplasty at 7 and 11 years to treat patellofemoral arthritis. At final follow-up, no component showed radiographic evidence of loosening, and no evidence of periprosthetic osteolysis was identified. Progressive loss of joint space was observed radiographically in the opposite compartment of nine knees (18%) and in the patellofemoral space of seven knees (14%). With revision or evidence of radiographic loosening as the end point, the authors reported a survival rate of 98.0% ± 2.0% at 10 years and of 95.7% ± 4.3% at 13 years. At 13-year follow-up, the survival rate was 100%, with aseptic loosening as the end point.

Berger RA, Rosenberg AG, Barden RM, Sheinkop MB, Jacobs JJ, Galante JO: Long-term follow-up of the Miller-Galante total knee replacement. *Clin Orthop Relat Res* 2001;388:58-67.

Of 172 Miller-Galante I total knee arthroplasties evaluated, the authors reported 21 revisions and 15 patellar revisions, 2 of which included femoral revisions attributable to abrasion. Six well-fixed femoral and tibial components were also revised to treat early instability (N = 2), pain (N = 1), periprosthetic fracture (N = 1), and infection (N = 2). No patients had aseptic loosening of the implant or osteolysis. With revision or component loosening as the end point, the authors reported a 10-year survivorship rate of 84.1% ± 4.1%. Of 109 Miller-Galante II total knee arthroplasties evaluated, the authors reported no component revisions, aseptic loosening, nor osteolysis. With revision or component loosening as the end point, the reported 10-year survivorship rate was 100%.

Fisher DA, Watts M, Davis KE: Implant position in knee surgery: A comparison of minimally invasive, open unicompartmental, and total knee arthroplasty. *J Arthroplasty* 2003;18(7 suppl 1):2-8.

The authors evaluated patients who underwent minimally invasive UKA, open UKA, or total knee arthroplasty. They reported that the total knee arthroplasty group had the smallest amount of implant variation and the greatest accuracy of placement and limb alignment. The two UKA groups had small but significant differences in postoperative alignment and tibial position. The authors concluded that UKA was less accurate than total knee arthroplasty in terms of implant placement and limb alignment and that minimally invasive UKA was not as accurate as open UKA in tibial placement or postoperative limb alignment.

Gioe TJ, Killeen KK, Hoeffel DP, et al: Analysis of unicompartmental knee arthroplasty in a community-based implant registry. *Clin Orthop* 2003;416:111-119.

The authors determined the long-term survival rates for UKA using data from a community implant and explant registry. These data were assessed and compared with data on total knee arthroplasty survival rates. The major reasons for revision for UKA included progression of arthritis in the uninvolved compartments (51.3% of patient), aseptic loosening (25.6%), and polyethylene wear (20.5%). With revision as the end point, the authors reported survival rates of 92.6% (range, 90.0% to 95.2%) at 5-year follow-up and 88.6% (range, 85.0% to 92.2%) at 10-year follow-up for UKAs, whereas primary total knee arthroplasties had a survival rate of 94.8% (range, 93.5% to 96.0%) at 10-year follow-up.

Hernigou P, Deschamps G: Patellar impingement following unicompartmental knee arthroplasty. *J Bone Joint Surg Am* 2002;84:1132-1137.

The authors reported that the patellofemoral joint was affected by degenerative changes and patellar impingement after UKA and that these complications were mutually exclusive and affected the functional outcome of the arthroplasty. Regarding symptoms and the need for revision, they also reported that patellar impingement affected the knee more severely.

Jenny JY, Boeri C: Accuracy of implantation of a unicompartmental total knee arthroplasty with two different instrumentations. *J Arthroplasty* 2002;17(8):1016-1020.

The authors adapted conventional instruments for tricompartmental total knee arthroplasty implantation for UKA implantation. They reported that although the radiographic accuracy of implant placement improved significantly using the new instrumentation, there was no significant difference in survival rates or clinical outcomes at 5-year follow-up for both groups.

Laskin RS: Unicompartmental knee replacement: Some unanswered questions. *Clin Orthop* 2001;392:267-271.

The author describes many of the benefits of UKA and provides some important guidelines to consider before performing UKA.

Ohdera T, Tokunaga J, Kobayashi A: Unicompartmental knee arthroplasty for lateral gonarthrosis: Mid-term results. *J Arthroplasty* 2001;16(2):196-200.

The authors of this study assessed 17 patients (average age, 64.5 years) who underwent UKA to treat lateral gonarthrosis at a minimum 5-year follow-up and reported that although five patients had slight osteoarthritic deterioration in the medial compartment, lateral compartment arthroplasty is a reliable and successful treatment option for patients with a low level of physical activity.

Repicci JA: Mini-invasive knee unicompartmental arthroplasty: Bone sparing technique. *Surg Technol Int* 2003;11:282-286.

The author describes a technique for UKA that includes limited surgical exposure, internal landmarks for prosthetic insertion, and pain management to facilitate outpatient status.

Romanowski MR, Repicci JA: Minimally invasive unicondylar arthroplasty: 8-year follow-up. *J Knee Surg* 2002;15:17-22.

The authors of this study performed 136 UKAs using a surgical technique that involved a limited medial parapatellar incision to reduce perioperative morbidity and bone preparation techniques to preserve bone for future arthroplasty procedures. At 8-year follow-up, they reported that 4% of patients (Ahlback stage 2 and 3) required revision. They concluded that minimally invasive UKA provides a low morbidity alternative treatment for patients with symptomatic medial compartment osteoarthritis.

Skyrme AD, Mencia MM, Skinner PW: Early failure of the porous-coated anatomic cemented unicompartmental knee arthroplasty. *J Arthroplasty* 2002;17(2):201-205.

The authors of this retrospective study analyzed the results of 26 porous-coated anatomic UKAs to determine the failure rate, mode of failure, and presentation of the failure. They reported a revision rate of 42%, with a mean revision time of 38.4 months. The most common mechanisms of failure included femoral loosening (55%), polyethylene wear (55%), loosening and polyethylene wear (72%), and fracture-dislocation of the femoral prosthesis (18%). The authors concluded that the porous-coated anatomic UKA requires regular patient assessment because of the high failure rate; if failure occurs, prompt revision is required to avoid the onset of osteolysis.

Svard UC, Price AJ: Oxford medial unicompartmental knee arthroplasty: A survival analysis of an independent series. *J Bone Joint Surg Br* 2001;83:191-194.

The authors report the outcome of a series of 124 Oxford meniscal-bearing UKAs that were done to treat osteoarthritis of the medial compartment. At 10-year follow-up, 94 knees were still at risk, and the cumulative survival rate was 95.0%, which is comparable to the survival rates reported by the manufacturers of the prosthesis and independent series assessing total knee replacement. The authors concluded that if patients are appropriately selected, then this type of implant can be a reliable treatment option for patients with anteromedial osteoarthritis of the knee.

Improvements in UKA Implant Design

Collier MB, Engh CA Jr, Engh GA: Shelf age of the polyethylene tibial component and outcome of unicondylar knee arthroplasty. *J Bone Joint Surg Am* 2004; 86-A:763-769.

The authors reported that shelf age accelerated the fatigue failure of polyethylene inserts that were sterilized with gamma irradiation in air and compromised the intermediate-term clinical outcomes of patients who underwent UKA. They concluded that continued attention to the relationship between shelf age and clinical performance of the polyethylene component is warranted with UKA implants.

Emerson RH Jr, Hansborough T, Reitman RD, Rosenfeldt W, Higgins LL: Comparison of a mobile with a fixed-bearing unicompartmental knee implant. *Clin Orthop Relat Res* 2002;404:62-70.

The authors of this study compared two matched groups of patients who underwent UKA; 51 received a fixed-bearing knee implant and 50 received a mobile-bearing implant. They reported that the fixed-bearing group had an average +2.6° of alignment and the mobile-bearing group had +5.5° of alignment. With component loosening and revision as an end point, the authors reported a 99% survival rate for the mobile-bearing group and a 93% survival rate for the fixed-bearing group at 11-year follow-up.

Controversies in UKA

Deshmukh RV, Scott RD: Unicompartmental knee arthroplasty for young patients. *Clin Orthop* 2002;404:108-112.

Although UKA is being used to treat younger patients, the authors caution for continued use of strict selection criteria and bone conserving techniques during surgery in this patient population.

Hallock RH, Fell BM: Unicompartmental tibial hemiarthroplasty: Early results of the UniSpacer knee. *Clin Orthop* 2003;416:154-163.

The authors present 1- and 2-year follow-up data on 67 patients (71 knees) who received the UniSpacer Knee System (four patients underwent bilateral knee surgery) and report that five implants (7%) had to be revised to total knee arthroplasty and 10 implants (14%) had to be revised to another UniSpacer Knee System implant.

Pennington DW, Swienckowski JJ, Lutes WB, Drake GN: Unicompartmental knee arthroplasty in patients sixty years of age or younger. *J Bone Joint Surg Am* 2003;85-A:1968-1973.

This retrospective study of 41 active patients 60 years of age or younger was conducted to evaluate the results of UKA. Two asymptomatic patients required revision of a modular tibial component because of substantial radiographic evidence of polyethylene wear. Another patient underwent revision total knee arthroplasty to treat continuing knee pain and a progressive tibial radiolucent line > 2 mm in width. Although nine patients experienced progression of arthritis in the unresurfaced compartments, none of these implants were revised, and no decreases in Hospital for Special Surgery scores were reported. An 11-year survivorship of 92% was reported.

Scott RD: Unispacer: Insufficient data to support its widespread use. *Clin Orthop* 2003;416:164-166.

The author concludes that fewer than 1% of patients with osteoarthritis are appropriate candidates for this particular implant and widespread use is unlikely because implantation is technically demanding.

Classic Bibliography

Ansari S, Newman JH, Ackroyd CE: St. Georg sledge for medial compartment knee replacement: 461 arthroplasties followed for 4 (1-17) years. *Acta Orthop Scand* 1997;68:430-434.

Barck AL: 10-year evaluation of compartmental knee arthroplasty. *J Arthroplasty* 1989;4:S49-S54.

Barrett WP, Scott RD: Revision of failed unicompartmental knee arthroplasty. *J Bone Joint Surg Am* 1987;69:1328-1335.

Berger RA, Nedeff DD, Barden RM, et al: Unicompartmental knee arthroplasty: Clinical experience at 6- to 10- year followup. *Clin Orthop* 1999;367:50-60.

Bert JM: 10-year survivorship of metal-backed, unicompartmental arthroplasty. *J Arthroplasty* 1998;13:901-905.

Broughton NS, Newman JH, Baily RAJ: Unicompartmental replacement and high tibial osteotomy for osteoarthritis of the knee: A comparative study after 5-10 years follow-up. *J Bone Joint Surg Br* 1986;68:447-452.

Capra SW Jr, Fehring TK: Unicondylar arthroplasty: A survivorship analysis. *J Arthroplasty* 1992;7:247-251.

Cartier P, Sanouiller JL, Grelsamer RP: Unicompartmental knee arthroplasty surgery: 10-year minimum follow-up period. *J Arthroplasty* 1996;11:782-788.

Emerson R, Potter T: The use of the McKeever metallic hemi-arthroplasty for unicompartmental arthritis. *J Bone Joint Surg Am* 1985;67:208-212.

Engh GA, McAuley JP: Unicondylar arthroplasty: An option for high-demand patients with gonarthrosis. *Instr Course Lect* 1999;48:143-148.

Gill T, Schemitsch EH, Brick GW, Thornhill TS: Revision total knee arthroplasty after failed unicompartmental arthroplasty or high tibial osteotomy. *Clin Orthop* 1995;321:10-18.

Heck DA, Marmor L, Gibson A, Rougraff BT: Unicompartmental knee arthroplasty: A multicenter investigation with long-term follow-up evaluation. *Clin Orthop* 1993;286:154-159.

Insall J, Aglietti P: A five to seven-year follow-up of unicompartmental arthroplasty. *J Bone Joint Surg Am* 1980;62:1329-1337.

Insall J, Walker P: Unicondylar knee replacement. *Clin Orthop* 1976;120:83-85.

Insall JN, Dorr LD, Scott RD, Scott WN: Rationale of The Knee Society clinical rating system. *Clin Orthop* 1989;248:13-14.

Jackson M, Sarangi PP, Newman JH: Revision total knee arthroplasty: Comparison of outcome following primary proximal tibial osteotomy or unicompartmental arthroplasty. *J Arthroplasty* 1994;9:539-542.

Karpman RR, Volz RG: Osteotomy versus unicompartmental prosthetic replacement in the treatment of unicompartmental arthritis of the knee. *Orthopedics* 1982;5:989-991.

Kozinn SC, Scott R: Unicondylar knee arthroplasty. *J Bone Joint Surg Am* 1989;71:145-150.

Larsson SE, Larsson S, Lundkvist S: Unicompartmental knee arthroplasty: A prospective consecutive series followed for six to 11 years. *Clin Orthop* 1988;232:174-181.

Laskin RS: Unicompartmental tibiofemoral resurfacing arthroplasty. *J Bone Joint Surg Am* 1978;60:182-185.

Levine WN, Ozuna RM, Scott RD, Thornhill TS: Conversion of failed modern unicompartmental arthroplasty to total knee arthroplasty. *J Arthroplasty* 1996;11:797-801.

MacIntosh DL: Hemi-arthroplasty of the knee using a space occupying prosthesis for painful varus and valgus deformities. *J Bone Joint Surg Am* 1958;40:1431.

Marmor L: Unicompartmental arthroplasty of the knee with a minimum ten-year follow-up period. *Clin Orthop* 1988;228:171-177.

Marmor L: Unicompartmental knee arthroplasty: Ten- to 13-year follow-up study. *Clin Orthop* 1988;226:14-20.

McKeever DC: Tibial plateau prosthesis. *Clin Orthop Relat Res* 1985;192:3-12.

Munk B, Frokjaer J: A 10-year follow-up of unicompartmental arthrosis treated with the Marmor method. *Ugeskr Laeger* 1994;156:4029-4031.

Murray DW, Goodfellow JW, O'Connor JJ: The Oxford medial unicompartmental arthroplasty: A ten-year survival study. *J Bone Joint Surg Br* 1998;80:983-989.

Padgett DE, Stern SH, Insall JN: Revision total knee arthroplasty for failed unicompartmental replacement. *J Bone Joint Surg Am* 1991;73:186-190.

Potter TA, Weinfeld MS, Thomas WH: Arthroplasty of the knee in rheumatoid arthritis and osteoarthritis: A follow-up study and implantation of the McKeever and MacIntosh prosthesis. *J Bone Joint Surg Am* 1972;54:1-24.

Psychoyios V, Crawford RW, O'Connor JJ, Murray DW: Wear of congruent meniscal bearings in unicompartmental knee arthroplasty: A retrieval study of 16 specimens. *J Bone Joint Surg Br* 1998;80:976-982.

Schai PA, Suh J, Thornhill TS, Scott RD: Unicompartmental knee arthroplasty in middle-aged patients: A 2- to 6- year follow-up evaluation. *J Arthroplasty* 1998;13:365-372.

Scott RD, Joyce MS, Ewald FC, Thomas WH: McKeever metallic hemi-arthroplasty of the knee in unicompartmental degenerative arthritis. *J Bone Joint Surg Am* 1985;67:203-207.

Scott RD, Cobb AG, McQueary FG, Thornhill TS: Unicompartmental knee arthroplasty: Eight- to 12-year follow-up evaluation with survivorship analysis. *Clin Orthop* 1991;271:96-100.

Scott RD, Santore RF: Unicondylar unicompartmental replacement for osteoarthritis of the knee. *J Bone Joint Surg Am* 1981;63:536-544.

Squire MW, Callaghan JJ, Goetz DD, Sullivan PM, Johnston RC: Unicompartmental knee replacement: A minimum 15 year followup study. *Clin Orthop Relat Res* 1999;367:61-72.

Stern SH, Becker MW, Insall JN: Unicondylar knee arthroplasty: An evaluation of selection criteria. *Clin Orthop* 1993;286:143-148.

Stockelman RE, Pohl KP: The long-term efficacy of unicompartmental arthroplasty of the knee. *Clin Orthop Relat Rel* 1991;271:88-95.

Tabor OB Jr, Tabor OB: Unicompartmental arthroplasty: A long-term follow-up study. *J Arthroplasty* 1998;13:373-379.

Weale AE, Murray DW, Crawford R, et al: Does arthritis progress in the retained compartments after Oxford medial unicompartmental arthroplasty? A clinical and radiological study with a minimum ten-year follow-up. *J Bone Joint Surg Br* 1999;81:783-799.

Weale AE, Newman JH: Unicompartmental arthroplasty and high tibial osteotomy for osteoarthrosis of the knee: A comparative study with a 12- to 17-year follow-up period. *Clin Orthop* 1994;302:134-137.

Chapter 7

Patellofemoral Arthroplasty

Jess H. Lonner, MD

Jo-ann Lee, MS

Joseph C. McCarthy, MD

Wayne B. Leadbetter, MD

Introduction

Isolated patellofemoral arthritis can be painful and debilitating, but often it can be treated effectively with nonsurgical interventions such as weight reduction, physical therapy, and judicious use of oral or injectable medications. However, when pain is refractory to these efforts, surgery may be considered. Several surgical options have been used for patellofemoral arthritis, including arthroscopic débridement and lavage, unloading procedures (Maquet tubercle elevation or Fulkerson tubercle anteromedialization), patellectomy, cartilage grafting techniques, patellar resurfacing, patellofemoral arthroplasty, and total knee arthroplasty. Specifically, patellofemoral arthroplasty has been used to treat isolated patellofemoral chondral degeneration. Results may be improved by (1) limiting the procedure to patients with arthritis that is strictly localized to the anterior compartment of the knee and without patellar malalignment; (2) accurately aligning and implanting the prosthesis and balancing the soft tissues to optimize patellar tracking; (3) using an implant that engages the patella within the trochlear groove, but which has limited constraint and a sagittal radius of curvature that mates well with the native distal femur; and (4) minimizing activities postoperatively that require repetitive patellofemoral loading in deep flexion.

Newer and improving designs, which have reduced the incidence of patellofemoral complications, as well as interest in less invasive alternatives to standard total knee arthroplasty, have stimulated considerable enthusiasm for patellofemoral arthroplasty.

Epidemiology

Chondromalacia patella has been observed in 40% to 60% of patients at autopsy, and in 20% to 50% of patients at the time of arthrotomy for other diagnoses. The prevalence of isolated patellofemoral arthritis is high, occurring in as many as 11% of men and 24% of women older than 55 years with symptomatic osteoarthritis of the knee and nearly 4% of patients with painless osteoarthritis of the knee. This gender predilection is undoubtedly related to the often subtle patellar malalignment and dysplasia that is common in women. The patellofemoral cartilage is also vulnerable to direct traumatic injury because of its unprotected location in the body.

Alternative Methods of Management
Nonsurgical Treatment

Conservative management is the mainstay of treatment of isolated patellofemoral arthritis; relatively few patients ultimately require surgical intervention. A directed therapy program emphasizing short arc quadriceps strengthening, isometrics, stretching of the lateral retinacular structures, and preservation of motion is frequently successful in mitigating symptoms. There is some evidence to suggest that vastus medialis obliquus dysfunction may be associated with patellofemoral pain, which reinforces the importance of a directed strengthening program. Additionally, considering the excessive loads to which the anterior compartment of the knee is exposed, a supervised program of weight reduction can also be beneficial. Avoiding provocative maneuvers such as ascending and descending stairs, squatting, jumping, and biking can help to minimize the loads on the patellofemoral joint and reduce the pain from arthritis. Hamstring tightness can increase patellofemoral forces; therefore, hamstring stretching may be helpful. Oral anti-inflammatory medications or analgesics and intra-articular injections of corticosteroids or hyaluronans may be effective adjuvant therapeutic options. Additionally, although data are lacking, patellar unloading sleeves or braces may play a role in the nonsurgical management of this condition. In patients who fail to respond to a minimum of 3 to 6 months of nonsurgical management, surgical intervention may be considered.

Arthroscopic Surgery

Arthroscopic options for patellofemoral chondromalacia and arthritis include lavage or débridement with or without marrow stimulation. Arthroscopic débridement and lavage may be advantageous in patients who have failed to respond to conservative management and continue to have recurrent effusions or mechanical catching by decreasing the debris load that may be a source of inflammatory mediators. Removal of an unstable chondral flap on the patella or trochlear groove may improve the mechanical symptoms. However, these interventions have varied results, and patients should be counseled regarding the likelihood of only partial and temporary symptomatic relief and the persistence of functional limitations. The poor intrinsic healing capabilities of articular cartilage limit the value of arthroscopic treatments of patellofemoral arthritis, particularly in the absence of mechanical symptoms.

Various technical modalities are available for débridement of chondromalacia, including mechanical shavers, thermal devices, and lasers. Although lasers have provided limited short-term symptomatic improvement, they have extremely worrisome potential complications, including extensive damage of the cartilage and necrosis of subchondral bone. Compared with mechanical débridement, radiofrequency ablation may have better short-term results; however, the long-term effects of thermal energy on articular cartilage have yet to be defined and it should be used with caution.

One study analyzed a series of 36 patients who underwent arthroscopic chondroplasty for isolated chondromalacia patella without patellar malalignment. Patients with traumatic chondromalacia had 60% good or excellent results compared with 41% good or excellent results in all other patients in the study. Lateral retinacular release, after chondral degeneration has already occurred, is often ineffective in resolving anterior knee pain. Another study used chondroplasty for varying degrees of chondromalacia of the patella to remove loose fibrillation, but not to penetrate through subchondral bone nor to débride intact cartilage. At a mean 40-month follow-up, good to excellent results were reported in 49% of patients and fair results were reported in 44% of patients. It was noted that 78% of patients were satisfied with the outcome and that the grade of chondromalacia did not correlate with the outcome. Marrow stimulation techniques, such as microfracture, have also fared relatively poorly in treating lesions of the patellofemoral articulation. The reparative fibrocartilage tissue, composed primarily of type I collagen, does not withstand well the excessive shear stresses common to the patellofemoral articulation.

Tibial Tubercle Unloading Procedures

Anteromedialization of the tibial tubercle is a time-tested and well-established procedure for the treatment of patellar maltracking associated with patellofemoral malalignment. Anteriorization of the tibial tubercle increases the lever arm for extensor mechanism function and reduces the patellofemoral joint reaction forces by increasing the angle between the patellar tendon and quadriceps tendon. Medializing the tibial tubercle improves the Q angle and thereby decreases the strong lateral vectors acting upon the patella. Combining these two components can therefore both improve patellar tracking and relieve pain associated with subchondral overload of the lateral patellar facet. The obliquity of the tibial tubercle osteotomy allows for adjustment in the extent of anteriorization, and bone graft is not necessary. The angle can be adjusted to accommodate varying degrees of subluxation and articular cartilage damage. Although excellent to good results have been reported in 89% of patients at a follow-up of more than 5 years, no patients achieved excellent results, and satisfaction was only 75% in the presence of Outerbridge grade III or IV chondromalacia.

Direct anteriorization of the tibial tubercle has also been recommended for patients with patellofemoral arthrosis when there is no patellar subluxation or malalignment. Symptom improvement with the classic Maquet osteotomy has been reported in 30% to 90% of patients. Biomechanical studies have demonstrated reductions in contact pressures; however, contact areas may shift proximally, paradoxically overloading the proximal portion of the patella in deep flexion. The optimal patient to benefit from a Maquet osteotomy is one with posttraumatic arthrosis or chondromalacia involving the inferior half of the patella. Patients with proximal arthrosis or diffuse patellofemoral arthrosis and those who have undergone multiple prior patellofemoral surgeries will have compromised outcomes. Its limited indications, unpredictable results, and risk of complications such as wound necrosis or osteotomy nonunion restrict the practical application of this procedure.

Cartilage Grafting

Autologous chondrocyte implantation for isolated patellar cartilage lesions has produced satisfactory results in approximately 75% of patients at 2- to 10-year follow-up. Its proponents advise that residual patellar malalignment is a common reason for failure of this technique; therefore, residual patellar malalignment should be addressed before or simultaneous with autologous chondrocyte implantation. Autologous osteochondral transplantation has been recommended for patients with patellofemoral lesions. Although the duration of follow-up is not clear, one study reported a 79% satisfactory rate among patients who underwent patellar and/or trochlear mosaicplasty.

Patellectomy

Patellectomy has been historically used to treat patients with debilitating patellofemoral arthrosis. Patellectomy has been shown experimentally to reduce extension power by 25% to 60%, with a concomitant requisite increase in quadriceps force of 15% to 30% to achieve adequate extension torque. Tibiofemoral joint reaction forces may increase as much as 250%, which explains the propensity for tibiofemoral arthrosis after patellectomy. Variable pain relief, residual quadriceps weakness, and secondary instability along with failure rates as high as 45% relegate patellectomy to being a salvage procedure for the rare patient who responds poorly to other more successful interventions. Additionally, the results of total knee arthroplasty can be compromised after patellectomy.

Total Knee Arthroplasty

Total knee arthroplasty is generally effective for elderly patients with isolated patellofemoral arthritis, yielding good and excellent results in 90% to 95% of patients at midterm follow-up; anterior knee pain, however, has been reported in as many as 7% to 19% of patients. In one study that compared total knee arthroplasty and tricompartmental arthrosis for the treatment of isolated patellofemoral arthrosis, Knee Society clinical scores, bipedal stair climbing capacity, and ability to rise from a seated position were all significantly better in the total knee arthroplasty group. Given its predictably good results, total knee arthroplasty is preferable to patellofemoral arthroplasty in the treatment of elderly patients with isolated patellofemoral arthrosis. However, in younger patients with isolated patellofemoral arthrosis, patellofemoral arthroplasty may be considered.

Anterior Compartment Resurfacing

Patellofemoral arthroplasty is a worthwhile option for young and middle-aged patients with localized patellofemoral arthrosis or severe recalcitrant chondromalacia. Early prosthetic designs resurfaced only the patella, using a metal implant. Although the patella is commonly more degenerated than the trochlea, results have been variable with this technique. The recognition that residual anterior knee pain may be related to trochlear chondromalacia led to the development of first-generation patellofemoral resurfacing arthroplasties using a polyethylene patellar component and metallic trochlear component.

Patellofemoral Arthroplasty

Patient Selection

The outcome of patellofemoral arthroplasty can be optimized by limiting its application to patients with isolated patellofemoral osteoarthrosis, posttraumatic arthrosis, or severe chondrosis (Outerbridge grade IV), and then only after an extended supervised program of nonsurgical treatment. Additionally, this option is best reserved for patients with severe pain and functional limitations and those who experience considerable dis-

comfort during prolonged sitting, stair or hill ambulation, or squatting. The procedure should not be used to treat patients with inflammatory arthritis or chondrocalcinosis involving the menisci or tibiofemoral chondral surfaces, nor should it be recommended to patients with inappropriate expectations. Alternative etiologies of anterior knee pain such as patellar tendinitis, synovitis, patellar instability, sympathetic mediated pain, or pain referred from the back or ipsilateral hip should be excluded.

Although it can be most effective for treating patellofemoral dysplasia, patellofemoral arthroplasty should be avoided in patients with considerable patellar maltracking or malalignment unless corrected preoperatively. This is not to say, however, that slight patellar tilt, observed on preoperative tangential radiographs or at the time of arthrotomy or trochlear dysplasia should be considered contraindications for this procedure. In such instances, a lateral retinacular release may be necessary at the time of arthroplasty. Persistent subluxation may cause pain and snapping and potentially wear of the prosthesis. Patients with excessive Q angles should undergo successful tibial tubercle realignment before patellofemoral arthroplasty. Additionally, identification of tibiofemoral arthrosis during prior arthroscopic procedures or at the time of the arthrotomy for patellofemoral arthroplasty should prompt the abandonment of patellofemoral arthroplasty. The presence of even focal grade III tibiofemoral chondromalacia can compromise the outcome after patellofemoral arthroplasty, although these patients will often acknowledge resolution of the most prominent component of pain.

As with other knee arthroplasty procedures, this treatment method should be restricted to patients willing to modify their activity levels to minimize stress overload and accelerated implant wear. Laborers and athletes who opt to continue their trade or aggressive recreational involvement are not ideal candidates for this procedure. Patients should be discouraged from activities that require excessive loading in deep flexion. Although there are intuitive concerns, there are no known data available to determine whether obesity or cruciate ligament insufficiency place patellofemoral arthroplasty at risk for failure.

Although there are no stringent age criteria for patellofemoral arthroplasty, it is an excellent alternative to total knee arthroplasty or patellectomy for patients younger than 55 years who have isolated anterior compartment arthrosis. Elderly patients may be better suited for total knee arthroplasty because of its remarkable track record and proven survivorship and because some degree of tibiofemoral chondromalacia is ubiquitous in more elderly patients, but the decision should be individualized for each patient.

Clinical Evaluation

Evaluation of the patient under consideration for patellofemoral arthroplasty should be thorough to confirm that the pain and chondral disease are, in fact, localized to the anterior compartment of the knee. This can usually be done by obtaining a detailed history of the problem and by performing a meticulous physical examination.

The key elements of the history that should be elaborated include whether there was previous trauma to the knee, a history of patellar dislocation, or prior patellofemoral problems. A history of recurrent atraumatic patellar dislocations may suggest considerable malalignment and may need to be corrected before considering patellofemoral arthroplasty. A clear description of the location of the pain is important because discomfort anywhere but directly retropatellar or just lateral or medial to the patella will not be relieved with a patellofemoral arthroplasty. Patellofemoral pain often is exacerbated by activities such as stair climbing and descent, ambulating on hills, standing from a seated position, sitting with the knee flexed, and squatting. Walking on level ground tends not to be as problematic. A description of anterior crepitus is common. After establishing the location and quality of pain, it is important to ascertain whether there were previous interventions, such as physical therapy, weight reduction, medications, injections, or surgery.

On physical examination, pain on patellar inhibition testing (retropatellar pain caused by active contraction of the quadriceps muscle while manually preventing proximal excursion of the patella), patellofemoral crepitus, and retropatellar knee pain with squatting are typical. Any associated medial or lateral tibiofemoral joint line tenderness should raise the suspicion of more diffuse chondral disease (even in the presence of relatively normal radiographs) and may be a contraindication to patellofemoral arthroplasty. It is also essential to rule out other potential sources of anterior knee pain, such as pes anserinus bursitis, patellar tendinitis, prepatellar bursitis, instability, or pain referred from the ipsilateral hip or back. Careful assessment of patellar tracking and the Q angle also are important. Because even subtle tracking abnormalities and malalignment can predispose patients to inferior outcomes (particularly with certain implant designs) in patients with high Q angles, a tibial tubercle realignment procedure (anteromedialization) should be performed before patellofemoral arthroplasty.

Generally, weight-bearing radiographs are appropriate diagnostic imaging studies. Weight-bearing AP and midflexion PA radiographs are critical to determine the presence of tibiofemoral arthritis. Mild squaring-off of the femoral condyles and even small marginal osteophytes may be accepted, provided the patient has no tibiofemoral pain with functional activities and on physical examination and that there is minimal chondral degeneration identified during arthroscopy or arthrotomy. Lateral radiographs will occasionally demonstrate patellofemoral osteophytes, but they usually are more useful in identifying patella alta or baja. Axial radiographs will demonstrate the position of the patella within the trochlear groove and the extent of arthritis, although it is not uncommon to have apparent patellofemoral joint space preservation with minimal or no osteophytes despite significant cartilage loss. Often subchondral sclerosis and facet flattening may be the only radiographic evidence of patellofemoral arthrosis (Figure 1). CT and MRI are not necessary for evaluating patellofemoral arthrosis, although they can be useful for assessing instability. Photographs from prior arthroscopic treatment will provide valuable information regarding the extent of anterior compartment arthrosis and the status of the tibiofemoral cartilage and menisci.

Surgical Technique

During arthrotomy, it is essential to avoid cutting normal articular cartilage or the menisci. Before proceeding with patellofemoral arthroplasty, the entire joint should be carefully inspected to make sure the tibiofemoral compartments are free of disease.

The trochlear component should be externally rotated parallel to the epicondylar axis to enhance patellar tracking. Osteophytes bordering the intercondylar notch should be removed. The trochlear component should maximize coverage of the trochlea, without extending beyond the mediolateral femoral margins anteriorly, encroaching on the weight-bearing surfaces of the tibiofemoral articulations, or overhanging into the intercondylar notch. During preparation of the recipient trochlear bed, excessive removal of subchondral bone should be avoided. The component edges should be flush with or recessed approximately 1 mm from the adjacent articular cartilage. The patella is resurfaced by the same principles observed in total knee arthroplasty, restoring the original patellar thickness and medializing the component. The exposed cut surface of the lateral patella that is not covered by the patellar prosthesis should be beveled to avoid the potentially painful articulation on the trochlear prosthesis.

Assessment of patellar tracking is performed with the trial components in place. Attention is paid to identify patellar tilt, subluxation, or catching of the components. Patellar tilt and mild subluxation usually can be addressed successfully by performing a lateral retinacular release. As stated earlier, more severe extensor mechanism malalignment (such as an excessive Q angle) should have been addressed preoperatively. With appropriate patient selection and surgical technique, proximal realignment at the time of surgery should be unneces-

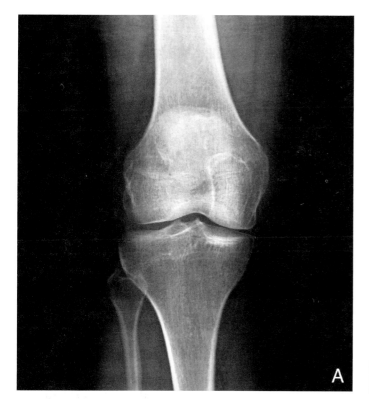

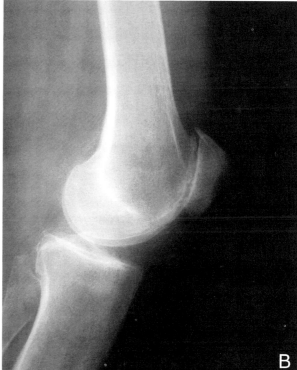

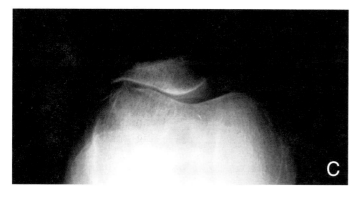

Figure 1 Weight-bearing AP **(A)**, lateral **(B)**, and axial **(C)** radiographs demonstrating advanced patellofemoral arthrosis with sparing of the tibiofemoral compartments.

sary in most patients, even in those with preoperative patellofemoral dysplasia and slight patellar tilt or subluxation (Figure 2).

Postoperative Management

Isometrics and range-of-motion exercises are started immediately. Use of a continuous passive motion machine during hospitalization (average, 2 to 3 days) may accelerate flexion recovery, but it is probably not necessary for all patients. Full weight bearing is permitted with support (crutches and a cane) until there is adequate recovery of quadriceps strength. Full recovery of quadriceps strength can take 6 months or longer, considering the often severe quadriceps atrophy that is encountered in patients with patellofemoral arthritis. Thromboembolism prophylaxis is used for 4 to 6 weeks. Use of perioperative antibiotics is advisable for 24 hours, and appropriate pre-

cautions regarding antibiotic prophylaxis for dental procedures or other interventions should be taken.

Clinical Results

With a few exceptions, the clinical results for patellofemoral arthroplasty have been relatively constant for two to three decades, despite differences in component design and variable indications for surgery. Most series have reported good and excellent results in approximately 85% of patients, although there have been some outliers. Most failures are related to uncorrected patellar malalignment or patellar maltracking resulting from component malposition. Geometric features of some trochlear components may predispose patients to patellofemoral complications such as pain, snapping, and subluxation. Radius of curvature, breadth, and degree of constraint of the trochlear component can impact patel-

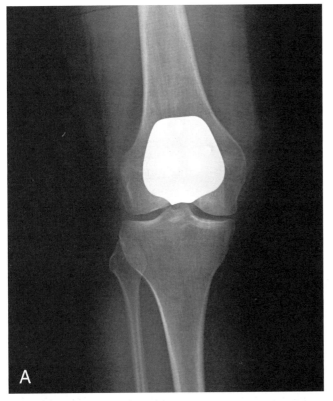

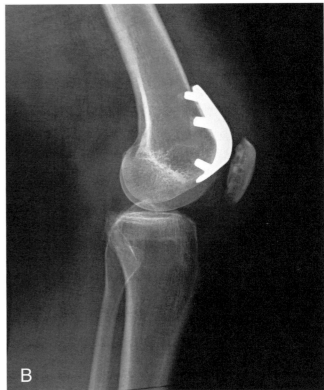

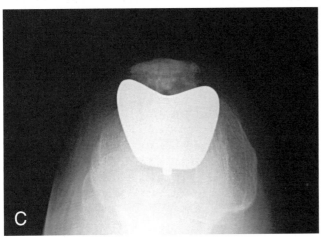

Figure 2 **A** through **C,** Postoperative radiographs after successful patellofemoral arthroplasty.

lar tracking and outcomes. Because improved implant designs have substantially reduced the incidence of patellofemoral complications, tibiofemoral arthritis is the major source of failure. In one reported series, less than 1% of patellofemoral arthroplasties failed because of loosening or wear of the implants, although follow-up in most series has averaged less than 7 years. In another series with a mean follow-up of 15.6 years (range, 10 to 21 years), 25% of patients who underwent isolated patellofemoral arthroplasty required secondary surgeries for progressive tibiofemoral arthritis, including 2 proximal tibial osteotomies and 10 total knee arthroplasties. Overall, 75% of the implants studied were still functioning well into the second decade after implantation.

Some designs have been particularly vulnerable to patellofemoral problems, resulting in secondary surgeries to correct maltracking or malalignment. In one study, 88% of patients with Richards type I or II patellofemoral arthroplasty had good or excellent results, but 70% had a residual extensor lag, which in most instances was quite subtle, at a mean 5.8-year follow-up. An aggressive preoperative quadriceps strengthening program should be instituted, particularly for patients with considerable muscle atrophy. Another study reported on 72 patients who underwent Richards type II and III patellofemoral arthroplasties with a multitude of concomitant surgical procedures, including unicompartmental arthroplasties, proximal tibial osteotomies, distal patellar realignments, or proximal patellar realignments. Two patients had lateral patellar subluxation, one had patella baja resulting in catching of the patella on the trochlea, and four had progressive tibiofemoral degeneration. Another study reported an 86% long-term success rate in 45 patients who underwent patellofemoral arthroplasty; however, secondary soft-tissue surgery was necessary in 18% of patients early on and revision of the patellofemoral arthroplasty was necessary to address catching, imbalance, or malposition in seven patients.

Results may be less predictable with some implant designs. A 55% unsatisfactory rate was reported in patients who underwent patellofemoral arthroplasty using the Lubinus implant (Link, Hamburg, Germany); revision was required in 21 knees (28%) at a mean follow-up of 7.5 years. Fifteen knees were successfully revised for maltracking (5 to total knee arthroplasty and 10 to a patellofemoral arthroplasty with a different geometry), and 5 knees were revised to total knee arthroplasty for progressive tibiofemoral osteoarthritis. Another study reported on 66 Autocentric (DePuy, Warsaw, IN) patellofemoral arthroplasties with 14 concomitant procedures, including 9 tibiofemoral osteotomies and 5 distal realignments. Fifteen percent were revised to total knee arthroplasty, although the precise reasons for doing so were not reported. The authors found the best results using this device in patients with patellar fracture or patellar subluxation. Patients with primary degenerative arthritis of the patellofemoral articulation tended to fail at a higher rate than those with underlying dysplasia or posttraumatic arthrosis, probably because of the subclinical presence of tibiofemoral degeneration at the time of arthroplasty or subsequent development of tibiofemoral arthritis. No instance of loosening in a cohort of cemented trochlear components was reported, but in 4 of 24 cementless implants, trochlear loosening occurred at a mean of 5.5 years after implantation. The authors concluded that trochlear components should be cemented.

One series reported a stratification of results depending on which of two disparate knee designs were used. The outcomes of 30 consecutive patellofemoral arthroplasties using the Lubinus implant were compared with those of 25 consecutive patellofemoral arthroplasties using the Avon (Stryker/Howmedica, Allendale, NJ) trochlear component and the NexGen (Zimmer, Warsaw, IN) all-polyethylene dome-shaped patellar component. Patients in each group had similar demographic characteristics, range of motion, and knee scores. The incidence of fair and poor results from patellofemoral dysfunction, subluxation, catching, and substantial pain was reduced from 17% with the first-generation design of the Lubinus prosthesis to less than 4% with the second-generation design of the Avon trochlear implant. The design features of the trochlear component that impacted the results included the sagittal radius of curvature, proximal extension, breadth, and constraint.

Summary

Patellofemoral arthroplasty can be an effective treatment alternative for patellofemoral arthritis resulting from primary osteoarthrosis, dysplasia, or posttraumatic arthrosis in patients younger than 55 or 60 years who have normal patellofemoral alignment and no considerable maltracking or subluxation. Patients who have had prior distal realignment procedures such as tibial tubercle anteromedialization or direct anteriorization may be candidates for patellofemoral arthroplasty if the maltracking and/or subluxation has been corrected.

Patellofemoral arthroplasty may provide patients with substantial pain relief of isolated patellofemoral arthrosis; however, the procedure is technically demanding. Residual instability may result in early implant failure, which highlights the importance of excluding patients with uncorrectable patellar instability or malalignment. Implant malposition, which may be hastened by particular implant designs, may also contribute to failures from maltracking and mechanical catching of the patella. Sparing of the tibiofemoral compartments, menisci, and cruciate ligaments allows preservation of a more kinematically sound knee joint than total knee arthroplasty. Patellofemoral arthroplasty is a particularly attractive treatment option for young, active patients, and it can be easily converted to total knee arthroplasty if necessary.

Although sparse, long-term data suggest that loosening of cemented trochlear and all-polyethylene patellar components is uncommon and that the number of patients who need additional surgery for progressive tibiofemoral arthritis may be only approximately 25% at a mean of 15 years after patellofemoral arthroplasty. With emerging implant designs, the incidence of anterior knee pain after patellofemoral arthroplasty should be comparable to that after total knee replacement surgery (approximately 4% to 7% of patients). Even small amounts of tibiofemoral cartilage loss may compromise the results enough to warrant restricting this procedure to younger patients. The predictable success of total knee arthroplasty makes it the preferable choice in elderly patients with isolated patellofemoral arthritis.

Annotated Bibliography

Alternative Methods of Management

Brittberg M, Tallheden T, Sjogren-Jansson E, et al: Autologous chondrocytes used for articular cartilage repair: An update. *Clin Orthop Relat Res* 2001;391:S337-S348.

In this study, good and excellent results were achieved at 2- to 10-year follow-up in a mean of 74% of patients who were treated with autologous chondrocyte implantation.

Hangody L, Fules P: Autologous osteochondral mosaic-plasty for the treatment of full-thickness defects of weight-bearing joints. *J Bone Joint Surg Am* 2003;85-A(suppl):25-32.

In this study, 79% of patients who were treated with autologous osteochondral transplantation of the patella and/or trochlea had good to excellent results at 10-year follow-up, whereas 92% of patients who were treated with femoral condylar implants had good to excellent results.

Minas T, Bryant T: The role of autologous chondrocyte implantation in the patellofemoral joint. *Clin Orthop Relat Res* 2005;436:30-39.

The authors of this study assessed 45 patients who underwent autologous chondrocyte implantation involving the patellofemoral articulation and reported that good or excellent results were achieved in 71% at a mean follow-up of 46 months (range, 2 to 7 years). The authors concluded that patellar realignment was crucial to achieving success.

Parvizi J, Stuart MJ, Pagnano MW, Hanssen AD: Total knee arthroplasty in patients with isolated patellofemoral arthritis. *Clin Orthop* 2001;392:147-152.

Although significant improvement in Knee Society pain and function scores was reported at a mean follow-up of 5 years after total knee arthroplasty was performed to treated isolated patellofemoral arthritis, 21 of 31 knees required lateral retinacular release; the incidence of residual anterior knee pain was 19%.

Witvrouw E, Cambier D, Danneels L, et al: The effect of exercise regimens on reflex response time of the vasti muscles in patients with anterior knee pain: A prospective randomized intervention study. *Scand J Med Sci Sports* 2003;13:251-258.

Reflex response times of the vastus medialis obliquus and vastus lateralis muscles were reported to not be changed after 5 weeks of open or closed kinetic chain exercises, but anterior knee pain decreased after both exercise programs.

Patellofemoral Arthroplasty

Kooijman HJ, Driessen APPM, van Horn JR: Long-term results of patellofemoral arthroplasty. *J Bone Joint Surg Br* 2003;85:836-840.

The authors reported the long-term results of patients who underwent patellofemoral arthroplasty using the Richards Mod II prosthesis; 86% of patients (45 knees) had excellent or good results at a mean follow-up of 17 years. Ten patients were converted to total knee arthroplasty after a mean follow-up of 15.6 years.

Lonner JH: Patellofemoral arthroplasty: Current concepts. *Univer Penn Orthop J* 2002;15:1-5.

This is a review of the current indications for and considerations regarding patellofemoral arthroplasty.

Lonner JH: Patellofemoral arthroplasty: Pros, cons, design considerations. *Clin Orthop Relat Res* 2004;428:158-165.

The author addresses the role of patellofemoral arthroplasty for the treatment of patellofemoral arthritis, discusses the outcomes of patellofemoral arthroplasty, and identifies trochlear design features that impact the results, such as the sagittal radius of curvature, trochlear constraint, breadth, and proximal extension. The reported incidence of patellofemoral complications was reduced from 17% with a first-generation implant to 4% with a second-generation implant.

Merchant AC: Early results with a total patellofemoral joint replacement arthroplasty prosthesis. *J Arthroplasty* 2004;19:829-836.

The author of this study presented the short-term results of patellofemoral arthroplasty. Of the 15 patients who were followed for an average of 3.75 years, 14 (93%) had excellent or good results and 1 had fair results according to the activities of daily living scale scores.

Smith AM, Peckett WRC, Butler-Manuel PA, Venu KM, d'Arey JC: Treatment of patellofemoral arthritis using the Lubinus patellofemoral arthroplasty: A retrospective review. *Knee* 2002;9:27-30.

In this study, the authors reported that good and excellent results were achieved in 45 knees (34 patients; 64%) treated with Libinus patellofemoral arthroplasty. Patellar maltracking was a common cause of failure.

Tauro B, Ackroyd CE, Newman JH, Shah NA: The Lubinus patellofemoral arthroplasty: A five to ten year prospective study. *J Bone Joint Surg Br* 2001;83:696-701.

In this study, 76 Lubinus patellofemoral arthroplasties were performed in 59 patients and followed for 7.5 years. Satisfactory clinical outcomes using the Bristol knee scoring system were satisfactory in only 45% of patients, with maltracking occurring in 32%.

Classic Bibliography

Arciero R, Toomey H: Patellofemoral arthroplasty: A three to nine year follow-up study. *Clin Orthop* 1988;236:60-71.

Argenson JN, Guillaume JM, Aubaniac JM: Is there a place for patellofemoral arthroplasty? *Clin Orthop* 1995;321:162-167.

Blazina ME, Fox JM, Del Pizzo W, Broukhim B, Ivey FM: Patellofemoral replacement. *Clin Orthop* 1979;144:98-102.

Burke DL, Ahmed AM: The effect of tibial tubercle elevation on patellofemoral loading. *Trans Orthop* 1980;5:162.

Cartier P, Sanouiller JL, Grelsamer R: Patellofemoral arthroplasty. *J Arthroplasty* 1990;5:49-55.

Dinham JM, French PR: Results of patellectomy for osteoarthritis. *Postgrad Med* 1972;48:590.

Federico DJ, Reider B: Results of isolated patellar debridement for patellofemoral pain in patients with normal patellar alignment. *Am J Sports Med* 1997;25:663-669.

Fulkerson JP, Becker GJ, Meaney JA, Miranda M, Folcik MA: Anteromedial tibial tubercle transfer without bone graft. *Am J Sports Med* 1990;18:490-496.

Fulkerson JP: Anteromedialization of the tibial tuberosity for patellofemoral malalignment. *Clin Orthop* 1983; 177:176-181.

Kaufer H: Mechanical function of the patella. *J Bone Joint Surg Am* 1971;53:1151.

Krajca-Radcliffe JB, Coker TP: Patellofemoral arthroplasty: A 2 to 18 year follow up study. *Clin Orthop* 1996; 330:143-151.

Laskin RS, Van Steijn M: Total knee replacement for patients with patellofemoral arthritis. *Clin Orthop* 1999; 367:89-95.

Maquet P: Advancement of the tibial tuberosity. *Clin Orthop Relat Res* 1976;115:225.

McAlindon RE, Snow S, Cooper C, Dieppe PA: Radiographic patterns of osteoarthritis of the knee joint in the community: The importance of the patellofemoral joint. *Ann Rheum Dis* 1992;51:844-849.

Osborne AH, Fulord PC: Lateral release for chondromalacia patellae. *J Bone Joint Surg Br* 1982;64:202-205.

Schonholtz G, Ling B: Arthroscopic chondroplasty of the patella. *Arthroscopy* 1985;1:92.

Vuorinen O, Paakkala T, Tuuturii T, et al: Chondromalacia patellae: Results of operative treatments. *Arch Orthop Trauma Surg* 1985;104:175.

Chapter 8

Minimally Invasive Total Knee Arthroplasty

Peter M. Bonutti, MD, FACS

Introduction

Minimally invasive total knee arthroplasty (TKA) is in its early development stages and is not widely used by surgeons. However, it is becoming more widely requested by patients. Although minimally invasive TKA is technically challenging, early results show that it provides benefits that may not be achieved with traditional TKA, including improved cosmesis, less pain, faster recovery, and improved quadriceps strength (Figure 1).

Growing Interest in Minimally Invasive Surgery

Surgeons are typically consistent in their choice of surgical approach and technique, which is largely based on personal preference, training, and proven success. Traditionally, patients do not have any input on which procedure or approach is used for their surgery, simply because they are not informed enough to inquire about or request any other options. Patients today are part of what may be called the information era, with a plethora of data available to them through press releases, advertising, and especially the Internet. Arthroplasty procedures are being compared with other minimally invasive procedures and in many situations minimally invasive surgery is being requested.

Interest in minimally invasive surgical techniques for hip, knee, and spine procedures is growing. It has recently been reported that on average, joint replacement surgeons estimate that 5% of procedures are currently being done with some form of minimally invasive surgery. This percentage is expected to double over the next year, and in 5 years it could become the most common approach.

Minimally invasive arthroplasty is clearly a more difficult procedure than traditional arthroplasty. There is an issue of patient preselection, reduced visualization of landmarks, instrumentation accuracy, and the ability of arthroplasty implants to be compatible with minimally invasive techniques. Certain minimally invasive approaches limit the application of cement technique that

is essential for implant fixation. Clearly, minimally invasive surgery requires increased surgical time, and is associated with a steep learning curve with greater risk for malalignment and surgical complications.

Traditional TKA—Survivorship Versus Function

TKA is a proven surgical procedure with a 10-year survivorship rate of greater than 90%. TKA also has significant advantages, including having consistent reproducible results, the ability to correct the mechanical alignment, and the ability to address all three knee compartments. Many surgeons, therefore, question the need to change a procedure with such a good long-term track record.

Although it may be difficult to significantly improve the long-term survivorship of TKA by changing to a minimally invasive procedure, doing so may have a significant impact on the short-term functional results. Traditional TKA exposure requires prolonged rehabilitation that may require up to 1 year for full recovery. There is a significant amount of pain associated with the procedure, and patients need extensive physical therapy, often for months after surgery to obtain optimal function. In addition, some patients require additional surgical procedures such as manipulations to obtain good outcomes. An evaluation of patient concerns before undergoing total hip and total knee arthroplasty identified that the two greatest concerns were pain immediately after surgery and the length of recovery.

Although many reports show excellent long-term survivorship of TKAs, further investigation with respect to patient satisfaction clouds the strong success rates that have been documented. Studies have described a discrepancy between how surgeons and patients perceive TKA outcomes. One study reported that concerns and priorities of surgeons and patients differ and that one third of patients who underwent TKA reported dissatisfaction when evaluated 12 months postoperatively. Another study concluded that surgeons are more satisfied than patients after TKA.

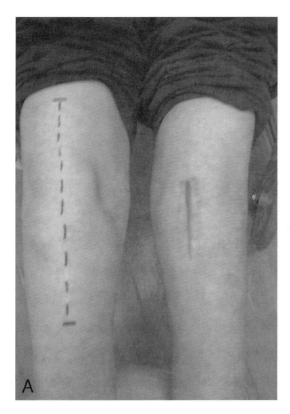

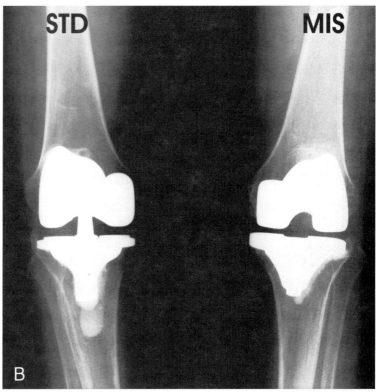

Figure 1 **A,** Photographs of standard TKA (*dashed line, left*) and minimally invasive TKA (*scar, right*) incisions. **B,** Radiograph of the same. STD = standard TKA, MIS = minimally invasive surgery TKA.

The Impact of Surgical Technique

The multiple reasons that exist for patient dissatisfaction are affected by the surgical approach used when performing TKA. The procedures are often done with large incisions (20 to 30 cm), and are not muscle sparing. Most significantly, the quadriceps mechanism is severed and the patella is everted, both of which are conditions that can contribute to permanent muscle damage. One study showed a permanent 30.7% isometric quadriceps strength loss after standard TKA. Patients have also been reported to have significant difficulty kneeling and squatting, going up and down inclines, and rising unassisted from a chair after standard TKA.

One recent study evaluated patients with isokinetic tests 2 years after successful TKA. Isometric peak extensor torque values were found to be reduced by up to 30.7%. This suggests that there is significant disruption of the quadriceps mechanism with traditional TKA and that these results may be permanent. This may be in large part related to surgical approach and could significantly contribute to postoperative functional deficiencies. Another study used a simple test of unassisted chair rise to evaluate quadriceps strength and function in patients who underwent TKA. Patients were asked to rise from a 16-inch chair without using their arms. At 3 months after TKA, only 40% of patients who under-

went traditional TKA could successfully perform the test ($P < 0.001$), at 6 months 64% could perform the test ($P = 0.001$), and at 1 year 72% could perform the test ($P = 0.002$). The findings from this simple test evaluating extensor mechanism function after TKA suggest that a functional deficit in the quadriceps may persist even 1 year after TKA and may remain evident to the patient during average daily activities. Studies that compared standard TKA and minimally invasive TKA report a statistically difference in quadriceps strength and recovery.

These deficiencies may be directly related to muscle damage to the quadriceps during TKA exposure and are the driving factors for the development of alternative surgical approaches to the knee, including minimally invasive approaches. The standard unicompartmental knee arthroplasty incision with an everted patella has been compared with a minimally invasive unicompartmental knee arthroplasty incision without patellar dislocation, and patients who underwent short incision unicompartmental knee arthroplasty have been reported to recover two times faster than those who underwent standard unicompartmental knee arthroplasty. These results challenged proponents of TKA to determine whether the same benefits could be realized for TKA if performed with a minimally invasive, muscle-sparing approach with a noneverted patella.

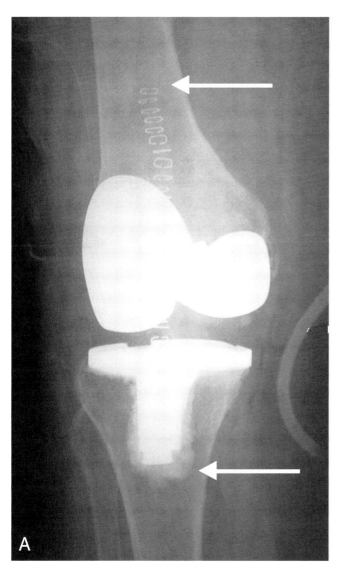

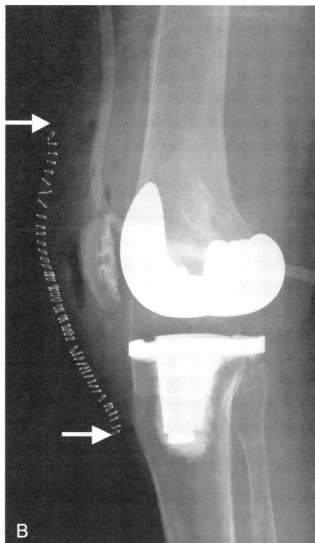

Figure 2 AP **(A)** and lateral **(B)** radiographs of a minimally invasive quadriceps-saving TKA showing rotational malalignment and collateral ligament imbalance. Arrows indicate the top and bottom of the incision and staple lines.

Minimally Invasive TKA–A Feasible Solution?

Orthopaedic surgeons first had to determine whether it would be possible to perform minimally invasive techniques for total knee replacement. As with all evolving surgical techniques, the limited surgical exposure of the minimally invasive procedure posed several challenges. The loss of landmark visibility inside the knee may reduce the ability to perform surgical releases, remove all necessary bone and tissue, achieve accurate bone cuts, and/or obtain optimal femoral and tibial component rotation. Extensive tension on the skin may cause wound necrosis. Moreover, reduced surgical exposure significantly limits existing instrumentation options. Implanting components with good cement pressurization technique is also more difficult to achieve accurately through the reduced incision and exposure.

These potential disadvantages affect instrument and implant design because surgeons must seek systems that are compatible with minimally invasive techniques. The design of these systems also poses an engineering challenge: to design implants and instruments that are streamlined and smaller, while maintaining, if not improving, implant longevity. For example, tibial components with a reduced keel may facilitate implantation; however, they may also increase the risk for failure of fixation when malalignment or cement pressurization is suboptimal, thereby increasing the risk of premature implant loosening (Figure 2).

There also may be significant limitations in patient selection. Early in the learning curve, minimally invasive techniques have had extremely limiting patient criteria, which include low body mass index, good preoperative range of motion, and minimal deformity. The initial suggested selection criteria for the quadriceps saving minimally invasive TKA approach include a patient with the following preoperative assessment: a minimum of 125° of flexion, less than 10° anatomic varus deformity, less than 15° anatomic valgus deformity, less than a 10° flexion contracture, and weight less than 180 lb. Given these stringent criteria, not only are few patients actually candidates for this approach, but it seems that surgeons are preselecting patients for the best results. However, the criteria have expanded as surgeon comfort has increased and instrumentation has improved. Clearly, patients with less deformity and good range of motion may have less difficulty with rehabilitation and better overall functional recovery than those with significant deformity, preoperative stiffness, or high body mass index. Most patients with end-stage TKA, however, have significant deformity, preoperative loss of motion, and elevated body mass index. Additionally, obese patients may benefit the most from the use of muscle sparing surgical techniques. Nonetheless, preselecting patients who are less difficult to treat is imperative in the early stages of a surgeon's learning curve.

In light of these challenges, minimally invasive TKA has several potential advantages, especially when compared with the traditional TKA surgical approach. The smaller incision is much less apparent on the leg than the full incision of a TKA. Because more than 61% of TKAs are performed on women, cosmesis has been a factor for patients requesting minimally invasive surgery. There is also less skin denervation (loss of sensation lateral to the incision) and possibly improved quadriceps strength. Blood loss and postoperative pain may be reduced significantly. Postoperative recovery is typically shorter with regard to length of hospitalization, physical therapy treatment, and overall return to functional activity. Long-term postoperative benefits may include improved strength and function, with the patient having an overall better perception of the outcome of the surgery.

A minimally invasive surgical technique has been developed that uses a modification of the midvastus approach with a noneverted patella (2-cm vastus medialis oblique [VMO] snip). This technique was used on 500 consecutive patients who underwent TKA, regardless of deformity, weight, or preoperative range of motion. This universal approach to the minimally invasive TKA challenge may be applicable to all patients who are TKA candidates (Figure 3). This approach is based on 10 features that allow a gradual, progressive approach to minimally invasive TKA (Table 1).

Transition to Minimally Invasive TKA

Minimally invasive TKA is clearly a more difficult procedure, with a potentially higher risk for complications than traditional TKA. The transition to a minimally invasive TKA technique is most successful when done as an evolutionary change, rather than a radical switch. Surgeons should gradually reduce incision length and develop muscle sparing approaches for appropriately selected patients. It is ideal to initially perform this procedure on patients who are generally female and have supple tissue, minimal deformity, less bulky quadriceps mechanics, and a good preoperative range of motion. Overall weight (body mass index) may not be a significant problem.

Although this approach recommends a gradual reduction of incision length, when making the incision shorter than as planned surgeons should remember that the incision can always be extended at any time during surgery, but it cannot be shortened. The goal is to have an incision length that approximates two times the length of the patella (approximately 6 to 12 cm). The location of the incision is flexible and has been described as either anterior, medial, lateral, or angled.

This evolutionary approach to minimally invasive TKA requires first becoming comfortable with the instrumentation. It is recommended that surgeons first perform a standard incision TKA with the new instruments to become comfortable with them. The next step is to perform a traditional TKA approach but without everting the patella, then progressing to muscle-sparing techniques, and finally to in situ bone cuts.

Several of the minimally invasive TKA approaches that have been described illustrate the evolution of the technique for those who use it. These approaches are classified based on quadriceps exposure as a 2-cm VMO split (mini-midvastus), a quadriceps-saving approach, a subvastus approach, and a direct lateral approach (Figure 4). Most recently, a direct lateral approach performed with computer-assisted navigation has been introduced. All of these approaches use a reduced incision length and a mobile skin window. They are all muscle-sparing approaches that avoid patellar eversion, require the use of downsized instruments, and use cemented implants.

The VMO split is described as an extensile universal approach, and the muscle split can be safely extended up to 8.8 cm. It is important to control flexion and extension with this approach and vary this during the procedure to create a mobile skin window. In situ bone cuts use the bone platforms to finish the bone cuts. The order of the bone cuts is tibia first, then femur, then patella (optional), but this can be varied for exposure.

The quadriceps-saving approach was introduced with the application of stringent criteria for patient preselection. The order of the bone cuts in this technique is patella first, femur second, and tibia third. Some have suggested this approach can be used for performing TKA on an outpatient basis.

A mini-midvastus approach dislocates the tibiofemoral joint before bone cuts, but does not evert the patella. The direct lateral approach is completely quadriceps sparing and fully computer navigated, using in situ bone

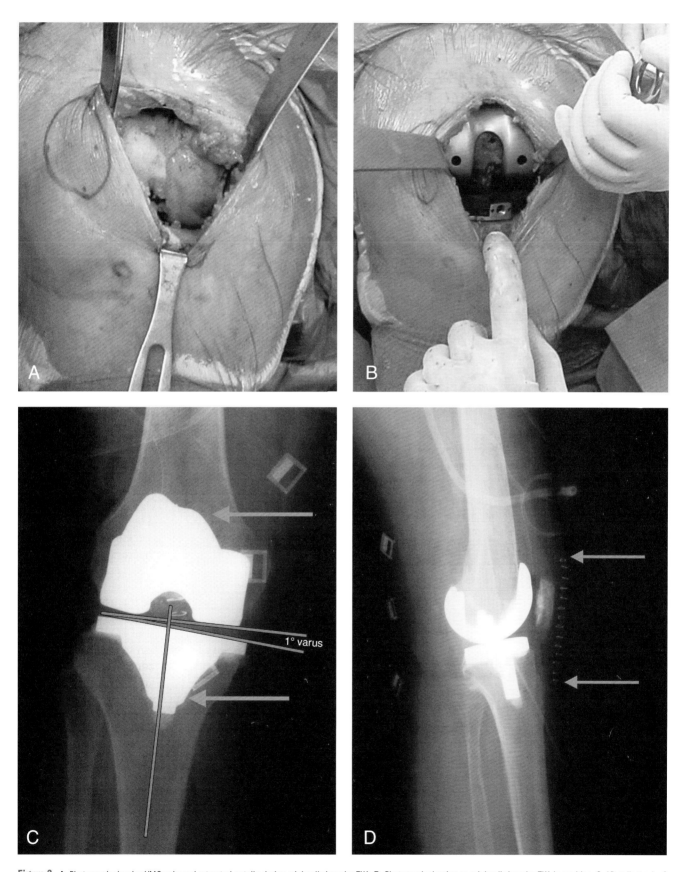

Figure 3   **A,** Photograph showing VMO snip and retracted patella during minimally invasive TKA. **B,** Photograph showing an minimally invasive TKA in position. **C,** AP radiograph of TKA. Arrows indicate the top and bottom of the incision and staple lines. **D,** Lateral radiograph of TKA. Arrows indicate the top and bottom of the incision and staple lines.

American Academy of Orthopaedic Surgeons

Table 1 | Ten Evolutionary Features of Minimally Invasive TKA

Decreases the skin incision length

Controls the flexion and extension of the leg to gain more exposure

Uses retractors symbiotically to achieve a mobile skin window

Uses quadriceps sparing approaches

Uses inferior and superior patellar releases to mobilize the patella

Avoids patellar eversion

In situ bone cuts are performed to avoid joint dislocation

Uses downsized instrumentation

Uses bone platforms to complete bone cuts

Possible use of the suspended leg approach to optimize exposure with gravity as an aid

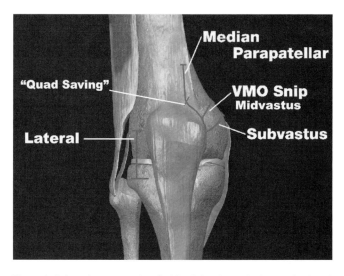

Figure 4 Schematic representation of minimally invasive surgical approaches based on quadriceps exposure.

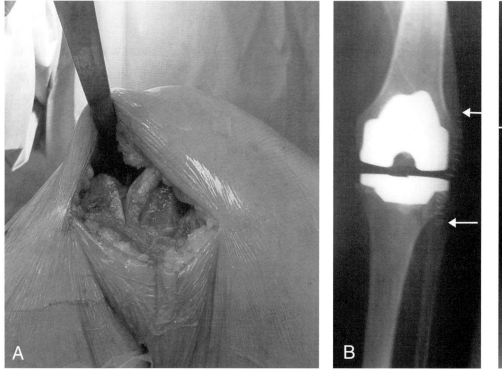

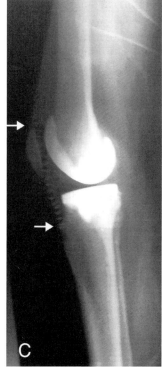

Figure 5 A, Photograph showing a minimally invasive direct lateral approach for TKA. AP **(B)** and lateral **(C)** radiographs of the same. Arrows indicate the top and bottom of the incision and staple lines.

cuts. This procedure requires a tibial component with a downsized keel (Figure 5).

All of these procedures require performing the skin incision with the knee in variable degrees of flexion, which stretches the skin. Exposure of the quadriceps mechanism through either mini-median parapatellar, mini-midvastus, or subvastus variations have been proposed, all with the goal of muscle sparing for decreasing

quadriceps trauma. The best approach is one that provides adequate exposure and that with which the surgeon is most comfortable.

Basic Concepts of Minimally Invasive TKA

As in all surgical procedures, the vascular anatomy must be considered. In an evaluation of the subvastus anatomy, nine variations of the neurovascular anatomy were

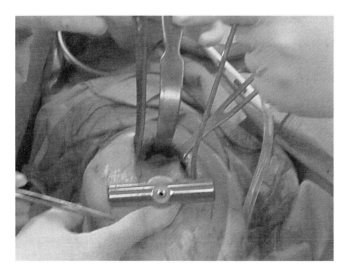

Figure 6 Photograph showing an minimally invasive VMO snip procedure. An elevated quadriceps mechanism is used to assess femoral rotation.

found. An anatomic study showed that subvastus approaches were associated with an increased risk of injury to the muscular-articular branch of the femoral artery and saphenous nerve. Additionally, significant mobilization can increase the risk of injury to the femoral artery and vein.

For all minimally invasive TKA approaches, however, the goal should be muscle sparing combined with avoidance of patellar eversion. The patella is mobilized and retracted laterally, which may decrease the stress to the patellar mechanism, especially when the quadriceps is tethered proximally by the tourniquet. Retracting rather than everting the patella may decrease the overall stress to the quadriceps mechanism, when combined with a muscle sparing approach, may improve functional recovery.

The principle of a mobile skin window is also important. In minimally invasive surgery, as the position of the knee moves through flexion and extension, the skin incision moves to expose a portion of the joint. Symbiotic use of retractors with mobile skin windows is an important factor in gaining selective exposure. Retracting medially will tighten the lateral skin and retracting laterally will tighten the medial skin. These techniques are facilitated with an adjustable leg holder that can control positions of flexion and extension during the procedure. Another option is the suspended leg technique, which is similar to that used in arthroscopy procedures. The leg is suspended over a padded bolster and left hanging, improving exposure to the posterior joint.

In addition to managing the mobile skin window, there are other recommendations for enhancing exposure to the joint. The order of the bone resection may help exposure, with each bone cut selectively opening up the next space. Anesthesia should optimize muscle relaxation and create greater mobility. Maximal flexion

of the knee before tourniquet inflation can assist with quadriceps mobilization.

Extramedullary tibial and intramedullary femoral instrumentation with downsized, soft-tissue friendly cutting blocks may significantly aid in gaining exposure. Because visual landmarks are reduced, assessing femoral rotation can be challenging (Figure 6). Identifying the epicondylar axis can also be difficult. Femoral rotation relies on clearly seeing landmarks such as Whiteside's line, the posterior condylar line, the tibial cut in flexion, and/or the grand piano sign during anterior femoral resection. The use of computer-assisted navigation can eliminate the need to violate the intramedullary canal. Computer-assisted navigation may further enhance implant alignment and position, although computer-assisted navigation currently is not ideal for minimally invasive surgery.

A purely lateral based approach has been recently developed that uses an incision smaller than 10 cm in length. This is a muscle sparing approach that penetrates the iliotibial band only and does not invade the quadriceps mechanism. The patella is not everted; with in situ bone cuts, the knee is not dislocated or subluxated during the procedure.

Clinical Results of Minimally Invasive TKA

The new minimally invasive TKA techniques have only short-term data reported to date, some with only months of clinical follow-up and few, if any, of the studies reporting data have gone through the peer review process. One recent presentation reported up to 4-year follow-up data (minimum follow-up, 2 years) for 216 minimally invasive TKA procedures performed on 70 men and 96 women (mean patient age, 72 years). The procedure used included a VMO snip with a noneverted patella, downsized instrumentation, and in situ bone cuts. There were no intraoperative conversions from minimally invasive surgery to the standard approach, and the incision length ranged from 6 to 12 cm. Postoperative clinical results showed that Knee Society scores averaged 95.8 (range, 70 to 100), overall Knee Society functional scores averaged 92.6 (range, 55 to 100), and radiographic results showed an average tibiofemoral alignment of 5.31° valgus (range, 0° to 9°) (Figure 7).

In the same study, there was a subgroup of 15 patients who had previously had a standard TKA done using a traditional approach. All 15 of these patients preferred the minimally invasive approach, and at follow-up all 15 patients reported that this knee felt stronger. These patients also reported that the minimally invasive TKA procedure reduced recovery time by 4 to 8 weeks.

Complications may occur with this procedure (Figure 8). Reoperations included six manipulations for range of motion less than 100°, two arthroscopic débridements (one for late onset of patellofemoral crepi-

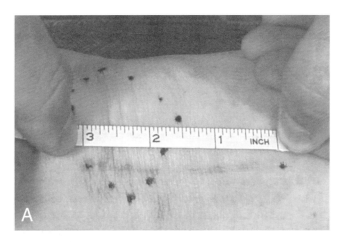

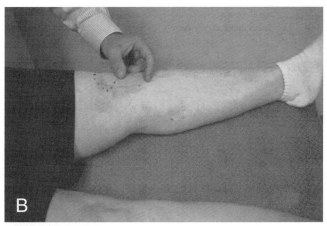

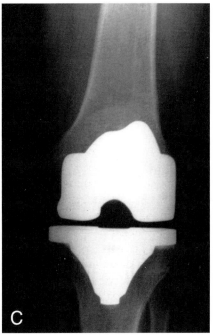

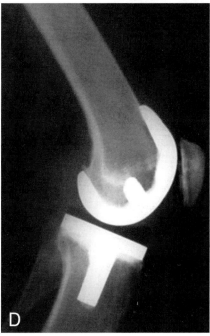

Figure 7 **A** and **B,** Photographs showing postoperative skin incision at 2-year follow-up. Postoperative AP **(C)** and lateral **(D)** radiographs of a patient who underwent minimally invasive TKA at 2-year follow-up.

tus and one for retained cement), and five repeat procedures, which is higher than the reoperation rates of most standard TKA series. The reoperations included one revised loose tibial component (possibly for poor cement technique and pressurization), one tibia with lateral overhang, one infection that developed after septicemia postcolonoscopy, and one suspected infection that was treated with synovectomy and polyethylene exchange (cultures were negative). There was also one traumatic medial collateral ligament/posterior cruciate ligament injury. Overall, 97% of patients reported satisfaction with the results.

Another clinical report evaluated 58 patients who underwent minimally invasive TKA procedures that used a quadriceps sparing approach. Fifteen of these patients were evaluated at greater than 6 months postoperatively and only three patients were evaluated at more than 1 year postoperatively. The average tourni-

quet time was 110 minutes, and the average length of hospital stay was 2.5 days. There were two intraoperative conversions to a more standard approach. Average tibial alignment was 2.5° of varus, which prompted instrumentation change. Medical complications included two arrhythmias, one pulmonary embolus, and one intraoperative myocardial infarct with right hemiparesis.

A later study by the same author reported on 70 patients who underwent minimally invasive TKA that used the same quadriceps sparing approach. In this study, the minimally invasive TKA procedure reported took twice as long as standard TKA. The average length of hospital stay was 4 days, and the complications were identical as those in the previous study, with peroneal nerve palsy as an additional intraoperative complication. Radiographic alignment showed 4° of tibiofemoral valgus alignment and a 2.5° tibiofemoral varus position. Anecdotally, a different surgeon was able to use the same instruments

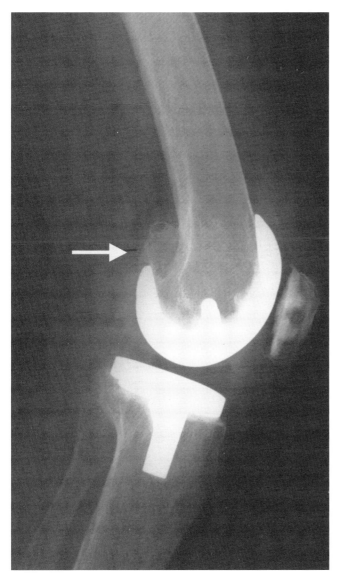

Figure 8 Lateral radiograph showing retained posterior osteophytes (*arrow*) in a patient who underwent minimally invasive TKA.

and surgical approach in highly selected patients and was able to perform minimally invasive TKA on an outpatient basis, suggesting that the recovery of patients after this procedure may have more to do with factors other than surgical technique and instrumentation (preoperative selection, prehabilitation, intraoperative and postoperative analgesia, injectable cocktails, analgesia in therapy, and immediate postoperative therapy).

Optimizing Minimally Invasive TKA

To date, only short-term and anecdotal results are available for minimally invasive TKA, and additional studies need to be performed. Clearly, a more rapid discharge of the patient from the hospital would be more cost-effective; however, this possibility must be weighed against the medical risks to the patient.

Rapid recovery is multifactorial and can be related to technique, which includes incision, muscle approaches, and soft-tissue disruption. It can also be related to surgical instruments, which are ideally soft-tissue friendly and accurate, and/or to implants, which can have downsized tibial keels and are adaptable to minimally invasive surgery. Recovery may also be related to patients and preoperative selection, motivation, and personal goals. Rehabilitation before surgery as well as immediately after surgery (starting the day of surgery) can be helpful. Pharmaceutical agents including injectable cocktails, nerve blocks, pain pumps, and narcotic medications may assist in reducing postoperative pain and, therefore, improve the ability of patients to recover. An important yet perhaps overlooked factor in patient recovery is the ability of the hospital and rehabilitation staff to motivate and educate the patient, thereby optimizing recovery.

The marriage of minimally invasive surgery with computer-assisted navigation may improve accuracy of bone cuts and enhance the ability to perform this surgery. Computer-assisted navigation allows statistically significant improvements in standing alignment, including femoral varus, valgus, and rotational alignment, and tibial slope, rotation, and varus, valgus alignment. It also reduces femorotibial mismatch and blood loss, with only a reported 13-minute increase in operating room time. Computer-assisted navigation, however, currently requires placement of implant trackers and surface mapping, which necessitates more extensive exposure.

Select clinical sites are using computer-assisted navigation with the median parapatellar and noneverted patellar approaches. The preliminary results have suggested excellent overall implant alignment. Although data on the first patients to undergo fully computer-assisted navigational minimally invasive TKA have been reported, only short-term data are currently available.

Summary

Overall, traditional TKA can lead to excellent improvement in pain and long-term survivorship. Patients' expectations and dissatisfaction with postoperative pain, prolonged recovery, and overall functional restrictions have piqued interest in minimally invasive techniques. Minimally invasive unicompartmental knee arthroplasty has been performed with excellent survivorship in selected studies; however, other studies have suggested minimally invasive unicompartmental knee arthroplasty may have reduced implant alignment and accuracy, resulting in a higher rate of revision.

Minimally invasive TKA, with the advantages of reduced skin incision, no patellar eversion, muscle-sparing approaches, in situ bone cuts, and downsized instrumentation may provide a better option. The procedure is technically demanding, with a significant learning curve and increased surgery time and risk of complications. Although short-term data suggest good results with a shorter recovery time, long-term data are needed to substantiate the advantages and success of using minimally invasive TKA techniques.

Annotated Bibliography

Growing Interest in Minimally Invasive Surgery

Bhattacharyya T, Tornetta P, Healy W, Einhorn T: The validity of claims made in orthopaedic print advertisements. *J Bone Joint Surg Am* 2003;85:1224-1228.

The authors of this article address the possibility that advertisements, especially those regarding joint arthroplasty, may not be substantiated by the findings in peer review literature.

Bullens PH, van Loon CJ, de Waal Malefijt MC, Laan RF, Veth RP: Patient satisfaction after total knee arthroplasty: A comparison between subjective and objective outcome assessments. *J Arthroplasty* 2001;16:740-747.

The authors of this study conclude that Knee Society scores may not accurately reflect patient satisfaction with TKA.

The Impact of Surgical Technique

Mahoney OM, McClung CD, dela Rosa MA, Schmalzried TP: The effect of total knee arthroplasty design on extensor mechanism function. *J Arthroplasty* 2002;17:416-421.

The authors of this study used a simple test of unassisted chair rise (rising from a chair without using arms) to assess the effect of TKA on the extensor mechanism function of patients. They found that patients who underwent TKA had significant delay in functional recovery of the quadriceps mechanism.

Price AJ, Webb J, Topf H, Dodd CA, Goodfellow JW, Murray DW: Rapid recovery after Oxford unicompartmental knee arthroplasty through a short incision. *J Arthroplasty* 2001;16:970-976.

The authors of this study compared performing unicompartmental knee arthroplasty through a standard incision with everted patella and through a short incision without everted patella. They found that the short incision healed two times faster than the standard approach and concluded that everting the patella may significantly affect postoperative recovery.

Silva M, Shepherd E, Jackson W, Pratt J, McClung C, Schmalzried T: Knee strength after total knee arthroplasty. *J Arthroplasty* 2003;18:605-611.

The authors identified a significant reduction in quadriceps strength (30.7%) measured isokinetically 2 years after traditional TKA exposure.

Minimally Invasive TKA–A Feasible Solution?

Bonutti PM, Kester M, Mont M: MIS total knee arthroplasty: Ten feature evolutionary approach. *Orthop Clin North Am* 2004;35:217-227.

The authors of this article present an evolutionary approach to minimally invasive TKA, the 10 features of which are listed in Table 1.

Laskin RS, Beksac B, Phongjunakorn A, et al: Minimally invasive total knee replacement through a mini-midvastus incision: An outcome study. *Clin Orthop Relat Res* 2004;428:74-81.

The authors of this study compared 51 consecutive patients who underwent primary tricompartmental minimally invasive TKA with 51 patients who underwent primary TKA using a standard incision. Short-term follow-up demonstrated that patients who underwent minimally invasive TKA had more rapid regaining of flexion, decreased need for analgesics, and achieved milestones permitting discharge 18% faster than the patients who underwent TKA using a standard incision.

Tria A: Advancements in minimally invasive total knee arthroplasty. *Orthopedics* 2003;26(suppl 8):S859-S863.

The author discusses experience using a quadriceps sparing minimally invasive approach to perform TKA in 120 patients. From early results, the author concludes that minimally invasive TKA produces better early motion, less blood loss, less pain, and a shorter hospital stay than standard TKA with no compromise in accuracy.

Tria A, Coon T: MIS TKA quad sparing approach. *Clin Orthop Relat Res* 2003;416:185-190.

The authors of this article delineate additional early clinical experience with minimally invasive TKA. They report that 70 patients underwent the procedure over a 9-month period and that early results indicate less intraoperative blood loss, shorter length of hospital stay, increased range of motion, and implant accuracy that is comparable to that of standard TKA.

Basic Concepts of Minimally Invasive TKA

Dalury DF: Does the midvastus approach compromise the vastus medialis obliquus? in *Proceedings of the 2004 Annual Meeting*. Rosemont, IL, American Academy of Orthopaedic Surgeons, 2004, p 454.

The author of this study reports that electromyographic intraoperative analysis cannot demonstrate muscle damage caused by surgical manipulation of the VMO during midvastus approach to the knee.

Scheibel M, Schmidt W, Thomas M: A detailed anatomical description of the subvastus region and its clinical relevance for the subvastus approach in total knee arthroplasty. *Surg Radiol Anat* 2002;24:6-12.

The authors conducted a study of vascular anatomy of the subvastus region and concluded that subvastus approaches may pose a greater risk for bleeding, arterial, and neurologic injury.

Clinical Results of Minimally Invasive TKA

Bonutti PM, McMahon M, Mont MA, Ragland P, Kester M: Minimally invasive total knee arthroplasty. *J Bone Joint Surg Am* 2004;86:26-32.

This prospective randomized study reports the short-term results of 166 patients who underwent minimally invasive TKA (216 knees). At a minimum 2-year follow-up (range, 2 to 4 years), the authors reported that 195 knees (97%) had good or excellent objective Knee Society scores and patient satisfaction indices. The authors also describe a lateral minimally invasive approach with computer navigation and compare minimally invasive and standard TKA approaches.

Haas S, Cook S, Beksac B: Minimally invasive total knee replacement through a mini-midvastus approach: A comparative study. *Clin Orthop Relat Res* 2004;428:68-73.

The authors of this article describe the clinically advantages of minimally invasive TKA.

Optimizing Minimally Invasive TKA

Bonutti PM, Kester M, Neal D: Use of suspended leg technique for minimally invasive total knee arthroplasty. *Orthopedics* 2003;26:899-903.

The authors of this article describe a novel approach to minimally invasive TKA with the leg suspended in a manner similar to that used in arthroscopic approaches.

Chauhan SK, Scott RG, Bredahl W, Beaver RJ: Computer-assisted knee arthroplasty versus a conventional jig-based technique. *J Bone Joint Surg Br* 2004;86: 372-377.

The authors report that computer-assisted navigation may improve accuracy during TKA and add only 13 minutes to the overall procedure.

Hozack WJ, Krismer M, Nogler M, et al (eds): *Minimally Invasive Total Joint Arthroplasty*. New York, NY, Springer-Verlag, 2004.

This textbook is dedicated exclusively to minimally invasive TKA. The knee section describes computer-assisted navigational approaches, VMO, quadriceps sparing, lateral approaches, and current and future technology.

Classic Bibliography

Cooper RE, Trinidad G, Buck W: Midvastus approach in total knee arthroplasty. *J Arthroplasty* 1999;14:505-508.

Dalury D, Jiranek W: A comparison of the midvastus and paramedian approaches for total knee arthroplasty. *J Arthroplasty* 1999;14:33-37.

Dickstein R, Heffes Y, Shabtai E, Markowitz E: Total knee arthroplasty in the elderly: patients' self-appraisal 6 and 12 months postoperatively. *Gerontology* 1998;44: 204-210.

Engh GA, Parks NL: Surgical technique of the midvastus arthrotomy. *Clin Orthop Relat Res* 1998;351:270-274.

Trousdale R, McGrory B, Berry D, Becky M, Harmsen W: Patients' concerns prior to undergoing total hip and total knee arthroplasty. *Mayo Clin Proc* 1999;74:978-982.

White RE Jr, Allman JK, Trauger JA, Dales BH: Clinical comparison of the midvastus and medial parapatellar surgical approaches. *Clin Orthop Relat Res* 1999;367: 117-122.

Chapter 9

Primary Total Knee Arthroplasty Outcomes

Khaled J. Saleh, MD, MSc (Epid), FRCSC, FACS

Kevin J. Mulhall, MD, MCh, FRCSI (Tr & Orth)

Aaron A. Hofmann, MD

Michael P. Bolognesi, MD

Richard S. Laskin, MD

Introduction

Whether to use cementless or cemented implant fixation has been debated since the first attempts at total knee arthroplasty (TKA). Many early prostheses were implanted without cement before cement became the main choice for fixation in total knee replacement. The proponents of cementless fixation have been motivated in part by the observation that cement failure caused by fragmentation and debonding can result in loosening of some cemented prostheses. The need for a treatment for the growing population of younger, more active patients has led to attempts to develop a more durable, secure, and biologically viable form of implant fixation. The proposed advantages of modern cementless fixation over cemented fixation include a more durable method of fixation, techniques that spare host bone, and the avoidance of cement-specific complications such as cement disease. Continued improvements in design and technique have allowed cementless fixation in TKA to become an established fixation solution for the treatment of patients with disabling degenerative knee disease.

Cementless TKA

Bone Ingrowth

Prolonged mechanical stability in cementless TKA relies on bone ingrowth into the porous surface of the implant. The ability to achieve bone ingrowth depends on several factors. Extensive basic science and clinical research has helped define these factors and delineate their importance with regard to successful cementless fixation. These factors include porous surface composition, the importance of pore size, relative lack of motion at the bone-implant interface, and intimate bone-implant apposition. Important factors for bone ingrowth include biologic ingrowth potential, which is affected by the patient's health, and the presence of factors that inhibit ingrowth, such as steroids or other medications or medical conditions.

Most modern porous surface preparations are composed of titanium and cobalt-chromium alloys. Animal studies have demonstrated that bone ingrowth occurs into both of these alloy materials. Despite this evidence, however, many surgeons have been hesitant to extrapolate animal bone ingrowth data to human applications because of possible species differences. One study compared titanium and cobalt-chromium alloy implants in human subjects. Identically structured cylinders were implanted in the load-bearing surface of distal femoral condyles of humans with osteoarthritis. The amount of bone ingrowth and the mineral apposition rate (a measurement of new mineralized bone laid down per unit of time) were quantified after explantation. The titanium implants had ingrowth almost double the amount measured in the implants with cobalt-chromium porous coatings. There were also differences noted in the direction of cancellous bone remodeling. The cancellous bone advanced toward the titanium but away from the cobalt-chromium, which suggests that titanium alloy may be more biocompatible than cobalt-chromium as a porous surface material.

Ceramic coatings, particularly hydroxyapatite, have been considered as a possible augment to porous-coating fixation in TKA components. It has been proposed that calcium phosphate (hydroxyapatite) can act as osteoconductive scaffolding and promote bone growth into the porous surface. Proponents believe this bone ingrowth can improve the initial stability of the component. One study compared human cancellous bone remodeling with titanium- and hydroxyapatite-coated implants. Hydroxyapatite-coated components showed an increase of 8% in bone ingrowth; however, a significantly lower bone mineral content at the implant interface was found. For both the titanium- and hydroxyapatite-coated implants, gaps ranging from 50 to 500 μm were filled with fibrous tissue, which suggests that hydroxyapatite-coated implants require precise surgical placement and intimate bone-implant contact. Early follow-up (2 to 5 years) of patients with hydroxyapatite-coated implants did not demonstrate a clear advantage over standard implants. Comparisons of hydroxyapatite-augmented implants and standard porous-coated implants demonstrated a slight increase in subsidence (using radiostereometric analysis) of the noncoated implants, but no significant clinical differences were measured at 2-year follow-up. A comparison of hydroxyapatite-coated implants and cemented implants showed increased initial migration of hydroxyapatite-coated implants, which stabilized at 3-month follow-up, and no difference in overall micromotion at 24-month follow-up.

The use of ceramic coating is not without risks. One study reported early implant failure (8 weeks), at which time the entire medial tibial plateau undersurface showed complete debonding of the hydroxyapatite. The marginal and equivocal improvements gained by the use of hydroxyapatite, coupled with its increased cost, have limited the widespread use of this technology in cementless TKA. Despite these concerns, a recent study reported favorable clinical and radiographic results at 6.6-year follow-up for the hydroxyapatite-coated Active Total Knee (Australia Surgical Design & Manufacture, Sydney, Australia). The 1,000 patients in this study had a cumulative survival of 99.14%, with only seven revisions. Another study of 138 hydroxyapatite-coated Insall-Burstein II knee implants reported a 95% survival rate at 13-year follow-up, with seven revision and no evidence of radiographic loosening.

There has been significant investigation to determine the optimal pore size for maximal bone ingrowth. One study evaluated cobalt alloy rods coated with cobalt alloy powder of four different particle sizes. Pore sizes ranged from 20 to 800 μm, and the surfaces had fully interconnecting voids. The rods were implanted into the lateral cortex of beagle femurs, and the rate of bone ingrowth and maximum fixation strengths attained were determined. Inferior mechanical strength and incomplete ingrowth of calcified tissue were observed at all time periods for the implants with pore sizes less than 50 μm. Rods with pore sizes of 50 to 400 μm showed ideal bone ingrowth that was determined to be complete at 8 weeks. Pore sizes larger than 400 μm correlated with the appearance of bone and fibrous tissue at 8 and 12 weeks. It was believed that the smaller pore size (50 to 400 μm) allowed bone to more quickly fill the pore spaces; therefore, the implant reached maximum fixation more rapidly. Thus, a 50- to 400-μm pore size was considered optimal for biologic fixation of porous-coated implants. Another study demonstrated that although a pore size of 100 μm allowed for bone ingrowth, a pore size of 150 μm was required for osteon formation. Human implant retrieval studies have shown that pore sizes of 400 to 600 μm allow for consistent bone ingrowth.

A microinterlock between the porous-coated implant and the host bone is required for bone ingrowth to occur. If excessive motion is present, bone ingrowth may not occur, and fibrous tissue ingrowth may occur instead. A study of porous-coated staple pullout strength in mongrel dogs reported that bone ingrowth can occur in the presence of some movement (up to 28 μm), whereas excess movement (150 μm or more) results in the attachment of connective tissue. In an attempt to minimize motion and maximize initial stability, current cementless TKA systems incorporate various forms of adjunctive fixation. Multiple studies have documented an improvement in initial implant stability by using screw fixation and press-fit stems and/or pegs.

Intimate bone-implant apposition is critical for the development of bone ingrowth. One study has shown that bone ingrowth does not occur when the distance between host bone and the porous coating was greater than 50 μm. The same group of researchers found that 76% of the surface area of the proximal tibia consisted of bone marrow space. These authors demonstrated that by placing morcellized autograft bone chips at the bone-implant interface, the cancellous bone porosity and the roughness of the resected proximal tibial plateau can be decreased. This technique immediately increases the contact between the host bone and porous coating and directly correlates with increased bone ingrowth. Surgical technique is very important in attaining this close contact and cannot be overlooked. The use of precision cutting instruments and a high degree of surgical skill are required for successful cementless knee implantation.

Component Design and Rationale

Cementless designs for total knee replacement incorporate the current understanding of the basic science principles involving bone ingrowth.

Femoral Component

Problems with femoral component fixation are rare because of the inherent three-dimensional structure of the distal femur and the use of femoral chamfer cuts, which together allow for a stable press-fit and the use of porous-coated femoral components in both hybrid and cementless TKA. Reproducible fixation to bone and good clinical results have been demonstrated in both of these application. The use of porous-coated pegs has been associated with some adverse changes and the loss of bone mineral density in the distal femur. A significant increase in the bone adjacent to the porous-coated fixation pegs resulted in stress shielding of the bone anteriorly as early as 1-year postoperatively and the development of a relative osteopenic area. Significant bone loss identified at the time of revision has correlated with these findings. The mismatch of bone density and resultant osteopenic stress riser in the distal femur caused by the pegs increased the possibility of a distal femoral periprosthetic fracture. Fixation pegs are helpful in maintaining rotational alignment, but they should be smooth and not porous coated. The use of a femoral component with a deep trochlear inset and generous radius profile has been shown to prevent excessive loads on the patellar component while simultaneously allowing good range of motion.

Tibial Component

The tibial component has given rise to the most significant challenge in obtaining lasting, secure fixation in cementless applications. Early designs were flat with short pegs and demonstrated difficulty in obtaining and maintaining fixation that often resulted in subsidence or liftoff of the tibial component. Biomechanical studies that involved loading these tibial components showed subsidence of the loaded side and liftoff of the opposite side. Improvement in component design, which included the addition of stems and screws, eliminated excess micromotion and added improved initial stability. The increased rigidity and improved stability of the newer designs decreased micromotion between the bone and the implant and, in turn, allowed for bone ingrowth. Adjunctive tibial screw fixation has not been free of adverse effects, however, and has been associated with osteolysis in some clinical studies. The screw hole and screw are thought to provide a conduit for polyethylene wear debris to the undersurface of the tibia. The incidence of this screw track osteolysis varies from 0 to 31% in large clinical series. One study hypothesized that component design, specifically the polyethylene attachment mechanism, was the main reason for the observed difference in the frequency of osteolysis among the various designs. One author attributed the lack of screw-associated osteolysis in his series (0 in 176 cementless TKAs) to an intimate screw hole and head fit, a secure tibial insert locking mechanism, and screw hole sealing from the plastic creep of the undersurface of the polyethylene inserts observed in postmortem retrievals. Porous-coating configuration and its effect of on osteolysis have also been studied. Smooth metal tracks between the patch porous coating on the undersurface of the tibial component of one implant design have been reported to apparently allow the migration of polyethylene debris from the joint area to the area surrounding the stem and screws. Approximately 20% of patients who underwent TKA with this design displayed evidence of osteolysis and bone loss at 2- to 4-year follow-up. Modification of this implant to a fully porous-coated design resulted in no evidence of osteolysis being reported at 4- to 8-year follow-up. These clinical data suggest that the undersurface of the tibial component should be fully porous coated. The proximal tibia displays asymmetric anatomy, with the medial plateau being larger than the lateral plateau. Maximum contact between the cortical and cancellous bone of the proximal tibia and the tibial component is desired. An asymmetric tibial component, with a larger medial side, may be advantageous in improving surface area contact between the resected tibial

surface and the tibial component. In one study, the increased coverage allowed for a more uniform load transmission to the cancellous bone of the proximal tibia and more surface area available for bone ingrowth, thereby improving fixation and clinical results.

Patellar Component

The cementless patella has presented a unique challenge for the proponents of cementless TKA. Early metal-backed designs demonstrated varying degrees of failure and success. Commonly reported modes of failure included wear or fracture of the polyethylene, dissociation of the polyethylene from the base plate, and dissociation of the base plate from the fixation pegs. Femoral and patellar component design and surgical technique all contributed to these failures. Box-shaped femoral components with a shallow trochlear groove were found to produce excessive forces at the patellofemoral joint. This problem was addressed with the development of a more curved femoral component with a deep trochlear groove that decreased the effective patellofemoral load, captured the patellar component, and allowed for a greater range of motion. On the patellar side, poor design factors included thin polyethylene, a metal endoskeleton for the polyethylene, and porous-coated peg fixation. The forces placed on the patella during activities of daily living alone exceed the yield point of polyethylene; therefore, some deformation will occur for all polyethylene designs. Design strategy must attempt to minimize the forces at the patellofemoral joint and maximize the patellar polyethylene thickness. Metal-backed patellae implanted using an onset technique (metal backing of the patellar component implanted flush with the cut surface of the patella) requires that the polyethylene be thin to maintain the overall patellar bone-implant construct thickness, which is effectively a setup for failure. An insetting technique allows for the use of thicker polyethylene and therefore a decrease in wear-related and fracture complications. Metal endoskeleton designs also have a decreased polyethylene thickness, which is most profound at the periphery, resulting in the same complications associated with thin polyethylene. Porous-coated pegs resulted in the same stress shielding complications as femoral components. One study noted bone ingrowth into the porous-coated pegs, with variable ingrowth into the plate portion of the patellar component. Peg fixation without plate fixation resulted in high eccentric shear forces at the peg-plate junction, with resultant failure at this junction. Studies have demonstrated excellent clinical results using newer designs of fully porous-coated metal-backed patellae. These include reports of no revisions of 451 inset metal-backed patellae at an average follow-up of 4 years, and a 95.1% survival rate at 10 years of 176 smooth-pegged metal-backed patellae.

Patient Selection

Traditional approaches toward patient selection have recommended that younger patients (younger than 60 years) should be considered candidates for cementless TKA. Older patients with presumed compromised bone strength are generally believed to be better served by cemented fixation. There are data in the literature, however, to support the use of cementless TKA in both younger and older patients. One study reviewed a series of 97 patients older than 65 years (average age, 71 years) who all underwent cementless TKA and followed-up for 31 months. The average Hospital for Special Surgery knee scores improved 44 points (from 55 to 99 at 2-year follow-up); knee flexion increased from 109° preoperatively to 123° at 2-year follow-up. Based on these early results, it was concluded that cementless TKA can be successful in patients older than 65 years and need not be reserved only for younger patients. Evaluating the pain relief response of a second-generation cementless knee implant, another study observed that age made no difference in ultimate pain relief obtained after cementless knee implantation.

A significant percentage of patients who require TKA are obese. There are no data to suggest that excessive weight should be considered an adverse risk factor for cementless TKA. One study evaluated 45 obese patients who underwent cementless TKA. This group was compared with a matched control group with respect to diagnosis, gender, age, and extent of preoperative deformity. At an average 7-year follow-up, no significant differences in the combined percentages of good and excellent clinical results were noted between the two groups.

Cementless TKA is not indicated for patients with significantly osteoporotic bone. Implant stability has been shown to be compromised by poor bone quality in biomechanical studies using synthetic models and cadaver bone. One study used a cadaveric tibial model to show that an increase in bone strength significantly reduced the degree of liftoff and micromotion of securely fixed tibial components. Another study recommended cementing all components in patients whose bone appeared soft and could be indented by thumb pressure over the central portion of the resected proximal tibia.

Concerns about compromised bone, implant fixation, and bone ingrowth has dissuaded many surgeons from considering cementless TKA for patients with inflammatory arthritis. Nonetheless, studies have demonstrated good to excellent results at short- and intermediate-term follow-up in patients with rheumatoid arthritis who underwent cementless TKA. One such study showed an improvement in knee scores from 32 to 88 over a 1- to 7-year follow-up period. Another study directly compared cementless with cemented fixation in a group of patients with rheumatoid arthritis. Good to excellent clinical results were reported for 91% of patients in the cementless TKA group versus 81% in the cemented TKA group at an average follow-up of 65 months.

Surgical Technique

Cementless TKA requires significant attention to surgical detail to obtain successful clinical results. Specific recommendations include the use of precision-cutting instrumentation, irrigation of all saw cuts, proximal tibia resection along the posterior slope, the use of autograft bone chips, and exacting patellar preparation. Precision-cutting instrumentation is essential for cementless TKA because it maximizes the intimate bone-implant apposition required for bone ingrowth. The cancellous surface irregularities that can be tolerated when using acrylic cement are not well tolerated during cementless fixation. The use of precision instrumentation with exacting tolerances, the use of new cutting blades for each patient, and meticulous surgical technique help make successful cementless TKA possible. Cementless TKA requires viable bone to attach to an implant's porous coating; therefore, specific protection against thermal necrosis (which occurs at 55°C) must be used routinely. Irrigation during bone resection maintains bone temperature at 38°C. Without irrigation, drilling or sawing maneuvers may increase the temperature of bone to as high as 170°C. Proximal tibia resection in line with the patient's natural posterior slope improves initial tibial component stability, protects against anterior subsidence, and allows the bone to be loaded in compression, perpendicular to the cancellous trabeculae. Mechanical testing has shown that proximal tibial bone resected parallel to the surface exhibited a 40% greater load-carrying capacity and 70% greater stiffness than bone resected perpendicular to the tibial long axis. The use of autograft bone chips as a low-viscosity biologic bone cement can be spread on the cancellous surfaces of the tibia, femur, and patella during implantation. This increases initial bone-implant contact and improves ultimate fixation. This slurry of bone acts like a grouting agent, filling in gaps within the cancellous bone and smoothing out small irregularities in the cut bone surface. Data indicate that the application of bone chips also increases the speed and amount of bone ingrowth by significantly increasing the mineral apposition rate and host bone available for ingrowth. Measured resection of the patella with component medialization and countersinking has produced excellent clinical results for certain cementless metal-backed patellar implants. This measured resection technique requires that only the thickness of bone that is removed be replaced; therefore overthickening of the patella is avoided. Improved patellar tracking can be attained by centering the component over the sagittal ridge, a position that is anatomically medial to the center of the patella.

Complications

Reported complications of cementless TKA have included metal-backed patellar failure, bone stress shielding, both of which were discussed previously, as well as osteolysis, component fracture, and failure of ingrowth.

Cementless methods of fixation have been plagued by complications secondary to osteolysis in the same way that cemented applications have been affected. Contact interfaces and surfaces of articulation are potential sources of wear debris regardless of fixation method. Risk factors for increased polyethylene wear of tibial inserts include heat-pressed manufacturing, increased crystallinity, thin (< 6 mm) insert constructs, poor locking mechanisms with resultant backside wear, and the use of excessively unconstrained and incongruent knee designs. The use of thin polyethylene tibial inserts and the abutment of the femoral component on a proud tibial insert spine have been implicated as the main contributors to the polyethylene wear debris and ultimate failure of the prostheses in one design. A high incidence of osteolysis with use of the Porous-Coated Anatomic knee (Biomet, Warsaw, IN) also has been well documented. One study reported specifically on the early delamination and surface failure of heat-pressed tibial inserts. The use of these heat-pressed tibial inserts and the nature of the unconstrained and incongruent design of the porous-coated anatomic knee were cited as the principal reasons for osteolysis in this type of knee implant. Screw-associated osteolysis is thought to occur when the screw hole and screw are able to provide a conduit for polyethylene wear debris to the undersurface of the tibia.

Component fracture in cementless TKA is exceedingly rare. Using cementless fixation, 37 instances of fractured femoral components have been reported, 36 of which involved the Ortholoc II femoral component (Wright Medical Technology, Arlington, TN). All fractures occurred at the junction of the beveled surfaces along the distal aspect of the component. More fractures were reported in smaller components and in components with a double layer (versus single layer) of sintered beads. All components demonstrated evidence of fatigue failure. It was theorized that the combination of the thinness of the metal at the beveled junctions, the decrease in thickness necessary to accommodate the porous coating, the notch effect of the beaded surface, and the weakened base metal secondary to bead sintering were collectively responsible for the component fracture sensitivity. Another report on a femoral component fracture cited regional osteonecrosis as the reason for this occurrence in a patient with a New Jersey low-contact stress knee implant. Osteonecrosis of the medial femoral condyle was believed to result in a loss of medial osseous support for the femoral component. This loss coupled with the adequate bone ingrowth of the

central and lateral flanges created a medial lever arm and led to subsequent fracture of medial flange.

Failure of ingrowth with cementless knee implantation has been reported frequently and has been a major deterrent to its widespread use. One study of 440 knee revisions that analyzed the method of failure reported that 13% of these revisions (37 knees) were the result of failure of ingrowth into a porous coated component. Another study of problems with cementless knee implants reported no femoral component loosening, a 21% rate of patellar component loosening, and an 8% rate of tibial component loosening. Other studies have reported clinical success in as high as 99.7% of patients who underwent implantation with the cementless technique, which likely reflects improvements in component design and implantation technique.

Implant Retrieval Studies

The results of implant retrieval studies are critical to understand the performance and behavior of cementless knee implants because they allow for the quantification of bone ingrowth as well as determination of appositional bone indices. Implant retrieval studies can be categorized as those evaluating malfunctioning components obtained at revision surgery and those analyzing well-functioning prostheses obtained postmortem. One study reported on 62 total knee components of various designs that were retrieved primarily at revision surgery at an average of 12 months postimplantation. Quantification analysis using a point-counting technique showed no more than 10% of porous coating ingrowth with bone in all components, and one third of the components exhibited only fibrous connective tissue ingrowth with no evidence of bone ingrowth. Another study evaluated 13 Miller-Galante I tibial components that were revised primarily to treat unexplained pain and found an average bone ingrowth of 9.5%. Preferential ingrowth was observed along the porous-coated fixation pegs. Deeper posterior resections and resections parallel to the tibia surface correlated with increased bone ingrowth (Figure 1).

The evaluation of well-functioning prostheses obtained at autopsy has provided more encouraging results. In a study in which five clinically successful porous-coated anatomic knee implants were evaluated histomorphometrically and histologically for bone ingrowth, the average bone ingrowth varied by component (patellae, 29%; tibias, 6%; and femora, 8%). Appositional bone averaged 53% at the patellar interface, 36% at the tibial interface, and 32% at the femoral interface. Another postmortem analysis of eight consecutively retrieved porous-coated Natural Knee (Sulzer Orthopaedics, Alton, England) tibial components revealed an average bone ingrowth of 6%; appositional bone averaged 73% (Figure 2). Higher percentages of bone in-

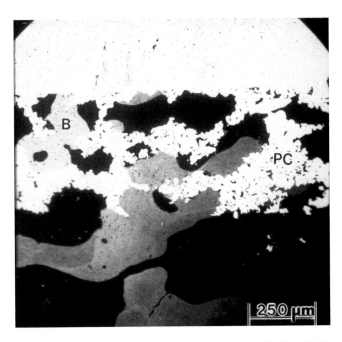

Figure 1 Backscatter electron imaging of host bone and implant interface. PC indicates porous coating and B indicates a region of bone ingrowth.

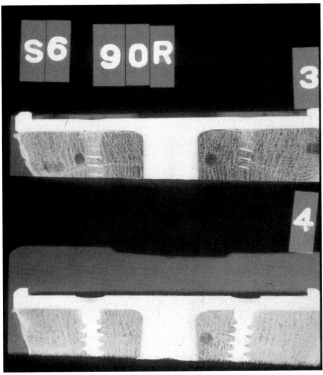

Figure 2 Cross-sectional microradiograph of a proximal tibia depicting intimate host bone implant apposition in a cementless tibial implant design augmented by screws.

growth (8% to 22%) were separately reported by the same author when analyzing 10 asymmetric tibial components removed for various reasons at 1 week to 48 months postimplantation. Eleven porous-coated metal-backed patellar components evaluated postmortem at the same institution demonstrated secure fixation, with appositional bone averaging 86% bone ingrowth averaging 13%. It was proposed that impaction of autograft bone chips through patellar reaming allowed for the higher rate of ingrowth. These studies of well-functioning implants suggest that small (6% to 22%) volume fractions of bone ingrowth into an implant's porous coating, coupled with significant appositional bone support, can yield successful clinical results.

Clinical Results

Several studies have evaluated the effectiveness of cementless TKA. Although many studies, generally with a follow-up of 5 years or less, described early clinical experience with specific designs, intermediate and long-term results provide more information regarding the durability and clinical success of any prosthetic design. Definitive long-term studies that support cementless fixation include a report of a single surgeon experience with the Ortholoc knee implant (Wright), which defines the 9- to 11-year follow-up of 163 patients and reports a 10-year component survivorship of 94.1%. Another single surgeon study describes the 10- to 14-year follow-up patients receiving the Natural Knee (Figure 3). Modified Hospital for Special Surgery knee scores were notable for a postoperative average of 97.8 points; average flexion was 120°. Implant survival was 93.4% (including

infection and simple polyethylene exchange) at 10-year follow-up, but femoral and tibial component interfaces had a 98% survival rate. Long-term data (7- to 12-year outcome analysis) are also available for cementless meniscal-bearing knee implants. At 12-year follow-up, an overall component survivorship of 95% has been reported.

More recently, the results were reported for a consecutive series of 114 porous-coated, cementless TKAs (Anatomic Graduated Components 2000, Biomet, Warsaw, IN) over a 2-year period. Only two tibial component revisions for loosening (one septic and one aseptic) were performed; no femoral or patellar component revisions were required. The cumulative component survival rate at 10- to 11-year follow-up was 97%. The flat-on-flat articulation of this implant did not result in catastrophic polyethylene wear or osteolysis. The 12- to 20-year follow-up (mean, 12.4 years) of 309 posterior cruciate ligament–retaining meniscal-bearing and rotating-platform New Jersey low contact stress total knee replacements reports good to excellent results in 97.9% of patients with primary posterior cruciate ligament–retaining meniscal-bearing prostheses and in 97.9% of those with primary rotating-platform prostheses. The survival rate of all components was greater than 97.4% using any mechanical reason for revision as an end point. A more recent study that assessed 184 total knee replacements reported an 18-year survival rate of

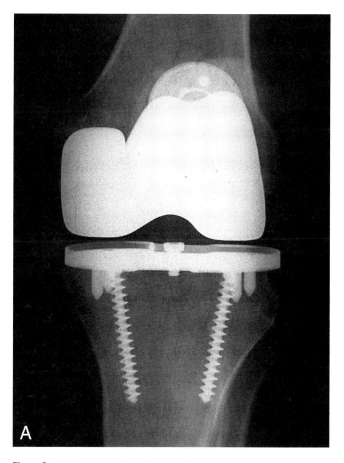
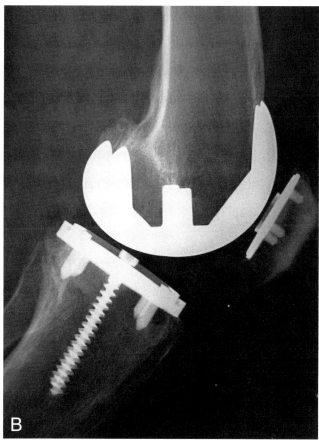

Figure 3 AP **(A)** and lateral **(B)** radiographs of a cementless total knee implant at 14-year follow-up. No significant radiolucencies are evident at the bone-prosthesis interface.

98.1%, with six revisions (five of which were done to treat infection).

Several studies have recently compared cementless and cemented designs in matched pair study designs. One such study reported the results of a consecutive series of 501 condylar primary total knee replacements (277 cemented and 224 cementless). Survivorship at 10 years was 95.3% and 95.6%, respectively. Clinical outcomes showed no significant differences between the two groups. A prospective study compared a group of 55 cementless Press Fit Condylar (PFC, Johnson & Johnson, Raynham, MA) TKAs with a matched group of 51 cemented PFC TKAs. The mean follow-up interval was 10 years. There was a notable increase in revision rate in the cementless PFC group, but postoperative knee scores were remarkably similar, with the cemented PFC group averaging 95 points and the cementless PFC group averaging 93 points. Cementless applications have also been compared with hybrid fixation. In one study, patients were randomized to undergo either cementless or hybrid fixation of cruciate–ligament retaining Miller Galante I knee arthroplasties. No significant differences were identified to warrant recommending one method of fixation over another.

The use of specific design qualities to attain biologic fixation has allowed cementless total knee replacement to be successful over the long term. The long term results are comparable to those for reported long-term cemented fixation clinical results. The ability to achieve these excellent survivorship results in younger, heavier, and often more active patients suggests that cementless biologic fixation should be considered as a viable treatment option along with cemented applications.

Cemented TKA

An ongoing debate exists on the decision to use cemented, cementless, or hybrid combinations of fixation methods for patients undergoing primary TKA. Mixed results on outcomes continue to be reported based on the method of fixation used. Although there are proponents for each approach, it is difficult to be dogmatic in recommending any one approach, even when taking into account different implants and patient populations. Data from large studies of patients from multiple sources (apart from studies of individual surgeons specializing in one technique, or in specific subgroups of surgical indications) and for all indications seem to demonstrate overall better results from cemented (in-

Table 1 | Summary of Effect Size Estimates

Measure	Years of Follow-up		
	0 to 2 **Effect Size**	2.1 to 5 **Effect Size**	> 5 **Effect Size**
Knee Society score	2.35	2.73	2.67
Hospital for Special Surgery score	3.91	3.01	2.67
Western Ontario and McMaster University Osteoarthritis index	1.62		
Medical Outcomes Society 36-Item Short Form score	1.27		

cluding hybrid) fixation. However, limitations in the current literature make it difficult to categorically claim better results for cemented fixation; other fixation methods have produced outcomes that are equivalent or better for some subgroups of patients.

TKA is a very effective procedure regardless of the method of fixation. TKA is associated with significant improvements in function and relief of knee pain and generally has a high patient satisfaction rating. However, as the number of TKAs continues to increase, ongoing high-quality analysis of the outcomes of all of these procedures will be needed.

Functional Outcomes

In a large and comprehensive meta-analysis of TKA outcome studies, it has recently been shown that the procedure is associated with very significant "effect sizes," which are essentially defined as the difference of the mean change for each outcome divided by the pooled standard deviation for each outcome; higher scores indicate better results (Table 1). The strongest evidence for positive results exists over a 2-year follow-up period; however, studies that extend to 5- and 10-year follow-ups show that similar positive results are maintained in the longer term. The actual effect sizes recorded were in the range of 2.35 to 3.91 for physician-derived measures (Knee Society scores and Hospital for Special Surgery scores) and 1.27 to 1.62 for patient-derived measures (The Western Ontario and McMaster University Osteoarthritis Index scores and Medical Outcomes Society 36-Item Short Form scores). However, few studies use multivariate models to associate outcomes with patient or implant characteristics. Therefore, the literature cannot support specific recommendations about which patients are most likely to benefit from TKA and what type of implant or implant fixation method is most beneficial.

For example, age, gender, and body mass index cannot be significantly correlated with TKA pain, satisfaction, or functional outcome. There is, however, an overall tendency for a higher body mass index to be associated with decreased functional outcome. Of more particular interest is the fact that current evidence regarding the type of prosthesis or the method of fixation cannot predict functional outcome. Although it is intuitive to believe that patient-related factors such as comorbidities, radiographic evidence of joint destruction, bone loss, extensor mechanism integrity, limited preoperative range of motion, alignment, the tibiofemoral angle, and ligament integrity must affect the outcome of surgery, there is currently no clear evidence to prove this. With few data available to differentiate functional outcomes based on fixation methods, much of the literature on this topic has focused on implant survival.

Survival of Cemented Versus Cementless Implants

Recent studies that have specifically compared cemented and cementless fixation have produced mixed results. An analysis of a prospective, randomized trial of 501 press-fit condylar TKA implants at a mean follow-up of 7.4 years showed a 10-year survival rate of 95.3% (95% confidence interval, 90.3 to 97.8) in the cemented fixation groups and 95.6% (95% confidence interval, 89.5 to 98.2) in the cementless fixation groups. However, another larger, retrospective, survivorship analysis of 11,606 TKAs (with overall implant survivorship of 91% at 10 years for 2,943 knees, 84% at 15 years for 595 knees, and 78% at 20 years for 104 knees) demonstrated survivorship levels of 92% for cemented prostheses compared with 61% for those fixed without cement—a highly significant difference. Such disagreements between studies regarding implant survivorship based on the fixation technique serve to emphasize the importance of high-quality studies and of large-scale arthroplasty registries.

Surgical Technique

Regardless of the fixation method chosen, the use of correct techniques to avoid complications and early failure are critical. It has been well demonstrated that alignment and correct balancing are crucial to the success of TKA. Accurate bone cuts also are critical. Although cemented components may accommodate slight imperfections more readily than cementless components, badly performed cuts can lead to malalignment that will negatively affect function and implant survivorship. Even with accurate cuts, it is important to ensure that components are fully seated because correct seating is easily obscured by the cement used for fixation. Varus-valgus alignment can be significantly affected by unequal medial-lateral cement mantles and poorly seated components. There is a tendency to place femoral components in relatively flexed positions if specific care is not taken to prevent this positioning with proprietary devices and simple techniques such as commencing component impaction from the posterior aspect to ensure adequate extension in component seating. When performing trial reductions, it is often worthwhile to widen fixation holes slightly (particularly on the tibia and patella) because it may be difficult during cement placement to determine if fixation pegs or stems of components are engaging holes correctly, thus allowing the correct orientation and seating of the components. It should also be noted that when definitive components are cemented in place, they may prove more stable and may seat better than the trial components, which are often slightly loose. Balance and stability should be rechecked at this point to allow further adjustments and the use of a larger size tibial component polyethylene thickness; the latter option is particularly relevant when using modular, metal-backed tibial components.

As has been the case for total hip arthroplasty, cementation techniques for TKA also have undergone generational development with improvements in the quality of component fixation to promote longevity. Poor cementing techniques have been related to early and continuous component migration, which is a positive factor in predicting aseptic loosening. The most useful tool in assessing component migration in TKA is roentgen stereophotogrammetric analysis using tantalum markers. Recent studies using roentgen stereophotogrammetric analysis have shown that improvements in cementing techniques can reduce migration values. It is advisable to use the third generation techniques of pulsatile lavage and injection of the cement, whether using specific cement guns or modified syringes. Other techniques described in recent publications include intraosseous suction or negative pressure intrusion in the proximal tibia, typically combined with standard third generation techniques. In clinical and cadaveric studies, the use of these techniques has produced significant improvements in cement penetration into the bony trabeculae of the tibial plateau and in the tensile and shear strengths of cement-bone composites. Although more difficult to clinically assess, work also has been done to improve femoral cementation techniques. One study that emphasized the importance of effective cementation of the posterior femoral condylar surfaces showed improved penetration depths, no gaps in the cement mantle on visual inspection, and no radiolucencies on radiographic evaluation when using cement injection. It is worth noting that if the knee is held in full extension while the cement is hardening (a technique that is typically used to compress components and possibly improve cement intrusion), it is possible to introduce posterior liftoff of either the tibial or femoral components and to cause varus or valgus malalignment, which may result in unacceptable outcomes.

Analysis of component design and the issue of whether to cement the stems of cemented implants continue to be debated in the literature. In a biomechanical cadaver study comparing surface with full tibial stem cementation, the investigators found no difference in micromotion with the use of either technique and found that the stability of the initial fixation using the surface cement technique was correlated to the depth of the cement penetration. Another study that used dual-energy x-ray absorptiometry scanning to assess the effects of cemented tibial stem design on stress shielding in the proximal tibia found that, at an average of 7 years after surgery, press-fit condylar prostheses (which have a single 4-cm stem) were associated with a significant reduction in bone density in the tibial metaphysis, whereas Miller-Galante I (Zimmer, Warsaw, IN) prostheses (which has four 0.5-cm pegs) were not. The authors suggested the use of shorter tibial stems or less cement with these implants.

Cemented TKA for Selected Diagnoses

A recent report published by the National Institutes of Health showed that patients with rheumatoid arthritis (RA) have more improvement following TKA than patients with osteoarthritis (OA). The exact reason for these results remains to be determined, but may be related to the poorer baseline function of RA patients. Registry data show good implant survivorship after TKA in patients with RA. Data from Sweden and Finland show patients with RA doing as well or better than patients with OA, although the Swedish registry did indicate that men with RA constitute a subgroup that is at increased risk for revision surgery, particularly because of infection. In the Finnish registry, 10-year survival for implants in TKA patients with OA was 94%, whereas patients with RA had an implant survival rate of 96% (not significantly different). Notably, there was no significant difference in implant survival regardless of whether cement was used for fixation. Good results have been achieved with cemented TKAs for patients with juvenile RA. Significant improvements in Knee Society scores, range of motion, pain, deformity, ambulation, and function have been reported for standard cemented implants and soft tissue at an average follow-up of 6 years, with acceptable implant survivorship rates in this young population. When using cementless techniques for patients with RA, cement will provide purchase for screws used in the typically soft bone and will provide initial component stability.

Outcomes also may be impacted for patients with diabetes mellitus who have TKA. A study of 363 TKAs in 291 patients with diabetes mellitus who had an average follow-up of 52 months showed that these patients had higher postoperative pain scores, more deep infections (1.2% versus 0.7%), and higher revision rates (3.6% versus 0.4%) when compared with a control group. Patients with diabetes mellitus may benefit from the use of antibiotic-laden cement.

A study of patients with ankylosing spondylitis who had a mean age of 55 years and who were reviewed at an average follow-up of 11.2 years showed that TKA using cemented implants provides excellent pain relief and good implant survival rates. However, these patients are at an increased risk for the development of stiffness and heterotopic bone formation (20%), and often do not achieve improved range of motion following surgery. Another study reported on TKA in patients who have clinically significant lymphedema. Although significant improvements in Knee Society functional and clinical scores were achieved, the gains were lower than found in groups with conventional indications for TKA. Furthermore, the total complication rate was 31%, including a 12% incidence of superficial infections, a 7% incidence of deep wound infections, and a 3.6% incidence of deep venous thrombosis. Similar mixed findings were reported in a recent retrospective study of 90 TKA patients with hemophilic arthropathy. Most of the patients were treated with cemented implants, although some cementless implants were used. Significant improvements in pain scores and clinical and functional Knee Society scores were achieved; however, there was a high complication rate, with 16% of the knees ultimately becoming infected. Antibiotic-laden cement was not used in this study. The 10-year implant survival rates were 83% based on component removal for any reason, and 77% for implant survival free of any infection.

Complications

Many complications of TKA are common to both cemented and cementless implants and are addressed in chapter 12. Traditionally, patient factors have been implicated in TKA complications; however, recent reports have found that the volume of patients treated by surgeons and institutions has a direct bearing on outcomes. Surgeons and institutions performing a large number of TKAs produce better functional outcomes and achieve lower rates of complications and mortality for their patients.

Although rare, recent reports of allergy to polymethylmethacrylate bone cement have been presented. Preoperative identification of this allergy should be made whenever possible. Some recent reports of cemented fixation have included an apparent lower incidence of periprosthetic fracture and two reports of significantly decreased postoperative wound drainage compared with cementless techniques. One study found that TKA for a valgus knee in patients with reduced bone mineral density predisposes the patient to fracture, whereas age, gender, and diagnosis did not.

Deep infection is a debilitating complication following TKA. The use of antibiotic-impregnated cement has recently attracted attention in the United States, although its use has been widespread in Europe for some time. Recent data, including basic science research and data derived from clinical trials and the arthroplasty registry, indicate that the use of antibiotic-impregnated cement is an effective strategy for reducing the risk of deep infection following TKA. Several prospective studies of cefuroxime-impregnated cement have demonstrated its usefulness both in fully cemented or hybrid applications. At 2-year follow-up, one randomized study found no infections in TKAs performed with antibiotic cement compared with an infection rate of 3.1% in TKAs performed using plain cement. Another randomized, blinded study found antibiotic-impregnated cement very effective in preventing infection at 4-year follow-up in patients with diabetes mellitus (0% versus 13.5% deep infection rate; $P = 0.021$). Concerns with the universal application of antibiotic-impregnated cement have involved possible allergic reactions, bacterial resistance, and cost. Current evidence, however, indicates that antibiotic-impregnated cement is beneficial to patients who have a moderate to high risk of infection.

Survivorship Analyses of Specific Implants

A large number of reports from studies on a single type of implant or from a single institution exist. Many of these reports provide information in a secondary manner on the method of implant fixation. For example, the Kaplan-Meier survival analyses have shown good medium- to long-term survival across a wide spectrum of cemented implants such as 98.86% survival at 15 years for the Anatomic Graduated Components system (Biomet, Warsaw, IN) (although 4.2% of the all-polyethylene patellar components were described as aseptically loose); 15-year implant survivorship (free of any component revision excluding infection) of 88.7% for the posterior cruciate retaining Kinematic I (Stryker, Kalamazoo, MI); a cumulative survival rate at 10 years of 95.5% for the Press-Fit Condylar knee (Johnson & Johnson, Warsaw, IN), 97% at 10 years for the Genesis I posterior cruciate ligament–retaining knee (Smith & Nephew, Memphis, TN), and 96.95% at 9 years for the Kinemax (Stryker) TKA (posterior cruciate ligament–retaining knee). Cemented Low Contact Stress (DePuy, Warsaw, IN) rotating-platform mobile-bearing TKAs also have produced typically good results. For example, one study of 119 rotating-platform mobile-bearing TKAs at 9- to 12-year follow-up showed that none required revision surgery (although some patients were lost to follow-up), and no patients had a prosthesis dislocation or periprosthetic osteolysis or loosening. More recent findings of increased gravimetric wear with rotating-platform total knee replacements compared with their fixed-bearing counterparts are discussed in chapter 11.

Other subgroups of cemented implants such as all-polyethylene tibial components are reported to provide good results. At intermediate-term follow-up, investigators have found no difference in the clinical performance or functional outcome between TKAs with metal-backed or all-polyethylene tibial components. A literature review of 5,950 TKAs that concentrated on implant survival rates found that all-polyethylene tibial components had significantly better survival than metal-backed tibial components (both nonstabilized and posterior stabilized components). This study also found no difference in survival between cemented posterior stabilized implants and implants that were not stabilized. Another study using roentgen stereophotogrammetric analysis showed that all-polyethylene tibial components had magnitudes of migration at least equal to or lower than metal-backed components, a good indicator of future survivorship.

Another study compared 334 cemented third-generation cruciate-retaining or posterior-stabilized TKAs. At 8-year follow-up, Kaplan-Meier implant survivorship was statistically similar with 95.9% survivorship for the cruciate-retaining TKAs and 99.5% for the posterior-stabilized TKAs. No differences were detectable in any of the outcomes analyzed.

Knee Registry Data

Large scale and national registries have become an important resource for assessing the performance of prostheses, particularly with regard to survivorship. More recently, improvements have been implemented in many of these databases so that more outcome information can be analyzed and reported. Most registry data suggest that overall revision rates for both cemented and cementless approaches are generally low (with implant survival averaging 95% to 99% at 5- to 7-year follow-up). Revision rates have gradually been improving over time. In a study derived from the Swedish Knee Registry, a cumulative revision rate of 25% after 18 years was found; however, the authors noted that the revision rate for newer procedures had decreased by 7% annually between 1976 and 1997.

One of the few registry reports from the United States on 5,760 TKAs done by 53 surgeons showed that cemented TKAs (in which all-polyethylene tibial implants fared best) had better survival rates than hybrid or ingrowth TKAs with a 10-year cumulative survival rate of more than 95%. These superior results for cemented TKAs also have been reported in recent data from the Swedish Knee Arthroplasty Register on 57,533 primary and revision TKAs. An increased risk of revision (1.4 times higher) has been found when using fully cementless techniques compared with cemented techniques ($P = 0.01$). The sole exception to this finding involved patients with RA who appear to do equally well with either type of fixation. These data have resulted in a decrease in the use of cementless prostheses in the

United States. There were no significant differences in the 10-year survival rates when comparing hybrid (cementless femoral component) to fully cemented components.

Another recent comprehensive report from the Norwegian Arthroplasty Register compared the survivorship of a number of popular prostheses from different manufacturers. The authors also reported outcomes based on the type of fixation used. Cement was used as the fixation method in 87% of the knees, 10% were hybrid, and 2% were cementless implants. With all revisions as the end point, no statistically significant differences in the 5-year survival rates were found in the cemented tricompartmental prosthesis brands: Anatomic Graduated Components, 97% (n = 279); Duracon (Stryker), 99% (n = 101); Genesis I, 95% (n = 654); Kinemax, 98% (n = 213); and Tricon (Smith & Nephew), 96% (n = 454). The bicompartmental (patella not resurfaced) Low Contact Stress prosthesis had a 5-year survival rate of 97% (n = 476). Despite the low number of cementless TKAs in the study, survival of cementless TKAs did not differ significantly from the cemented components.

The results of all the registry studies, regardless of the fixation method, showed that the most important negative factors in implant survival were patient age of 60 years or younger, male gender, and posttraumatic degenerative joint disease.

Summary

Based on the results of 10-year follow-up studies, the current literature supports either cemented or cementless approaches to fixation using modern techniques and developments in TKA. However, the preponderance of data appears to support cemented fixation as a standard for all indications, although it may ultimately be proved that cementless fixation has some advantages in particular subpopulations. More longer-term studies are needed to definitively determine which patients with given sets of characteristics would benefit most from TKA, and then to determine which implant, techniques, and fixation method are most appropriate in each set of circumstances.

Annotated Bibliography

Cementless TKA

Akizuki S: Fixation of a hydroxyapatite-tricalcium phosphate coated cementless knee prosthesis: Clinical and radiographic evaluation seven years after surgery. *J Bone Joint Surg Br* 2003;85:1123-1127.

In this study, 30 patients underwent TKA with the Miller-Galante II implant. Both the femoral and tibial components were plasma-sprayed with hydroxyapatite-tricalcium phosphate. The authors reported that this coated prosthesis showed good early fixation that was maintained at 7-year follow-up with good clinical and radiographic outcomes.

Berger RA, Lyon JH, Jacobs JJ, et al: Problems with cementless total knee arthroplasty at 11 years follow-up. *Clin Orthop Relat Res* 2001;392:196-207.

One hundred two patients with 131 consecutive cementless TKAs that retained the posterior cruciate ligament were followed up prospectively. At an average 11-year follow-up, the authors reported that cementless fixation yielded mixed results: cementless femoral fixation typically had excellent outcomes, but metal-backed patellar components had a 48% patellar revision rate. The rate of aseptic loosening for patients with cementless tibial components was 8%; the authors also reported a 12% incidence of small osteolytic lesions in this patient population. Based on these results, the authors abandoned cementless fixation in patients requiring TKA.

Buechel FF: Long-term follow-up after mobile-bearing total knee replacement. *Clin Orthop Relat Res* 2002;404: 40-50.

Clinical and radiographic analyses were done and survivorship rates were assessed in a series of 309 patients who underwent cementless posterior cruciate-retaining meniscal-bearing and rotating-platform total knee replacement. At 10- to 20-year follow-up (mean, 12.4 years), good to excellent results were reported in 97.9% of patients with primary posterior cruciate-retaining-bearing prostheses and in 97.9% of those with primary rotating-platform prostheses.

Cross MJ, Parish EN: A hydroxyapatite coated total knee replacement: Prospective analysis of 1000 patients. *J Bone Joint Surg Br* 2005;87:1073-1076.

One thousand patients who received a hydroxyapatite coated cementless total knee implant were followed for an average of 6.6 years. The authors reported that Knee Society scores improved from 96 to 180 and that only seven patients required revision (four because of septic loosening).

Fehring TK, Odum S, Griffin WL, Mason JB, Nadaud M: Early failure in total knee arthroplasty. *Clin Orthop Relat Res* 2001;392:315-318.

This study was conducted to assess the mechanisms of failure in patients who underwent revision surgery within 5 years of their index TKA. Of the 440 patients studied, 279 (63%) had revision surgery within 5 years of the index procedure, only 3% of whom (eight of the 279 patients) required revision surgery because of aseptic loosening of a cemented implant. The authors concluded that if all of the implants in the early failure group would have been cemented routinely and balanced carefully, the number of early revisions would have decreased by approximately 40%, and the overall failures would have been reduced by 25%.

Hofmann AA, Evanich JD, Ferguson R, et al: Ten- to 14-year clinical follow-up of the cementless Natural Knee system. *Clin Orthop Relat Res* 2001;388:85-94.

The authors of this study assessed 176 knees that were implanted with a cementless total knee implant. Average follow-up was 12 ± 1 years. Knee function was improved significantly. Knee scores improved to 97.8 ± 4.7 points and knee range of motion averaged 0° ± 2° to 120° ± 10° at last follow-up. Implant survival was 93.4% (including infection and simple polyethylene exchanges) and 95.1% (excluding infection and simple polyethylene exchanges) at 10-year follow-up. The authors concluded that these long-term results compared favorably with those of cemented systems.

Khaw FM, Kirk LM, Morris RW, Gregg PJ: A randomized, controlled trial of cemented versus cementless press fit condylar total knee replacement: Ten-year survival analysis. *J Bone Joint Surg Br* 2002;84:658-666.

A consecutive series of 501 cemented (219 patients, 277 implants) or cementless (177 patients, 224 implants) total knee replacements was assessed at a mean follow-up of 7.4 years (range, 2.7 to 13.0 years) to determine the 10-year implant survival rate, which was 95.3% (95% confidence interval 90.3 to 97.8) and 95.6% (95% confidence interval 89.5 to 98.2) in the cemented and cementless groups, respectively. The authors concluded that survivorship of the press-fit condylar total knee implant was good regardless of the method of fixation, which led them to question the use of more expensive cementless implants to treat this patient population.

Oliver MC, Keast-Butler OD, Hinves BL, Shepperd JA: A hydroxyapatite coated Install-Burnstein II total knee replacement. *J Bone Joint Surg Br* 2005;87:478-482.

The authors reported the clinical and radiographic outcomes of a consecutive series of 138 hydroxyapatite-coated total knee replacements with a mean 11-year follow-up (range, 10 to 13 years). Radiographic assessment revealed no implant loosening. Seven prostheses were revised, resulting in a cumulative survival rate of 93% at 13-year follow-up.

Parker DA: Long-term follow-up of cementless versus hybrid fixation for total knee arthroplasty. *Clin Orthop Relat Res* 2001;388:68-76.

In this prospective study, 99 patients (100 knees) with OA were randomized to undergo either cementless or hybrid fixation of cruciate-retaining Miller-Galante-I TKAs. Of 67 patients available for follow-up, 39 underwent revision surgery at an average 6.9 years postoperatively. The main reason for revision surgery was failure of metal-backed patellas with 25 knees revised at an average of 7.4 years, and the second most common reason was tibial polyethylene failure. The survival rate was 60% at 14-year follow-up for all knees, and 85% when failures resulting from metal-backed patellar components and infection were excluded, with no significant difference between the two groups. The authors concluded that elimination of poor design features related to the patellofemoral articulation and the use of thin tibial polyethylene, cruciate-retaining TKAs can yield good durable results, whether cementless or hybrid fixation is used.

Schroder HM: Cementless porous-coated total knee arthroplasty: 10-year results in a consecutive series. *J Arthroplasty* 2001;16:559-567.

The author assessed 114 Anatomic Graduated Components 2000 porous-coated, cementless TKAs performed consecutively in 102 patients. The cumulative prosthesis survival rate after 10- to 11-year follow-up was 97%. When pain and radiographic loosening also were considered, the success rate was 87%. Cementless insertion of a nonmodular, porous-coated total knee implant resulted in a long-term durable bone-prosthesis interface. The flat-on-flat articulation did not result in catastrophic polyethylene wear or osteolysis within the first 10 years.

Whiteside LA: Long-term follow-up of the bone ingrowth Ortholoc knee system without a metal-backed patella. *Clin Orthop Relat Res* 2001;388:77-84.

In this study, 265 Ortholoc-I femoral and tibial components (202 patients) were implanted using bone ingrowth technique. Of the 184 knees (165 patients) available for 15- to 18-year follow-up, one knee was revised because of loosening and five knees were revised because of infection. The overall survival rate at 18 years was 98.6%. The authors concluded that total knee replacement with bone ingrowth technique was a reliable and effective means of treating patients with end stage arthritis of the knee.

Cemented TKA

Back DL, Cannon SR, Hilton A, Bankes MJ, Briggs TW: The Kinemax total knee arthroplasty: Nine years' experience. *J Bone Joint Surg Br* 2001;83:359-363.

The authors reported on 422 primary cemented Kinemax (posterior cruciate retaining) TKAs by 31 different surgeons. Significant improvements were recorded in the mean Knee Society scores and range of motion. Cumulative implant survival was 99% at 5 years and 96.95% at 9 years.

Banwart JC, McQueen DA, Friis EA, Graber CD: Negative pressure intrusion cementing technique for total knee arthroplasty. *J Arthroplasty* 2000;15:360-367.

This cadaveric study compared negative pressure intrusion cementation of the tibial baseplate using a suction cannula in the proximal tibia with standard third-generation positive pressure intrusion. Although no differences were noted on radiographs or direct cement depth measurement analysis, scanning electron micrography revealed that the negative pressure specimens had fewer voids in the cement-bone composite and narrower empty spaces between bone and cement.

Bourne RB: Prophylactic use of antibiotic bone cement: An emerging standard in the affirmative. *J Arthroplasty* 2004;19:69-72.

This review article discusses preclinical testing; randomized, clinical trials; national joint arthroplasty data; and personal experience and concludes that the use of antibiotic-impregnated bone cement is indicated to reduce the risk of deep infection following both primary and revision total joint arthroplasty.

Bozic KJ, Kinder J, Meneghini RM, Zurakowski D, Rosenberg AG, Galante JO: Implant survivorship and complication rates after total knee arthroplasty with a third-generation cemented system: 5 to 8 years followup. *Clin Orthop Relat Res* 2005;430:117-124.

This report of 334 primary TKAs (186 cruciate-retaining and 148 posterior-stabilized) showed no differences in any of the outcome measurements analyzed between patients who had cruciate-retaining or posterior-stabilized implants. Kaplan-Meier implant survivorship, using revision for any reason and revision for aseptic loosening as end points, were 95.9% and 99.5% respectively at 8 years.

Forster MC: Survival analysis of primary cemented total knee arthroplasty: Which designs last? *J Arthroplasty* 2003;18:265-270.

This literature review analyzed implant survivorship data from 5,950 primary cemented fixed bearing condylar-type TKAs. No difference was exhibited overall in survival between posterior stabilized and nonstabilized implants; however, the subgroup of all-polyethylene nonstabilized tibial components was associated with significantly better survival than other implant types.

Furnes O, Espehaug B, Lie SA, Vollset SE, Engesaeter LB, Havelin LI: Early failures among 7,174 primary total knee replacements: A follow-up study from the Norwegian Arthroplasty Register 1994-2000. *Acta Orthop Scand* 2002;73:117-129.

This report compares survival rates among different prostheses, types of fixation, and whether the patella was resurfaced. No significant differences were found in the 5-year survival rates in a range of cemented prostheses regardless of the fixation method used.

Gioe TJ, Killeen KK, Grimm K, Mehle S, Scheltema K: Why are total knee replacements revised? Analysis of early revision in a community knee implant registry. *Clin Orthop Relat Res* 2004;428:100-106.

This study reports on 5,760 TKAs from a community joint implant registry in the United States. Cumulative implant survival rates were best for cemented TKAs compared with cementless or hybrid fixation methods.

Hervey SL, Purves HR, Guller U, Toth AP, Vail TP, Pietrobon R: Provider volume of total knee arthroplasties and patient outcomes in the HCUP-nationwide inpatient sample. *J Bone Joint Surg Am* 2003;85-A:1775-1783.

This study analyzed the relationship between volume and outcome of TKAs based on the 1997 Healthcare Cost and Utilization Project Nationwide Inpatient Sample. The authors performed logistic and multiple regression models on a target population of 277,550 patients, adjusting results for potential confounding factors. Only surgeons performing at least 15 procedures per year and hospital volumes of at least 85 per year were significantly and linearly associated with lower mortality rates. The authors propose volume standards to decrease patient mortality following TKA.

Kane RL, Saleh KJ, Wilt TJ, Bershadsky B: The functional outcomes of total knee arthroplasty. *J Bone Joint Surg Am* 2005;87:1719-1724.

The authors present a comprehensive structured literature review of the functional outcomes of TKA. Sixty-two studies met inclusion criteria and showed that TKA leads to substantial functional improvement based on an 'effect size' calculation devised by the authors. However, few studies were found to use sufficient scientific methodology to investigate specific associations between outcomes and patient characteristics.

Kane RL, Saleh KJ, Wilt TJ, et al: Total Knee Replacement. Rockville, MD, Agency for Healthcare Research and Quality, 2003.

This important report, published by the National Institutes of Health, contains valuable analyses and information regarding recent literature on primary TKA.

Labutti RS, Bayers-Thering M, Krackow KA: Enhancing femoral cement fixation in total knee arthroplasty. *J Arthroplasty* 2003;18:979-983.

The authors emphasize the importance of good cementation technique in avoiding early loosening. With particular focus on the posterior femoral condylar surfaces, they demonstrated greater penetration depths and fewer gaps in the cement mantle on visual inspection or less radiolucency on radiographic evaluation with cement injection versus noninjected cement. Statistical significance was not achieved in this study.

Meding JB, Reddleman K, Keating ME, et al: Total knee replacement in patients with diabetes mellitus. *Clin Orthop Relat Res* 2003;416:208-216.

At an average follow-up of 52 months, the authors compared 363 TKAs in 291 patients with diabetes mellitus to all other TKA patients. The average preoperative and postoperative pain scores were higher in patients with diabetes. Type I diabetes was associated with lower postoperative function scores and higher rates of deep infection. The revision rate (including infections) was higher in patients with diabetes (3.6% versus 0.4%).

Parvizi J, Duffy GP, Trousdale RT: Total knee arthroplasty in patients with ankylosing spondylitis. *J Bone Joint Surg Am* 2001;83-A:1312-1316.

This study reports on 30 cemented TKAs in 20 patients (average age, 55 years) with ankylosing spondylitis at an aver-

age follow-up of 11.2 years. Significant improvements were obtained in average Knee Society pain score; less improvement was found in function scores. Postoperatively, 20% of patients developed heterotopic bone formation. The average arc of motion showed improvement on only 1.9°. One revision surgery was required for a loose patellar component.

Robertsson O, Knutson K, Lewold S, Lidgren L: The Swedish Knee Arthroplasty Register 1975-1997: An update with special emphasis on 41,223 knees operated on in 1988-1997. *Acta Orthop Scand* 2001;72:503-513.

Results from the Swedish Knee Arthroplasty Register reflect increasing use of cemented implants, higher cumulative revision rates with cementless fixation, and improving implant survivorship on the whole for TKAs since the inception of the registry. This is a comprehensive study with data on implant types, indications, and patient characteristics.

Shrader MW, Morrey BF: Primary TKA in patients with lymphedema. *Clin Orthop Relat Res* 2003;416:22-26.

This retrospective study of 83 TKAs in 63 patients with significant lymphedema who had a minimum follow-up of 2 years found significant improvement in the Knee Society score and knee function score. The total complication rate of 31% was greater than in patients without lymphedema, with 10 superficial wound infections (12%), 6 deep infections (7%), and 3 patients (3.6%) who developed deep venous thrombosis.

Thomas A, Rojer D, Imrie S, Goodman SB: Cemented total knee arthroplasty in patients with juvenile rheumatoid arthritis. *Clin Orthop Relat Res* 2005;433:140-146.

Seventeen cemented TKAs using off-the-shelf posterior cruciate substituting implants and a routine lateral retinacular release in patients with juvenile RA were reviewed at a mean follow-up of 74 months. Knee Society scores improved from a mean of 38.9 ± 23.9 points to 81.9 ± 16.6 points. Both range of motion and ambulation scores improved significantly.

Classic Bibliography

Amstutz HC, Campbell P, Kossovsky N, et al: Mechanism and clinical significance of wear debris-induced osteolysis. *Clin Orthop Relat Res* 1992;276:7-18.

Armstrong RA, Whiteside LA: Results of cementless total knee arthroplasty in an older rheumatoid arthritis population. *J Arthroplasty* 1991;6:357-362.

Bachus KN, Hofmann AA, Dauterman LA: Canine and human cancellous bony ingrowth into cobalt chrome and titanium porous coated implants: A backscattered electron microscopic analysis. *Trans Orthop Res Soc* 1988;13:308.

Bayley JC, Scott RD, Ewald FC, et al: Failure of the metal-backed patellar component after total knee replacement. *J Bone Joint Surg Am* 1988;70:668-674.

Bayley JC, Scott RD: Further observations on metal-backed patellar component failure. *Clin Orthop Relat Res* 1988;236 :82-87.

Bloebaum RD: Porous-coated metal-backed patellar components in total knee replacement: A postmortem retrieval analysis. *J Bone Joint Surg Am* 1998;80:518-528.

Bloebaum RD, Bachus KN, Jensen JW, et al: Postmortem analysis of consecutively retrieved asymmetric porous-coated tibial components. *J Arthroplasty* 1997;12: 920-929.

Bloebaum RD, Bachus KN, Mitchell W, et al: Analysis of the bone surface area in resected tibia: Implications in tibial subsidence and fixation. *Clin Orthop Relat Res* 1994;309:2-10.

Bloebaum RD, Bachus KN, Momberger NG, et al: Mineral apposition rates of human cancellous bone at the interface of porous coated implants. *J Biomed Mater Res* 1994;28:537-544.

Bloebaum RD, Nelson K, Dorr LD, et al: Investigation of early surface delamination observed in retrieved heat-pressed tibial inserts. *Clin Orthop Relat Res* 1991; 269:120-127.

Bloebaum RD, Rhodes DM, Rubman MH, et al: Bilateral tibial components of different cementless designs and materials: Microradiographic, backscattered imaging, and histologic analysis. *Clin Orthop Relat Res* 1991; 268:179-187.

Bloebaum RD, Rubman MH, Hofmann AA: Bone ingrowth into porous-coated tibial components implanted with autograft bone chips: Analysis of ten consecutively retrieved implants. *J Arthroplasty* 1992;7:483-493.

Bobyn JD, Pilliar RM, Cameron HU, et al: Osteogenic phenomena across endosteal bone-implant spaces with porous surfaced intramedullary implants. *Acta Orthop Scand* 1981;52:145-153.

Bobyn JD, Pilliar RM, Cameron HU, et al: The optimum pore size for the fixation of porous-surfaced metal implants by the ingrowth of bone. *Clin Orthop Relat Res* 1980;150:263-270.

Boublik M, Tsahakis PJ, Scott RD: Cementless total knee arthroplasty in juvenile onset rheumatoid arthritis. *Clin Orthop Relat Res* 1993;286:88-93.

Branson PJ, Steege J, Wixson RL, et al: Rigidity of initial fixation in non-cemented total knee tibial components, in *Proceedings of the 33rd Annual Meeting*. Rosemont, IL, Orthopaedic Research Society, 1987, p 293.

Buechel FF: Cementless meniscal bearing knee arthroplasty: 7- to 12-year outcome analysis. *Orthopedics* 1994; 17:833-836.

Buechel FF, Pappas MJ: Long-term survivorship analysis of cruciate-sparing versus cruciate-sacrificing knee prosthesis using meniscal bearings. *Clin Orthop Relat Res* 1990;260:162-169.

Bugbee WD, Ammeen DJ, Park NL, Engh GA: 4 to 10-year results with the anatomic modular total knee. *Clin Orthop Relat Res* 1998;348:158-165.

Cameron HU, Pilliar RM, Macnab I: The effect of movement on the bonding of porous metal to bone. *J Biomed Mater Res* 1973;7:301-311.

Carlsson L, Regner L, Johansson C, et al: Bone response to hydroxyapatite-coated and commercially pure titanium implants in the human arthritic knee. *J Orthop Res* 1994;12:274-285.

Colizza WA, Insall JN, Scuderi GR: The posterior stabilized total knee prosthesis: Assessment of polyethylene damage and osteolysis after a ten-year minimum follow-up. *J Bone Joint Surg Am* 1995;77:1713-1720.

Collier JP, Mayor MB, McNamara JL, Surprenant VA, Jensen RE: Analysis of the failure of 122 polyethylene inserts from uncemented tibial components. *Clin Orthop Relat Res* 1991;273:232-242.

Cook SD, Thomas KA: Fatigue failure of noncemented porous-coated implants: A retrieval study. *J Bone Joint Surg Br* 1991;73: 20-24.

Cook SD, Thomas KA, Haddad RJ Jr: Histologic analysis of retrieved human porous-coated total joint components. *Clin Orthop Relat Res* 1988;234:90-101.

Diduch DR, Insall JN, Scott WN, Scuderi GR, Font-Rodriguez D: Total knee replacement in young active patients: Long-term follow-up and functional outcome. *J Bone Joint Surg Am* 1997;79:575-582.

Duffy GP: Cement versus cementless fixation in total knee arthroplasty. *Clin Orthop Relat Res* 1998;356:66-72.

Ebert FR, Krackow KA, Lennox DW, et al: Minimum 4-year follow- up of the PCA total knee arthroplasty in rheumatoid patients. *J Arthroplasty* 1992;7:101-108.

Engh CA, Hooten JP Jr, Zettl-Schaffer KF, et al: Evaluation of bone ingrowth in proximally and extensively porous-coated anatomic medullary locking prostheses retrieved at autopsy. *J Bone Joint Surg Am* 1995;77:903-910.

Evanich CJ, Tkach T, von Glinski S, et al: 6- to 10-year experience using countersunk metal-backed patellas. *J Arthroplasty* 1997;12:149-154.

Firestone TP, Teeny SM, Krackow KA, et al: The clinical and roentgenographic results of cementless porous-coated patellar fixation. *Clin Orthop Relat Res* 1991;273: 184-189.

Font-Rodriguez DE, Scuderi GR, Insall JN: Survivorship of cemented total knee arthroplasty. *Clin Orthop Relat Res* 1997;345:79-86.

Gill GS, Chan KC, Mills DM: 5 to 18-year follow-up study of cemented total knee arthroplasty for patients 55 years old or younger. *J Arthroplasty* 1997;12:49-54.

Heck DA, Robinson R, Partridge C: Patient outcomes after knee replacement. *Clin Orthop Relat Res* 1998;356: 93-110.

Hofmann AA: Cementless total knee arthroplasty in patients over 65 years old. *Clin Orthop Relat Res* 1991;271: 28-34.

Hofmann AA: Response of human cancellous bone to identically structured commercially pure titanium and cobalt chromium alloy porous-coated cylinders. *Clin Mater* 1993;14:101-115.

Hofmann AA: The cementless alternative to TKA. *Orthopedics* 1996;19: 789-791.

Hofmann AA, Bachus KN, Bloebaum RD: Comparative study of human cancellous bone remodeling to titanium and hydroxyapatite coated implants. *J Arthroplasty* 1993;8:157-166.

Hofmann AA, Bachus KN, Wyatt RWB: Effect of the tibial cut on subsidence following total knee arthroplasty. *Clin Orthop Relat Res* 1991;269:63-69.

Hofmann AA, Bloebaum RD, Bachus KN: Progression of human bone ingrowth into porous-coated implants. *Acta Orthop Scand* 1997;68:161-166.

Hofmann AA, Bloebaum RD, Rubman MH, et al: Microscopic analysis of autograft bone applied at the interface of porous-coated devices in human cancellous bone. *Int Orthop* 1992;16:349-358.

Hofmann AA, Murdock LE, Wyatt RWB, Alpert JP: Total knee arthroplasty: two- to four-year experience using an asymmetric tibial tray and a deep trochlear-grooved femoral component. *Clin Orthop Relat Res* 1991;269:78-88.

Huang C-H, Yang C-Y, Cheng C-K: Fracture of the femoral component associated with polyethylene wear and osteolysis after total knee arthroplasty. *J Arthroplasty* 1999;14:375-379.

Hulbert SF, Klawitter JJ, Talbert CD, et al: *Research in Dental and Medical Materials.* New York, NY, Plenum Press, 1969.

Hungerford DS, Krackow KA, Kenna RV: Cementless total knee replacement in patients 50 years old and under. *Orthop Clin North Am* 1989;20:131-145.

Jones GB: Arthroplasty of the knee by the Walldius prosthesis. *J Bone Joint Surg Br* 1968;50:505-510.

Jones LC, Hungerford DS: Cement disease. *Clin Orthop Relat Res* 1987;225:192-206.

Jones SM, Pinder IM, Moran CG, et al: Polyethylene wear in uncemented knee replacements. *J Bone Joint Surg Br* 1992;74:18-22.

Kim Y-H, Oh J-H, Oh S-H: Osteolysis around cementless porous-coated anatomic knee prostheses. *J Bone Joint Surg Br* 1995;77:236-241.

Knutson K, Lewold S, Robertsson O, Lidgren L: The Swedish knee arthroplasty register: A nation-wide study of 30,003 knees 1976-1992. *Acta Orthop Scand* 1994;65: 375-386.

Kobs J, Lachiewicz P: Hybrid total knee arthroplasty: Two- to five-year results using the Miller-Galante prosthesis. *Clin Orthop Relat Res* 1993;286:78-87.

Krackow KA: Uncemented total knee arthroplasty: A two to eight years survey and analysis of multi-center, multi-system results. *Am J Knee Surg* 1988;1:42.

Krause WR, Bradbury DW, Kelly JE, et al: Temperature elevations in orthopaedic cutting operations. *J Biomech* 1982;15:267-275.

Laskin R, Bucknell A: The use of metal-backed patellar prostheses in total knee arthroplasty. *Clin Orthop Relat Res* 1990;260:52-55.

Leach RE, Baumgard S, Broom J: Obesity: Its relationship to osteoarthritis of the knee. *Clin Orthop Relat Res* 1973;93:271-273.

Lee R, Volz R, Sheridan D: The role of fixation and bone quality on the mechanical stability of tibial knee components. *Clin Orthop Relat Res* 1991;273:177-183.

Lewis PL, Rorabeck CH, Bourne RB: Screw osteolysis after cementless total knee replacement. *Clin Orthop Relat Res* 1995;321:173-177.

Lombardi AV, Engh GA, Volz RG, et al: Fracture/dissociation of the polyethylene in metal-backed patellar components in total knee arthroplasty. *J Bone Joint Surg Am* 1988;70:675-679.

Miura H, Whiteside LA, Easley JC, et al: Effects of screws and a sleeve on initial fixation in uncemented total knee tibial components. *Clin Orthop Relat Res* 1990; 259:160-168.

Mont MA, Becher OJ, Lee CW, et al: Patellofemoral complications after total knee arthroplasty: A comparison of modular porous-coated anatomic with Duracon prostheses. *Am J Orthop* 1999;24:241-247.

Mont MA, Mathur SK, Krackow KA, et al: Cementless total knee arthroplasty in obese patients: A comparison with a matched control group. *J Arthroplasty* 1996;11: 153-156.

Nelissen RG, Valstar ER, Rozing PM: The effect of hydroxyapatite on the micromotion of total knee prostheses: A prospective, randomized, double-blind study. *J Bone Joint Surg Am* 1998;80:1665-1672.

Nilsson KG, Cajander S, Karrholm J: Early failure of hydroxyapatite-coating in total knee arthroplasty: A case report. *Acta Orthop Scand* 1994;65:212-214.

Nilsson KG, Karrholm J, Carlsson L, et al: Hydroxyapatite coating versus cemented fixation of the tibial component in total knee arthroplasty: Prospective randomized comparison of hydroxyapatite- coated and cemented tibial components with 5-year follow-up using radiostereometry. *J Arthroplasty* 1999;14:9-20.

Nilsson KG, Karrholm J, Ekelund L, et al: Evaluation of micromotion in cemented vs. uncemented knee arthroplasty in osteoarthrosis and rheumatoid arthritis: Randomized study using roentgen stereophotogrammetric analysis. *J Arthroplasty* 1991;6:265-278.

Onsten I, Nordqvist A, Carlsson AS, et al: Hydroxyapatite augmentation of the porous coating improves fixation of tibial components: A randomised RSA study in 116 patients. *J Bone Joint Surg Br* 1998;80:417-425.

Peters PC, Engh GA, Dwyer KA, et al: Osteolysis after total knee arthroplasty without cement. *J Bone Joint Surg Am* 1992;74:864-876.

Petersen MM, Olsen C, Lauritzen JB, et al: Changes in bone mineral density of the distal femur following uncemented total knee arthroplasty. *J Arthroplasty* 1995;10: 7-11.

Pilliar RM, Lee JM, Maniatopoulos C: Observations on the effect of movement on bone ingrowth into porous-surfaced implants. *Clin Orthop Relat Res* 1986;208:108-113.

Plante-Bordeneuve P, Freeman MAR: Tibial high-density polyethylene wear in conforming tibiofemoral prostheses. *J Bone Joint Surg Br* 1993;75:630-636.

Rader CP, Lohr J, Wittmann R, et al: Results of total arthroplasty with a metal-backed patellar component: A 6-year follow-up study. *J Arthroplasty* 1996;11:923-930.

Rand JA: Comparison of metal-backed and all-polyethylene tibial components in cruciate condylar total knee arthroplasty. *J Arthroplasty* 1993;8:307-313.

Regner L, Carlsson L, Karrholm J, et al: Ceramic coating improves tibial component fixation in total knee arthroplasty. *J Arthroplasty* 1998;13:882-889.

Ring PA: Uncemented surface replacement of the knee joint. *Clin Orthop Relat Res* 1980;148:106-111.

Robinson EJ, Mulliken BD, Bourne RB, et al: Catastrophic osteolysis in total knee replacement: A report of 17 cases. *Clin Orthop Relat Res* 1995;321:98-105.

Rosenberg AG, Andriacchi TP, Barden R, et al: Patellar component failure in cementless total knee arthroplasty. *Clin Orthop Relat Res* 1988;236:106-114.

Ryd L: Micromotion in knee arthroplasty: A roentgen stereophotogrammetric analysis of tibial component fixation. *Acta Orthop Scand Suppl* 1986; 220:1-80.

Ryd L, Lindstrand A, Stenstrom A, et al: Porous coated anatomic tricompartmental tibial components: The relationship between prosthetic position and micromotion. *Clin Orthop Relat Res* 1990;251:189-197.

Scuderi G, Insall J, Windsor R, Moran M: Survivorship of cemented knee replacements. *J Bone Joint Surg Br* 1989;71:798-803.

Stuchin SA, Ruoff M, Matarese W: Cementless total knee arthroplasty in patients with inflammatory arthritis and compromised bone. *Clin Orthop Relat Res* 1991;273: 42-51.

Stulberg SD, Stulberg BN, Hamati Y, et al: Failure mechanisms of metal-backed patellar components. *Clin Orthop Relat Res* 1988;236:88-105.

Sumner DR, Kienapfel H, Jacobs JJ, et al: Bone ingrowth and wear debris in well-fixed cementless porous-coated tibial components removed from patients. *J Arthroplasty* 1995;10:157-167.

Sumner DR, Turner TM, Dawson D, et al: Effect of pegs and screws on bone ingrowth in cementless total knee arthroplasty. *Clin Orthop Relat Res* 1994;309:150-155.

Tsao A, Mintz L, McRae C, et al: Failure of the porous-coated anatomic prosthesis in total knee arthroplasty due to severe polyethylene wear. *J Bone Joint Surg Am* 1993;75:19-26.

Vigorita VJ, Minkowitz B, Dichiara JF, et al: A histomorphometric and histologic analysis of the implant interface in five successful, autopsy-retrieved, noncemented porous-coated knee arthroplasties. *Clin Orthop Relat Res* 1993;293:211-218.

Volz RG, Nisbet JK, Lee RW, et al: The mechanical stability of various noncemented tibial components. *Clin Orthop Relat Res* 1988;226:38-42.

Wada M, Imura S, Bo A, et al: Stress fracture of the femoral component in total knee replacement: A report of 3 cases. *Int Orthop* 1997;21:54.

Walldius B: Arthroplasty of the knee using an endoprosthesis. *Clin Orthop Relat Res* 1996;331:4-10.

Whiteside LA: Cementless total knee replacement: Nine to eleven year results and ten year survivorship analysis. *Clin Orthop Relat Res* 1994;309:185-192.

Whiteside LA: Effect of porous-coating configuration on tibial osteolysis after total knee arthroplasty. *Clin Orthop Relat Res* 1995;321:92-97.

Whiteside LA: Four screws for fixation of the tibial component in cementless total knee arthroplasty. *Clin Orthop Relat Res* 1994;299:72-76.

Whiteside LA: The effect of patient age, gender, and tibial component fixation on pain relief after cementless total knee arthroplasty. *Clin Orthop Relat Res* 1991;271:21-27.

Whiteside LA, Fosco DR, Brooks JG: Fracture of the femoral component in cementless total knee arthroplasty. *Clin Orthop Relat Res* 1993;286:71-77.

Yoshii I, Whiteside L, Milliano M, et al: The effect of central stem and stem length on micromovement of the tibial tray. *J Arthroplasty* 1992;7:433-438.

Chapter 10

Total Knee Arthroplasty in Outliers

Jess H. Lonner, MD

Robert E. Booth, Jr, MD

Introduction

Predictable and sustainable pain relief and functional improvement are obtainable after total knee arthroplasty in over 90% of patients for 10 to 15 years postoperatively. Most total knee arthroplasties are performed for patients with primary degenerative osteoarthritis, minimal deformity, and reasonable motion, and standard techniques and instrumentation can be used. Although basic principles can be followed for most patients, there are outliers, which are patients with unique challenges such as extra-articular deformity, posttraumatic arthrosis, and neurologic conditions such as Parkinson's disease, recurvatum, and neuropathic arthritis who require modifications of the technique or prosthesis to correctly perform total knee arthroplasty and optimize results. Although the average age of patients undergoing total knee arthroplasty is 65 to 75 years, young and elderly patient populations also present unique challenges. In such instances, simply following a menu of standard steps is an inadequate approach to total knee arthroplasty. In essence, customizing the surgical approach, technique, and implant selection may be necessary for these unique challenges.

Extra-articular Deformity

It is common for the arthritic knee to be associated with a variable degree of localized deformity at the knee joint and soft-tissue contracture on the concavity of the deformity or laxity on the convexity. These conditions are generally addressed with adjustment of the intra-articular resection and soft-tissue release. Extra-articular deformity, however, may create a more complex scenario that cannot be treated with standard methods. These deformities include those that result after fracture malunion, periarticular osteotomy, or deformity resulting from metabolic diseases such as osteomalacia, rickets, or Paget's disease. Smaller deformities and those closer to the hip can usually be effectively treated with intra-articular bone resection perpendicular to the mechanical axis of the lower extremity and soft-tissue releases. Extra-articular deformities in excess of 10° in

the coronal plane or 20° in the sagittal plane can create a complex imbalance of the collateral ligaments if the deformity is addressed simply by modifying the intra-articular bone resection and soft-tissue releases. To avoid these problems and to reduce the need for constrained implants, corrective osteotomy before or simultaneous with total knee arthroplasty may be necessary (Figure 1). An alternative intervention is to use a modified intra-articular osteotomy that is perpendicular to the mechanical axis, but which avoids the attachments of the collateral ligaments. This may entail a limited resection of one condyle, leaving a gap that can be filled with bone graft, cement, or unicondylar wedges. This technique, however, may alter joint line position, particularly when involving the femoral condyles, and it is unclear whether the structural support in these situations would be adequate or whether the oblique shear forces of the bone-cement interfaces may compromise the stability of the implant and make it vulnerable to early failure.

The determination regarding whether a corrective osteotomy is necessary should be made with preoperative planning, using a weight-bearing full-length radiograph of the limb. Drawing the mechanical axis and the planned level of resection will help to identify whether a perpendicular resection would compromise the integrity of the insertion or origin of the collateral ligaments (Figure 2). In general, the need for corrective osteotomy depends not only on the extent of the deformity, but also on the location of the deformity relative to the knee joint. Deformities that are farther from the knee joint may be less in need of corrective osteotomy than those that are closer to the knee joint. Surgical approach will often depend on whether there is preexisting hardware that needs to be removed. Choices of fixation of the osteotomy will depend on the location of the osteotomy, bone quality, and surgeon experience. Alternatives include use of a compression plate, locked intramedullary nail, or long press-fit or cemented stem extension. There is concern that rotational stability with a press-fit stem may be inadequate, but planar oblique metaphyseal or diaphyseal osteotomies may be more

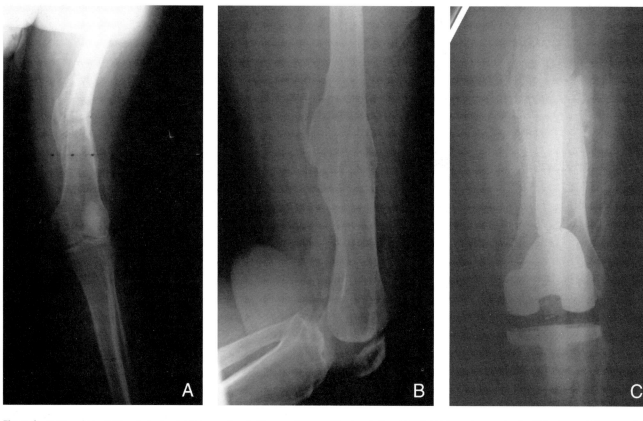

Figure 1 AP **(A)** and lateral **(B)** radiographs of right lower extremity 30 years after closed treatment of a midshaft right femur fracture showing 25° valgus malalignment of the femoral diaphysis and degenerative arthritis of the knee. **C,** Postoperative radiograph after simultaneous oblique planar corrective osteotomy of the femoral malunion and total knee arthroplasty. Rigid fixation was achieved with a press-fit stem with correction of the mechanical axis.

amenable to fixation with press-fit stems because they have more inherent rotational stability than wedge osteotomies. The risks of corrective osteotomy and total knee arthroplasty include fracture, nonunion, and arthrofibrosis as well as other potential complications typical of knees that have undergone multiple surgical procedures, such as wound healing problems, infection, patellofemoral dysfunction, and early mechanical failure. One study reported healing of all but 1 osteotomy in 11 patients treated with simultaneous femoral osteotomy and total knee arthroplasty, and restoration of the mechanical axis of the limb to within 2° of normal in each patient. Improvements in knee scores and functionality as well as an absence of instability and a minimal risk of complications were typical.

Distal Femoral or Proximal Tibial Osteotomies

Corrective osteotomy is indicated for patients with isolated medial or lateral compartmental arthritis, particularly young patients with high physical demands and some degree of deformity. Nonetheless, the extent and duration of pain relief vary, and tend to deteriorate by 7 to 10 years after surgery. Considering the limited success of periarticular osteotomy, some patients may ultimately require conversion to total knee arthroplasty. Al-

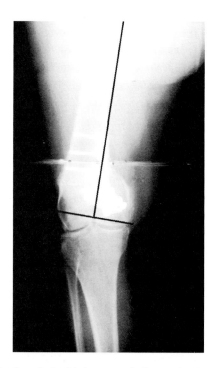

Figure 2 AP radiograph of a right lower extremity 7 years after distal femoral varus osteotomy shows considerable extra-articular malalignment of the supracondylar region of the distal femur with degenerative arthritis. Planning the level of femoral osteotomy 90° to the mechanical axis of the femur (*black lines*) shows that standard resection would compromise the attachment of the lateral collateral ligament.

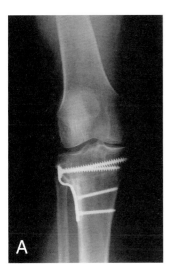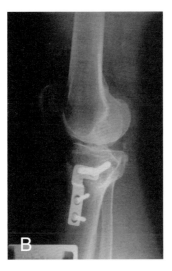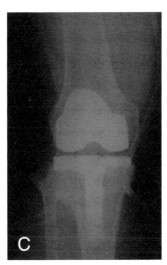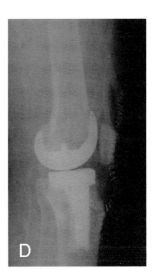

Figure 3 AP **(A)** and lateral **(B)** radiographs of a right knee after proximal tibial osteotomy shows deformity of the joint line with degenerative arthritis and retained plates. **C** and **D,** Postoperative radiographs after total knee arthroplasty and hardware removal illustrate the complexity of the procedure; a modified skin incision was used that included an L-shaped incision for hardware removal followed by a curvilinear incision that extended from the apex of the L-shaped incision and left a 7-cm bridge to avoid skin necrosis. A lateral tibial augment was used to treat bony deficiency, and a short cemented stem was used to support the implant and bypass the screw holes.

though the outcomes of total knee arthroplasty after conversion of the failed proximal tibial osteotomy have been reported extensively, there are fewer data available regarding conversion from failed distal femoral osteotomy. Nonetheless, there are several variables that complicate the facility with which total knee arthroplasty can be performed. The position of the skin incision must be taken into account. Transverse incisions can be safely bisected at a 90° angle; other curvilinear incisions make the approach for total knee arthroplasty far more complex. Strategies to minimize wound necrosis should be used, including allowance of a 6-cm bridge or in patients with multiple scars, using the lateral most incision that would not compromise the approach to the knee. Hardware may intrude into the canals and may need to be removed for placement of the total knee arthroplasty. At times all or some of the hardware may be left in place; however, this would prevent the use of intramedullary alignment systems. Extramedullary instrumentation can be useful and is accurate when appropriately used. Modifying the specific type of implant may also be necessary. The presence of screw holes in the tibial or femoral metaphyses or diaphyses may mandate the use of stemmed implants, particularly if metaphyseal bone quality is compromised. Additionally, periarticular deformity and translation of the shaft relative to the metaphysis may make it difficult to use standard implants. The use of offset stems or customized components with offset tibial keels may be necessary. Compromised intra-articular bone support may require the use of augments or cancellous bone graft (Figure 3).

Total knee arthroplasty after proximal tibial osteotomy has a potential for increased failure resulting from malalignment, compromised osseous support, extensor mechanism disruption, or infection. The preoperative evaluation for the possibility of an occult infection should be considered in patients who had previous osteotomy using an external fixator because of the risk of contaminated pin tracts. Serologic tests to determine the erythrocyte sedimentation rate and C-reactive protein level or white blood cell labeled bone scanning should be considered before knee replacement surgery; antibiotics should be mixed with cement when implanting the total knee arthroplasty. Patella baja and infrapatellar scarring, which are particularly common when the limb is immobilized after proximal tibial osteotomy, may make the exposure of the knee joint more difficult and renders the patellar tendon vulnerable to avulsion during surgery. The attachment of the patellar tendon should be protected in these instances. Tibial tubercle osteotomy or a quadriceps release may be useful to facilitate exposure and protect the patellar tendon during surgery, particularly when there is contracture of the infrapatellar tendon and patella baja. Proximalization of the tibial tubercle can be done to restore patellar height, but carries a risk of nonunion or displacement. Technically, the procedure is more demanding and failures have been reported from instability, patellar tendon avulsion, malalignment, and radiolucencies.

After varus-producing femoral osteotomy, resecting the distal femur perpendicular to the mechanical axis may result in compromise of the lateral collateral ligament attachment on the lateral femoral epicondyle. This may mandate the use of a semiconstrained or even a hinged implant, but a corrective osteotomy simultaneous with or before total knee arthroplasty may be necessary. Additionally, the extra-articular varus deformity of the femur that accompanies distal femoral varus osteotomies can create a situation in which the anatomic axis of the femur intersects the lateral femoral condyle rather than the intercondylar notch. If using an intramedullary alignment guide, the starting hole may need to be placed through the lateral femoral condyle rather than the intercondylar notch. Otherwise, it is not uncommon for the femoral component to be placed in a malaligned position. This malalignment and translocation of the femoral metaphysis presents a challenge if using a femoral stem because the prosthesis may overhang laterally (Figure 4). It may be prudent to use a short, thin, cemented stem so that the implant can be translated medially to avoid lateral overhang. One recent series reported on 11 total knee arthroplasties that were performed after distal femoral osteotomy. The authors found a high incidence of femoral varus malalignment (particularly when intramedullary instrumentation was used) and component lucencies. Additionally, knee scores were inferior to those reported in most series on primary total knee arthroplasty. As a result of the extra-articular deformity, ligamentous instability was common, requiring the use of constrained total knee arthroplasties in many patients.

Posttraumatic Arthritis

The tendency for the development of posttraumatic arthritis can be substantial in a relatively short period after tibial plateau fracture. Using survivorship analysis in the evaluation of 693 proximal tibial fractures, one study reported the incidence of posttraumatic arthrosis of the knee to be 16% at 5 years after fracture, 32% at 10 years, and 49% at 15 years.

The incidence of posttraumatic arthrosis after distal femur fractures is considerably lower, but it can occur with residual fracture malalignment or intra-articular step-off. One study reported that only 3 patients of 52 followed for 2 to 20 years after open reduction and internal fixation of intra-articular fractures of the distal femur had posttraumatic arthrosis, and no patient in this series required total knee arthroplasty during the follow-up period. In this series, however, no patient had intra-articular step-off of greater than 2 mm or residual malalignment greater than 8°, highlighting the importance of anatomic fracture reduction to minimize the risk of joint degeneration. In another series, a mean 13-year interval was observed between periarticular fracture and total knee arthroplasty, which provides evidence of the tolerance of articular cartilage to prolonged abnormal and excessive loading.

After intra-articular or periarticular fracture around the knee, malalignment, osseous defects, multiple incisional scars, arthrofibrosis, joint instability, retained hardware, and perhaps occult infection may individually or in concert need to be considered when planning and performing a total knee arthroplasty. Ultimately, this complex set of confounding variables contribute to a complication rate that may exceed 57%, with a high rate of failure resulting from infection, wound breakdown, instability, mechanical failure, stiffness, and patellar maltracking. Adherence to sound principles of surgical approach, soft-tissue balancing, and correction of limb malalignment are of paramount importance. Compromised bone support has been a common source of aseptic loosening in patients with posttraumatic arthritis. Stems can help to unload the compromised osseous support of the tibial or femoral metaphysis and can limit the risk of component subsidence (Figure 5). Cementless implants, especially after tibial plateau fracture, should be avoided because bone ingrowth with cementless arthroplasties may be inadequate, particularly because fibrous nonunions may be present. Fracture malunion may preclude the use of intramedullary alignment systems and extramedullary alignment jigs, and surgeons should become familiar with these instruments and use them during these surgical procedures (Figure 6). A 26% incidence of mechanical failure reported in one series was likely related to implant or limb malalignment. Restoring compromised osseous support is critical to avoiding premature subsidence or loosening of the prosthesis. Deficient bone should be excised and supplemented with bone graft or metallic augments; stem augmentation should be used liberally.

Wound problems have been reported in 6% of patients in one series, and this incidence could likely be reduced with adherence to specific surgical principles. Minimal skin bridges of 6 cm should be left between surgical scars if possible. Otherwise, previous surgical incisions should be used so as not to compromise wound healing. Deep flaps should be made beneath the deep fascia to avoid compromising the plexus of vessels feeding the adipose tissue and skin through the deep fascia. Additionally, the most lateral incision should be used without compromising exposure because most deep perforating vessels arise medially. Plastic surgery consultation should be sought in the event that there is adequate concern regarding the ability to safely approach the knee. Consideration should be given to rotational flaps, soft-tissue expanders, or a so-called sham incision before proceeding with arthroplasty.

When total knee arthroplasty is performed to treat patients with posttraumatic arthritis, septic failure can occur with a relatively high frequency, and a preoperative workup should be performed to exclude the possibility of occult infection. These tests should include serologic studies that assess the erythrocyte sedimentation rate and noncardiac C-reactive protein level as well as aspiration of the joint with culture and white blood cell count of fluid (white blood cell labeled scanning may occasionally be of value). Additionally, cement should be mixed with antibiotic powder during implantation to

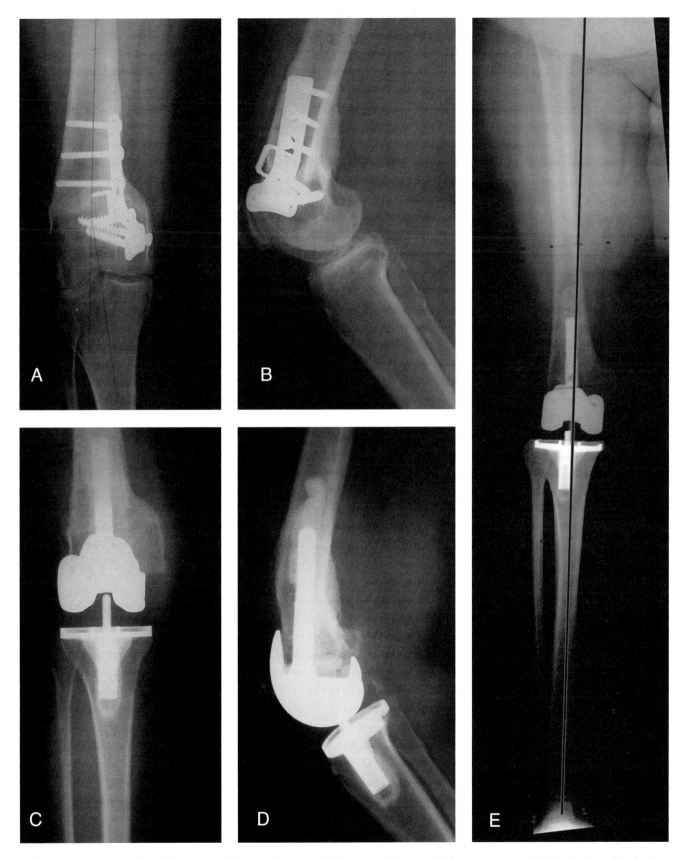

Figure 4 AP **(A)** and lateral **(B)** radiographs of a right knee showing advanced arthritis 7 years after right distal femoral osteotomy with retained hardware. Note the extra-articular deformity AP **(C)** and lateral **(D)** radiographs after total knee arthroplasty and hardware removal. Treatment involved use of a 20-mm medial augment with a skim cut of the lateral femoral condyle so as not to compromise the origin of the lateral collateral ligament and to avoid the need for corrective osteotomy. **E,** Full-length radiograph of the right lower extremity shows restoration of the mechanical axis (*vertical line*).

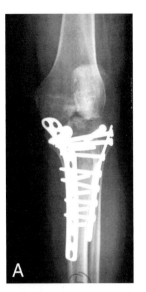
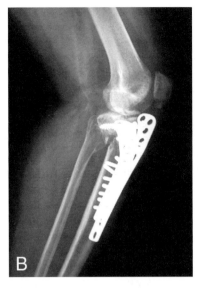
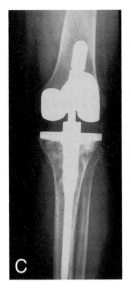
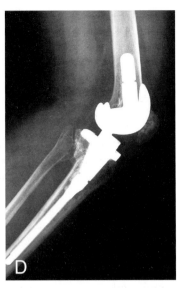

Figure 5 AP **(A)** and lateral **(B)** radiographs of a left knee after open reduction and internal fixation of a comminuted tibial plateau fracture. AP **(C)** and lateral **(D)** radiographs after conversion to a total knee arthroplasty with removal of hardware. Because of the compromised integrity of the medial collateral ligament and fibrous nonunions of the tibial metaphysis, a stemmed NexGen Legacy Constrained Condylar Knee implant (Zimmer, Warsaw, IN) was used.

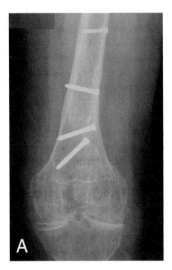
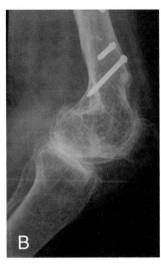
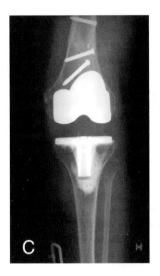
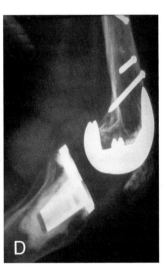

Figure 6 AP **(A)** and lateral **(B)** radiographs of a knee 40 years after open reduction and internal fixation of distal femur fracture with multiple retained screws, which are buried by subsequent bony overgrowth. Hardware removal clearly would be difficult in this situation. AP **(C)** and lateral **(D)** radiographs showing successful total knee arthroplasty with retained hardware. Extramedullary instrumentation was necessary with hardware retention.

help reduce the risk of postoperative infection, even in patients with no prior infection.

Patellar tendon avulsions or intraoperative lacerations have been reported in several series, and care must be taken during surgery to protect the extensor mechanism. Patellar maltracking is another reported complication that may be related to soft-tissue imbalance, or it may be related to difficulties in achieving appropriate rotational alignment of the tibial or femoral components in the setting of posttraumatic deformity and fracture malunion.

In one series, statistically significant improvements in Knee Society scores were found at a mean follow-up

of 46 months after total knee arthroplasty performed to treat patients with posttraumatic arthrosis of fracture of either the proximal tibia or distal femur. However, excellent or good functional scores were reported in 58% of patients and excellent or good clinical scores were reported in 71% of patients; complications occurred in 57% of patients, including aseptic failure (26%), septic failure (10%), patellar tendon rupture (3%), and wound breakdown requiring wound débridement and muscle flap coverage (6%). Component malalignment, occult infection, compromised osseous support, and multiple scars led to a large percentage of these complications. The authors recommended the judicious use of stem augmentation and correction of malunited fractures, either through modification of intra-articular resection or corrective osteotomy. The authors found a 26% incidence of accelerated mechanical failure as a result of component or limb malalignment. Another report of 62 total knee arthroplasties performed after fracture of the tibial plateau found a significant improvement in Knee Society pain and function scores at a mean follow-up of 4.7 years, but intraoperative complications occurred in 10% of patients and postoperative complications in 26%. Additionally, a 21% revision rate was reported, including manipulation in five knees, wound revision in three knees (with a local gastrocnemius flap in one), and five revisions. Deep infections occurred in two knees. Patellar avulsion occurred intraoperatively in one patient and collateral insufficiency occurred postoperatively in one patient. The incidence of postoperative complications such as scarring, malalignment, wound problems, and sepsis also remains elevated after posttraumatic arthritis related to distal femur fractures.

Parkinson's Disease

Parkinson's disease is manifested by loss of motor coordination, muscle tremors, spasticity, and occasionally mental impairment as a result of the degeneration of the substantia nigra of the basal ganglia. Total knee arthroplasty in patients with Parkinson's disease can provide considerable pain relief and significant improvement in function, but the results are inferior to those achieved in patients without Parkinson's disease. Although studies have shown reasonable outcomes, physical recovery can be prolonged and there is a higher tendency for mental confusion in the perioperative period; therefore, postoperative narcotics should be used sparingly. Additionally, ambulatory capacity will vary among patients, depending on the severity of Parkinson's disease; thus, functional recovery can vary. Those patients with considerable hamstring spasm may be particularly vulnerable to compromised functional outcomes and limited extension. Preoperative neurologic evaluation should be completed to ensure reasonable medical control, and a neurologic consultation should be sought within the immediate postoperative period. Patients with Parkinson's disease will have significantly increased functional capacity, decreased pain, and decreased length of stay following primary total knee arthroplasty with optimal use of medications and when neurologic intervention is sought during the perioperative period, compared with patients whose Parkinson's disease is not treated perioperatively.

Recurvatum

Genu recurvatum of more than 5° in the arthritic knee has been reported to occur in 0.5% to 1% of patients who are candidates for total knee arthroplasty. The eti-ology of substantial recurvatum is varied, but the implications and complexities of total knee arthroplasty and its outcomes can be substantial. Common causes of recurvatum such as the mild hyperextension deformity that often accompanies the idiopathic valgus knee deformity of rheumatoid or degenerative arthritis, or iatrogenic deformity from malunion and anterior slope of the proximal tibia after proximal tibial osteotomy are not contraindications to surgery, but can make performing total knee arthroplasty more challenging. Alternatively, patients who lack quadriceps strength because of underlying neuromuscular conditions such as poliomyelitis are at particular risk for compromised outcome and failure after total knee arthroplasty. The patient with substantial recurvatum and degenerative arthritis of the knee should therefore be evaluated for the possibility of an undiagnosed neuromuscular disorder. In patients with paralysis of the quadriceps muscle, total knee arthroplasty is generally contraindicated because of the high risk of failure from instability and recurrent recurvatum postoperatively.

Preoperative examination must also assess the posture of the foot and ankle. Patients who chronically lock the knee in hyperextension to ambulate may have a concomitant ipsilateral equinus contracture that may need to be corrected before total knee arthroplasty to minimize the ongoing tendency of hyperextension of the knee after surgery. A more constrained implant or hinged implant may be necessary to address the hyperextension instability that is common in these patients, particularly those with a paralytic etiology of recurvatum. In patients with paralytic or paretic conditions of the knee, it may be desirable to leave the knee in slight hyperextension, which may allow patients to continue to ambulate by compensating for the quadriceps weakness by swinging the knee into hyperextension to lock it so that it does not buckle during heel strike or the stance phase of gait. Patients with considerable extensor mechanism weakness should be counseled preoperatively that a postoperative brace might be necessary to allow them to ambulate without drop lock buckling. Although intentionally leaving the limb with 5° to 10° of residual recurvatum and laxity in extension may be desirable for those with quadriceps paresis for functional reasons, it may predispose patients to instability and loosening.

When the recurvatum is not associated with paresis or paralysis of the quadriceps, accurate balancing of the flexion and extension spaces is paramount. Correcting extension laxity is important for preserving the longevity of the implant and for minimizing the risk of recurrent recurvatum. The extension gap can be decreased to equal the flexion gap by underresecting the distal femur, using augments on the distal femur to lower the joint line (in which instance use of a stem is advisable), transferring the collateral ligaments proximally and posteriorly, or plicating the posterior capsule. The latter two options are difficult, whereas results with the former two are generally more reproducible and pose less risk for recurrent deformity. If posterior cruciate ligament–retaining implants are used, then resection or release of the posterior cruciate ligament with an implant of appropriate topography can render the flexion space slightly larger in size, which may equalize the flexion/extension spaces. An additional alternative is to resect additional bone from the posterior femoral condyles and use a smaller femoral component. In other words, the options involve either reducing the extension space or increasing the flexion space to balance the flexion and extension gaps.

Neuropathic Arthropathy

Neuropathic arthropathy, commonly referred to as Charcot arthropathy, is a degenerative condition of the joint accompanied by varying degrees of joint destruction and fragmentation that results from impaired proprioception and compromised periarticular sensation. It can be associated with diseases such as diabetes mellitus, tabes dorsalis from tertiary syphilis, congenital indifference to pain, syringomyelia, and vitamin B_{12} deficiency. The joint initially appears swollen and unstable, but the extent of joint destruction often far exceeds the tolerable degree of pain. An inability to sense or respond to alterations in joint loads or microtrauma may account for the significant destruction of the knee joint in these patients. The knee joint is perhaps the most frequently affected large joint in the setting of neuropathic disease. Patients with neuropathic joints should be evaluated for the etiology of this particular problem, including serologic tests for syphilis, glucose levels, vitamin B_{12} levels, and thiamine levels. The true cause of the neuropathic arthropathy often may be elusive.

Traditionally, neuropathy of the knee was considered a contraindication to total knee arthroplasty, and bracing or fusion was recommended. However, as the staging of Charcot arthropathy has become better understood and surgical techniques and design of modern prostheses have evolved, better outcomes are achievable with total knee arthroplasty. The deformity, bone loss, and instability of the neuropathic knee present technical challenges, which should be addressed with stem extensions to offset the insufficient metaphyseal bone, with metallic augments or bone graft to address bone loss, and occasionally with semiconstrained or hinged implants to address significant ligamentous instability. Additionally, many early failures were associated with undetected neurosyphilis, but this incidence has declined with improvements in antibiotics and neurosyphilis detection. Neuropathic knee arthrosis is currently most often the result of diabetes mellitus, and treatment results in this segment of the patient population are far superior to those with neurosyphilis.

Charcot arthropathy can be divided into stages. The earlier inflammatory and fragmentation stages are inopportune times to perform total knee arthroplasty; the surgery is best postponed until the reconstructive or coalescence stages of the disease process. Total knee arthroplasty can provide excellent pain relief but variable improvement in joint function in patients with Charcot arthropathy of the knee. At 7.9-year follow-up (range, 2 to 15 years), significant improvements in Knee Society pain and function scores and range of motion in 29 patients who underwent total knee arthroplasty for Charcot arthropathy were reported. Augments or bone grafting were used commonly, as were stem extensions and semiconstrained or hinged implants. Complications included periprosthetic fracture, aseptic loosening, and instability. Nonetheless, the results of total knee arthroplasty were only slightly inferior to those performed for patients with other diseases.

Young Patient Population

Highly active and athletically oriented young patients are at risk for a variety of ligamentous and chondral injuries that may promote degenerative arthritis in this patient population. Total knee arthroplasty is particularly challenging in young patients with degenerative arthritis. These patients tend to be more active than their elderly counterparts, subject the implants to greater cyclical loads, and thereby risk early failure. Because of their higher activity levels, young patients with degenerative arthritis have unique treatment challenges after knee replacement surgery that are not necessarily relevant to elderly patients who undergo total knee arthroplasty or other young patients with inflammatory arthritis. Although total knee arthroplasty is not desirable in the young active patient population, with some patients other nonsurgical or surgical alternatives are no longer viable or they have failed. Multiple scars, arthrofibrosis, malalignment, or prior surgical deformities from osteotomy or trauma create a technically challenging and potentially compromised environment for total knee arthroplasty. One series reported the results of patients 55 years of age or younger who underwent total knee arthroplasty for osteoarthrosis at a mean follow-up of 8 years; the average Hospital for Special Surgery knee score improved from 55 to 92. The authors reported an overall anticipated 18-year survival rate of 94%, although when patellar revision or spacer exchanges were included in failures, the expected survivorship was reduced to 87% at 18 years. In this series, activity level improved in all but two patients. In another series that reported the results of patients 40 years of age or younger who underwent total knee arthroplasty for degenerative osteoarthritis at a mean follow-up of 7.9 years, the average Knee Society knee scores increased from 47 to 88 points and function scores increased from 45 to 70 points. Overall, Knee Society knee scores were considered good or excellent in 82% of patients, but postoperative function scores were good or excellent in only 40% of knees. If workers' compensation cases were excluded, Knee Society knee scores were good or excellent in 91% of patients and function scores were good or excellent in 50% of patients. The aseptic failure rate in this patient population was 13% at 8-year follow-up and occurred more commonly in patients who underwent multiple prior surgeries, such as osteotomies.

An additional complex subset of patients in the younger age group is made up of patients who are involved in workers' compensation claims; these patients have been shown to do relatively poorly despite reasonable objective findings. In one series evaluating the impact of workers' compensation claims, of 42 patients undergoing total knee arthroplasty, the results at a mean follow-up of 80 months were significantly worse in those patients receiving compensation compared with those who were not receiving compensation despite similar objective parameters in range of motion, stability, and radiographic alignment.

Elderly Patient Population

As the population continues to age, active and healthy patients older than 80 years are more frequently undergoing total knee arthroplasty. There is concern that even healthy octogenarians and nonagenarians present too great of a surgical risk because of limited reserves to withstand the physiologic stress of total knee arthroplasty. Nonetheless, the disabling pain of arthritis often interferes with the quality of life of these elderly patients, making total knee arthroplasty a reasonable consideration. Several studies have reported excellent results in patients in their 80s and 90s with limited complications. One study found that octogenarians had better relief of pain after total knee arthroplasty than younger patients, and improvements in pain and functionality were more predictable in elderly patients. The need for an assisted ambulatory device after surgery decreased in one series from 74% of nonagenarian patients to 51% after total knee arthroplasty. The primary complication reported in octogenarians and nonagenarians is confusion. This condition can be minimized by limiting narcotic analgesics, reducing the tendency for fat embolism by using extramedullary instrumentation or evacuating and decompressing marrow contents from the intramedullary canal if intramedullary instrumentation is used, expediting the surgical procedure, correcting anemia, treating hypoxia, and potentially by avoiding bilateral total knee arthroplasty. For most patients in this population, confusion is transient and resolves in a matter of days. Other postoperative medical complications such as urinary retention, cardiac events, pulmonary embolism, gastrointestinal bleeding, or ileus are

rare and also tend to resolve without permanent sequelae. The mortality rate among octogenarians and nonagenarians after total knee arthroplasty ranges from 0 to as high as 3.6%.

Summary

In the performance of total knee arthroplasties, just as in any human endeavor, there is a Gaussian distribution of precipitating pathologies as well as the surgical skills to address them. Standard or cookbook surgical approaches are unlikely to routinely produce the anticipated good results from total knee arthroplasty, particularly when applied to patients with any of the unique conditions previously described. Although average techniques typically yield average results, outliers thus treated will have uncertain results that may defy successful revision.

The first obligation of the orthopaedic surgeon is to identify the uniqueness of a special situation. Then a plan should be formulated to address its particular challenges (structural, biologic, neurologic, or sociologic). Although fostered by standardized instruments and codified surgical techniques, the temptation must be resisted to reduce outliers to the mean or to a final common pathway. In essence, customizing total knee arthroplasty to the less common but special conditions encountered will optimize its results.

Annotated Bibliography

Extra-articular Deformity

Lonner JH, Siliski JM, Lotke PA: Simultaneous femoral osteotomy and total knee arthroplasty for treatment of osteoarthritis associated with severe extra-articular deformity. *J Bone Joint Surg Am* 2000;82:342-348.

At a mean follow-up of 46 months, mean Knee Society function scores increased from 22 to 81, knee scores from 10 to 87, and arc of motion from 56° to 89° in 11 patients treated with simultaneous corrective femoral osteotomy and total knee arthroplasty. Mechanical alignment was restored to within 2° of normal with each patient, and all but one osteotomy healed.

Wang JW, Wang CJ: Total knee arthroplasty for arthritis of the knee with extra-articular deformity. *J Bone Joint Surg Am* 2002;84-A:1769-1774.

In this study, 15 total knee arthroplasties were performed in patients with degenerative arthritis with associated extra-articular deformities of the femur or tibia. The average angle of the femoral deformity was 15.1° in the coronal plane and 8.1° in the sagittal plane; the average tibial deformity was 19° in the coronal plane. Each patient was treated with intra-articular bone resection perpendicular to the mechanical axis and soft-tissue balancing without a need for corrective osteotomy. All implants were either posterior cruciate retraining or substituting; additional constraint was not required. At a mean follow-up of 38 months, the average Knee Society knee score improved from 22 to 92 and the average function score improved from 28 to 87.

Distal Femoral or Proximal Tibial Osteotomies
Nelson CL, Saleh KJ, Kassim RA, et al: Total knee arthroplasty after varus osteotomy of the distal part of the femur. *J Bone Joint Surg Am* 2003;85-A:1062-1065.

Total knee arthroplasty was performed in 11 knees after distal femoral osteotomy. The average patient age was 44 years, and the mean follow-up was 5 years. Mean Knee Society knee scores increased from 35 to 84 and function scores increased from 49 to 68. A constrained implant was necessary in 5 of 11 knees. Mean radiographic alignment was 3° of valgus, with a range of 1° to 6° valgus at latest follow-up. The authors noted that the surgery was technically demanding and associated with a tendency to place the femoral component in relative varus angulation (< 5° of valgus).

Parvizi J, Hanssen AD, Spangehl MJ: Total knee arthroplasty following proximal tibial osteotomy: Risk factors for failure. *J Bone Joint Surg Am* 2004;86-A:474-479.

In this study, 166 total knee arthroplasties were performed after prior proximal tibial osteotomy, and patients were followed for a mean of 15 years. A high rate of radiographic evidence of loosening (8% of patients) was observed at a mean 6-year follow-up. Male gender, increased weight, young age at the time of total knee arthroplasty, coronal laxity, and preoperative limb malalignment were considered risk factors for early failure.

Posttraumatic Arthritis
Saleh KJ, Sherman P, Katkin P, et al: Total knee arthroplasty after open reduction and internal fixation of fractures of the tibial plateau. *J Bone Joint Surg Am* 2001; 83-A:1144-1148.

The authors conducted a retrospective analysis of 15 total knee arthroplasties performed an average of 39 months after open reduction and internal fixation of a fractured tibial plateau. At an average follow-up of 6 years, the average Hospital for Special Surgery knee score improved from 51 to 80. Range of motion increased from a mean of 87° preoperatively to 105° postoperatively, but there was a high incidence of infections (20%) and patellar tendon disruptions (13%).

Weiss NJ, Parvizi J, Hanssen AD, Trousdale RT, Lewallen DG: Total knee arthroplasty in post-traumatic arthrosis of the knee. *J Arthroplasty* 2003;18(3 suppl 1):23-26.

In this study, 78% of patients who underwent total knee arthroplasty after prior tibial plateau fracture and 52% who underwent total knee arthroplasty after prior femoral fracture had good or excellent results. Complications included patellar tendon rupture, wound necrosis or dehiscence, stiffness, deep infection, and instability. Fifty-two percent of patients who underwent total knee arthroplasty after prior femoral fracture had acceptable restoration of limb alignment, correction of deformity, and adequate tibial and femoral component position-

ing compared with 77% of those who underwent total knee arthroplasty after prior tibial fracture.

Weiss NG, Parvizi J, Trousdale RT, Bryce RD, Lewallen DG: Total knee arthroplasty in patients with a prior fracture of the tibial plateau. *J Bone Joint Surg Am* 2003;85-A:218-221.

The authors of this study reviewed 62 total knee arthroplasties that were performed after prior fracture of the tibial plateau. At a mean follow-up of 4.7 years, significant improvement was noted in Knee Society scores, but 13 reoperations were necessary, including manipulation under anesthesia (5 knees), wound revision (3 knees), and component revision (5 knees). A 10% intraoperative complication rate and a 26% postoperative complication rate were reported.

Parkinson's Disease
Mehta S, Van Kleunen JP, Booth RE Jr, Lotke PA, Lonner JH: Total knee arthroplasty in patients with Parkinson's disease, in *Proceedings of the 71st Annual Meeting.* Rosemont, IL, American Academy of Orthopaedic Surgeons, 2004, p 448.

The authors of this study reported that patients with Parkinson's disease who had a neurologic consultation either preoperative or immediately postoperatively had a shorter length of stay (2.5 days shorter), a 19-point increase in Knee Society pain scores, and a 19-point increase in Knee Society function scores when compared with patients who underwent delayed neurologic consultation.

Recurvatum
Giori NJ, Lewallen DG: Total knee arthroplasty in limbs affected by poliomyelitis. *J Bone Joint Surg Am* 2002;84-A:1157-1161.

The authors reported that quadriceps strength affected outcomes in patients with poliomyelitis who underwent total knee arthroplasty. Knee Society pain and clinical scores were reported to have improved in limbs that had at least antigravity quadriceps strength before surgery; however, declining Knee Society function scores were noted in a large percentage of patients regardless of quadriceps strength.

Meding JB, Keating EM, Ritter MA, et al: Total knee replacement in patients with genu recurvatum. *Clin Orthop* 2001;393:244-249.

In this study, 57 total knee arthroplasties were performed in 53 patients with at least 5° of hyperextension deformity. The average recurvatum was 11°, but no instances of neuromuscular etiology were identified preoperatively. At a mean follow-up of 4.5 years, postoperative knee extension averaged 0° (range, 10° of hyperextension to 10° flexion contracture). Using a posterior cruciate ligament–retaining implant in all patients, only 3.5% of knees (two patients) had hyperextension deformities after surgery (10° each). No revisions were necessary.

Neuropathic Arthropathy

Parvizi J, Marrs J, Morrey BF: Total knee arthroplasty for neuropathic (Charcot) joints. *Clin Orthop* 2003;416: 145-150.

The authors of this study reviewed 40 total knee arthroplasties that were performed in 29 patients with Charcot arthropathy and reported the results at a mean follow-up of 8 years. Significant improvements were noted in Knee Society pain and function scores and range of motion. Metal augments, bone grafting, and stems were necessary for a large percentage of patients. Despite the success reported, six reoperations were necessary to treat periprosthetic fractures, aseptic loosening, instability, and infection.

Young Patient Population

Lonner JH, Hershman S, Mont M, Lotke PA: Total knee arthroplasty in patients 40 years of age and younger with osteoarthritis. *Clin Orthop* 2000;380:85-90.

At a mean follow-up of 8 years, the authors of this study reported that in 32 total knee arthroplasties performed for osteoarthritis, Knee Society knee scores increased from 47 to 88 points and function scores increased from 45 to 70 points. Knee Society knee scores were considered good or excellent in 82% of patients and function scores were considered good or excellent in 40%. Excluding patients receiving workers' compensation, knee scores were good or excellent in 91% of patients, but function scores were only good or excellent in 50%. There was an aseptic failure rate of 12.5% at 8-year follow-up.

Elderly Patient Population

Berend ME, Thong AE, Faris GW, Newbern G, Pierson JL, Ritter MA: Total joint arthroplasty in the extremely elderly: Hip and knee arthroplasty after entering the 89th year of life. *J Arthroplasty* 2003;18:817-821.

In this study, 101 total hip or total knee arthroplasties were performed in 83 patients who were 89 years of age or older. Thirty-one percent of patients died at a mean follow-up of 2.5 years (3.6% died within the first 2 months after surgery). Excluding deaths, the perioperative medical complication rate was 14%; complications included decubitus ulcer, urinary tract infection, cardiopulmonary events, and perforated bowel.

Joshi AB, Gill G: Total knee arthroplasty in nonagenarians. *J Arthroplasty* 2002;17:681.

In this study, 20 total knee arthroplasties were performed in 18 patients who were 90 years of age or older. One postoperative death occurred within 90 days of surgery. At 62-month follow-up, only one surgical complication (wound dehiscence) was reported, but 26% of the surviving patients had medical complications, and the average length of hospital stay was 10 days. Although pain relief was typical and Knee Society knee scores were excellent in all patients, none of the patients had excellent function scores.

Pagnano MW, McLamb LA, Trousdale RT: Total knee arthroplasty for patients 90 years of age and older. *Clin Orthop* 2004;418:179-183.

The authors of this study performed 51 total knee arthroplasties in 41 patients who were 90 years of age or older. Clinical and functional outcomes were excellent at a minimum follow-up of 2 years, with the average Knee Society pain score improving from 29 to 87. One early postoperative death occurred; transient postoperative confusion, urinary retention, new onset of atrial fibrillation, upper gastrointestinal bleeding, ileus, pneumonia, and electrolyte imbalance were common complications in the early postoperative period.

Classic Bibliography

Belmar CJ, Barth T, Lonner JH, Lotke PA: Total knee arthroplasty in patients 90 years of age and older. *J Arthroplasty* 1999;14:911-914.

Chow GH, Hohl M: Osteoarthritis of the knee following tibial plateau fracture: A survivorship analysis, in *Proceedings of the 1992 Annual Meeting*. Park Ridge, IL, American Academy of Orthopaedic Surgeons, 1992, p 65.

Diduch DR, Insall JN, Scott WN, et al: Total knee replacement in young active patients. Long term follow up and functional outcome. *J Bone Joint Surg Am* 1997;79: 575-582.

Duffy GP, Trousale RT: Total knee arthroplasty in patients with Parkinson's disease. *J Arthroplasty* 1996;11: 899-904.

Hosick WB, Lotke PA, Baldwin A: Total knee arthroplasty in patients 80 years of age and older. *Clin Orthop* 1994;(299):77.

Lonner JH, Pedlow FX, Siliski JM: Total knee arthroplasty for posttraumatic arthrosis of the knee. *J Arthroplasty* 1999;14:969-975.

Mont MA, Meyerson JA, Krackow KA, Hungerford DS: Total knee arthroplasty in patients receiving workers' compensation. *J Bone Joint Surg Am* 1998;80:1285-1290.

Siliski JM, Mahring M, Hofer HP: Supracondylar-intercondylar fractures of the femur. *J Bone Joint Surg Am* 1989;71:95-104.

Vince KG, Insall JN, Bannerman CE: Total knee arthroplasty in the patients with Parkinson's disease. *J Bone Joint Surg Br* 1989;71:51.

Younger AS, Duncan CP, Masri BM: Surgical exposures in revision total knee arthroplasty. *J Am Acad Orthop Surg* 1998;6:55-64.

Zicat B, Rorabeck CH, Bourne RB: Total knee arthroplasty in the octogenarian. *J Arthroplasty* 1993;8:395.

Chapter 11

Revision Total Knee Arthroplasty

Khaled J. Saleh, MD, MSc (Epid), FRCSC, FACS

Kevin J. Mulhall, MD, MCh, FRCSI (TR & Orth)

Issada Thongtrangan, MD

Robert L. Barrack, MD

Introduction

As total knee arthroplasty (TKA) is increasingly performed in a younger and more active population with a longer life expectancy, the number of TKA revisions will inevitably increase as time-dependent implant failures occur. Although 19,138 TKA revision procedures were performed in the United States in 1995, a marked growth in this incidence can be expected in the coming years.

TKA revision procedures are typically more complex than primary TKA procedures. They are associated with greater potential complications for the patient, less favorable implant survival profiles, and greater surgical complexity and expense. It is therefore necessary to optimize patient-, surgeon-, and implant-dependent factors to obtain the best possible results.

It is of critical importance at the outset to determine the specific etiology of failure in each patient. This is facilitated with a thorough patient assessment, including physical examination and judicious use of ancillary tests. The appropriate steps in the process then include careful preoperative planning and determination of technical issues and the need for any special instrumentation, specific implants, and other supplementary reconstructive materials such as grafts. The surgeon must be able to perform adequate exposures and safe extraction of components while preserving the extensor mechanism and native bone. Reconstruction can then proceed according to the principles of restoring stability, kinematics, and the joint line while restoring or replacing bone loss and obtaining stable well-aligned components.

Patient Evaluation

History

Because certain patient characteristics are associated with greater risks of both aseptic and septic failure and with potential complications to the revision procedure, the initial history should focus on identifying these factors. Conditions such as diabetes mellitus, rheumatoid arthritis, immunosuppression, and prolonged steroid treatment have all been associated with a higher incidence of infection and wound-healing problems. An increased risk of deep infection occurs in those with renal failure, diabetes, acquired immunodeficiency syndrome (with a CD4 cell count < 200/μL), psoriasis, rheumatoid arthritis, or systemic lupus erythematosus. Multiple previous knee operations may predispose patients to higher rates of infection and implant failure. Preoperative stiffness, which often limits range of motion postoperatively, should be discussed with the patient as a potential problem. However, it is notable that patients with long-standing disease are more often satisfied with their outcomes than patients with a short duration of disease.

The history should elicit the location, character, severity, and timing of symptoms as well as identify the precipitating or alleviating factors of pain. The relationship of any symptoms to the original surgery should also be established. This information can then be used to accurately direct further investigations. For example, continuation or progression of preoperative pain combined with a stiff knee may indicate an extrinsic etiology, pain since arthroplasty combined with pain at rest may suggest infection, start-up or activity-related pain of recent onset may imply aseptic loosening, and difficulty rising from a chair or negotiating stairs in the presence of good knee motion may suggest tibiofemoral instability. However, if the stiffness has gradually occurred since the time of arthroplasty and is accompanied by pain, there should always be a high index of suspicion of the presence of deep periprosthetic infection.

Physical Examination

Physical examination in patients undergoing TKA revision begins with inspection, with assessment of previous incisions and any skin lesions or vascular changes. Active and passive ranges of motion are recorded, and special attention should be given to the extensor mechanism. Any quadriceps lag and fixed flexion contractures are documented, as is quadriceps strength. Patellar clunking, patellar subluxation, and poor patellar tracking are all common forms of failure that can be detected during physical examination. An effusion or any painful areas should also be documented.

Stability to varus-valgus and anteroposterior stress should be evaluated, as should any rotational instability. Overall alignment of the limb and rotational deformity, if noted, should be carefully evaluated to determine the source of the deformity. Assessment of anteroposterior stability with the knee flexed deserves special emphasis because flexion instability is a frequent cause of painful knee dysfunction. It may be useful to assess the knee with the patient in a sitting position with the foot resting on the floor. The patient is often more relaxed in this position and marked posterior sag often can be observed, particularly in patients with failed cruciate ligament–retaining prostheses (Figure 1). The foot is stabilized, and anterior and posterior drawer tests with the patient sitting can be performed. Standard anterior and posterior drawer tests are then performed along with a quadriceps active test and the posterior sag sign is assessed at 60° hip and 90° knee flexion. Finally, the neurologic and vascular status of the limb should be assessed and compared with that of the contralateral limb.

As pain from hip or spine pathology may commonly radiate to the knee, every knee examination should be accompanied by a thorough spine and hip examination and additional studies when appropriate. For patients with pain referred from the hip joint, an intra-articular injection of local anesthetic into the hip joint is often extremely helpful in differentiating the pain source. Bursitis of the iliotibial or pes anserinus bursa tends to cause localized pain and may respond to anesthetic and steroid injection.

Finally, the patient's mental health, employment status, and environment may be contributing factors to a poor outcome and should be evaluated. A disparity between the patient's subjective level of symptoms and objective physical findings may result from referred pain or may be magnified for secondary gain. Any legal issues involved should also be noted and preferably resolved before any proposed surgery.

Diagnostic Investigations

Laboratory

Routine blood tests should be part of the workup of all patients before TKA revision surgery. The possibility of infection should always be suspected when evaluating any painful, loose knee arthroplasty. Although individually nonspecific and nondiagnostic, an elevated white blood cell count, erythrocyte sedimentation rate, or C-reactive protein level raises the index of suspicion of an infected TKA. The most important test in determining the presence of deep periprosthetic infection is an aspirate of synovial fluid for leukocyte differential count and culture. Synovial fluid samples with a leukocyte count less than 2,000/μL and a differential with fewer than 50% polymorphonuclear cells have a 98% negative predictive value for the absence of infection. Gram-positive stains of revision aspirate do not have adequate sensitivity (14.7%) to be

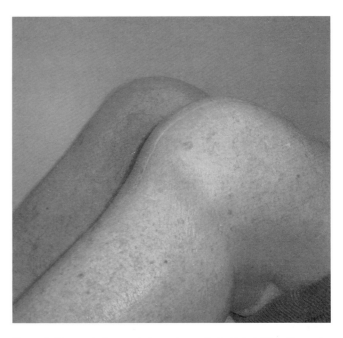

Figure 1 Photograph shows posterior sag in a patient with instability with a posterior cruciate-retaining primary knee arthroplasty.

helpful in identifying periprosthetic infection and do not rule out the presence of infection. Although there are instances in which surgeons are clearly comfortable that no infection exists, it is recommended that aspiration be routinely performed and repeated if necessary before a TKA revision is undertaken in patients in whom any doubt exists. It is important that all antibiotics be discontinued at least 4 to 6 weeks before the aspiration. Intraoperative frozen section, demonstrating 10 or more polymorphonuclear leukocytes per high power field, is also sensitive and specific in the diagnosis of infection and should be performed at the time of TKA revision when there is any suspicion of infection (Figure 2).

Recently, interleukins (cytokines) and tartrate resistant acid phosphatase concentrations in synovial fluid aspirates have been shown to be significantly higher in patients undergoing TKA revision compared with those undergoing primary TKA. Although such findings are of interest, it remains to be determined what role these and other immunologically based findings will have in the diagnostic armamentarium.

Imaging Studies

Appropriate radiographs are mandatory for TKA revision assessment and procedural planning. Weight-bearing long leg AP, lateral, and skyline patellar views are often useful. These views are used for sizing, bone stock assessment, implant position, and alignment. In assessing bone stock, femoral osteolysis is usually most severe adjacent to the femoral condyles. On the AP radiograph, severe osteolytic bone destruction appears as a radiolucency, often with a sclerotic border expanding toward the cortical margins of

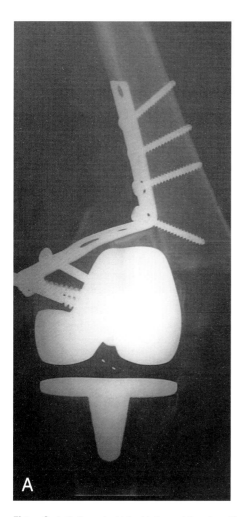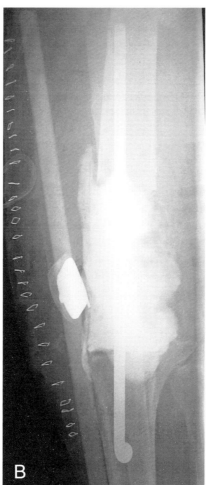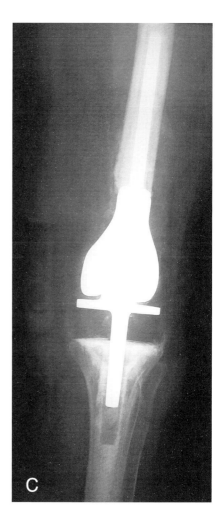

Figure 2 **A,** Radiograph obtained before revision of an elderly patient with failure of internal fixation for periprosthetic fracture. Erythrocyte sedimentation rate and C-reactive protein levels were elevated preoperatively, which increased suspicion of superimposed infection. During revision surgery, purulent material was found and frozen section analysis confirmed infection. Because of extensive bone loss of the distal femur secondary to ununited fracture and infection and the patient's advanced age, a two-stage revision was performed, with resection of the infected, largely necrotic distal femur and placement of a fixed antibiotic spacer **(B)**. The patient was treated with additional parenteral antibiotics for 6 weeks at which point all markers were normal. The knee was then reconstructed using a distal femoral replacement and antibiotic laden cement **(C)**. There was no recurrence of infection at 1-year follow-up.

the metaphyseal bone. On the lateral radiograph, a sclerotic rim of bone often demarcates these lesions.

Radiographs typically underestimate the actual bone loss found intraoperatively. Osteolytic lesions in the distal femur up to 36 mm may even be missed entirely on routine films; therefore, investigators have recommended oblique radiographs in follow-up, particularly in patients with posterior-stabilized implants (Figure 3). Radiographs of the contralateral knee can also help in the assessment of joint line height using the fibular head and femoral epicondyles as corresponding reference points. Additional radiographs such as varus/valgus stress views may also occasionally be indicated when immobility is a concern.

Patients can report a painful knee after TKA when a diagnosis of implant loosening is clinically suspected but not confirmed on standard radiographs. Additional relevant imaging studies should be directed by positive physical or radiographic findings. Technetium Tc 99m (^{99m}Tc)

screening is occasionally used, but tends to be more instructive when negative and thus refuting a diagnosis of deep infection or aseptic loosening. It is important to remember that increased scan activity may persist for prolonged periods after arthroplasty, particularly in patients with cementless prostheses; therefore, the value of ^{99m}Tc screening in the first 12 months after arthroplasty is questionable and rarely of much use. Indium-111 leukocyte scanning may provide additional information in patients with suspected infections; it is a sensitive but only moderately specific diagnostic tool. False-positive results can occur in association with rheumatoid arthritis, massive osteolysis, and up to 14 months after undergoing cementless TKAs. False-negative results may occur with chronic and indolent infections. Combined techniques using ^{99m}Tc screening, indium-111 leukocyte scanning, and sulfur-colloid imaging appear to increase the accuracy of radiographic imaging tests.

Fluoroscopic examinations in various planes may help delineate any mechanical problems. Several studies have proposed the additional value and even the superiority of fluoroscopy over plain radiography for assessing radiolucencies in TKAs. The advantage of using this adjunct technique is that loosening can be excluded with greater confidence and workup can subsequently be directed toward other potential sources.

CT may be useful in detecting malrotation of the femoral component by using the epicondylar axis as a landmark. The role of CT in the detection of osteolysis is still debatable; however, periprosthetic osteolytic lesions seem to be better detected using three-dimensional CT.

Traditional MRI is often nondiagnostic because of significant metal artifact. In one series, 41 patients with persistent pain after TKA had MRI scans that were tailored to reduce metallic susceptibility artifact. The findings led to surgical or other therapeutic interventions in 20 patients and influenced clinical treatment in all patients. This suggests that optimized MRI, in which the metallic artifact is diminished, can be a clinically useful adjunct to traditional imaging techniques in the evaluation of patients with painful TKA.

Modes of Failure

There is obviously a wide spectrum of causes of failure in TKA. Failure may occur early or late after implantation, and such failures may be multifactorial or related to specific factors, which can in turn be patient-, surgeon-, and/or procedure-related. A recent retrospective review determined that more than half of the revisions in a single series were performed less than 2 years after the primary TKA.

Aseptic Loosening

Surgical technique, poor patient selection, poor compliance, poor implant design factors, or combinations of these factors can ultimately lead to aseptic loosening. An accurate diagnosis as to the precise mechanism underlying loosening will help minimize the risk of a recurrence of the same mechanism of failure after the TKA revision procedure. Good quality plain radiographs are imperative for assessment of these patients and will often reveal the diagnosis after critical analysis. Current radiographs should be sequentially compared with previous films to establish any change in prosthesis position, progressive radiolucencies, polyethylene wear, or radiographic signs of infection. In one series, radiographs were diagnostic in 91% of patients, demonstrating complete radiolucencies (80%), polyethylene wear (43%), component breakage (5%), metallic debris (3%), patellar subluxation or dislocation (4%) (Figure 4), and osteolysis (4%).

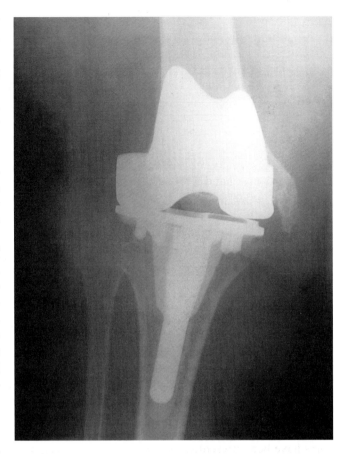

Figure 3 Radiograph showing gross osteolysis on the femoral side largely obstructed by the femoral component but appreciated on the medial side with lysis of the condyle and subsidence of the articular aspect of the component approximately to the level of the epicondyle.

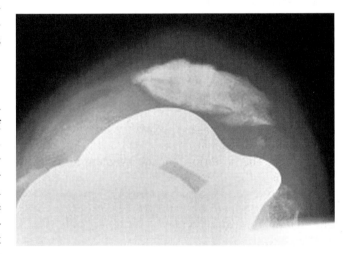

Figure 4 Radiograph showing patellar subluxation that required complete revision of femoral and tibial components to correct malalignment.

Deep Infection

Once the fixation status of a symptomatic TKA has been established, the most critical next step is differentiating aseptic from septic loosening. It has been found that revision procedures are associated with up to three times the rate of infection encountered in primary TKA. Although the problem of infection in TKA is discussed in chapter 15, it must be emphasized that with compromised tissues and host, extensive hardware and allograft use, and prolonged surgical time, the issue of infection is of critical importance in TKA revision surgery. Because surgical duration longer than 2.5 hours has been found to significantly increase the risk of infection, it is essential to perform these complex procedures with clear and adequate planning and the necessary expertise on hand to expedite the procedures.

Flexion Instability

Flexion instability seems to be an underrecognized cause of persistent pain and functional problems in patients who have undergone posterior cruciate ligament–retaining TKA. The patient with flexion instability commonly has a TKA implant that is radiographically well aligned and well fixed, that is stable to varus and valgus stress in full extension, and has an excellent arc of motion. Careful examination of the degree of AP laxity, particularly in flexion, is important if the diagnosis of flexion instability is suspected, as discussed previously. The typical patient with flexion instability has pain, recurrent swelling, generalized knee tenderness, and a sense of instability about the knee. When those symptoms have been present since the index TKA, it suggests that the flexion gap was left unbalanced. An excessive flexion gap may result from numerous technical errors, including overresection of the posterior femoral condyles (from undersizing the femoral component) and excessive tibial slope. The functional effect of each of these technical errors can be magnified when coupled with a tibial component that is flat in the sagittal plane.

Flexion instability may also occur in patients in whom the TKA functioned well for a period but subsequently have the typical constellation of pain and problems suggestive of flexion instability. This instability may be the result of failure of the posterior cruciate ligament, often through attrition and/or posterior polyethylene wear. The posterior cruciate ligament in these patients may be intrinsically weak secondary to age-related degenerative changes, or it may have been weakened after inadvertent iatrogenic injury or from the reactivation of rheumatoid disease. Finally, TKAs that are too tight in flexion early after surgery may progress to rupture the posterior cruciate ligament, which can lead to an improvement in flexion but also to flexion instability.

Flexion instability after primary posterior cruciate ligament–retaining TKA can be addressed successfully by revision of the TKA to a posterior-stabilized implant. However, because balance of the flexion and extension spaces confers stability to these knees, careful attention must be given to balance of the flexion and extension gaps at the time of the revision procedure. It has been found that the posterior-stabilized TKA facilitates balancing of the flexion and extension spaces and thus is the implant of choice when revising a posterior cruciate ligament–retaining TKA for flexion instability. Revision procedures that included only insertion of a thick tibial polyethylene have been unreliable because insertion of a thick liner does not address the underlying imbalance between the flexion and extension gaps. Although it has been suggested that polyethylene exchange can be an effective, low morbidity procedure to treat certain types of prosthetic knee instability, it is associated with reported failure rates of 29% and 36% at 5-year follow-up. The use of thick spacers to address this problem is not recommended because of the potentially high failure rate, except perhaps in older, low-demand patients with late rather than early TKA failure (Figures 5 and 6).

Malalignment

The rotational and axial alignment of TKA components are critical in preventing exaggerated polyethylene wear, patellofemoral complications, and ultimately implant failure. Component positioning and soft-tissue balance are critical for the alignment of medial and lateral compartments and in flexion and extension so that lift-off and edge loading of the femur on the polyethylene does not occur. CT has been used to determine that 69.2% of patients having a primary posterior-stabilized TKA had a correlation between condylar lift-off and malalignment of the femoral component. It has been reported that placing the femoral component parallel to the transepicondylar axis lessens the incidence of femoral condylar lift-off, thus potentially reducing polyethylene wear by reducing eccentric edge loading. A knee wear simulator has been used to show that a model of 3° varus malalignment caused higher wear rates than a high-intensity loading group, emphasizing the importance of alignment to wear and failure. Malalignment may also have other implications. For example, internal rotation malalignment of the tibial component has been found to directly correlate with anterior knee pain postoperatively. It is therefore essential that surgeons are capable of achieving correct alignment with the particular implant of choice to avoid excessive wear.

Reflex Sympathetic Dystrophy

Reflex sympathic dystrophy (RSD) is a relatively uncommon complication of TKA (0.8% of patients); patients with RSD typically have excessive pain, marked limitation of flexion, and cutaneous hypersensitivity. The classic posttraumatic RSD findings of objective vasomotor changes and radiographic osteopenia are difficult to interpret in patients who have had TKA. ^{99m}Tc scanning

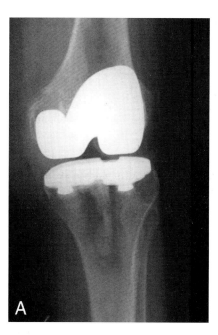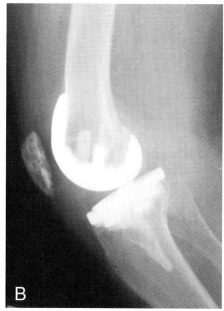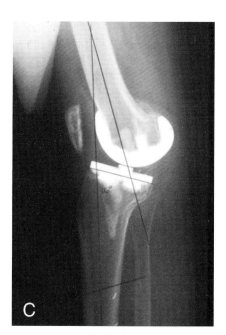

Figure 5 AP **(A)** and lateral **(B)** radiographs of a symptomatic TKA. The patient had full active extension. **C,** Lateral radiograph during stance phase revealed recurvatum deformity at stance phase. Observation of gait revealed hyperextension.

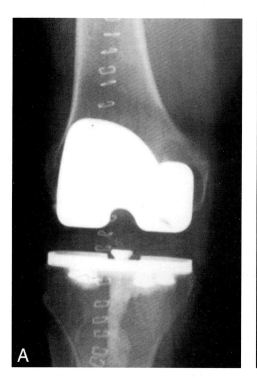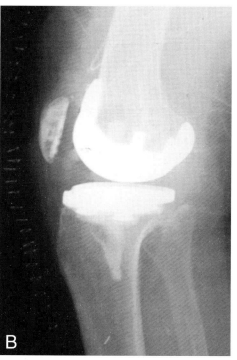

Figure 6 A and **B,** Radiographs showing isolated liner exchange used to block hyperextension and relieve symptoms. This is an example of one of the few indications for isolated liner exchange in an older, less active patient. In general, isolated liner changes have been associated with a high rate of failure.

usually is not helpful in diagnosing RSD in patients who have undergone TKA. Lumbar sympathetic block is useful for diagnosis and treatment. In patients with persistent RSD, lumbar sympathectomy may be indicated. No surgical intervention is indicated for the extremity for coexisting mechanical dysfunction of the TKA before the symptoms of RSD are controlled.

Arthrofibrosis and Other Causes of Postoperative Stiffness

The causes of arthrofibrosis after TKA are multifactorial. Limited range of motion preoperatively appears to predispose patients to having problems with motion postoperatively. Patients with preoperative knee flexion of less than 75° have been reported to gain less flexion postoperatively than patients whose preoperative flexion was greater than 75°. Patients with a previous femoral fracture or a knee fixed in extension preoperatively may have underlying quadriceps contracture and scarring, which, if left uncorrected, can markedly limit motion postoperatively.

Poor flexion and extension may result from inadequate release or recession of a tight posterior cruciate ligament. Another pitfall when selecting a posterior cruciate ligament–retaining component is lack of posterior slope. This will cause tightening of the posterior cruciate ligament in flexion if the rollback mechanism functions according to design.

Other situations can include anterior tilt of the tibial component, resulting in posterior impingement against the femoral component, which is associated with limited range of motion and anterior lift-off of the tibial component and late loosening. Posterior tilt of the femoral component alters the contact areas and can produce prominence of the anterior flange, increased patellofemoral wear, trochlear flange impingement, and limitation of motion. Anterior displacement or oversizing of the femoral component can displace the extensor mechanism ventrally, which limits knee motion. Posterior displacement of the femoral component with notching of the anterior cortex can cause not only supracondylar fracture but also a knee tight in flexion with limited motion. Internal rotation of the femoral component can lead to lateral subluxation or dislocation of patella that, in turn, can cause pain and limitation of flexion. External rotation of the femoral component has been recommended to enhance ligament balancing in flexion and to facilitate optimal patellar tracking.

An elevated joint line results in relative patella infera, with premature patellar contact with the intercondylar notch region in flexion creating tightness in the extensor mechanisms. This can be a common cause of anterior knee pain after TKA. Generally, joint elevation less than 8 mm is associated with improved knee scores, better range of motion, and less patellofemoral pain in patients who have undergone TKA.

Manipulation under anesthesia should be considered if an unsatisfactory range of motion has reached a plateau in the first 3 months after TKA. Tethered patellar syndrome, arthrofibrosis, and patellar malalignment problems can be diagnosed and treated arthroscopically with removal of fibrous bands or lateral release. Arthroscopy also can be helpful in other conditions, such as retained cement, polyethylene wear, loose bodies, and subclinical infections. Poor results are reported with arthrolysis and isolated exchange of tibial insert in patients with stiff knees after TKA; however, better results have been observed in the relief of painful and stiff TKAs by performing full TKA revision with a posterior-stabilized condylar prosthesis.

When performing a revision TKA for malpositioned components with stiffness and revising adequate implant balancing, release of all potential soft-tissue contractures is essential. Particular attention should be directed to possible quadriceps tendon and vastus intermedius adhesions to the femur and suprapatellar pouch, medial and lateral gutters, collateral ligaments, and lateral patellar retinaculum. Attempts should be made to achieve the perfect balance of flexion-extension gap as well as medial and/or lateral structures. In most patients, when both components are revised, a posterior cruciate ligament–substituting design should be used.

Extensor Mechanism

Rates of patellofemoral complications reported in the literature range from 5% to 55% of patients, and patellofemoral complications are an indication for up to 29% of all TKA revision procedures. Patellar instability has been implicated as the cause of up to 29% of all secondary TKA procedures. Patellofemoral instability has also been associated with subluxation, dislocation, aseptic loosening, and component wear and failure. Factors associated with patellofemoral instability include extensor mechanism imbalance, asymmetric patellar resection, and component malposition.

An additional potential complication relating to the extensor mechanism is soft-tissue impingement at the undersurface of the junction of the patellar component and quadriceps mechanism. A fibrous nodule may form at this junction and enter the trochlear notch during knee flexion. As the knee proceeds into extension, the nodule catches on the femoral component causing pain, a snapping sensation, and instability. This phenomenon has been described as the patellar clunk syndrome. If conservative therapy fails, then consideration should be given to performing arthroscopic or open débridement (Figure 7).

The ultimate potential complication related to the extensor mechanism is complete failure: either iatrogenic failure resulting from intraoperative injury (particularly at the patellar tendon insertion for which extreme care must always be taken in the revision scenario) or postoperative failure with sudden onset of weakness or inability to extend the knee and difficulty ambulating (Figure 8, *A*). A variety of repairs have been reported for these injuries, but results are typically poor because of their technically demanding and complicated nature. Allograft reconstruction is often ultimately required, and although associated with acceptable results for difficult repairs, the best approach remains vigilance and avoidance of this major complication (Figure 8, *B* and *C*).

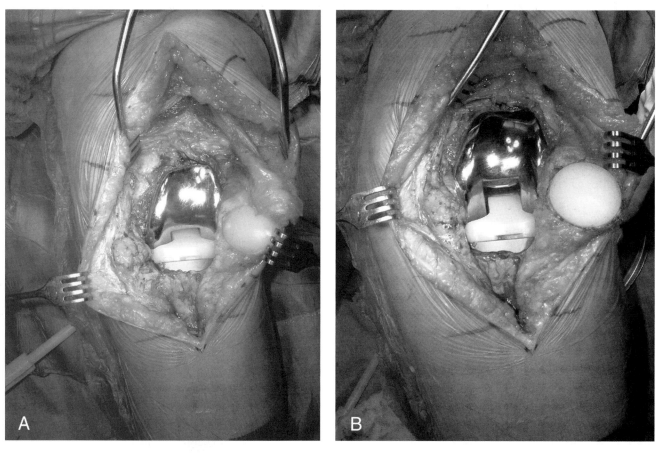

Figure 7 **A,** Intraoperative photograph showing a fibrous nodule at the junction of patella and quadriceps tendon that resulted in a painful clunk syndrome. **B,** Intraoperative photograph showing the knee after resection of the nodule, which led to complete resolution of the painful symptoms.

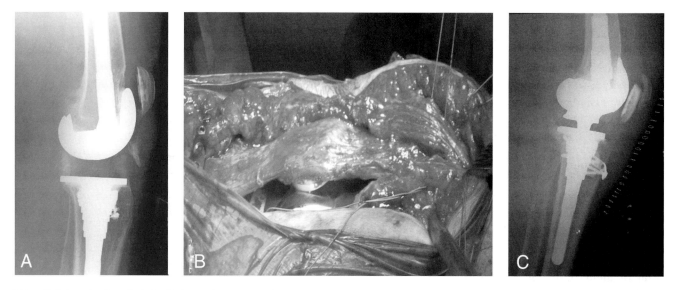

Figure 8 **A,** Lateral radiograph obtained before revision surgery showing patella alta secondary to patellar tendon rupture. The patient also had gross medial collateral ligament insufficiency. **B,** Intraoperative photograph showing allograft reconstruction of the extensor mechanism: tibial fixation (left), allograft patella (center), and proximal suturing of allograft to native quadriceps in extension (right). **C,** Postoperative radiograph showing a well-fixed new extensor mechanism in the appropriate position with a rotating hinge implant to further compensate for an absent medial collateral ligament.

Preoperative Planning and Surgical Technique

Surgical Exposure

Primary wound healing is essential to the success of any TKA procedure. Delay in wound healing predisposes the artificial joint to bacterial colonization and infection. In addition to delay in wound healing and wound sloughing, drainage that persists for more than 7 days has been associated with 17% to 50% of deep TKA infections. The skin arterioles of the anterior knee arise from the terminal branches derived from the patellar arterial ring. This cutaneous vascular network has already been compromised by the primary TKA and is at further risk if surgical exposure is not performed atraumatically. Minimizing injury to the subfascial dermal plexus by minimizing flap elevation, avoiding excessive retraction, and using blunt dissection techniques will decrease the risk of skin necrosis, especially for at-risk groups. Before arthrotomy, patellar blood supply should also be assessed. The standard midline parapatellar approach sacrifices the three medial genicular arteries. If a lateral retinacular release has been performed during the primary procedure as well, the superior lateral genicular and possibly the inferior lateral genicular artery will also be compromised. Additionally, the lateral meniscectomy during the initial operation would have sacrificed the anterior recurrent tibial artery and possibly the inferior lateral genicular artery, leaving the patella partially devascularized (Figure 9). Special approaches that may be required in TKA revision include quadriceps snip (Figure 10), modified V-Y turndown (Figure 11), and tibial tubercle osteotomy (Figure 12).

Implant Inspection

A thorough assessment of all components provides information for determining the mechanism of failure of the previous arthroplasty (Figure 13). Malalignment, joint line elevation, and soft-tissue imbalance must be corrected at revision. Inspection will often provide information as to which of these factors is present or confirm suspicions raised during preoperative planning. Scratches or burnishing in the trochlear groove should prompt evaluation of the patellofemoral articulation (Figure 14). Implant design (metal-backed patella), malrotation of the femur, or an oversized femoral component may have led to abnormal patellofemoral mechanics and subsequent failure. Damage to the condyles of the femoral component usually indicates third body wear or metal-on-metal articulation secondary to polyethelene insert failure. Post wear in posterior-stabilized implants implies an alignment, rotational, or stability problem (Figure 15).

Recent studies concerning revisions of both cemented and cementless TKAs have shown that femoral components should not be retained when revising loose tibial components, regardless of fixation or apparent

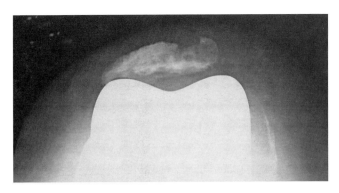

Figure 9 Radiograph showing osteonecrosis of the patella with secondary fracture.

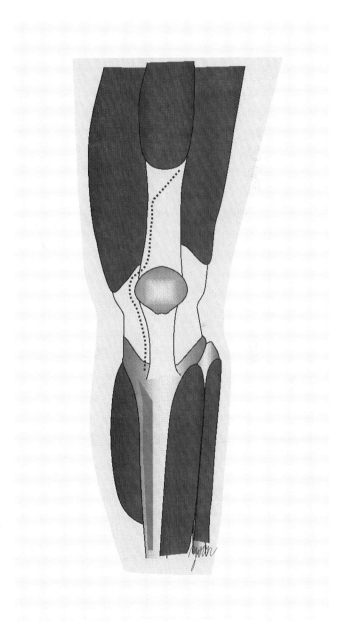

Figure 10 Diagram of the quadriceps snip technique of improving surgical access. (Reproduced with permission from Kassim RA, Saleh KJ, Badra ML, Yoon P: Exposure in revision total knee arthroplasty. *Semin Arthoplasty* 2003;14(3).)

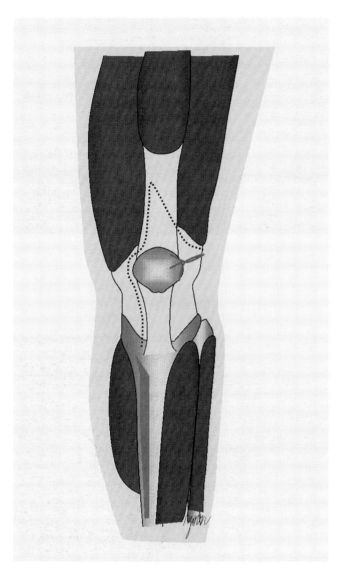

Figure 11   Illustration of modified V-Y turndown technique for use in more complex cases, with an effort being made to preserve patellar vascularity. (Reproduced with permission from Kassim RA, Saleh KJ, Badra ML, Yoon P: Exposure in revision total knee arthroplasty. *Semin Arthroplasty* 2003;14(3).)

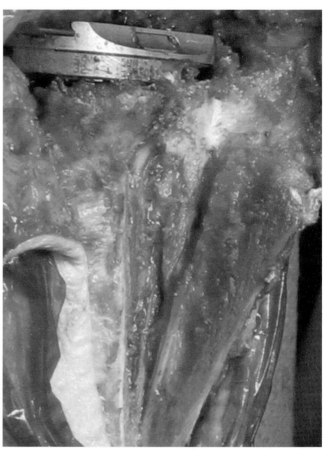

Figure 12   Intraoperative photograph showing a tibial tubercle osteotomy (hinged on an intact lateral soft-tissue sleeve) performed for obtaining access to the intramedullary stem.

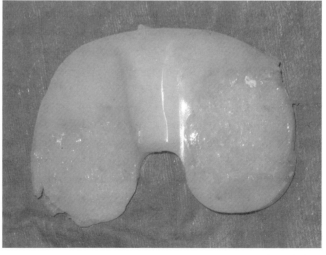

Figure 13   Photograph of a polyethylene component retrieved at revision TKA showing severe wear secondary to malalignment during the primary procedure.

lack of femoral wear or osteolysis. Such retention was associated with an unacceptably high failure rate in one study.

Implant Removal

Implant removal may be difficult if the components are not loose. The goal is to remove the components while maintaining the existent bone stock. Scar-tissue débridement is undertaken to fully expose the metal-bone interface and to remove residual polyethylene, metal, and polymethylmethacrylate debris.

The tibial polyethylene component is usually removed first to create more space and facilitate further dissection. Removal of the tibial polyethylene component in the modular situation is easily accomplished us-

ing an extractor or an osteotome introduced between the metal-polyethylene interface. If the tibial component is all-polyethylene, a reciprocating saw is applied at

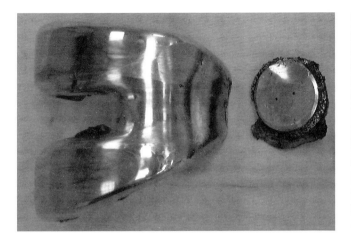

Figure 14 Photograph of a retrieved femoral component showing burnishing caused by wear from failed metal-backed patellar component that necessitated revision of all components.

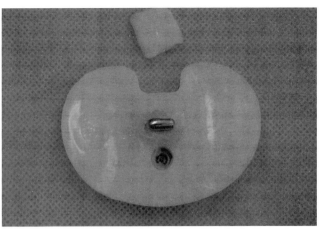

Figure 15 Photograph of a retrieved tibial component of a posterior cruciate ligament–substituting implant showing a broken post.

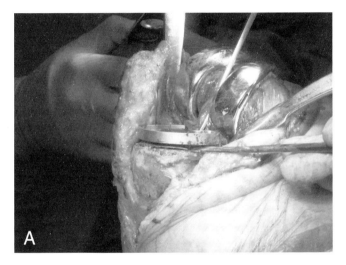

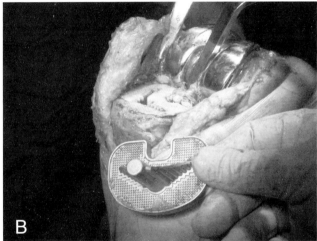

Figure 16 **A,** Intraoperative photograph showing accurate placement of osteotome in the implant-cement interface when removing tibial components. **B,** Intraoperative photograph showing successful removal of a tibial component without causing any bone loss and leaving behind cement mantle.

the cement-polyethylene interface to separate the tray from its tibial peg. The polyethylene stem can then be resected under direct vision with a high-speed burr. Removal of the cemented or cementless metal-backed tibial component requires circumferential dissection to accurately identify the metal-cement-bone or metal-bone interfaces, respectively. If the tibial component is a cemented metal-backed tray, then the osteotome is advanced between the metal-cement interface (Figure 16). If the tibial component is a cementless metal-backed tray, then the osteotome is advanced between the metal-bone interface. Care must be taken not to apply pressure against the bone with the osteotome because this can lead to bone depression and possible fracture. Cutting instruments must always be applied against the component at the interfaces. If the bone stock and the

bone quality are good, stacked osteotomes can be used to further dissociate the component.

The same principles for tibial component extraction apply to extraction of the femoral component. The posterior femoral condyles must also be cleared of host bone before extraction. This technique can be interrupted at the femoral fixation pegs as well as at the tibial central peg. The osteotome may have to be used again circumferentially around these fixation devices. Implant removal can be extremely difficulty if a well-fixed cementless or fully cemented stemmed component exists. In this situation, a high-speed diamond tip drill may be needed to remove the component piecemeal.

If patellar component extraction is also required, removal of the patellar polyethylene component is usually easier with an oscillating saw or with an osteotome, depending on the quality of the bone. Patellar extraction may be difficult in patients with a well-fixed, metal-backed patellar implant. A powered surgical instrument can aid in the extraction of such a component.

Preparation and Assessment of the Knee for Reconstruction

Once the implants are removed, all residual membrane and pseudocapsule are removed sharply and with curets. Care should be taken in removing membrane from the popliteal area to avoid significant potential complications because there have been reports of significant vascular complications related to anatomically variant arteries in this location.

Clearance of this tissue is important to remove debris, a potential stimulus to inflammation, and potential soft-tissue blocks to motion. Cement and metallic debris are usually embedded on all bone surfaces, and débridement requires the use of high-speed burrs and curets without sacrificing existing bone stock. Copious irrigation of the joint will remove any residual cement or debris that might impede maximum fixation of the new cement-bone interfaces. Once all the surfaces have been cleansed, the bone and soft-tissue deficits are evaluated and a final decision is made as to precisely which prosthesis is required.

Ligament Integrity

Competence of the medial collateral ligament and lateral collateral ligament along with the adequacy of the bone stock to which they are attached is crucial. To a large extent, collateral ligament integrity dictates the type of prosthesis that should be used in the reconstruction. Secondary to asymmetric bone loss and component loosening or settling, ligaments are stretched or torn on the convex side and contracted on the concave side.

If both collateral ligaments are intact and there is little bone loss, a primary posterior cruciate ligament–stabilizing prosthesis may be used. In most revision procedures, however, modular implants are used because they provide options for intramedullary fixation, various augments for bone deficits, and potentially differing degrees of constraint. If ligament asymmetry is present, initial balancing should be performed by subperiosteal release on the contracted side as in a primary TKA procedure. If balancing is unsuccessful in either the medial or lateral plane, the degree of constraint must be increased by implanting a constrained condylar prosthesis. In the uncommon instance where there is complete absence of a collateral ligament, use of a rotating hinge-type prosthesis will be necessary (Figure 17).

Bone Defects

Bone loss is common in TKA revision and usually occurs in specific patterns. Bone defects are a consequence of several factors: implant malalignment with bone collapse, migration of implants and aseptic loosening, iatrogenic bone loss during implant removal, stress shielding, osteolysis, and osteonecrosis.

Several classification systems have been introduced to describe and develop treatment protocols for patients with distal femoral and proximal tibial bone defects. Bone defect assessment is based on the defect size, defect location, containment of the defect, and defect symmetry or disparity (whether it involves one or both condyles or plateaus).

The Anderson Orthopaedic Research Institute Bone Defect Classification describes three types of defect based on the radiographic status of the metaphyseal bone of the distal femur and proximal tibia. Femoral defects are denoted by F (FI, FII, or FIII) and tibial defects are denoted by T (TI, TII, or TIII). The metaphyseal region in this classification is defined as bone distal to the femoral epicondyles of the femur and proximal to the tibial tubercle for tibial defects.

Type I defects have intact metaphyseal bone with structurally sound cancellous bone. The cancellous bone does not crush easily. In addition, type I defects have no component subsidence. Type II defects involve damaged metaphyseal cancellous bone with subsidence of the component or joint line alteration attributable to bone loss. Small osteolytic defects may be present distal to the epicondyles. On the femoral side, these defects may be divided into type IIA, when a single condyle is involved, and type IIB, when both condyles are affected. Type III defects have deficient metaphyseal bone that compromises a major segment of the condyle or plateau. When this occurs in the femur, the bone is deficient at or above the level of the epicondyles with subsidence of the femoral component to that level. An important aspect of the usefulness of this classification system is that it helps guide treatment according to the type of defect identified.

Bone Defect Reconstruction

There are many reconstructive options available for the management of bone defects, including morcellized bone grafts, cement fill (with or without screws), various structural bone grafts, augments and stems on modular devices, customized bone-substituting implants, or often combinations of these alternatives. The ultimate choice for specific patients will be determined by the availability of devices and graft materials, experience and preference of the surgeon, and patient-related factors, such as activity levels and life expectancy. Preoperative planning is therefore critical and, as has been discussed previously, it should be reiterated that although good quality plain radiographs or fluoroscopic images are fundamental in planning, they typically underestimate the actual bone deficit found at the time of revision.

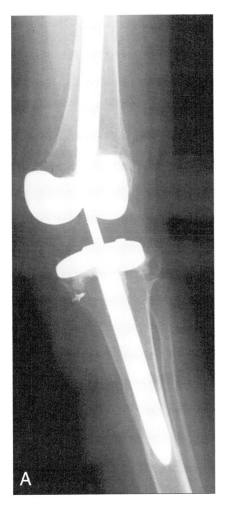
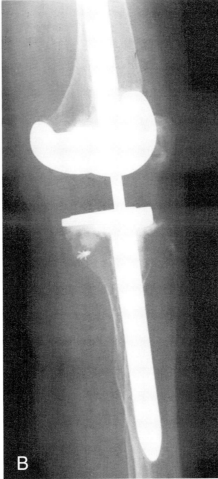
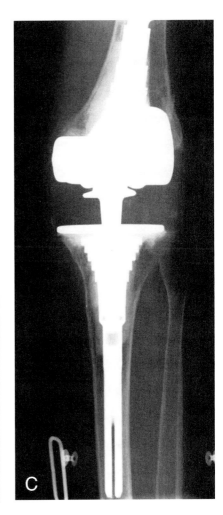

Figure 17 AP **(A)** and lateral **(B)** radiographs of a TKA revision performed for medial collateral ligament insufficiency. Residual valgus laxity is apparent. **C,** Postoperative radiograph after conversion to a rotating-hinge implant resulting in resolution of instability.

It is usually preferable to restore bone stock in active or young patients, whereas the use of augments on modular devices or bone-replacing implants may be more appropriate in elderly, sedentary patients. Furthermore, it is advisable to retain as much of the remaining bone as possible; certainly, no more than 10 mm of bone from either femur or tibia should be resected because the strength of the cancellous bone decreases as bone is resected into the metaphysis. Additionally, loss of femoral bone can make restoration of the joint line more difficult.

In addressing specific bone defects, a graduated approach may be adopted. Small, cystic bone defects (types I and II) can be packed with cancellous autograft or allograft or filled with cement. With limited collapse of a femoral condyle or tibial plateau (type II and type III defects), metal augmentations of the revision components may suffice. Distal and posterior femoral joint line augments are extremely useful in restoring balanced flexion and extension gaps and the joint line, and tibial plateau wedge augments can restore bone loss and alignment. However, if augments are used, it is usually advisable to add intramedullary stems to the components for additional fixation and alignment.

For larger defects (type III), impacted morcellized and/or structural allografting is useful. Because areas of morcellized bone graft do not initially provide mechanical support, stemmed components are recommended to share load with the intact diaphyseal bone until sufficient rigidity develops in the metaphysis with graft incorporation. Massive segmental bone loss on the femoral or tibial side may be addressed using large structural allografts with stemmed implants (again for stability and load sharing to allow healing of the graft) (Figure 18). Alternatively, in elderly patients with segmental defects, hinge-type prostheses provide excellent stability and defect correction with rapid rehabilitation. Large bulk allograft may be used when there is loss of one or both condyles or when a large contained defect is present in which a large femoral head allograft can be placed to

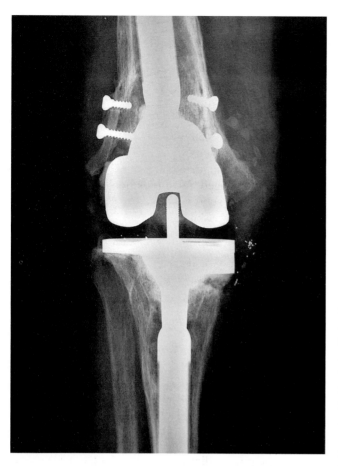

Figure 18 Radiograph showing the use of techniques to address bone loss: structural allografting of a deficient distal femur and metal augmentation to compensate for a deficient medial proximal tibia.

give stability to the reconstruction. A distal femoral allograft rarely is necessary, but it can be used for massive metaphyseal and diaphyseal bone loss when there is no native bone stock available for reconstruction.

Bone Grafting
Bone grafting in the setting of revision TKA is designed to replace lost native bone stock, thus providing a solid base for the revision implants and reconstituting bone to facilitate any future revisions if required.

Structural bone grafting in TKA revision, in contrast to total hip revision, has good results at short- to medium-term follow-up. An examination of radiographs of nine TKAs having structural grafts in situ for an average of 41 months demonstrated no radiolucent lines and no component loosening, with all grafts intact without collapse. Histologic sections of specimens from the same patients showed callus formation at the cortical margins of the allograft; and although there was no trabecular collapse, there was no revascularization of allograft evident. Remnants of the subchondral plate of the allografts lacked any host ingrowth, emphasizing the importance of clearing cartilage and subchondral plate

from allografts to maximize the potential for host ingrowth. In a series of 13 distal femoral allografts used for reconstruction of large uncontained defects, another group found that by 1 year all allografts had achieved incorporation or union to host bone. No collapse had occurred, and there were no instances of sepsis. Longer-term review of structural allografts has shown a survival rate of 72% (95% confidence interval; range, 69% to 75%) at 10-year follow-up. Impaction grafting is another alternative to structural allograft, the promising short- to medium-term results of which have reported as the technique gains popularity. Impaction grafting is similar in principle to that used in revision hip arthroplasty, with use of morcellized bone and mesh for treating uncontained defects.

Cementing of Bone Defects
In selected patients, cement or cement with screw augmentation may be used to fill bony defects. Cement filling alone is an acceptable option for femoral reconstruction when the trial component is stable to varus and valgus stressing, even though one or both of the distal condyles may not have flush contact with the component. The chamfer cuts in this procedure provide stability and should be flush with the component. Metal augments to the distal femur also may be used.

The use of a screw-cement construct to confer stability when the femoral chamfer cuts do not provide stability and one distal femoral condyle is deficient has been reported. A titanium screw is placed in the distal femoral condyle and left proud so that it can reinforce the cement and support the deficient condyle. The screw should be inserted to such a depth that it does not contact the prosthesis. Biomechanical testing of this technique for a tibial wedge defect reconstruction found it to have 30% less deflection than cement alone.

Augments
The use of modular augments has enhanced the ability of surgeons to flexibly and quickly address bone loss that previously would have required a custom prosthesis, large cement volumes, or the time-consuming fashioning of bone graft. Almost all manufacturers now offer revision systems with modular augments for reconstruction. Modular augmentation of the femoral component in TKA revision has three major objectives: (1) filling bony defects with biomechanically stable components to allow weight bearing and functional motion, (2) creation of equal flexion and extension spaces to provide ligamentous stability, and (3) restoration of a nearly anatomic joint line. Because femoral bone loss typically occurs on the posterior or distal surfaces, posterior and distal augments are most frequently used. Augmentation of the distal femur will decrease the extension space and lower the joint line. Augmentation of the posterior condyles decreases the flexion space. Bone

loss on the tibia affects the extension and flexion spaces and the joint line equally. The use of a posterior augment on the lateral femoral condyle will help ensure relative external rotation of the femoral component to improve patellofemoral mechanics. Restoration of the anteroposterior and mediolateral dimensions of the femur in conjunction with a nearly anatomic joint line results in balanced soft tissues with ligamentous stability throughout the range of motion.

Biomechanical testing and validation of augments and wedges has centered on their use in the treatment of tibial defects, with few data available regarding the use of femoral augments. An analysis of different techniques for reconstruction of medial tibial plateau bony defects in cadaveric specimens demonstrated that metal wedge augments provide significant improvement in stability compared with cement alone while maintaining surgical flexibility. Clinical series have demonstrated successful medium-term outcomes with cemented tibial wedges. It has also been demonstrated that step-shaped reconstructions provide more rigid support and significantly decreased shear forces at the augment-cement interface and the cement-bone interface than wedge reconstructions.

Component Selection

Prosthesis selection in TKA revision is based on the degree of constraint and mode of fixation (cemented or cementless and stemmed or unstemmed). Most surgeons undertaking TKA revision use cemented components with or without press-fit stems.

Constraint

TKA prosthetic design is a balance between conformity and constraint, which relies on the simultaneous interaction of the supporting soft tissues and the contoured prosthetic surface. It is preferable to use the least constrained prosthesis. Therefore, in most revision procedures, a posterior-stabilized articulation can be used. However, if there is functional loss of the medial collateral ligament or lateral collateral ligament, if the flexion and extension spaces cannot be balanced, or if a severe valgus deformity is present, then use of a constrained condylar prosthesis may be desirable.

Posterior-stabilized implants, with their conforming articulation and spine-and-cam mechanism, provide adequate stability when the collateral ligaments are intact. Although this spine-and-cam mechanism acts as a mechanical posterior cruciate ligament, it provides no varus or valgus restraint. It is for this reason that modular revision implant systems have been designed to allow interchange of posterior-stabilized and constrained polyethylene inserts. If a constrained articulation is needed, then it simply can be inserted onto the tibial tray.

Constrained condylar components are selected for patients with extreme collateral ligamentous injury or when a marked flexion-extension gap mismatch is present that cannot be managed by proper component selection and orientation. Hinged constrained devices are not commonly required and are reserved for patients with severe posterior capsular insufficiency and uncontrolled hyperextension.

Reported indications for using a second-generation modular rotating-hinge implant have included aseptic loosening of a hinged prosthesis, loosening and bone loss associated with chronic extensor mechanism disruption, component instability with chronic medial collateral ligament disruption, and comminuted distal femur fracture. Early clinical and radiographic results have been comparable with those of TKA using a standard condylar revision design, which suggests that second-generation modular rotating hinge components can be used successfully in selected patients undergoing salvage TKA revision. Other designs such as the total condylar constrained knee prosthesis were intended to provide greater stability and constraint with a nonlinked implant. Despite concerns that the increase in constraint would lead to accelerated component loosening and wear, there are recent reports of an 80% survival rate at an average follow-up of 15.3 years.

Custom prostheses are rarely used for TKA revision, but there are three indications to be considered: (1) when the bone is so oversized or undersized that standard components simply will not fit; (2) when stems are needed to enhance fixation, but the bone shape precludes the use of standard devices (adjacent fracture malunion, offset stem); and (3) when the size or location of bone loss cannot be accommodated by standard augments.

Intramedullary Stems

The use of intramedullary stems in TKA revision provides fixation of components into diaphyseal bone, which, in turn, provides stability to the reconstruction (Figures 19 and 20). Axial alignment is reproduced, and the stems partially relieve stresses on the deficient metaphyseal bone or allograft. Stems physiologically transfer surface or joint loads into the medullary canal and are recommended to stabilize large bone defects requiring augmentation or structural bone grafting. Stems are also necessary to bypass perforations by at least 4 cm. When intramedullary stems are to be used, the femoral and tibial intramedullary canals are sequentially reamed by hand, which obviates the need for aggressive reaming that can potentially cause cortical perforations. The issue that has produced much recent interest is that of whether to use cemented or hybrid stem fixation (cemented condylar elements with cementless stem). Clinical outcomes for both methods have been recently reported.

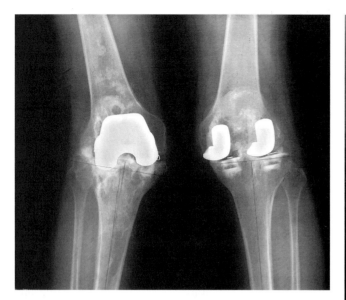

Figure 19 AP radiograph of failed bilateral knee arthroplasties with marked associated bone loss and deformity.

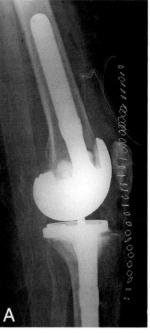
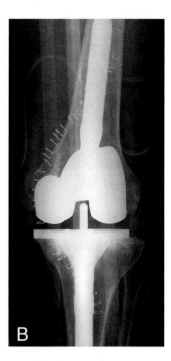

Figure 20 **A** and **B,** Radiographs after revision showing several elements of successful reconstruction. Augments were used on the distal femur to compensate for bone loss and restore gap balance in flexion and extension. Stems were used with the increased constraint of the construct (cementless stems in this patient). The joint line and accurate alignment have been restored. Skin staples show the use of a previous incision to minimize compromise of wound vascularity.

One proposed advantage of the cementless technique is that it allows for easier removal of components and debris should a subsequent revision be necessary. Disadvantages can be encountered in femoral shaft obliquity because of a healed fracture, previous fracture, or osteotomy, or excessive bowing of the tibia or femur. Passage of a large canal-filling stem can be difficult if not impossible in such patients.

As with metal augments, nearly all biomechanical testing of stems has been performed on the tibia, with subsequent rationale carried over to femoral reconstruction. It has been determined that a 70-mm stem used in the tibia bears 23% to 38% of an applied axial load. Strain distributions for various stems have also been measured, showing stress shielding of the proximal tibia, with the distance of the shielding equivalent to the length of the stem. This raises concerns that the stress shielding may result in bony resorption and late component failure.

When large press-fit stems are used, the position of the femoral implant is dictated by the axis of the distal femur. Instances occur, such as in patients with a previous healed fracture, in which the mediolateral or AP position of the implant is not appropriate because of malalignment in the distal femur. Offset stems have been introduced to address some of these mismatches between components and anatomy. These stems are modular and allow for shifting of the condyles relative to the stem in the mediolateral and AP directions. Offset stems also may be used to help adjust the flexion and extension spaces. The flexion space is increased if the stem shifts the femoral component anteriorly. Conversely, a posterior shift decreases the flexion space.

Although cemented fixation of the condylar elements of the components in revision TKA is generally accepted and yields reliable results, the issue of whether to use cement in fixation of the intramedullary stems remains controversial. Some general principles guiding this choice include the use of cemented stems in patients with extremely osteoporotic, capacious canals or in those in whom use of a press-fit stem will induce malalignment, and the use of cementless stems in patients in whom cement extrusion into fracture or osteotomy sites or into a structural allograft-host bone interface should be avoided.

Alignment of the Component

Because restoration of limb alignment is essential to the outcome of a TKA revision procedure, it is critical to restore the mechanical axis. The cutting jigs for most TKA revision systems generally use intramedullary alignment guides and allow distal femoral cuts to be made at 5° to 7° of valgus and the tibial cut at 0° to the horizontal. Most long-stem femoral components currently come in only 5° valgus orientation, necessitating a similar cut on the femur.

When making the bone cuts, it is essential to remove as little bone as possible and simultaneously restore the mechanical axis. There are two methods commonly used for restoration of axial alignment. After removal of the failed implant and cement, the intramedullary alignment device with the distal femoral cutting guide attached is inserted until the cutting slot removes a small portion of the distal femur. The relationship between the cutting block and the intramedullary alignment device (usually 5° to 7° of valgus) reestablishes the correct axial alignment. However, if the medial collateral ligament is thought to be functionally incompetent, the femur should be cut in slightly less than the normal 5° to 7° valgus. This results in a relative varus alignment of the mechanical axis, which protects the incompetent medial collateral ligament. The proposed cut may reestablish a flat bony surface on only one of the condyles and may not remove bone from both condyles. The other condyle may require additional trimming to allow the placement of augments or bone graft. The cut femoral surface provides a reference line that is parallel and often proximal to the desired joint line.

The second method for axial alignment involves the use of revision systems with cutting slots in the trial components. In this instance, the intramedullary stem of the trial component recreates the axial alignment. The trial component with the stem is advanced until bone is encountered and pinned in place. The bone cuts then are performed through the slots on the trial component. The cutting slots correspond to the modular augments available in the revision system.

Several authors have reported a correlation between clinical result and prosthesis alignment. Not only is axial alignment important for function and outcome, rotational alignment is crucial for patellofemoral mechanics and the balancing of flexion and extension gaps.

To avoid problems with malrotation during TKA revision, anatomic landmarks and reference lines are used to guide femoral component placement. Several anatomic references have been described. The posterior condylar line, surgical epicondylar axis, and the Whiteside axis are commonly used in primary TKA for femoral alignment. These landmarks are typically absent in the TKA revision setting, except the surgical epicondylar axis, which remains available for rotational referencing in nearly all TKA revisions. This axis is defined by a line connecting the peak of the lateral epicondyle and the sulcus between the two prominences of the medial epicondyle.

Trial Reduction and Soft-Tissue Balancing

Once soft-tissue and bone abnormalities have been corrected, the prosthetic components are assembled and a trial reduction is performed. The definitive size of the components is only appreciated during the trial reduction and is combined with soft-tissue balancing and joint line restoration.

The tibial and femoral trial components are put in place with the appropriate trial polyethylene insert, and

adjustments to ligament tension are made to balance the flexion and extension gaps. Although the goal is to achieve a flexion gap equal to the extension gap, this is often difficult to achieve in TKA revision surgery. The knee is initially balanced in flexion with the trial components in place. Balancing may require soft-tissue release (partial or complete) or lengthening on the tight side and a thicker polyethylene insert to balance the knee on the opposite side, keeping in mind that stability in extension with laxity in flexion will require posterior femoral condylar augmentation.

Once the knee is balanced in flexion, the problem of soft-tissue balancing becomes more manageable. Varying the thickness of the polyethylene tibial insert in flexion also affects the extension space, whereas augmenting the femur distally only affects the extension space. If the knee is too loose in extension, the solution requires distal femoral augmentation using metal augmentation, cement spacers, or modular implants, which would concomitantly lower the joint line and potentially create patella alta. If the knee is too tight in extension, the solution requires distal femoral resection or reduction in distal femoral augmentation, which would elevate the joint line and can potentially create patella baja. Therefore, surgeons have the option of using a thicker polyethylene tibial insert and/or a larger femoral component with distal femoral augments to restore the proper joint level and balance the flexion and extension gaps.

Soft-tissue balancing using ligamentous augment and advancement techniques is still controversial in TKA revision. A host of ligamentous and capsular ligamentous advancement techniques, even augmentation substitution techniques, have been reported. Although some of these techniques may seem applicable in exceptional instances, caution is advised and problems should be anticipated. The most common issues are whether there is adequate bone surface and whether there is enough internal space to permit harvesting and fixation of such elements. In particular, intramedullary stems and intercondylar housings occupy substantial space at the distal femur. It may be very difficult, if not impossible, to achieve proper fixation of the reconstruction element.

Joint Line Restoration

In TKA revision, ascertaining the proper level of the joint line is more difficult. Preoperative radiographs of the contralateral side can be obtained to determine the proper position of the joint line. The joint line lies approximately 1 cm proximal to the fibular head, 2.5 cm distal to the medial femoral epicondyle, or 1 cm distal to the lateral epicondyle. Elevation of the joint line is reported to occur relatively commonly in patients undergoing TKA revision (up to 79% of patients). Based on prospectively collected Knee Society clinical rating scores, it has been shown that excessive elevation, particularly

8 mm or more, results in significantly poor clinical outcomes. This complication may be avoided by taking particular care to restore distal femoral length. Improper positioning of the new joint line during revision surgery can also lead to patellar problems. Patellar subluxation will occur in the final phases of knee extension if the joint line is erroneously displaced distally (patella alta). Similarly, if the joint is displaced proximally (patella baja), impingement of the revised patellar component against the tibial component will occur. This will result in diminution of flexion, increased wear of the patellar implant, and increased incidence of anterior knee pain.

Patellar Tracking

After restoring the joint line, it is crucial that surgeons ensure proper patellar tracking. Internal rotation of the femoral or the tibial component will cause lateral subluxation of the patella. Medialization of the femoral or the tibial component can also contribute to patellar maltracking. The corollary of this is that medialization of the patellar component improves tracking and avoids lateral impingement of the lateral patellar facet against the lateral femoral condyle. If the positioning of all components is satisfactory and the patella still tracks laterally, a lateral retinacular release should be performed.

An important consideration when performing a lateral release is preservation of the superior lateral geniculate artery (assuming previous procedures did not sacrifice this artery). This artery can be found within the subsynovial fat at the inferior margin of vastus lateralis. The release is performed in the coronal plane, distal to the superior lateral geniculate artery and just lateral to the patella, extending as far as the joint line. The release is performed proximal to the superior lateral geniculate artery in an oblique (45° anteriorly) fashion. On rare occasions (for example, patients with patellar dislocations), a distal realignment may be necessary.

Patellar Revision

The patella may present difficulties in decision making in TKA revision surgery, and it has been the topic of much recent analysis. The options in patellar revision vary from retention of minimally worn, stable, and well-aligned, all-polyethylene components; revision; patellaplasty; reconstruction with bone graft; osteotomy; and, less commonly, patellectomy. It has been further suggested that metal-backed buttons should be removed regardless of wear or fixation and replaced with an all-polyethylene domed patellar component. This may be a point for debate, but metal-backed implants should certainly be viewed with a low threshold for revision.

Patellaplasty (resection of the patellar component and leaving the intact bony shell) has been used when remaining patellar thickness is less than 10 to 12 mm, which is the reported limit to replacement. The hope

here is that the patella will gradually become covered with soft tissue and thus function reasonably with minimal discomfort. Patellaplasty has been used when severe bone loss precludes reimplantation of a new patellar component, but relatively few such reports are available and outcomes are variable. Anterior knee problems have been reported at high rates, ranging from 20% to 45%. Reviews of patients with severely deficient patellae who underwent revision TKA have concluded that patellar component resection at time of revision TKA is preferable to formal patellectomy. It has been reported that patellaplasty is an acceptable option in patients with a bone-deficient patella, although anterior knee symptoms persisted in almost one third of patients. In one direct comparison of patients having patellar revision or patellaplasty, the latter had more difficulty with climbing stairs and kneeling and also lower postoperative Knee Society scores. A multicenter study of patients who underwent patellaplasty, patellar revision, and patellectomy with a minimum 2-year follow-up demonstrated that the revision group fared the best, followed by the patellaplasty group; the patellectomy group fared the worst.

Because restoring patellar thickness could improve strength and diminish extensor lag, attention has turned to reconstituting the bone-deficient patella. Newer techniques such as bone grafting, trabecular metal shell resurfacing, and osteotomy techniques show promise with good short-term results. Some of these interventions, however, seem to carry an increased risk of patellar fracture.

Restoration of patellar thickness is associated with better outcomes, probably because of improved extensor mechanism biomechanics. Despite increasing interest in trying to restore bone deficiency, the optimal solution for patients with a bone-deficient patella is currently unproved and patellaplasty remains an acceptable option in selected patients.

Salvage Procedures and Knee Arthrodesis

Patients who have undergone several attempts at TKA revision may ultimately be left with the dilemma of choosing between amputation, pseudarthrosis, or arthrodesis.

Amputation or permanent resection arthroplasty results in a poor overall outcome, with a low likelihood of ambulation; given the currently available techniques in TKA revision surgery, amputation or permanent resection arthroplasty can and should be avoided in most patients. However, these options may be appropriate in patients with life-threatening infection, irreparable soft-tissue deficiency, or severe bone loss.

Knee arthrodesis is an option that, although not usually indicated if a revision procedure is possible, can at least result in a stable, pain-free limb and allow independent ambulation in some patients. The techniques of knee arthrodesis include external fixation using compression with pin frame or fine wire devices and internal fixation using either intramedullary nail or plate fixation. Although the severity of bone loss is a critical factor in determining the prospects of success with fusion procedures, relative indications have been extended with the advent of ring fixator devices.

Although associated with satisfactory fusion rates in selected patients, dual-plating techniques are not commonly used in revision TKA. This probably reflects the unsuitability of this approach in patients with significant bone loss and also the extent of exposure typically required.

The stated advantages of external fixation arthrodesis include the technical ease of application, it provides compression when sufficient bone substance remains, and a one-stage procedure may be possible in patients with active infection. However, disadvantages include patient discomfort, cumbersome devices, and a relatively high incidence of complications relating primarily to pin tract infections. Additional reported difficulties include achieving rigid fixation in the presence of severe bone loss, particularly with traditional devices. This has been addressed recently with the use of ring fixators. Proponents of ring fixators claim that ring fixator techniques are particularly useful in patients with extensive bone loss, significant limb shortening, axial deformity, active infection, or a previous failed arthrodesis. Problems associated with patient tolerance and complication rates, however, present obstacles to its more widespread use.

In addition to having the highest reported fusion rates, the advantages of intramedullary nail arthrodesis include immediate weight bearing and provision of prolonged rigid fixation without a cumbersome external fixation device. However, a potential disadvantage in patients with infection is the need for a two-stage procedure. Modular titanium intramedullary nails have been reported to have lower nonunion and complication rates that traditional intramedullary nails. Newer intramedullary nail designs combine the advantages of intramedullary fixation, compression, and alignment with an interlocking capability that allows the use of shorter rods.

Postoperative Care

Rehabilitation of patients who have undergone revision TKA is crucial to the final outcome. Rapid postoperative mobilization is helpful to minimize postoperative complications associated with inactivity, such as thromboembolic disease, urinary retention, gastrointestinal ileus, and pneumonia. Continuous passive motion is commonly used, but there is no general consensus regarding its true long-term benefits. Although some surgeons routinely use continuous passive motion in the initial period after TKA revision, others do not recommend its routine use, but rather prefer allowing early active range of motion to be initiated by the physiotherapists and patients. If anterior skin integrity is an issue, then initial immobilization in extension may be considered with a waiting period of 2 days before the use of continuous passive motion. In general, patients must be educated on the importance of the rehabilitation exercises to restore full extension and flexion past 90°.

The amount of weight bearing is individualized based on the quality of fixation and the strength of the patient's remaining condylar and metaphyseal bone. Weight bearing is protected until union of the allograft is radiographically evident, usually at 3 to 4 months postoperatively in patients with extensive structural allograft or impaction grafting. Active extension is prohibited in patients with extensive exposure of the extensor mechanism, including those who have undergone V-Y turndown and tibial tubercle osteotomy to prevent rupture of the extensor mechanism. Gradual active extension exercise is permitted at 6 weeks postoperatively in these patients. The end result of rehabilitation following extensile approaches, however, is not clear. The only study that appears to specifically address the natural history after extensile approaches in TKA revision analyzed the results and range of motion in 123 revision TKAs with a mean follow-up of 30 months. Equally satisfactory outcomes were encountered in patients who had standard exposure and quadriceps snip, whereas those with quadriceps turndown and tibial tubercle osteotomy had equally inferior outcomes.

Clinical Results

Although many reports of revision TKA outcomes are on small series or experience with particular implants and are therefore limited by study design shortfalls, these reports represent the current knowledge base and standards in clinical outcomes of TKA revision practice. The problems with revision TKA outcome studies to date include the heterogeneity of TKA revisions and the lack of universally accepted assessment criteria and measures. This was addressed in a recent comprehensive report from the National Institutes of Health. In response to these shortcomings, a comprehensive prospective clinical study of the outcomes of TKA revision surgery is currently underway with a multicenter group, the North American Knee Arthroplasty Revision Study Group.

It is clear, however, that the results of TKA revision procedures have not been as satisfactory as those of primary TKA, with good TKA revision results varying from 76% to 89% of patients. Uniformly poor results have been reported in patients who underwent TKA revision for unexplained pain. Actual failure rates typically approximate to 1% of patients per year, with short-term (< 5 year) failure rates up to 10% or more being reported. The overall complication rate for TKA revisions is also high (up to 30% of patients), of which wound complications are the most common.

In a study comparing the overall outcome after salvage revision TKA (secondary to excessive bone loss, enlarged flexion gap, collateral ligament insufficiency, or extensor mechanism insufficiency), a significant difference in flexion range of motion was found when comparing hinged and nonhinged designs (96.5° versus 107.5°, respectively), but no significant difference was found in a variety of outcome measures. The authors concluded that in salvage TKA the implant design does not significantly affect the overall functional outcome.

Modular systems for TKA revision have become increasingly popular, but reports on these systems are also variable (for example, an 84% rate of excellent or good results and an 8% rate of early failure have been reported). In a recent report on a series of TKA revisions using cemented long-stem prostheses, the 10-year survival rate (no revision or removal for any reason) was 96.7%. The 11-year component survival rate with revision as the end point was 95.7%. There is considerable variety in the recent literature concerning systems using cementless stems, with reported failure rates ranging from 10% to 16% at approximately 5-year follow-up. Another study has reported better outcomes, with a 93.5% survival rate at 8.6-year follow-up, but this study compared an all cobalt-chromium implant and a more commonly used titanium TKA system. As a result, the issues of stem use and fixation for TKA revision remain unresolved, despite there being proponents for both approaches; additional analysis is therefore warranted.

Summary

Short-term reports on the outcome of revision TKA have indicated that generally good results can be obtained at 5-year follow-up. Mid- or long-term results, however, are not as well documented. The results of surgery appear to be closely related to the technical demands placed on surgeons because of bone loss, ligamentous instability, and varying levels of compromise of the extensor mechanism. In addition, an important element of surgical judgment is required regarding the use of bone graft, cement, modularity, and prosthetic constraint that is not necessarily reflected in the reports of the outcomes of various procedures and implants. Because of the large number of factors that require stratification, each treatment group for any one series is usually too small for any definitive conclusion or comparison to be made. Well-designed, comprehensive outcomes analyses are required to make definitive judgments regarding the best interventions regarding patients requiring TKA revision and to help determine the indications and timing of such interventions.

Annotated Bibliography

Patient Evaluation

Mason JB, Fehring TK, Odum SM, Griffin WL, Nussman DS: The value of white blood cell counts before revision total knee arthroplasty. *J Arthroplasty* 2003;18(8):1038-1043.

In an analysis of 86 patients who underwent revision TKA (55 for aseptic and 31 for septic TKA failure) and had preoperative aspirations of the knee, it was found that aspirates with a white blood cell count of 2,500/mL and 60% polymorphonuclear cells are highly suggestive of infection.

Nadaud MC, Fehring TK, Fehring K: Underestimation of osteolysis in posterior stabilized total knee arthroplasty. *J Arthroplasty* 2004;19(1):110-115.

Using cadaveric femurs and posterior-stabilized femoral components, the authors demonstrated that osteolytic lesions of 36 mm are not easily discernible on standard AP and lateral radiographs, but are visible on oblique radiographs. The authors recommended routine radiographic surveillance of patients who have undergone TKA using standard and oblique views.

Modes of Failure

Fehring TK, Odum S, Griffin WL, Mason JB, Nadaud M: Early failures in total knee arthroplasty. *Clin Orthop* 2001;392:315-318.

In this study, the causes for failure in 440 TKA revisions were reviewed. The authors found that 63% of patients had TKA revision within 5 years of their index TKA (38% because of infection, 27% because of instability, and 13% because of failure of ingrowth of a porous-coated implant). The authors concluded that use of cemented components and correct balancing of all the early failure could have reduced revisions by 40% and overall failures by 25%.

Sharkey PF, Hozack WJ, Rothman RH, Shastri S, Jacoby SM: Why are total knee arthroplasties failing today? *Clin Orthop* 2002;404:7-13.

The authors conducted a retrospective review of TKA revisions to reveal reasons for failure; in the order of prevalence, reasons included polyethylene wear, aseptic loosening, instability, infection, arthrofibrosis, malalignment or malposition, deficient extensor mechanism, osteonecrosis in the patella, periprosthetic fracture, and isolated patellar resurfacing. More than half of the TKA revisions in the early group were done less than 2 years after the index procedure, most commonly for infection (25.4% compared with 7.8% of late presenters).

Preoperative Planning and Surgical Technique

Barrack RL, Rorabeck C, Partington P, Sawhney J, Engh G: The results of retaining a well-fixed patellar component in revision total knee arthroplasty. *J Arthroplasty* 2000;15(4):413-417.

The results of patients retaining a well-fixed patellar component were compared with those of patients who underwent revision to a cemented all-polyethylene component, and the authors reported that retention had equivalent short-term results to those obtained when the patellar component was revised.

Bradley GW: Revision total knee arthroplasty by impaction bone grafting. *Clin Orthop* 2000;371:113-118.

In this study, cemented and cementless techniques with impaction grafting were used during revision TKA for 21 patients, with follow-up ranging from 6 to 62 months. One failure was reported, and the average improvement in combined Knee Society knee and function scores was 87 points.

Clatworthy MG, Ballance J, Brick GW, Chandler HP, Gross AE: The use of structural allograft for uncontained defects in revision total knee arthroplasty: A minimum five-year review. *J Bone Joint Surg Am* 2001; 83-A(3):404-411.

In this prospective review, with 96.9-month independent follow-up of 29 knees after structural allografting significant improvements were noted in Hospital for Special Surgery score and range of movement (23% of patients had re-revision at a mean of 70.7 months, resulting in a survival rate of the allografts of 72% at 10 years).

Conditt MA, Stein JA, Noble PC: Factors affecting the severity of backside wear of modular tibial inserts. *J Bone Joint Surg Am* 2004;86(2):305-311.

In this study, 124 polyethylene tibial inserts of 12 different designs were retrieved at the time of TKA revision. Stereomicroscopy demonstrated moderate-to-severe backside wear in all designs, independent of the capture mechanism.

Hanssen AD: Bone-grafting for severe patellar bone loss during revision knee arthroplasty. *J Bone Joint Surg Am* 2001;83-A(2):171-176.

The author describes a new technique of patellar bone grafting of deficient patellae during TKA revision. At a mean follow-up of 36.7 months, the Knee Society function and pain scores had improved significantly, and midterm clinical results indicated that this new technique was potentially useful.

Lonner JH, Lotke PA, Kim J, Nelson C: Impaction grafting and wire mesh for uncontained defects in revision knee arthroplasty. *Clin Orthop* 2002;404:145-151.

In a review of 17 TKA revisions with large uncontained defects treated with impaction allografting and wire mesh containment, the authors showed that Knee Society clinical and function scores increased from an average of 47 to 95 points and 48 to 73 points, respectively, with no failures reported.

Mackay DC, Siddique MS: The results of revision knee arthroplasty with and without retention of secure cemented femoral components. *J Bone Joint Surg Br* 2003; 85(4):517-520.

The survival rate of 67 TKA revisions for aseptic loosening with and without the retention of secure, cemented femoral components were compared; the authors reported that re-revision occurred in 28% of the retention group and in 7% of the fully revised group, indicating that retention of femoral components cannot be recommended even when conditions appear to be suitable.

Nelson CL, Lonner JH, Lahiji A, Kim J, Lotke PA: Use of a trabecular metal patella for marked patella bone loss during revision total knee arthroplasty. *J Arthroplasty* 2003;18(7 suppl 1)37-41.

The authors of this study evaluated short-term results following patellar resurfacing with a trabecular metal patellar shell for patients with marked patellar bone loss. Twenty consecutive patients were evaluated at a mean 23-month follow-up; good or excellent results were reported in 17 of 20 patients. Complications included three patients with polar patellar fractures postoperatively.

Rorabeck CH, Mehin R, Barrack RL: Patellar options in revision total knee arthroplasty. *Clin Orthop* 2003; 416:84-92.

The authors recommend retention of well-fixed, minimally worn, all-polyethylene cemented patellar buttons, removal of metal-backed buttons, and use of all-polyethylene domed patellar components for revision when more than 8 mm of the patella remains. Otherwise, patellaplasty is indicated, with the awareness that anterior knee pain, subluxation, and poor functional results are likely.

Siddique MS, Rao MC, Deehan DJ, Pinder IM: Role of abrasion of the femoral component in revision knee arthroplasty. *J Bone Joint Surg Br* 2003;85(3):393-398.

In this assessment of 60 TKA revision procedures done to treat patients with failed porous-coated anatomic TKA, the authors reported that 42% of the retention group failed at mean 2.1 years compared with 15% of the full revision group at mean 6.8 years. A complete change of primary bearing surfaces at the time of revision was recommended.

Werle JR, Goodman SB, Imrie SN: Revision total knee arthroplasty using large distal femoral augments for severe metaphyseal bone deficiency: A preliminary study. *Orthopedics* 2002;25(3):325-327.

The use of large (30-mm) metal distal femoral augments to compensate for severe bone deficiencies were reviewed and improvements in Hospital for Special Surgery and Knee Society scores and range of motion and no failures were reported at a mean 37-month follow-up.

Salvage Procedures and Knee Arthrodesis

Incavo SJ, Lilly JW, Bartlett CS, Churchill DL: Arthrodesis of the knee: Experience with intramedullary nailing. *J Arthroplasty* 2000;15(7):871-876.

In this retrospective review of 22 patients who underwent knee arthrodesis using different intramedullary nail designs, the authors reported that infection after TKA was the most common indication for the procedure, fusion occurred in all patients, and four patients required additional surgery. The authors recommended the use of customized intramedullary nail designs.

Postoperative Care

Cushner FD, Foley I, Kessler D, Scuderi G, Scott WN: Blood management in revision total knee arthroplasty. *Clin Orthop* 2002;404:247-255.

This retrospective analysis of aseptic TKA revisions showed that patient age did not influence hemoglobin level or transfusion rates; patients with preoperative hemoglobin levels less than 13 g/dL were found to be significantly more likely to require a transfusion.

Clinical Results

Babis GC, Trousdale RT, Morrey BF: The effectiveness of isolated tibial insert exchange in revision total knee arthroplasty. *J Bone Joint Surg Am* 2002;84-A(1):64-68.

The authors of this article assessed 56 isolated tibial insert exchanges (mean patient age, 66 years) that were required because of wear or instability; patients were followed for an average of 4.6 years. The authors reported that 25% of patients subsequently required re-revision at a mean follow-up of 3 years and that the cumulative survival rate at 5.5-year follow-up was 63.5%.

Barrack RL, Brumfield CS, Rorabeck CH, Cleland D, Myers L: Heterotopic ossification after revision total knee arthroplasty. *Clin Orthop* 2002;404:208-213.

In this consecutive series of 135 TKA revisions with a minimum 2-year follow-up, The incidence of heterotopic ossification was noted to be 23% before TKA revision and 56% subsequently, which resulted in lower functional scores but not decreased range of motion. The only significant risk factor was the presence of infection (76% of patients); gender, body mass index, surgical time or approach, or previous surgery were not determined to be significant risk factors.

Barrack RL, Lyons TR, Ingraham RQ, Johnson JC: The use of a modular rotating hinge component in salvage revision total knee arthroplasty. *J Arthroplasty* 2000; 15(7):858-866.

A second-generation modular rotating hinge design was used for 16 salvage TKA revisions (because of aseptic loosening of a hinged prosthesis, loosening and bone loss associated with chronic extensor, or medial collateral ligament mechanism disruption) and the outcomes were compared with those of patients who underwent TKA revision using a standard condylar revision design. The authors found comparable short-term clinical and radiographic results for the two groups.

Brooks DH, Fehring TK, Griffin WL, Mason JB, McCoy TH: Polyethylene exchange only for prosthetic knee instability. *Clin Orthop* 2002;405:182-188.

Although the authors believed that isolated polyethylene exchange can be effective in revision of some unstable TKAs, they reported a 29% failure rate in 16 knees with this treatment method at 4-year follow-up, indicating that this treatment should be used only with selected patients.

Bugbee WD, Ammeen DJ, Engh GA: Does implant selection affect outcome of revision knee arthroplasty? *J Arthroplasty* 2001;16(5):581-585.

The authors compared 42 TKA revisions with implants designed for primary TKA, 42 TKA revisions with modified primary components, and 55 TKA revisions with modular components specifically designed for revision arthroplasty and found that superior results were achieved with the modular components specifically designed for revision arthroplasty.

Christensen CP, Crawford JJ, Olin MD, Vail TP: Revision of the stiff total knee arthroplasty. *J Arthroplasty* 2002;17(4):409-415.

The authors of this study evaluated range of motion after TKA revision in a consecutive series of patients with pain and limited range of motion at an average 37.6-month follow-up. The average range of motion increased from 39.7° preoperatively to 83.2° postoperatively, and all patients were satisfied with the outcomes.

Fehring TK, Odum S, Olekson C, Griffin WL, Mason JB, McCoy TH: Stem fixation in revision total knee arthroplasty: A comparative analysis. *Clin Orthop* 2003;416: 217-224.

This study of 113 TKA revisions with 202 metaphyseal engaging stems (107 cemented and 95 press-fit) revealed that 93% of the cemented stems were radiographically stable and 7% were possibly loose, whereas only 71% of the cementless stems were categorized as stable, 19% were possibly loose, and 10% were definitely loose.

Gofton WT, Tsigaras H, Butler RA, Patterson JJ, Barrack RL, Rorabeck CH: Revision total knee arthroplasty: Fixation with modular stems. *Clin Orthop* 2002;404: 158-168.

The authors conducted a prospective review of 91 consecutive TKA revisions using a modular all cobalt-chromium stemmed revision knee system and hybrid stem fixation at a mean follow-up of 5.9 years. They reported that fixation with modular stems resulted in significant improvement in pain scores, function, range of motion, and total Knee Society score. Kaplan-Meier survivorship was reported to be 93.5% at 8.6 years.

Whaley AL, Trousdale RT, Rand JA, Hanssen AD: Cemented long-stem revision total knee arthroplasty. *J Arthroplasty* 2003;18(5):592-599.

The authors of this study reported that 38 fully cemented posterior-stabilized stemmed TKA revisions with a mean 10.1-year follow-up demonstrated significant improvements in

Knee Society pain and function scores, and a satisfactory 10-year survival rate (96.7%).

Classic Bibliography

Barrack RL, Matzkin E, Ingraham R, et al: Revision knee arthroplasty with patella replacement versus bony shell. *Clin Orthop* 1998;356:139-143.

Barrack RL, Smith P, Munn B, Engh G, Rorabeck C: Comparison of surgical approaches in total knee arthroplasty. *Clin Orthop* 1998;356:16-21.

Elia EA, Lotke PA: Results of revision total knee arthroplasty associated with significant bone loss. *Clin Orthop* 1991;271:114-121.

Engh GA, Ammeen DJ: Bone loss with revision total knee arthroplasty: Defect classification and alternatives for reconstruction. *Instr Course Lect* 1999;48:167-175.

Fehring TK, McAvoy G: Fluoroscopic evaluation of the painful total knee arthroplasty. *Clin Orthop* 1996;331:226-233.

Haas SB, Insall JN, Montgomery W III, Windsor RE: Revision total knee arthroplasty with use of modular components with stems inserted without cement. *J Bone Joint Surg Am* 1995;77:1700-1707.

Laskin RS: Management of the patella during revision total knee replacement arthroplasty. *Orthop Clin North Am* 1998;29(2):355-360.

Lonner JH, Siliski JM, Scott RD: Prodromes of failure in total knee arthroplasty. *J Arthroplasty* 1999;14:488-492.

Partington PF, Sawhney J, Rorabeck CH, Barrack RL, Moore J: Joint line restoration after revision total knee arthroplasty. *Clin Orthop* 1999;367:165-171.

Rand JA: Modular augments in revision total knee arthroplasty. *Orthop Clin North Am* 1998;29:347-353.

Rorabeck CH, Smith PN: Results of revision total knee arthroplasty in the face of significant bone deficiency. *Orthop Clin North Am* 1998;29:361-370.

Sculco TP, Choi JC: The role and results of bone grafting in revision total knee replacement. *Orthop Clin North Am* 1998;29:339-346.

Vyskocil P, Gerber C, Bamert P: Radiolucent lines and component stability in knee arthroplasty.: Standard versus fluoroscopically-assisted radiographs. *J Bone Joint Surg Br* 1999;81:24-26.

Waldman BJ, Mont MA, Payman KR, et al: Infected total knee arthroplasty treated with arthrodesis using a modular nail. *Clin Orthop* 1999;367:230-237.

Whiteside LA: Cementless fixation issues in revision total knee arthroplasty. *Instr Course Lect* 1999;48:177-182.

Chapter 12

Complications After Total Knee Arthroplasty

Giles R. Scuderi, MD

Robert T. Trousdale, MD

Stiffness

A stiff total knee replacement can be painful and lead to decreased use and disability. Walking on a level surface requires 65° of knee flexion, rising from the seated position or climbing stairs requires 70° of flexion, and descending stairs requires 90° of flexion. Stiffness, or loss of motion, following total knee replacement can be caused by patient factors, technical errors, local knee variables, and postoperative complications. The results of nonsurgical treatment or surgical intervention are dependent on the cause of stiffness (Table 1).

One of the most important patient variables is the preoperative range of motion. A knee that is stiff preoperatively may have restricted motion postoperatively because of contracture of the extensor mechanism and capsular fibrosis. Another patient variable is body habitus. An obese patient with pendulous thighs may have posterior soft-tissue impingement as the knee flexes. A recent review reported factors related to a lower postoperative range of motion in a group of patients with varus alignment to include female gender, an extreme varus alignment preoperatively, and young age. In a group of patients with valgus knees, factors related to limited flexion included young age and limited intraoperative extension. However, the principal predictive factor of the postoperative range of motion was the preoperative range of motion. Patients with posttraumatic arthritis are susceptible to postoperative stiffness. Additional factors influencing postoperative range of motion are patient compliance with the rehabilitation program and tolerance to pain. A patient who does not actively participate in a physiotherapy program will likely develop arthrofibrosis and limited motion.

There are several technical factors that influence postoperative range of motion, including overstuffing of the patellofemoral joint, mismatch of the flexion and extension gaps, inaccurate ligament balancing, component malposition, oversized components, joint line elevation, and excessive tightening of the extensor mechanism at the time of closure. Overstuffing of the patellofemoral joint can be caused by anteriorization of the femoral

component, underresection of the patella, creating a thicker bone component composite, and choosing a femoral component that is too big. Besides impacting patellofemoral kinematics, an oversized femoral component will lead to a narrow flexion space that can further impact knee motion. Failure to create equal and balanced flexion and extension will result in limited range of motion. The flexion gap may be smaller than the extension gap if insufficient bone is resected from the posterior condyles or if the distal femoral condyles are overresected. To stabilize the knee in extension, a thicker tibial component, which may be too big for the flexion gap, may be erroneously selected. This may limit flexion because of an extended posterior condylar offset and tightness of the supporting ligaments in flexion. The solution to this situation would be to either downsize the femoral component and accept the thicker tibial component or augment the distal femur and select a thinner tibial component. In contrast, failure to correct a preoperative flexion contracture or overresection of the posterior condyles may result in a residual postoperative flexion contracture with loss of extension, especially if a thicker tibial component is implanted to provide stability in flexion. In knees with a severe preoperative flexion contracture, the deformity is corrected with a posterior capsular release and resection of additional bone from the distal femur. Removal of posterior femoral osteophytes and release of the deep medial collateral ligament, the semimembranosus tendon, and the pes anserinus tendon in patients with a severe fixed varus deformity and the attainment of a good intraoperative range of motion improves the ability to achieve a good postoperative range of motion. Appropriate ligament releases, along with proper bone resection, create equal, rectangular, and symmetric flexion and extension gaps. The rotational position of the femoral component has been shown to affect the kinematics of the knee and in turn affect motion. Positioning the femoral component along the epicondylar axis creates a rectangular flexion gap, reduces lift-off, and improves flexion.

Ligament balancing must also take into account the posterior cruciate ligament. Failure to balance or release

Table 1 | Factors Affecting Stiffness After Total Knee Arthroplasty

Patient Factors

Preoperative range of motion
  Body habitus
  Female gender
  Extreme varus alignment preoperatively
  Young age
  Limited intraoperative extension
Postoperative range of motion
  Patient compliance with rehabilitation
  Pain tolerance

Technical Factors

Postoperative range of motion
  Overstuffing of the patellofemoral joint
  Mismatch of the flexion and extension gaps
  Inaccurate ligament balancing
  Component malposition
  Oversized components
  Joint line elevation
  Excessive tightening of the extensor mechanism at closure
Postoperative complications
  Infection
  Delayed wound healing
  Hemarthrosis
  Component failure
  Periprosthetic fracture
  Reflex sympathetic dystrophy
  Heterotopic ossification (severe)

a tight posterior cruciate ligament with a cruciate-retaining prosthesis will result in limited flexion. Conversely, a cruciate-retaining knee with flexion instability because of an incompetent posterior cruciate ligament will have limited flexion, which is the result of a paradoxic roll forward of the femoral component with earlier posterior impingement and tightening of the extensor mechanism from anterior femoral displacement. Excessive elevation of the joint line with a cruciate-retaining knee prosthesis may lead to patella infera that is associated with patellar pain and limited motion. An anterior or cephalad slope on the resected tibia will also limit flexion.

The environment in which the prosthesis is implanted will also impact the postoperative range of motion. Arthrofibrosis with limited motion can be a biologic complication that is independent of surgical and patient variables. The knees of some patients have overactive fibroblasts that generate excessive scar tissue with intra-articular adhesions. Patients who form keloids, as

well as those with juvenile rheumatoid arthritis and anklyosing spondylitis, may be at a higher risk of developing intra-articular adhesions.

Postoperative complications that alter the rehabilitation program may also impact the range of motion. Infection, delayed wound healing, hemarthrosis, component failure, or periprosthetic fracture may necessitate a period of immobilization, which in turn can lead to a loss of motion. Reflex sympathetic dystrophy is a noteworthy complication that creates a myriad of problems, but one of the most significant is loss of motion. Heterotopic ossification, when severe, may also result in a stiff knee.

The best management of postoperative stiffness is prevention by providing thorough preoperative patient education, aggressive postoperative rehabilitation, and avoidance of technical errors. Evaluation of a patient with a stiff total knee replacement starts with a complete history, review of the medical records, thorough physical examination, and radiographic analysis. CT may be helpful in determining the rotational position of the components. An aspiration and blood tests, including a complete blood cell count, erythrocyte sedimentation rate, and C-reactive protein level, will help rule out an infection.

Early treatment for patients with less than 3 months of stiffness includes an aggressive physiotherapy program with adequate analgesia. In some patients, dynamic splinting may be helpful. Closed manipulation under general anesthesia, with complete muscle relaxation, can also improve motion in selected patients. When patients present in the first 6 weeks with range of motion less than 90° or less than that achieved during the procedure, a manipulation should be contemplated. After induction of general anesthesia and complete muscle relaxation, the patient is placed in the supine position on the operating table. The ipsilateral hip is flexed to 90° while the surgeon applies pressure to the lower leg. This maneuver should be performed gently and in a sustained manner to disrupt the adhesions. Forceful manipulation of the knee may result in fracture or disruption of the extensor mechanism. Caution should be taken when trying to manipulate the knee into extension for a flexion contracture to avoid resulting in a femoral supracondylar fracture.

For patients with knees that are chronically stiff for more than 3 months, the treatment plan is more difficult because of maturation of the adhesions and soft-tissue contracture. Surgical options include arthroscopic arthrolysis, open arthrolysis, and component revision. Arthroscopic arthrolysis and posterior cruciate ligament resection in a tight cruciate-retaining knee with manipulation provides variable results. Although the improvement of range of motion with this technique was reported to occur in only 43% of patients, another study reported an average 30.6° of improvement in knee

Table 2 | Factors Affecting Instability After Total Knee Arthroplasty

Ligament imbalance

Component malalignment

Component failure

Implant design

Mediolateral instability (symmetric)

Bone loss from overresection of the distal femur

Bone loss from femoral component loosening

Soft-tissue laxity of the medial and lateral collateral ligaments

Connective tissue disorders (rheumatoid arthritis or Ehlers-Danlos syndrome)

Mediolateral instability (asymmetric)

Inaccurate femoral or tibial bone resection

Bone loss from femoral or tibial component loosening

Collateral ligament imbalance (underrelease, overrelease, or traumatic disruption)

range of motion. Open arthrolysis involves a radical débridement, release of a tight posterior cruciate ligament if present, lateral retinacular release, and quadricepsplasty. A pie crust quadricepsplasty followed by a gradual manipulation has been recommended. A quadriceps snip at the time of exposure will also have the same benefit. Modular implants were designed so that the tibial polyethylene component could be exchanged without removing the core components in the event a mechanical failure occurred. Occasionally, in well-fixed and well-aligned knees with a flexion contracture and limited range of motion, it may be appealing to exchange the tibial component to a thinner size; however, it has been reported that isolated tibial exchange, arthrolysis, and débridement do not provide a reliable treatment for knee stiffness. Revision total knee replacement is indicated for patients with component malposition or failure, incorrect component sizing, joint line displacement, or inadequate bone resection. When performing a revision arthroplasty, it may be necessary to perform a quadriceps snip, V-Y quadricepsplasty, or tibial tubercle osteotomy to gain exposure. When deciding to perform a revision total knee replacement it is most important to know the reason for failure and loss of motion. Failure to correctly identify the cause of failure may result in a recurrence of the problem.

Instability

One of the most common causes of aseptic failure following total knee replacement is instability. Significant symptomatic instability occurs in approximately 1% to 2% of patients undergoing primary total knee replacement. Although this rate is low, symptomatic instability accounts for 10% to 20% of all revisions when the re-

sults of several studies are evaluated. Instability may occur in the mediolateral plane (axial instability) or the anteroposterior plane (flexion instability) (Table 2).

Axial Instability

Axial instability can be caused by ligament imbalance, component malalignment, component failure, or implant design. There have been reports of patients with instability in whom the collateral ligaments are intact and competent, but because of implant failure, loosening, or subsidence, the tension in the soft-tissue sleeve is altered, resulting in knee instability. In these patients, revision should be directed toward reestablishing the flexion and extension gaps by addressing the bone loss on the femur or tibia. Because the soft-tissue envelope and collateral ligaments are still present, ligament reconstruction or a constrained implant may not be necessary.

Ligament imbalance may also be the result of inappropriate soft-tissue balancing caused by either inadequate release or overrelease of a contracted collateral ligament when correcting fixed axial deformities. In both instances, an asymmetric extension gap is created, resulting in instability. Another iatrogenic cause of axial instability is inadvertent damage to the medial collateral ligament during surgery. This can occur when cutting the proximal medial tibia or posterior femoral condyle. When intraoperative damage to the medial collateral ligament occurs, primary repair of the ligament or reattachment of the ligament to the bone and postoperative bracing has been recommended. In a study of 16 knees with either an intraoperative disruption of the medial collateral ligament or an avulsion from the bone that were treated using this technique, there were no reported instances of postoperative instability. However, most studies advocate the use of a constrained prosthesis rather than primary repair of the medial collateral ligament. A constrained implant provides more predictable stability if this situation occurs.

Mediolateral instability can be asymmetrical or symmetrical. Several variables result in a symmetric axial instability, including bone loss from overresection of the distal femur or femoral component loosening and soft-tissue laxity of the medial and lateral collateral ligaments, which may or may not be associated with hyperextension. Connective tissue disorders such as rheumatoid arthritis or Ehlers-Danlos syndrome may result in a generalized ligamentous laxity, which if not addressed at the time of total knee replacement may result in persistent instability. Asymmetric axial instability may be the result of inaccurate femoral or tibial bone resection; bone loss or subsidence associated with a loose femoral or tibial component; and collateral ligament imbalance, either from underrelease, overrelease, or traumatic disruption.

Critical to the course of treatment is determination of the cause of failure, which can be determined through a thorough history and meticulous physical examination. Radiographs with stress views or dynamic fluoroscopy may be helpful in determining the degree of instability. The cause of instability must be corrected at the time of revision arthroplasty; otherwise, it may recur. Symmetrical instability in both flexion and extension may be addressed with revision to a thicker tibial component. Asymmetric instability resulting from improper bone cuts or bone loss usually requires augmentation of the bone deficiency with modular augments or bone grafts. Augmentation is directed toward reestablishing the joint line and appropriate tension in the soft-tissue envelope.

Flexion Instability

Flexion instability is the result of a flexion gap that is larger than the extension gap. This instability may occur in several scenarios. In preparing the femur, anteriorization of the femoral component or downsizing the femoral component may create a flexion gap, which is larger than the extension gap. When the flexion space is larger than the extension space and a tibial polyethylene component that only fills the extension space is selected to prevent a flexion contracture, the knee will be poorly balanced and unstable in flexion. This condition can occur with the use of both cruciate-retaining and posterior-stabilized implants.

Acute posterior dislocation occurs in approximately 0.15% of knees following total knee replacement with a posterior-stabilized prosthesis. Factors that may influence this rate include the design of the femoral cam and tibial post mechanism, the number of available femoral component sizes, and the nature of the soft-tissue releases performed to correct fixed deformities. One study noted that patients with an above average range of motion postoperatively have a greater risk of dislocation; however, this may be the result of suboptimal intraoperative soft-tissue balancing. Possible mechanisms for dislocation in a posterior-stabilized prosthesis have been identified. In slight flexion a hamstring contracture or posteriorly directed force may result in the femoral cam riding up and over the tibial post if the polyethylene insert is relatively thin and does not fill the flexion gap. The implant design also influences the degree of instability, especially when the femoral cam is designed to ride up the tibial spine as the knee flexes, creating a short jump distance. Another mechanism may occur in patients in whom an extensive lateral release has been performed to correct a valgus deformity. In these patients, a rotatory dislocation may occur with the knee in flexion. There have also been reports of tibial post fracture, which may be the result of flexion instability or create instability. A loose flexion space will cause increased stress on the tibial post because, as the knee flexes, the femoral cam impacts the tibial post. If the knee is unstable, the stress on the polyethylene tibial post may exceed the material properties, resulting in breakage of the post and additional instability.

Flexion instability in patients with posterior cruciate-retaining total knee implants is less dramatic than in patients with posterior-stabilized implants, but it can be just as disabling. With an improved understanding of flexion instability, the overall incidence may be higher in patients with posterior cruciate-retaining prostheses than in those with posterior-stabilized prostheses. Flexion instability in patients with posterior cruciate-retaining implants may report a variety of nonspecific but significant symptoms, including anterior knee pain, a sense of instability, and recurrent joint swelling. Physical findings may include effusion, soft-tissue tenderness of the pes tendons and retinacular tissues, above-average motion, and posterior instability as demonstrated by a positive posterior drawer or sag sign. Symptomatic flexion instability in patients with posterior cruciate-retaining total knee implants may occur in the early postoperative period or it may be delayed. Early failure is likely the result of inadequate flexion and extension gap balancing, which is most commonly caused by inadequate balancing of the posterior cruciate ligament. Symptoms may also present after a period of relatively good function, in which instance late rupture or attenuation of the posterior cruciate ligament is a likely cause. It is unknown whether techniques that have been described to assist in the intraoperative balancing of the posterior cruciate ligament to optimize femoral rollback and kinematics of posterior cruciate-retaining prostheses place the posterior cruciate ligament at risk for late failure. Failure to adequately release the posterior cruciate ligament can certainly limit flexion and may contribute to postoperative stiffness or polyethylene wear. Overrelease of the posterior cruciate ligament may lead to an incompetent ligament, with paradoxic roll forward of the femur in flexion and flexion instability. The use of video fluoroscopy has demonstrated highly variable and erratic kinematics in cruciate-retaining prostheses. Therefore, it appears that accurately recreating optimal tension in the posterior cruciate ligament is important in maintaining stability. The surgical technique used to implant these devices is critical for achieving a successful outcome. In particular, the creation of balanced flexion and extension gaps is paramount in avoiding flexion instability.

Few published reports exist about the results of treatment for symptomatic flexion instability. After the posterior dislocation of a posterior-stabilized prosthesis, nonsurgical treatment that includes cast or brace immobilization for approximately 3 to 4 weeks followed by quadriceps strengthening may be associated with a successful outcome. In separate studies, approximately two thirds of patients with acute dislocations were reported to be successfully managed without surgery. If recurrent dislocations occur, then revision surgery with exchange of a modular polyethylene insert to a thicker insert should be considered. One study reported successful results in three patients who were treated with polyethylene exchange. If symmetric flexion and extension gaps cannot be created during the polyethylene exchange, then use of a constrained articulation is recommended because it provides greater margin of safety in a given situation than a posterior-stabilized prosthesis. In some instances, this may require removal of well-fixed components and complete revision.

The treatment of symptomatic flexion instability in patients with posterior cruciate-retaining prostheses is clearer because of the generally poor outcomes of nonsurgical treatment or simple polyethylene exchange in these patients. One study reported poor results in all patients with cruciate-retaining prostheses who were treated either nonsurgically or with polyethylene exchange alone. Similarly, only one of three patients (33%) treated with polyethylene exchange in another study improved. In this series, revision to a posterior-stabilized prosthesis was much more successful with marked improvements seen in 19 of 22 patients (86%). Another study also reported good results in six patients who underwent revision to a posterior-stabilized prosthesis. It is apparent that in patients with cruciate-retaining prostheses and symptomatic flexion instability, revision total knee replacement with a thicker anterior augmented or deep dished congruent cruciate-retaining articulation may be adequate, but revision to a posterior-stabilized prosthesis or constrained implant is the definitive solution.

Neurovascular Injury

Nerve injury after a total knee replacement is relatively uncommon. A prevalence of 0.3% in a series of approximately 9,000 patients who underwent total knee replacement has been reported. Nerve injury during total knee replacement can occur from direct compression or from realignment of a limb, especially a limb that is in valgus and flexion before surgery. Risk factors for nerve palsy after total knee replacement include severe valgus and flexion deformities, preoperative neuropathy, tourniquet use longer than 120 minutes, and postoperative bleeding complications (Table 3). For patients with severe valgus and flexion deformities, once the lateral soft tissues are released and the limb is realigned, the peroneal nerve can be tethered at the fibular head. Some authors have reported rates of peroneal nerve injury in patients with severe valgus deformities of up to 3% to 4%, which rises to 8% to 10% for those who have undergone correction of a severe flexion contracture of more than 60°. Routine exposure of the peroneal nerve dur-

Table 3 | Factors Affecting Neurovascular Injury After Total Knee Arthroplasty

Severe valgus and flexion deformities
Preoperative neuropathy
Tourniquet use > 120 minutes
Postoperative bleeding complications
Epidural anesthesia

ing correction of the valgus flexion deformity is probably not necessary, but after correction of a valgus deformity neurovascular status should be carefully assessed. Routine splinting during the perioperative period of the limb in a slight amount of flexion (approximately 25°) is also reasonable in these patients who are at risk for nerve injury.

The use of epidural anesthesia may also be a mild risk factor for development of peroneal palsy. In one study of 31 patients who experienced peroneal nerve palsy after total knee replacement, the authors suggested that the use of epidural anesthesia for postoperative pain control potentially could lead to decreased limb sensation, thereby leaving the limb in an unprotected state and potentially placing the nerve at risk for a compression injury.

If peroneal palsy does develop, the initial treatment should be an ankle-foot orthotic device and observation. If recovery does not occur, late decompression of the nerve and/or restoration of a dorsiflexion by muscle transfer can be performed. Persistent foot drop in which the patient does not tolerate an ankle-foot orthotic device is the primary indication for a decompression and/or muscle transfer procedure.

Vascular injury at the time of knee arthroplasty is also relatively uncommon. It is important before arthroplasty to document the vascular status of the limb. The prevalence of popliteal artery injury is relatively rare for multiple reasons. Popliteal vessels are not tethered at the level of the joint line. Furthermore, with knee flexion, which occurs during most of the procedure, the vascular bundle moves in a posterior direction. The popliteal artery is approximately 9 mm posterior to the posterior aspect of the tibial plateau at 90° of flexion. It is important to remember that the popliteal artery lies anterior to the popliteal vein, and thus would more likely be injured by a saw blade or scalpel when surgically approached from the front of the knee. An MRI study documented that the popliteal artery is located just lateral to the midline at the level of the tibial plateau. Hyperflexion can produce kinking of the vessel, and hyperextension can produce tenting of the popliteal artery. The authors recommended placing posterior retractors just medial to the midline to avoid injury to the popliteal artery. If in doubt as to the integrity of the

Table 4	Factors Affecting Wound Complications After Total Knee Arthroplasty

Systemic Factors

Type II diabetes mellitus
Severe vascular disease
Rheumatoid arthritis
Medication use (infliximab and corticosteroids)
Tobacco use
Nutritional status
Albumin level < 3.5 g/dL
Total lymphocyte count < 1,500/μL
Perioperative anemia
Obesity

Local Factors

Previous surgical incisions
Deformity
Skin adhesions secondary to previous surgery or trauma
Local blood supply

Surgical Technique

Length of skin incisions
Large subcutaneous skin flaps
Preservation of the subcutaneous fascial layer
Optimizing arthroplasty techniques

Postoperative Factors

Avoiding the development of postoperative hematoma
Avoiding knee flexion past 40° during the first 3 to 4 days
The use of nasal oxygen for the first 24 to 48 hours in high-risk patients
The use of tissue expanders preoperatively to facilitate incision healing

popliteal artery, it is worthwhile to let the tourniquet down after the bony cuts have been made and assess whether there is extreme bleeding. If popliteal arterial injury does occur, prompt consultation with a vascular surgeon and immediate repair is indicated. Popliteal artery injury potentially can lead to very serious complications, including acute ischemia, compartment syndrome, and potential amputation.

Wound Complications

Proper wound healing is critical for a successful total knee replacement. Initial efforts should be focused on prevention of wound complications. The knee generally has a plentiful blood supply both medially and laterally. Factors influencing wound complications fall into one of four categories: systemic factors, local factors, surgical technique factors, and postoperative factors (Table 4). Systemic factors that are important can be easily ascer-

tained by a thorough history and physical examination. Systemic illnesses such as type II diabetes mellitus, severe vascular disease, or rheumatoid arthritis should be optimized before surgery. Medications such as infliximab and corticosteroids that can affect wound healing should be discontinued if possible. Cigarette smoking inhibits skin microcirculation, and cessation of smoking 3 to 4 weeks before surgery may be beneficial. The patient's nutritional status may also play an important role in wound healing. Albumin levels lower than 3.5 g/dL and total lymphocyte counts less than 1,500/μL may make a patient more prone to wound failure. Perioperative anemia and marked obesity have also been thought to play a role in wound healing. Obese patients may require more vigorous skin retraction, and some series that have assessed total knee arthroplasty in obese patients have demonstrated increased wound drainage postoperatively.

Local factors also play an important part in healing. Previous incisions, deformity, skin adhesions secondary to prior surgery or trauma, and local blood supply are all important factors. Many local factors may not be able to be modified.

Modifying surgical techniques, however, can help maximize wound healing potential. In the present era of using smaller skin incisions, it is important to handle the skin gently, avoiding large subcutaneous skin flaps, especially laterally; preserving the subcutaneous fascial layer is also important. Optimizing arthroplasty techniques to keep the lateral release rate low is important because lateral release will decrease skin oxygen tension at the lateral wound edge. If the patient has had previous skin incisions, using the most acceptable medial incision is reasonable because laterally the skin's oxygen tension decreases. Keeping skin bridges between old incisions greater than 5 to 6 cm and avoiding crossing old incisions at angles less than 60° is also helpful.

Postoperative factors that affect wound healing include avoiding the development of a postoperative hematoma. The use of a tourniquet, time to tourniquet release, and the use of drains postoperatively remain controversial. In patients at risk for wound problems, knee flexion greater than 40° during the first 3 to 4 days postoperatively should be avoided because researchers have shown a decrease in oxygen skin tension as knee flexion increases. The use of nasal oxygen for the first 24 to 48 hours in high-risk patients may also be helpful.

The best form of treatment of a wound complication is prevention. In patients at risk, tissue expanders have been used preoperatively to facilitate the healing of an incision. Despite the best surgical efforts, wound complications can still occur and may include serous drainage, hematoma, superficial necrosis, or full-thickness tissue necrosis. A tense hematoma, serous drainage, or superficial necrosis with drainage that lasts for longer than 4 days after total knee arthroplasty is probably best treated with aggressive surgical débridement. Watching drainage or observing a tense hematoma that compromises the skin or limits range of motion is probably not in the patient's best interests. Watching the drainage for more than 3 to 5 days probably puts the implant at risk for deep periprosthetic infection. Full-thickness necrosis is the most serious wound complication, and by definition it involves deep penetration of the soft tissues. Aggressive surgical débridement and coverage of the defect with a local flap, gastrocnemius flap, or free flap (depending on the size and location of the deformity) is warranted. Small defects may be treated using local or gastrocnemius flaps, whereas soft-tissue deficits greater than 15 to 20 cm^2 may be treated using a free flap. Although the outcome of total knee arthroplasty after a flap has been placed may be less satisfactory than in patients who do not experience wound complications, reliable salvage of the implant and the knee can be obtained.

Summary

Patients with a stiff total knee replacement can experience symptoms including pain, decreased use, and disability. This loss of motion can be caused by a variety of factors, such as technical errors, local knee variables, and postoperative complications. The cause of stiffness typically determines whether nonsurgical or surgical treatment is indicated.

Although the results of total knee replacement are highly successful at long-term follow-up, failures do occur. One of the more frequent causes of failure is instability (axial instability or flexion instability). Although acquired ligamentous incompetence can occur, particularly in patients with cruciate-retaining prostheses, many instances of flexion instability likely result from an intraoperative failure to create symmetric, balanced flexion and extension spaces. In primary total knee replacement, use of a well designed posterior-stabilizing prosthesis or cruciate-retaining prosthesis with creation of symmetric, balanced flexion and extension gaps should minimize the incidence of postoperative instability. When symmetric flexion and extension spaces cannot be produced intraoperatively in either complex primary or revision procedures, use of a more constrained articulation such as a constrained condylar type prosthesis or hinged prosthesis may be required.

Neurovascular injury during total knee arthroplasty is rare. Using careful surgical technique and appropriate preoperative and postoperative measures, the rate of injury to the neurovascular structures should be less than 1%. If injury to the popliteal artery does occur, prompt recognition and repair will result in successful limb salvage for most patients. Most peroneal nerve injuries will be secondary to a stretch neurapraxia and best treated with immediate knee flexion and an ankle-foot orthotic device if ankle dorsiflexion is lost.

Wound complications are not always avoidable after total knee arthroplasty. Despite meticulous surgical technique and appropriate wound closure, wound failure can occur. The key to prevention of these complications is identifying patients at risk and optimizing the perioperative medical problems. When wound failure does occur, aggressive surgical treatment is indicated. With this approach, the implant can usually be retained with an acceptable long-term result.

Annotated Bibliography

Stiffness

Babis GC, Trousdale RT, Pagnano MW, Morrey BF: Poor outcomes of isolated tibial insert exchange and arthrolysis for the management of stiffness following total knee arthroplasty. *J Bone Joint Surg Am* 2001;83:1534-1536.

The authors of this study found that isolated tibial exchange, arthrolysis, and débridement do not provide a reliable treatment for knee stiffness.

Dennis DA: The stiff total knee arthroplasty: Causes and cures. *Orthopedics* 2001;24(9):901-902.

The author reports that pie crust quadricepsplasty followed by a gradual manipulation may assist in gaining motion during an open lysis of adhesions.

Lo CS, Wang SJ, Wu SS: Knee stiffness on extension caused by an oversized femoral component after total knee arthroplasty. *J Arthroplasty* 2003;18:804-808.

The authors report that in addition to impacting patellofemoral kinematics, an oversized femoral component will lead to a narrow flexion space that can further impact knee motion.

Ritter MA, Harty LD, Davis KE, Meding JB, Berend ME: Predicting range of motion after total knee arthroplasty. *J Bone Joint Surg Am* 2003;85:1278-1285.

The authors of this study found that factors related to a lower postoperative range of motion in a group of patients with varus alignment included female gender, an extreme varus alignment preoperatively, and young age.

Scuderi GR, Komistek RD, Dennis DA, Insall JN: The impact of femoral component rotational alignment on condylar lift off. *Clin Orthop Relat Res* 2003;410:148-154.

Positioning the femoral component along the epicondylar axis was reported to create a rectangular flexion gap, reduce lift-off, and improve flexion.

Instability

Brooks DH, Fehring TK, Griffin WL, et al: Polyethylene exchange only for prosthetic knee instability. *Clin Orthop Relat Res* 2002;405:182-188.

The results of this study suggest that polyethylene exchange can be an effective, low morbidity procedure to treat certain types of prosthetic knee instability.

Clarke HD, Scuderi GR: Flexion instability in primary total knee replacement. *J Knee Surg* 2003;16:123-128.

The authors of this study report that when the flexion space is larger than the extension space and a tibial polyethylene component that only fills the extension space is selected to prevent a flexion contracture, the knee will be poorly balanced and unstable in flexion. This can occur with both cruciate-retaining and posterior-stabilized implants.

Engh GA, Koralewicz LM, Pereles TR: Clinical results of modular polyethylene insert exchange with retention of total knee components. *J Bone Joint Surg Am* 2000; 82:516-523.

The authors report that when components are well fixed and well aligned, modular tibial polyethylene exchange provides a treatment alternative to complete revision for patients with instability.

Leopold SS, McStay C, Klafeta K, Jacobs JJ, Berger RA, Rosenberg AG: Primary repair of intraoperative disruption of the medial collateral ligament during total knee arthroplasty. *J Bone Joint Surg Am* 2001;83:86-91.

The authors of this study report that intraoperative repair of the medial collateral ligament with postoperative bracing in a cruciate-retaining prosthesis can provide a successful treatment option.

Mauerhan DR: Fracture of the polyethylene tibial post in a posterior cruciate substituting total knee arthroplasty mimicking patella clunk syndrome: A report of 5 cases. *J Arthroplasty* 2003;18:942-945.

The author reports the findings on a small series of five patients with symptoms of a patellar clunk syndrome but who actually had a fracture of the tibial post that caused subluxation of the femur on the tibia. The diagnostic characteristics that help differentiate between these two conditions are discussed.

Puloski SKT, McCalden RW, MacDonald SJ, Rorabeck CH, Bourne RB: Tibial post wear in posterior stabilized total knee arthroplasty: An unrecognized source of polyethylene debris. *J Bone Joint Surg Am* 2001;83A: 390-394.

The authors of this study found that although tibial post wear may be a source of polyethylene debris, wear patterns depend on post-cam mechanics, post location, and post geometry.

Scuderi GR: Revision total knee arthroplasty: How much constraint is enough? *Clin Orthop Relat Res* 2001; 392:300-305.

The author reports that in most patients with intact and balanced collateral ligaments, a posterior stabilized articulation will provide stability; however, in patients with medial collateral insufficiency, lateral collateral insufficiency, and inability to balance the flexion and extension gaps, a constrained articulation should be used.

Sharkey PF, Hozack WJ, Rothman RH, Shastri S, Jacoby SM: Why are total knee arthroplasties failing today? *Clin Orthop* 2002;404:7-13.

The authors report that instability is a common cause of aseptic failure in total knee arthroplasty.

Neurovascular Injury

Clarke HD, Schwartz JB, Math KR, Scuderi GR: Anatomic risk of peroneal nerve injury with the "pie crust" technique for valgus release in total knee arthroplasty. *J Arthroplasty* 2004;19(1):40-44.

The authors report that at the level of a standard tibial retraction the peroneal nerve is an average of 1.49 cm (range, 0.91 to 2.18 cm) from the posterolateral tibial bone.

Berger L, Antbock W, Lange A, Winkler H, Klein G, Engh A: Arterial occlusion after total knee arthroplasty. *J Arthroplasty* 2002;17:227-229.

The authors of this article discuss arterial injury after total knee arthroplasty.

Wound Complications

Riss MD: Skin necrosis after total knee arthroplasty. *J Arthroplasty* 2002;17(4 suppl 1):74-77.

The author provides a complete discussion of how to treat skin loss after total knee arthroplasty.

Classic Bibliography

Adam RF, Watson SF, Jarratt JW, et al: Outcome after flap coverage for exposed total knee arthroplasties: A report of 25 cases. *J Bone Joint Surg Br* 1994;76:750-753.

Asp JP, Rand JA: Peroneal nerve palsy after total knee arthroplasty. *Clin Orthop Relat Res* 1990;261:233-237.

Benowitz NL, Jacob P III: Daily intake of nicotine during cigarette smoking. *Clin Pharmacol Ther* 1984;35:490-504.

Bocell JR, Thorpe CD, Tullos HS: Arthroscopic treatment of symptomatic total knee arthroplasty. *Clin Orthop Relat Res* 1991;271:125-134.

Dennis DA: Wound complications in total knee arthroplasty. *Instr Course Lect* 1997; 46:165-169.

Dennis DA, Komistek RD, Stiehl JB, et al: Range of motion following total knee arthroplasty: The effect of implant design and weight bearing conditions. *J Arthroplasty* 1998;13: 748-752.

Dickhaut SC, DeLee JL, Pase CP: Nutritional statistics: Importance in predicting wound healing after amputation. *J Bone Joint Surg Am* 1984;66:71.

Diduch DR, Scuderi GR, Scott WN, et al: The efficacy of arthroscopy following total knee replacement. *Arthroscopy* 1997;13:166-171.

Farrington WJ, Charnley GJ, Harries SR, et al: The position of the popliteal artery in the arthritic knee. *J Arthroplasty* 1999;14:800-802.

Fehring TK, Valadie AL: Knee instability after total knee arthroplasty. *Clin Orthop Relat Res* 1994;299:157-162.

Galinat BJ, Vernance JV, Booth RE, Rothman RH: Dislocation of the posterior stabilized total knee arthroplasty. A report of two cases. *J Arthroplasty* 1988;3:363-367.

Garvin K, Scuderi GR, Insall JN: The evolution of the quadriceps snip. *Clin Orthop Relat Res* 1995;321:131-137.

Gold DA, Scott SC, Scott WN: Soft tissue expansion prior to arthroplasty in the multiply operated knee: A new method of preventing catastrophic skin problems. *J Arthroplasty* 1996;11:512.

Holt BT, Parks NL, Ensh GA, et al: Comparison of closed reduction drainage and no drainage after primary total knee arthroplasty. *Orthopedics* 1997;20:1121.

Horlocker TT, Cabanela ME, Wedel DJ: Does postoperative epidural analgesia increase the risk of peroneal nerve palsy after total knee arthroplasty? *Anesth Analg* 1994;79:495-500.

Idusuyi OB, Morrey BF: Peroneal nerve palsy after total knee arthroplasty: Assessment of predisposing and prognostic factors. *J Bone Joint Surg Am* 1996;78:177-184.

Johnson DP, Eastwood DM: Lateral patellar release in knee arthroplasty: Effect on wound healing. *J Arthroplasty* 1992;7(suppl):427-431.

Krackow KA, Jones MM, Teeny SM, et al: Primary total knee arthroplasty in patients with fixed valgus deformity. *Clin Orthop* 1991;273:9-18.

Laubenthal KN, Smidt GL, Kettlekamp DB: A quantitative analysis of knee motion during activities of daily living. *Phys Ther* 1972;52:34-43.

Lombardi AV, Mallory TH, Vaughn BK, et al: Dislocation following primary posterior stabilized knee arthroplasty. *J Arthroplasty* 1993;8:633-639.

Lonner JH, Pedlow FX, Siliski JM: Total knee arthroplasty for post-traumatic arthrosis. *J Arthroplasty* 1999;14:969-975.

Markovich G, Door LD, Klein NE, et al: Muscle flaps in knee arthroplasty. *Clin Orthop Relat Res* 1995;321:122.

Montgomery RL, Goodman SB, Csongradi J: Late rupture of the posterior cruciate ligament after total knee replacement. *Iowa Orthop J* 1993;13:167-170.

Ninomiya JT, Dean JC, Goldberg VM: Injury to the popliteal artery and its anatomic location in total knee arthroplasty. *J Arthroplasty* 1999;14:803-809.

Pagnano MW, Hanssen AD, Lewallen DG, Stuart MJ: Flexion instability after primary posterior cruciate retaining total knee arthroplasty. *Clin Orthop Relat Res* 1998;356:39-46.

Ritter MA, Faris PM, Keating EM: Posterior cruciate ligament balancing during total knee arthroplasty. *J Arthroplasty* 1988;3:323-326.

Rosenberg AG, Verner JJ, Galante JO: Clinical results of total knee revision using the Total Condylar III prosthesis. *Clin Orthop* 1991;273:83-90.

Rush JH, Vidovich JD, Johnson MA: Arterial complications of total knee replacement: The Australian experience. *J Bone Joint Surg Br* 1987;69:400-402.

Schmalzried TP, Noordin S, Amstutz HC: Update on nerve palsy associated with total hip replacement. *Clin Orthop Relat Res* 1997;344:188-206.

Scott RD, Thornhill TS: Posterior cruciate supplementing total knee replacement using conforming inserts and cruciate recession. Effect on range of motion and radiolucent lines. *Clin Orthop* 1994;309:146-149.

Stern SH, Insall JN: Total knee arthroplasty in obese patients. *J Bone Joint Surg Am* 1990;72:1400.

Stiehl JB, Komistek RD, Dennis DA, et al: Fluoroscopic analysis of kinematics after cruciate retaining knee arthroplasty. *J Bone Joint Surg Br* 1995;77:884-889.

Waslewski GL, Marson BM, Benjamin JB: Early incapacitating instability of posterior cruciate ligament retaining total knee arthroplasty. *J Arthroplasty* 1998;13:763-767.

Weiss AP, Krackow KA: Persistent wound drainage after primary total knee arthroplasty. *J Arthroplasty* 1993;8:285-289.

Williams RJ, Westreich GH, Siegel J, Windsor RE: Arthroscopic release of the posterior cruciate ligament for stiff total knee arthroplasty. *Clin Orthop Relat Res* 1996;331:185-191.

Wong R, Lotke P, Ecker M: Factors influencing wound healing after total knee arthroplasty. *Orthop Trans* 1986;10: 497.

Chapter 13

Osteonecrosis of the Knee

Michael A. Mont, MD

Jess H. Lonner, MD

Phillip S. Ragland, MD

Joseph C. McCarthy, MD

Introduction

Osteonecrosis of the knee is an uncommon disease that occurs at nearly 10% of the incidence of osteonecrosis of the hip. First described in the 1960s, it represents two distinct disorders: spontaneous osteonecrosis of the knee (SPONK) and secondary osteonecrosis of the knee. These two entities can be differentiated by the age of the patient at presentation, associated risk factors, location, and treatment options (Table 1). It is imperative that these two disorders not be confused with other disorders of the knee such as osteochondritis dissecans, bone bruises, or transient osteopenia of the knee because treatment methods are quite different for these disorders; therefore, orthopaedic surgeons should have a clear understanding of the clinical profile, diagnostic methods, and treatment options for these two disorders.

SPONK typically occurs in female patients older than 55 years and involves one condyle, most commonly the medial femoral condyle. However, less often the lateral femoral condyle or the tibial plateaus can be involved. These patients have no associated risk factors for osteonecrosis, and the disease is typically unilateral (> 95% of patients). Secondary osteonecrosis of the knee usually occurs in a younger patient population (45 years of age or younger), involves multiple compartments, is commonly bilateral (> 80% of patients), and has associated risk factors for osteonecrosis such as sickle cell anemia, corticosteroid exposure, and alcohol use.

Etiology and Pathogenesis

The exact etiology of these two disorders is currently unknown. It been hypothesized that SPONK is the result of minor trauma in osteoporotic bone that results in subchondral fluid accumulation, intraosseous edema, and resultant ischemia. However, up to 10% of patients diagnosed with SPONK report no history of trauma. The two predominant hypotheses regarding the etiology of secondary osteonecrosis are (1) vascular interruption of the subchondral microcirculation secondary to emboli or microthrombi and (2) posttraumatic osteonecrosis. It is believed that these mechanisms lead to intramedullary edema, elevated intraosseous pressures, and ultimately ischemia. The most common risk factor associated with secondary osteonecrosis is corticosteroid use, which may increase the size of marrow fat cells causing the elevated pressures and subsequent edema. Likewise, the pathophysiology related to the other risk factors associated with secondary osteonecrosis of the knee (Gaucher's disease, dysbarism [caisson disease], hypercoagulability, alcohol abuse, and sickle cell anemia) is unknown but likely similar in mechanism to that seen for osteonecrosis of the hip.

Clinical Features

Patients with SPONK are typically females older than 55 years who report the sudden onset of pain localized to the medial femoral condyle. This pain is commonly exacerbated by weight bearing or stair climbing and can occur at night. On physical examination, an effusion may be present that causes pain and decreased range of motion.

Patients with secondary osteonecrosis of the knee are typically females younger than 55 years; however, this disease can occur at any age (mean age, fourth decade of life). These patients typically report longstanding, generalized, nonspecific pain in the affected joint(s) and have at least one of the associated risk factors. Multiple joints can be affected; the lesions occur in the epiphysis, diaphysis, or metaphysis; and multiple condyles are usually involved. Pain occurs directly over the bony structures involved. The tibia is involved in addition to the femur in approximately 20% of patients. Additionally, signs and symptoms associated with the systemic disorders associated with secondary osteonecrosis of the knee should be considered when performing a clinical evaluation of these patients.

Differential Diagnosis

Disorders to consider in the differential diagnosis of osteonecrosis of the knee are osteochondritis dissecans, primary osteoarthritis, meniscal pathology, bone bruises,

Table 1 | Comparison of SPONK and Secondary Osteonecrosis

	SPONK	Secondary Osteonecrosis
Age (years)	Typically > 55	Typically < 55
Sex (males:females)	1:3	1:3
Associated risk factors	None	Corticosteroids, alcohol abuse, systemic lupus erythematosus, etc
Other joint involvement	Rare	Approximately 75%
Laterality	99% unilateral	Approximately 80% bilateral
Condylar involvement	One (usually medial femoral condyle or either tibial plateau	Multiple
Location	Epiphyseal to the subchondral surface	Diaphyseal, metaphyseal, epiphyseal
Symptoms	Commonly sudden onset of pain and increased pain with weight bearing or stair climbing and at night	Usually long-standing, insidious pain; the patient may have symptoms and signs of an underlying disorder such as systemic lupus erythematosus
Examination	Pain localized to affected area; small synovitis or effusion may occur; ligaments are stable; range of motion may be limited by pain or effusion	Pain is difficult to localize; ligaments are stable; range of motion is grossly intact, but may be limited by pain

and pes anserine bursitis. Osteochondritis dissecans is more common in men, usually located in the lateral condyle, and patients are typically adolescents (15 to 20 years of age). Patients with osteoarthritis report a slower onset of pain, and radiographic changes are detected in the cartilage before the bone. Meniscal pathology can be present with similar signs and symptoms of osteonecrosis, but it has a different radiographic appearance. However, some patients with osteonecrosis may have meniscal tears that are directly visible during arthroscopy. These patients report persistent pain following meniscectomy. Additionally, in patients with pain after yttrium-aluminum-garnet laser arthroscopic meniscectomy, further evaluation for osteonecrosis of the knee should be considered. Patients with pes anserine bursitis have pain on the medial aspect of the knee, but this pain is usually well below the joint line and is relieved with a subcutaneous injection of lidocaine. Finally, bone bruises and osteopenia of the knee (bone marrow edema syndrome) are transient disorders, which usually resolve within 6 months.

Diagnosis
Radiography
In older patients with idiopathic knee pain or younger patients with risk factors associated with osteonecrosis, weight-bearing AP and lateral radiographs of the knee should be obtained. Additionally, skyline and Merchant views can be helpful in identifying medial condylar and patellar lesions.

In the early stages of the disease process, radiographs may appear normal. However, as the disease progresses, flattening or a radiolucency bordered by a sclerotic halo may be identified in the weight-bearing portion of the affected condyle. In the late stages of the disease, subchondral collapse with secondary osteoarthritic changes may be seen (Figure 1). As previously stated, SPONK lesions are typically seen on the medial femoral condyle, and lesions of secondary osteonecrosis can be intramedullary or either in the medial or lateral condyle. A prognostic significance of radiographic findings has been reported in patients with osteonecrosis of the knee using the ratio formed by the product of the area of the lesion (greatest diameter in AP and lateral radiographs) and the width of the necrosis and the width of the entire condyle. Patients with a ratio greater than 50% typically have a poor prognosis and require prosthetic replacement.

Magnetic Resonance Imaging
The sensitivity of MRI allows detection of osteonecrosis before plain radiography and allows physicians to determine the size and location of the lesion more precisely than radiography. SPONK lesions are typically solitary, in the medial condyle, appearing as an area of low-signal intensity with a rim of high-signal intensity caused by edema on T2-weighted MRI scans (Figure 2). In T1-weighted MRI scans, SPONK lesions appear as an area of low-signal intensity entrapped by an area of high-signal intensity. The lesions of secondary osteonecrosis have similar features, but are often multifocal serpiginous lesions involving the medial or lateral condyle and can frequently appear in the metaphysis, diaphysis, or epiphysis (Figure 3).

Bone Scanning
Historically, bone scanning has been used to identify SPONK lesions. Bone scanning, however, has a sensitiv-

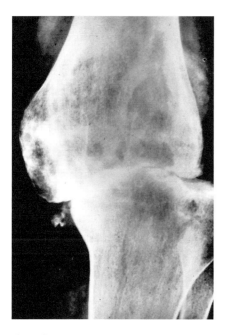

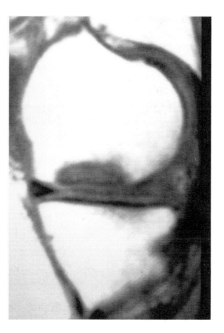

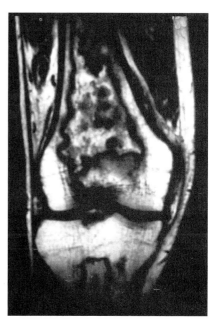

Figure 1 AP radiograph of a knee with secondary osteonecrosis showing sclerotic changes and loss of joint space seen in late stage disease.

Figure 2 MRI scan showing a unilateral SPONK lesion.

Figure 3 MRI scan showing the characteristic appearance of secondary osteonecrosis of the knee.

ity of only 60% to 80% for lesions of secondary osteonecrosis of the knee.

Staging

A staging system for SPONK was first described in 1979. In this system, patients with pain but no abnormalities on plain radiographs were classified as stage I (initial). In stage II (avascular), evidence of flattening is visible, with the lesion appearing as a radiolucent oval shadow with surrounding osteosclerosis. In stage III (developed), subchondral collapse has occurred, and a calcified plate with a clear sclerotic halo is visible. Finally, in stage IV (degenerative), sclerotic changes with osteophyte formation and deformity are present. This staging system was modified to include five categories. In this modified system, stage I SPONK is normal appearing, stage II consists of flattening of the convex portion of the condyle, stage III appears as a radiolucency with bony reaction, stage IV lesions are seen as a calcified plate or flap fragment with a radiolucency surrounded by a sclerotic halo, and stage V lesions have joint space narrowing, tibial or femoral subchondral sclerosis, and osteophyte formation.

For secondary osteonecrosis, a staging system has been described for the knee that is a modification of the Ficat and Arlet staging system for osteonecrosis of the hip. Stage I has no changes on radiography but MRI results or scintigraphy are positive. In stage II, sclerotic or cystic changes or both are present on plain radiographs, with a normal appearing contour to the distal segment of the femur and proximal tibia. In stage III, subchondral collapse

and flattening of the condyles (crescent sign) is evident. In stage IV, joint space narrowing and degenerative changes on the opposite side of the joint are evident.

Nonsurgical Treatment

In the initial report of outcomes of treatment modalities for what is now known as SPONK, recommended treatment consisted of conservative management (analgesics, weight-bearing precautions, physical therapy, osteotomy, arthrotomy, and prosthetic replacement). With the development of more sensitive diagnostic modalities such as MRI and scintigraphy, the distinction of the two disorders (SPONK and secondary osteonecrosis of the knee) became apparent, resulting in a change in the indications for different treatment modalities.

For both disorders, nonsurgical management consists of oral medication (a trial of narcotic analgesics and nonsteroidal anti-inflammatories), protected weight bearing, and physical therapy (such as quadriceps strengthening). Several reports have shown excellent results using nonsurgical management for patients with SPONK lesions; however, the results for secondary osteonecrosis have been poor.

One study reported good results in 9 of 12 patients with small SPONK lesions. Similar results were reported in a prospective study, with good or excellent results noted in 18 of 22 knees (80%) with nonsurgical treatment of idiopathic osteonecrosis of the knee.

In another study, successful clinical outcomes were reported at a mean follow-up of 8 years in 8 of 41 (20%) initially symptomatic knees treated nonsurgically. In a

Table 2 | Comparison of Treatment Options for SPONK and Secondary Osteonecrosis

Condition	Treatment Options
SPONK	Osteotomy, unicondylar arthroplasty, total knee arthroplasty
Secondary osteonecrosis	Arthroscopy, core decompression, osteochondral allograft/autograft, total knee arthroplasty

subset of 26 patients who received nonsurgical management matched to a cohort of 26 patients treated surgically for secondary osteonecrosis of the knee, only a 23% survival rate was reported in the nonsurgical group. Thus, it is recommended that nonsurgical management be reserved for patients with SPONK lesions and not for patients with secondary osteonecrosis of the knee.

Surgical Treatment

Various surgical modalities are available for management of osteonecrosis of the knee (Table 2). These include arthroscopic débridement, osteochondral allografts, osteotomy, core decompression, and prosthetic replacement.

Arthroscopic Débridement

Patients with SPONK frequently have meniscal pathology, but repair has been shown to have no impact on the natural course of the disease. This was shown in a study that reported that despite good results in 4 of 5 patients with osteonecrosis of the knee, arthroscopy had no effect on the long-term outcome. Furthermore, several studies have shown arthroscopy to be a causative factor in the pathogenesis of osteonecrosis. This has been hypothesized to be the result of direct trauma or increased intraosseous pressure incurred during the procedure. Thus, arthroscopy has variable results at best, but is likely not indicated in management of patients with SPONK lesions. This is because osteonecrosis of the knee is a disorder of osseous tissue, and soft-tissue repair or débridement therefore has no effect on that pathogenesis of the disease. Arthroscopy, however, is recommended for use as a diagnostic modality to assess the integrity of the femoral condyles in early stage secondary osteonecrosis of the knee and thus determine the presence of collapse or erosive changes that are not apparent on plain radiographs.

Osteochondral Allograft

Several studies have reported the results of using osteochondral allograft techniques for osteonecrosis of the knee. The authors of one such study used fresh, nonfrozen osteochondral allograft in 24 knees and reported good or excellent results in 10 of 15 knees (66%) with posttraumatic osteonecrosis, 1 of 6 knees (15%) with spontaneous osteonecrosis, and 0 of 3 knees with steroid-induced osteonecrosis. The authors concluded that failures in steroid-associated necrosis were because of the effect of corticosteroids on vascularization of the allograft. Another study reported good or excellent results in 12 of 17 knees (70%) with secondary osteonecrosis at a mean follow-up of 4.2 years (range, 2 to 9 years). Nonetheless, the multiple condylar nature of secondary osteonecrosis likely does not lend itself to optimum outcome for this treatment modality, and in light of the superior results of conservative management for SPONK lesions, the use of osteochondral allograft for this disease requires further investigation.

High Tibial Osteotomy

Because SPONK lesions are often solitary lesions that are isolated to the medial condyle, osteotomy is a potential treatment modality. Satisfactory results have been reported using high tibial osteotomy to treat patients with SPONK. One group of authors used high tibial osteotomy in 37 knees in which drilling and grafting techniques were used adjunctively in 23 knees and reported good or excellent results in 35 of 37 knees at 2 to 8.5 year follow-up; disappearance of the necrotic lesion occurred in 13 knees, and radiographic improvement was observed in 17 knees. In another series, grafting and osteotomy were used in 21 of 31 patients with SPONK; osteotomy was used in 10 patients. Good or excellent results were reported in 27 knees at a mean follow-up of 6.2 years. Based on these results, high tibial osteotomy may be a reasonable option for the treatment of patients with SPONK. The results of high tibial osteotomy for secondary osteonecrosis have been less encouraging and its use in this patient population is not recommended because of the multiple condylar nature and common bilaterality of this disease.

Core Decompression

The subchondral location of SPONK lesions does not make this disease amenable to treatment with core decompression. Results of using core decompression to treat patients with secondary osteonecrosis, however, have been promising. In a study comparing core decompression and conservative management in the treatment of 45 patients with secondary osteonecrosis (79 knees), a 74% success rate (34 of 47 knees) was reported in the core decompression group compared with an 82% success rate (26 of 32 knees) in the conservative management group at a mean follow-up of 11 years. The authors concluded that core decompression is a reasonable treatment option for patients with Ficat and Arlet stage

I and II lesions and that it offers a minimally invasive procedure with limited morbidity. Core decompression should be considered for patients with tibial and femoral lesions once the lesions have been appropriately localized using MRI. A percutaneous approach using 3 to 6 mm of trephine under fluoroscopic guidance into the area of the lesions is recommended. For femoral lesions, a medial or lateral entry point proximal to the metaphyseal flare may be used. For tibial lesions, a point medial to the tibial tubercle may be used, but care must be taken to avoid the medial saphenous nerve. The trephine is inserted into cortical bone under fluoroscopic control and is advanced to subchondral bone. For both approaches, patients should ambulate postoperatively with crutches or a cane at 50% weight bearing for 6 weeks followed by full weight bearing.

Prosthetic Replacement

Patients with late-stage disease have limited options for treatment and are therefore candidates for prosthetic knee replacement. The unicondylar profile of SPONK lesions makes unicondylar replacement an option for these patients. Although the use of unicondylar knee replacement is controversial, good or excellent results have been reported in 30 of 34 knees (89%) at a mean follow-up of 5.5 years. Unicondylar replacement is not recommended for patients with secondary osteonecrosis, however, because of the bicondylar nature of the disease.

The results of total knee arthroplasty have been variable for patients with SPONK. In one study that compared 32 knees with SPONK to 63 osteoarthritic knees, no statistically significant difference in the outcome of total knee arthroplasty was found for the two groups. However, another study predicted a 68% survivorship rate in 29 patients with SPONK who underwent total knee arthroplasty. In light of these variable results, further investigation of total knee arthroplasty for the treatment of patients with SPONK is required.

Historically, the results of total knee arthroplasty in patients with secondary osteonecrosis have been disappointing. One study reported a 55% survivorship of total knee arthroplasty in patients younger than 50 years with a history of corticosteroid use. The results were poorer for patients with systemic lupus erythematosus, with only a 44% survivorship in these patients being reported. These results are unsatisfactory considering the multiple reports showing an overall success rate of greater than 90% for total knee arthroplasty.

In a more recent study on the use of total knee arthroplasty to treat 30 patients with osteonecrosis of the knee (32 knees; 22 patients had secondary osteonecrosis of the knee and 8 patients had SPONK), good or excellent results were reported at a mean follow-up of 108 months (range, 48 to 144 months) in 31 of 32 knees

(97%). The authors concluded that cemented prostheses with proper use of augmented stems improves the outcome of total knee arthroplasty in patients with osteonecrosis of the knee.

Summary

Osteonecrosis of the knee includes two separate disorders: SPONK and secondary osteonecrosis of the knee. These disorders are differentiated by location, joint involvement, age of onset, and treatment options. Early diagnosis and treatment are essential to optimize outcome. Therefore, physicians should have a high index of suspicion in patients with characteristic symptoms of the two disorders. Currently, several joint preserving treatment modalities are being used that have shown promising results in the treatment of patients with early-stage disease. However, further investigation regarding the etiology and pathogenesis of osteonecrosis is necessary to improve treatment outcomes.

Annotated Bibliography

Etiology and Pathogenesis

Berger CE, Kroner A, Kristen KH, Minai-Pour M, Leitha T, Engel A: Spontaneous osteonecrosis of the knee: Biochemical markers of bone turnover and pathohistology. *Osteoarthritis Cartilage* 2005;13(8):716-721.

The results of this study showed increased focal degradation of type 1 cartilage in patients with SPONK.

Clinical Features/Differential Diagnosis/Diagnosis/Staging

Ragland PS, Dolphin MS, Etienne G, Mont MA: Diagnosis and treatment of osteonecrosis of the knee. *Tech Knee Surg* 2004;3(3):163-169.

The authors present a thorough discussion of osteonecrosis of the knee and provide a useful treatment algorithm for patients with SPONK.

Nonsurgical Treatment

Mont MA, Baumgarten KM, Rifai A, Bluemke DA, Jones LC, Hungerford DS: Atraumatic osteonecrosis of the knee. *J Bone Joint Surg Am* 2000;82:1279-1290.

The authors found that only 20% of symptomatic knees treated nonsurgically had successful outcomes; they concluded, therefore, that nonsurgical management should only be used in patients with asymptomatic knees.

Surgical Treatment

Mont MA, Rifai A, Baumgarten KM, Sheldon M, Hungerford DS: Total knee arthroplasty for osteonecrosis. *J Bone Joint Surg Am* 2002;84:599-603.

The authors of this study reported a 97% success rate at 9-year follow-up in patients who were treated with total knee arthroplasty using cemented prostheses and ancillary stems.

Classic Bibliography

Aglietti P, Insall JN, Buzzi R, et al: Idiopathic osteonecrosis of the knee: Etiology, prognosis and treatment. *J Bone Joint Surg Br* 1983;65:588-597.

Ahlbäck S, Bauer GCH, Bohne WH: Spontaneous osteonecrosis of the knee. *Arthritis Rheum* 1968;11:705-733.

Lotke PA, Ecker ML: Current concepts review: Osteonecrosis of the knee. *J Bone Joint Surg Am* 1988;70:470-473.

Mont MA, Tomek IM, Hungerford DS: Core decompression for avascular necrosis of the distal femur: Long-term followup. *Clin Orthop* 1997;334:124-130.

Ritter MA, Eizember LE, Keating EM, et al: The survival of total knee arthroplasty in patients with osteonecrosis of the medial condyle. *Clin Orthop* 1991;267:108-114.

Chapter 14

Osteolysis in Total Knee Arthroplasty

Sanaz Hariri, MD

William J. Maloney, MD

Harry E. Rubash, MD

Introduction

Periprosthetic osteolysis after total knee arthroplasty (TKA) is a well-recognized intermediate to long-term complication. Over the past four decades, the prevalence of osteolysis following TKA has increased. As with osteolysis after total hip arthroplasty (THA), development of osteolysis after knee replacement surgery is related to at least three factors: generation of wear debris, access of that debris to bone, and the biologic reaction to the wear debris. Although occurring more commonly in association with loose components, osteolysis can occur with stable cementless implants and less commonly with stable cemented implants. It is important, therefore, that orthopaedic surgeons have a thorough understanding of the etiology, incidence, clinical presentation, radiographic diagnosis, location, and treatment of osteolysis and be familiar with current thought regarding minimizing its development.

Etiology

The chief culprit in osteolysis is often particulate debris. There are many potential sources of particulate debris, including polyethylene, metal, and cement. Polyethylene sources include the tibial bearing surface, tibial post, backside of the tibial insert (the nonbearing portion), and polyethylene patellar component. Metallic debris can result from complete wear-through of the polyethylene, failure of a locking mechanism, and loose screws. Loosening of the implant may lead to cement debris.

Articular Wear

There are two primary active failure modes of polyethylene in TKAs: delamination and adhesive-abrasive wear. Delamination starts as a subsurface crack that extends to the surface, and a large (> 0.5 mm) piece of polyethylene may move into the joint (Figure 1). In adhesive wear, implant motion and the orientation and strain hardening of the implant surface result in the removal of small (usually a few micrometers or less) polyethylene debris (Figure 2). Abrasive wear occurs when hard aspirates on the femoral surface and hard third-body particles (such as bone chips and cement particles) cut the polyethylene surface.

In addition to wear, creep and plastic deformation change the contour of the polyethylene surface over time. Creep accumulates during the first 2 years after surgery, leading to permanent deformation of the insert. Plastic deformation is a transient phenomenon that occurs when the joint is loaded. These two mechanisms do not lead to the generation of polyethylene debris and must be distinguished from the mechanisms of wear.

A method to quantify the wear of retrieved polyethylene tibial inserts (metrologic method) has been developed that compares digitized surface maps of worn and unworn articular surfaces to calculate the volume and linear penetration of the wear. This method has been used to analyze inserts tested on a knee simulator. The metrologic calculation of wear strongly correlated with the gravimetric calculation (calculating insert weight loss with corrections for fluid absorption). Nonetheless, analysis of polyethylene wear in vivo remains a challenge.

Access of the wear particles to the implant-bone interface and periprosthetic bone is affected by implant design and surgical technique. In general, access to bone is more of an issue with cementless than cemented components. Wear debris can gain access to periprosthetic bone through screw holes in the tibial baseplate and regions of the implant-bone interface that lack bone ingrowth. Incomplete porous coatings also provide an access channel for wear debris.

Histologic studies of interface membranes in revision TKA revealed sheets of histiocytes and occasional giant cells; however, necrosis, lymphocytes, plasma cells, and polymorphonuclear leukocytes were not found in significant quantities. Polyethylene and metal debris measuring smaller than 10 μm were found within the histiocytes. Most of the polyethylene debris was less than 1 to 3 μm. Larger birefringent polyethylene debris (10 to 75 μm) was found within foreign-body giant cells.

Polyethylene wear debris triggers a cellular release of chemical mediators that in turn stimulates an osteolytic response. Macrophages phagocytose less than

10 μm of diameter wear particles generated by abrasive-adhesive wear. These activated macrophages then release interleukin (IL)-1β, which stimulates osteoclastic cell formation and increases osteoclastic activity. These activated osteoclasts release tartrate-resistant acid phosphatase (TRAP) during the bone resorptive process. One study compared the IL-1β and TRAP concentrations in synovial fluid aspirations in osteoarthritic knees of patients awaiting a primary TKA and in patients awaiting revision TKA. IL-1β and TRAP concentrations were found to be greater in knees scheduled to undergo revision arthroplasty than in osteoarthritic native knees, presumably because of the polyethylene debris found within the patients awaiting TKA revision.

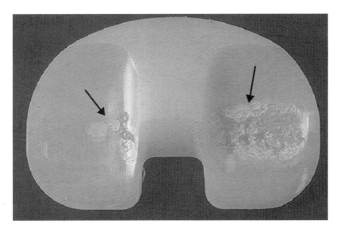

Figure 1 Photograph showing grossly visible delamination (*arrows*) on the articular surface of a polyethylene tibial insert retrieved during revision TKA. (*Reproduced with permission from Muratoglu OK, Vittetoe DA, Rubash HE: Damage of implant surfaces in total knee arthroplasty, in Callaghan JJ, Rosenberg AG, Rubash HE, Simonian PT, Wickiewicz TL (eds): The Adult Knee. Philadelphia, PA, Lippincott Williams & Wilkins, 2002, p 298.*)

Although the local effects of particulate debris have been detailed, the systemic effects are less clear. One study analyzed postmortem and biopsy specimens of patients with total joint arthroplasties, 10 of whom had had primary TKAs for a mean in situ duration of 84 months. Patients who had prostheses had a greater concentration of particles, predominantly polyethylene, than the control groups, particularly in the lymph nodes. However, only 2 of the 10 patients with primary TKAs had evidence of metallic wear in the liver or spleen compared with 7 of the 8 patients with revised THAs and 2 of the 11 patients with primary THAs. The clinical significance of these findings is undetermined.

Polyethylene Fragmentation

Research over the past decade has demonstrated the importance of manufacturing technique, sterilization methods, packaging, and shelf life on wear performance. It is now known that polyethylene sterilized with gamma radiation and stored in oxygen with a long shelf life is associated with higher prevalence of osteolysis. Oxidized polyethylene has a lower resistance to wear, thus increasing the particle load.

Backside Wear

Backside polyethylene wear is defined as the polyethylene deformation between the tibial insert and base plate. Modularity has been associated with a higher prevalence of osteolysis, most likely because it can result in a higher particle load from backside wear.

A recent study found that polyethylene thickness and type of locking mechanism influenced backside deformation. All 106 tibial inserts that were retrieved exhibited both articular and backside deformation. The

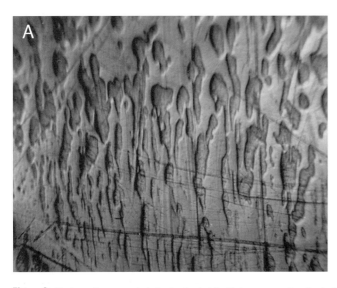

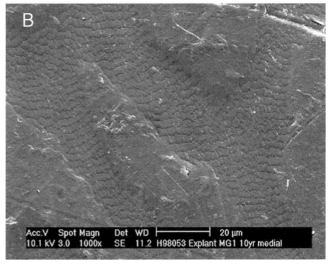

Figure 2 Electron microscope photographs showing the likely precursors to adhesive/abrasive wear on polyethylene tibial inserts: striated (lace) morphology **(A)** and surface ripples **(B)** (original magnification × 1000). (*Reproduced with permission from Muratoglu OK, Vittetoe DA, Rubash HE: Damage of implant surfaces in total knee arthroplasty, in Callaghan JJ, Rosenberg AG, Rubash HE, Simonian PT, Wickiewicz TL (eds): The Adult Knee. Philadelphia, PA, Lippincott Williams & Wilkins, 2002, p 302.*)

mean backside deformation score was reported to be 33% greater for implants from patients with osteolysis than for implants from patients without osteolysis.

Box-Post Impingement

Impingement can occur between the posterior cruciate ligament (PCL)-substituting post and the metal femoral intercondylar box. A recent study analyzed 16 PCL-substituting TKAs that were revised because of aseptic loosening and osteolysis and reported that 12 retrieved knee implants had damage to the lateral and medial side walls of the post. Another recent study found that all 23 of the retrieved TKAs implanted for a mean of 35.6 months had evidence of post damage, an average of 39.9% of the post surface showed some evidence of deformation (predominantly adhesive wear), and seven posts (30%) showed severe damage with gross loss of polyethylene, two of which required revision because of wear (one because of isolated post wear and the other because of severe post wear with subsequent fracture).

Metal Debris

Metal particles accelerate polyethylene wear via a third-body mechanism and are often synergistic with polyethylene when stimulating macrophages. Sources of metal debris include failure of the metal-backed patellar components, impingement of a tibial pin and clip on the femoral implant, and corrosion at the tibial screw-base plate interface. An early study found metal corrosion at the screw-base plate interface and at the entry sites of screws into the tibial metaphysis in all revision patients. The corrosion resulted in very fine metal particles, particularly abundant in those with loosened tibial components. Intracellular metal particles were found in histiocytes and averaged less than 3 μm.

Cement Debris

Osteolysis used to be primarily attributed to "cement disease." Although polymethylmethacrylate can fragment and cause inflammatory and foreign-body reaction to its wear debris that can lead to osteolysis, it is now clear that cement debris is only one (and not even the most significant) of several particulate debris types leading to osteolysis.

Incidence

Cemented TKAs

Just as with THAs, osteolysis around TKAs occurs in cemented as well as cementless components. However, osteolysis occurs much less frequently in the knee than the hip. In a retrieval study of failed TKAs, particles from the TKA tissues (mean size, 1.7 μm) were greater than three times larger than previously characterized particles from failed THAs (mean size, 0.5 μm). This size disparity may be attributable to the differences in joint conformity and wear patterns between the two types of articulations. The larger TKA debris likely results in a diminished mediator release, and thus a decreased incidence of osteolysis and aseptic loosening in knees as compared with hips. The radiolucencies in the knee typically start at the periphery of the implant-bone interface and work their way around the tibial or femoral component. Osteolysis has been reported less frequently in cemented than cementless TKAs.

A recent study assessed 193 cemented modular Insall-Burstein II (Zimmer, Warsaw, IN) posterior-stabilized cemented total knee prostheses in 131 patients. Evidence of osteolysis was detected on radiographs in the proximal tibia in eight knees in six patients; however, no clinical or radiographic loosening of the tibial components was detected.

Another recent study compared 172 cemented Miller-Galante I (MGI, Zimmer) TKAs in 155 patients with 109 cemented Miller-Galante II (MGII, Zimmer) TKAs in 92 patients at an average follow-up of 11 and 9 years, respectively. The 10-year survivorship was 84% for the MGI TKAs (largely because of patellofemoral complications) and 100% for the MGII TKAs. Neither model had evidence of aseptic loosening or osteolysis. All radiolucencies were less than 1 mm. Wear was not a cause of failure in either of the TKAs. The authors postulated that the cement (via its stabilizing fixation and blockage of particle access to the cement-bone interface) and the relatively unconstrained articular surface (resulting in more of a rolling than a sliding motion on the polyethylene surface) minimizes polyethylene wear and therefore osteolysis.

Another recent study followed 334 third-generation cemented NexGen (Zimmer) TKAs in 287 patients for 5 to 8 years. The survivorship in terms of revision for any reason and revision for aseptic loosening were 95.9% and 99.5%, respectively. Only one patient had a progressive radiolucency attributable to osteolysis; 21% of the PCL-retaining implant group and 22% of the PCL-stabilized implant group had nonprogressive tibial radiolucencies of 1 mm.

Nonetheless, there are reports of radiographically significant osteolysis in cemented TKAs. For example, in a study of intermediate and long-term results of the modular cemented PCL-substituting Insall-Burstein II prosthesis, radiographic evidence of osteolysis was found in 17 of the 128 knees assessed (16%). Osteolysis was defined in this study as the presence of a radiolucency with a minimum diameter of 10 mm in at least one dimension and of 5 mm in diameter in the second dimension, loss of trabeculation, and the presence of a sclerotic rim. Twenty-three osteolytic lesions were identified in the 17 knees with radiographic evidence of osteolysis. The average diameter of the lesion was 17 mm (range, 5 to 39 mm; average area and SD, 2.4 +/– 1.9 cm^3).

A study of 2,016 cemented primary TKAs (Press-Fit Condylar modular system, DePuy, Warsaw, IN) found an 8.3% prevalence of wear-related failure correlating to five variables: patient age, patient gender, polyethylene sheet vendor, polyethylene finishing method, and polyethylene shelf age. Noting the frequent changes in specific polyethylene manufacturing details during the life of this implant, the authors emphasized the potential deleterious effects that small changes in the manufacturing process may have on osteolysis and thus the ultimate outcome of a prosthesis despite an initially favorable survivorship.

Cementless TKAs

The incidence of osteolysis in cementless total knees is much higher than in cemented total knees. Although osteolysis in cemented TKAs is often associated with unstable components, osteolysis in cementless TKAs is often associated with a stable component.

The results of the first large-scale study of osteolysis around TKAs were published in 1992. The Synatomic and Arizona prostheses (DePuy) were assessed and osteolysis was defined as a lytic osseous defect extending beyond the limits of that potentially caused by loosening of the implant alone, absence of cancellous bone trabeculae, and geographic demarcation by a shell of bone. In this series of 174 consecutive cementless TKAs, 27 (16%) of the implants showed radiographic evidence of osteolysis at an average 35-month follow-up. Fifteen (56%) of these 27 implants had to be revised at an average of 45 months postoperatively, although none was revised primarily because of osteolysis. When the components associated with osteolysis were examined intraoperatively, 9 of 15 tibial implants and 1 of 2 femoral implants were found to be unstable, which may have been attributable to design defects in the prostheses. For example, the high peak of the central tibial eminence of the polyethylene combined with flexion of the femoral implant likely contributed to excessive tibial eminence wear and particulate-driven osteolysis.

In a more recent study of 125 cementless PCL-retaining MGI TKAs at a minimum 14-year follow-up, it was reported that 21% of the tibial trays and 17% of the femoral components showed radiographic evidence of osteolysis. No knee had to be revised because of osteolysis. It was noted that specific design features of the MGI TKA may have led to the high rate of osteolysis, including a titanium femoral component, flat-on-flat articulation, polyethylene irradiation in air, and screw holes serving as conduits for the debris. However, the rate of osteolysis reported in this study is remarkably higher than that found in the previously mentioned study of MGI TKA. The use of cement as opposed to a cementless technique may account for the difference in osteolysis rates.

Screw Fixation

The use of screws in tibial base plate fixation is another factor affecting the rate of osteolysis. The interface between the screw head and the polyethylene insert undersurface generates polyethylene debris. Furthermore, the screw holes provide access tracts for debris into the tibial metaphyseal cancellous bone. Thus, the cement mantle is only protective if not violated by screw holes. Other concerns include fretting at the screw head-base plate junction and micromotion between the screws and cement.

Periprosthetic Fractures

Most lytic lesions occur around well-fixed implants. However, there have been a few reports of catastrophic TKA failures caused by osteolysis. Catastrophic TKA failures occur because patients are rarely symptomatic when they have osteolysis. Thus, careful review of radiographs for evidence of osteolysis and developing a plan to monitor and address these lesions are important to halt progression to catastrophic TKA failure.

Clinical Presentation

Patients can remain clinically asymptomatic despite extensive bone loss. Occasionally, however, osteolysis of the knee is associated with reports of swelling or late instability rather than pain. Wear particles can result in synovitis that causes an effusion. The synovitic process can affect knee stability, especially with PCL-retaining implants, because it can result in damage to the PCL. On physical examination, patients often have palpable synovial thickening and mild or moderate effusion. A knee effusion postoperatively should trigger an investigation for osteolysis. In one series, knees with osteolysis had an average of 3.9° of flexion contraction compared with 0.9° in those without osteolysis. Patients with knee instability have accelerated polyethylene wear, which causes osteolysis.

The clinical presentation of osteolysis in the knee is different than that in the hip. The hip, a nonsubcutaneous joint, is less accessible and can rarely be examined as well as the knee. Thus, bogey synovitis often associated with massive wear or debris in the knee can be palpated, and the patient will become symptomatic. The correlation between knee scores and osteolysis, however, is unclear.

Although periprosthetic bone loss may be caused by aseptic osteolysis, the possibility of infection as the cause must always be ruled out via clinical and laboratory investigation, with knee aspiration as the diagnostic gold standard.

Radiographic Diagnosis

Because it is difficult to measure polyethylene wear in the knee, the first radiographic sign of significant wear may be osteolysis (Figures 3 and 4). Three factors in particular make osteolysis occurring around TKA prostheses difficult to identify radiographically. First, the complex geometry of knee implants and the distal femur and proximal tibia can make recognition and quantification of osteolysis difficult. Also, osteolysis after TKA typically occurs in the thick, relatively radiolucent cancellous bone of the distal femur and proximal tibia. Not only does the implant obscure the bone, but also because cancellous bone is less radiodense, bone loss is less obvious. Radiographs thus typically underestimate osteolysis. Furthermore, stress shielding of the distal femur may be difficult to differentiate from osteolysis.

Radiographically apparent osteolysis can be classified into two major categories: focal or expansile. In focal osteolysis, there is a border of sclerotic bone that surrounds the area of osteolysis. In expansile osteolysis, there is no such border, presumably because the ability of bone to contain the process of debris migration is overwhelmed. The adjacent cortical shell may fracture in patients with expansile osteolysis.

Radiographic diagnosis of osteolysis is particularly important because neglected asymptomatic osteolysis can progress to catastrophic TKA failure. In contrast, early recognition of osteolysis can be addressed with relatively simple solutions, such as bone grafting through a cortical window with or without concurrent liner exchange.

Although AP and lateral radiographs may suffice for assessing PCL-retaining implants, the condylar pillars of bone are obscured in posterior-stabilized implants on routine radiographs because of the box. A recent cadaver study demonstrated that osteolytic lesions could be much more easily detected on the oblique views than on the standard AP and lateral views. This was particularly true in lesions less than 3.8 mm in diameter. The authors encouraged using oblique radiographs to evaluate femoral bone stock in patients with eccentric polyethylene wear, chronic synovitis with recurrent effusions, and osteolysis around the tibial component and for defining a lesion before surgical intervention for osteolytic wear-related problems. Three-dimensional imaging modalities (CT and MRI) with metal suppression technology appear to be the future of improved osteolysis detection.

Because of radiographic diagnostic limitations, synovial fluid aspiration has been proposed as another, albeit more invasive, method for assessing wear. In one recent study, knees were aspirated and the polyethylene particles were isolated and analyzed with a scanning electron microscope. The authors proposed that aspiration of the knees of patients with well-functioning prostheses and analysis of particle size, shape, and concentration may be used to compare wear in newer models with that of older established prostheses.

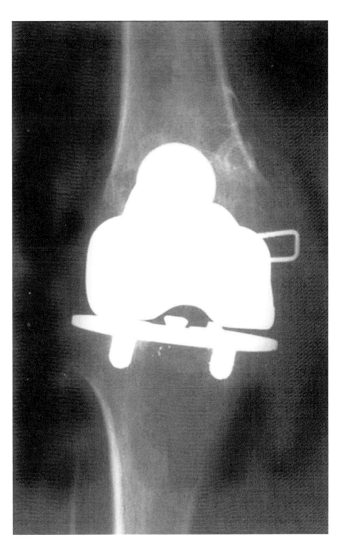

Figure 3 Radiograph showing a lytic bone lesion beneath the TKA tibial base plate. *(Reproduced with permission from Muratoglu OK, Vittetoe DA, Rubash HE: Damage of implant surfaces in total knee arthroplasty, in Callaghan JJ, Rosenberg AG, Rubash HE, Simonian PT, Wickiewicz TL (eds): The Adult Knee. Philadelphia, PA, Lippincott Williams & Wilkins, 2002, p 302.)*

In light of the above challenges to the radiographic diagnosis of osteolysis, surgeons should identify patients who are most susceptible to osteolysis so that they may be especially vigilant in assessing their radiographs. Knowledge of the most common anatomic locations of osteolysis is also helpful in the identification of osteolysis.

Location of Osteolysis

In patients with loose cemented implants, osteolysis usually begins at the loose interfaces and extends into the cancellous bone. One study reported the common locations of osteolysis in patients with well-fixed implants. Distal femur osteolysis, best seen on lateral plain radiographs, most commonly occurs at the posterior condyles and the region beneath the collateral ligaments in the

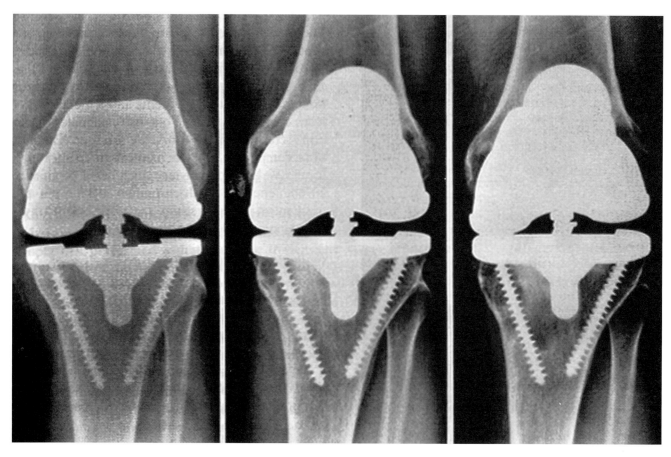

Figure 4 Sequential radiographs obtained immediately postoperatively **(A)**, 47 months postoperatively **(B)**, and 59 months postoperatively **(C)** illustrate advancing osteolytic lesions along both the implant-bone and screw-bone interfaces. *(Reproduced with permission from Peters PC Jr, Engh GA, Dwyer KA, Vinh TN: Osteolysis after total knee arthroplasty without cement. J Bone Joint Surg Am 1992;74:866.)*

femoral condyles. Osteolysis of the posterior condyles typically appears as a reduced radiodensity on lateral radiographs with scalloped ill-defined borders. Osteolysis of the femoral condyles typically has a flame-shaped radiolucency extending proximally into either condyle on AP radiographs.

Tibial osteolysis often occurs along access tracks to cancellous bone (for example, along screws or tibial stems) or around the periphery of well-fixed implants. Evidence of osteolysis may be seen along the medial and lateral borders of the tibial component on AP radiographs and along the anterior and posterior borders on lateral views. When examining the patella, the most common locations of osteolysis are around the implant margins or at the implant-bone or cement-bone interfaces on either the patellar skyline or lateral knee radiographs.

Risk Factors

Several demographic and physical patient factors affect osteolysis. It has been reported that more active patients with older prostheses tended to have a higher rate of osteolysis. This finding is particularly significant because

the population of patients undergoing TKA has changed dramatically over time. Many patients who undergo TKA today expect to return to active lifestyles. Higher activity creates greater wear volume that, in turn, increases the likelihood of osteolysis.

Although early studies did not find patient weight, gender, or age to be risk factors for osteolysis, more recent studies have arrived at different conclusions. In a study of Press-Fit Condylar (PFC, Johnson and Johnson, Warsaw, IN) modular prostheses, 1,287 patients underwent TKA. At 5-year follow-up, 94 had wear-related failure and 14 more had major osteolysis or wear-related revision. Five variables significantly correlated with wear-related failure: patient age (5% decrease in likelihood of wear-related TKA failure with every 1-year increase in patient age), patient gender (men were 2.8 times more likely than women to have wear-related TKA failure), polyethylene vendor, polyethylene finishing method (polycarbonate tumbling decreased wear-related failures), and polyethylene shelf age (the likelihood of wear-related failure increased 187% for every 1-year increase in shelf life). These findings emphasized the fact that relatively small changes in polyethylene manufacturing can have a significant effect on wear. The study did not, however, find a correlation between polyethylene thickness and wear-related events. It should also be noted that these inserts were gamma sterilized in air.

Asymmetric polyethylene damage and wear are more common in knees with osteolysis. Patients who have undergone bilateral TKA are at greater risk for implant loosening and osteolysis compared with those who have undergone unilateral TKA. In regard to polyethylene characteristics, heat-pressed (PCA, Howmedica, Rutherford, NJ) and carbon-reinforced (Zimmer) polyethylene have demonstrated higher wear rates. On the tibial side, an insecure locking mechanism between the tibial tray and polyethylene insert (leading to micromotion between these two components), an imperfect tibial tray surface finish, and access routes for particles to the tibial cancellous bone (such as screw holes) predispose patients to osteolysis. On the femoral side, titanium components are a risk factor for osteolysis.

Intraoperative Assessment and Management of Osteolysis

Defect Classification

Because preoperative assessment often underestimates the extent of bone loss, intraoperative inspection is the most accurate method of assessing bone stock. Defects are described in terms of size, location, and depth. An ideal classification system would be objective and reproducible, have therapeutic and prognostic importance, and take into consideration the quality of the remaining bone and its vascularity. Although such a classification system is yet to be developed, the Anderson Orthopaedic Research Institute bone defect classification system provides some guidelines for bony defect management.

In type I defects, the metaphyseal bone is intact and cancellous bone graft or cement may be used to fill the defect. In type II defects, the metaphyseal bone loss compromises implant support, requiring cement fill, augments, or bone graft to restore a reasonable joint line level. In type III defects, there is a deficient metaphyseal segment in either the condyle or the plateau. When revised, they require long-stemmed revision implants plus bone grafting or a custom or hinged component.

A classification system of bony defects found at the time of knee revision surgery and a surgical treatment algorithm have been described that separates defects into major and minor categories and then further subcategorizes them as contained or uncontained. Minor defects are less than 1 cm^3 and are below the level of the epicondyles. Major defects are greater than 1 cm^3 and are above the level of the epicondyles. Contained defects have cancellous bone loss only. Uncontained defects have both cancellous and cortical bone loss; thus, a portion of the implant is unsupported. Dissociations of the condyles are classified as uncontained.

Defect Management

Bone defects are managed using a combination of allograft bone chips, structural grafts, and metal augments. In general, bone defects at the level of the distal femur or proximal tibia can be managed with metal augments. Larger defects usually require grafting. Contained defects can be treated with impaction grafting of allograft bone chips and can be performed in the presence of well-fixed implant components. Commercially available bone substitutes may be helpful in containing the intra-articular communication with the bone defect once it has been packed with bone chips. Uncontained defects are generally managed with structural allografts. Femoral head allografts usually suffice for management of larger defects, although a distal femoral or proximal tibial allograft may be necessary in some patients. Tibial and femoral extension stems should be used when grafting has been performed to help stress-protect the graft. Less commonly, patients with severe bone loss and associated collateral ligament loss will require a rotating hinge prosthesis. In these patients, the bone defects can usually be managed with the implant and do not require grafting.

General guidelines for defect management have been described. Contained defects should be filled with cancellous grafts because they revascularize more rapidly than structural grafts. Restoration of structural stability is the goal of treatment in patients with uncontained defects, which are characterized by loss of cortical, structurally supportive bone. Modular augments are needed to bypass the defects; structural allografts are used in patients in whom bone loss is too extensive. Structural allograft does not fully revascularize, however, and may eventually collapse.

Published results of the treatment of large osteolytic defects at the time of revision surgery are limited. In a minimum 5-year follow-up study on revision TKAs, one study reported a fairly high failure rate. Overall, revisions that required bulk structural allografts failed less frequently (19.2%) compared with those that were managed without grafts (42.9%). Of the 24 knees revised for osteolysis and wear, only one required re-revision for a wear-related complication. Another recent study specifically addressed the outcome of revision surgery in which large osteolytic defects were managed. Only 3 of the 28 patients who underwent TKA revision were considered to be candidates for impaction grafting around well-fixed implant components. In the remaining 25 patients, 8 required bulk structural grafts and 15 had impaction grafting of allograft bone chips. Short- to intermediate-term follow-up demonstrated stable radiographs in 25 of 28 knees. One patient (two knees) who was asymptomatic had radiographs that demonstrated progressive radiolucencies around the tibial component after isolated tibial revision. There was one clinical failure as a result of infection and extensor mechanism insufficiency.

Component Revision Timing and Options

Few data exist to help surgeons guide the management of distal femoral or proximal tibial osteolysis at the time of TKA revision. Although not always the case, osteolysis in association with cemented components is usually associated with a loose implant. In contrast, severe osteolysis can develop after cementless TKA in association with osseointegrated cementless components.

When osteolysis is present and the implants are well fixed, the decision to perform surgery is based on the degree of bone loss and patient symptoms. The decision to recommend revision surgery is more difficult in patients who are asymptomatic. In addition to the degree of bone loss, other factors to take into account include patient age and activity level, patient comorbidities, and the risk for the development of a pathologic fracture. No objective data exist to guide optimal timing for surgical intervention.

When the implants are stable, surgeons have a choice to graft the osteolytic lesion and exchange the tibial insert or revise the component. Again, few data are available to direct treatment. Tibial polyethylene insert exchange with impaction grafting of lytic lesions can be successful provided the implant is otherwise well aligned and the knee can be made ligamentously stable with a new insert. It is important to remember that the PCL can be damaged as part of the synovitic process. As a result, a standard tibial insert may not be sufficient to provide stability, and a PCL-substituting implant may be needed, which requires femoral revision. Although most knee replacement systems offer a more constrained tibial insert for their cruciate-retaining designs, the actual impact these more constrained inserts have on articular stability varies significantly.

Knees that exhibit early wear-related failure likely have technical or implant-related factors that contributed to the failure process. In such instances, revision surgery should be considered. In contrast, patients who functioned well for many years and then had wear-related failure are reasonable candidates for an insert exchange, provided the implants are well fixed.

Minimizing Osteolysis
Technical Factors

Technical issues that affect knee alignment and ligament balancing can impact wear by reducing stresses at the polyethylene tray and the implant-bone interfaces. Perfect alignment is difficult to achieve. Slight malalignment may not represent a functional problem for the patient, but it can result in increased stresses in the polyethylene and potentially accelerate wear. Ligament balancing and implant design act in concert to dictate

knee stability. A tight flexion gap most commonly associated with underrelease of the PCL in cruciate-retaining knee replacement systems or oversizing of the femoral component can lead to accelerated polyethylene wear posteromedially. Patients with a loose flexion gap and minimally conforming implants are prone to increased anteroposterior translation of the femur on the tibia during gait (paradoxical motion). Translation of the femur on the tibia increases shear stresses in the polyethylene and may accelerate wear.

Furthermore, the surgeon should avoid overall hyperextension with flexion of the femoral component and excessive posterior slope of the tibial component in a posterior-stabilized system. The tibial polyethylene insert should be at least 10 mm thick to minimize contact stress. Cam-post mechanisms should allow for some hyperextension without excessive impingement or torsional constraint.

Polyethylene Sterilization

The polyethylene sterilization process is another factor that can affect wear. Traditional polyethylene is sterilized using gamma irradiation in air. The radiation promotes cross-linking, which improves wear resistance. However, this process also leads to the formation of free radicals that may oxidize, adversely affecting the polyethylene mechanical properties. Polyethylene strength and ductility is reduced while its modulus is increased, predisposing it to delamination and pitting. In the mid-1990s, there was a shift to gamma sterilization in inert environments (nitrogen, argon, or vacuum) to minimize oxidation during gamma irradiation in air.

Shelf Life

The mechanical toughness of polyethylene sterilized by gamma irradiation in air decreases with increasing shelf life. In a study that investigated the effect of shelf life on polyethylene degradation, 188 Synatomic TKA implants (DePuy) sterilized by gamma irradiation in air were assessed. Clinical failure was defined as component retrieval resulting from polyethylene degradation. Patients were classified based on shelf storage duration. The mean shelf life of the six prostheses requiring revision for polyethylene degradation was 8.4 years. Another study found a significant inverse linear correlation between polyethylene shelf life and time to revision in 75 unicondylar knee replacements performed with polyethylene gamma irradiated in air. A significant step toward minimizing polyethylene wear is to minimize the length of insert shelf life.

Backside Wear

To minimize backside wear, locking mechanisms have been developed that minimize relative motion during off-axis loading, and base plates have been developed that are made of harder materials. For example, titanium alloys have lower hardness and therefore their surface is more easily damaged and less wear-resistant than cobalt-chromium alloys.

One study examined 124 polyethylene tibial inserts retrieved during TKA revision at an average of 50.7 months (range, 0 to 180 months). The inserts were assessed for pitting (shallow surface voids) and burnishing (highly polished surfaces). Three different types of locking mechanisms were retrieved: (1) linear capture using a tongue and groove with tracks that run anterior to posterior or medial to lateral and augmented with a locking pin; (2) peripheral capture using a snap fit with beveled edges along either the entire periphery or a segment of the periphery; and (3) central captured with a mushroom-shaped pin and immobilized with a peripheral flange to prevent rotation around the pin. Components with a linear tongue-and-groove mechanism had more severe burnishing than the other types of locking mechanisms. However, although cobalt-chromium should theoretically be more wear resistant than titanium, the cobalt-chromium alloy base plates exhibited more severe pitting than titanium base plates. The authors did not discuss the potential reasons for this finding.

Another study also found evidence of considerable micromotion in an analysis of retrieved implants using a broad variety of contemporary locking mechanisms. The authors concluded by calling for development of better locking mechanisms to minimize polyethylene wear debris generation.

When designing implants, it must also be considered that design factors at the articulation of the femur and the tibial insert can also affect backside wear by transmitting forces to other articulating surfaces. For example, a highly conforming femur-tibial insert geometry may inhibit anteroposterior or mediolateral motion at this articulation. Shear forces are then transferred to the tibial base plate-tibial insert interface, promoting backside wear.

Conformity

Conformity decreases polyethylene insert wear and fatigue because it allows distribution of weight-bearing contact stresses over a larger area. In the hip, the acetabular cup and femoral head are almost fully conforming. However, through the flexion range of the knee, the radius of the femoral component does not always match the radius of the tibial component. A study that varied the conformity ratios and the loads on a joint found that stress calculations were much higher at 1,000 N (standing) on a flat inlay component when compared with 6,000 N (running) on a conforming component. A small increase in conformity had a greater effect on stress parameters than a relatively large load increase.

A study that isolated and analyzed wear particles obtained from TKA revisions compared nonheat-pressed PCL-retaining prostheses, and found that the group of 14 prostheses with relatively congruent surfaces had fewer particles, smaller particles, and less surface damage than the group of 19 prostheses with relatively flat nonconforming surfaces. Increasing conformity decreases the magnitude of stresses on the polyethylene and increases stability. However, increasing conformity also limits range of motion, increases stress on the ligaments and tibial base plate fixation, and increases susceptibility to three-body abrasion from entrapped cement particles and particles of worn polyethylene.

Mobile-Bearing Prosthesis

There are two ways to reduce inlay stress on the polyethylene insert: load changes (force and activity restrictions) and conformity changes (design changes). Stress parameters are more sensitive to the conformity changes. However, increasing conformity reduces polyethylene stress but increases stress at the tibial fixation interfaces. The mobile-bearing designs attempt to address this tradeoff. One of the theoretic advantages of mobile meniscal-bearing prostheses is that the articular surfaces of the components can be congruent over the entire range of motion, increasing contact areas and therefore decreasing contact stresses on the polyethylene insert. Furthermore, the flat-topped tibial plates under the free sliding menisci should transmit only minimal tensile and shear stresses to the underlying bone, thereby diminishing the risk of tibial base plate loosening.

However, a study comparing the prevalence of osteolysis after failed TKA with mobile-bearing prostheses and fixed-bearing prostheses found that the prevalence of osteolysis was significantly higher in the mobile-bearing group (47% versus 13%). The possible reasons for this unexpected finding were discussed, noting that excision of the posterior femoral osteophytes is commonly performed in knee arthroplasty, but the Low Contact Stress (LCS) system (DePuy) uses an extra posterior femoral condyle cut to increase the range of motion. This extra cut exposes cancellous bone surface not covered by the prosthesis, providing an access tract for particles into the bone-implant interface. Furthermore, the LCS system may produce an increased number of smaller particles because of its greater conformity and greater undersurface wear. Increasing conformity leads to smaller particulate debris, and these smaller particles are more biologically active, inducing more significant cellular reaction, osteolysis, and aseptic loosening.

However, several other long-term studies show a low incidence of osteolysis in the LCS system. In one study, at a mean 4.5-year follow-up, there were overall good results in approximately 72% of patients with TKA without any change in component position and alignment, osteolysis, or cement-bone radiolucency during follow-up. In another study (mean follow-up, 12.4 years), good to excellent results were seen in 97.9% of patients with the LCS system. Massive osteolysis was not observed in any of the patients whose knees had not undergone previous surgery. However, at an average 10.2-year follow-up, osteolysis was found in 1.8% of the patients with multiple previous knee surgeries. These patients required bone grafting of contained defects. Another study (9- to 12-year follow-up) of 114 patients who underwent TKA with an LCS system reported an increase in the average Hospital for Special Surgery knee rating from 57 points (range, 28 to 80 points) preoperatively to 84 points (range, 59 to 97 points) at the final follow-up evaluation. No periprosthetic osteolysis or evidence of loosening on follow-up radiographs was found.

Polyethylene Cross-Linking

Significant advances have been made in the preparation and sterilization of polyethylene inserts in regard to wear resistance. A new technique of polyethylene preparation consists of radiation cross-linking to reduce wear and subsequently melt-annealing to reduce the concentration of residual free radicals that lead to polyethylene oxidative degradation. These components have been compared with conventional inserts that do not undergo this process. When both components were artificially aged (aggressively oxidized in an air convection oven at 80°C for 35 days) and then placed on a test machine for 5 million cycles to stimulate gait, the aged conventional inserts showed subsurface cracks that propagated to the articulating surface and began to delaminate at 5 million cycles. None of the aged highly cross-linked tibial inserts showed any subsurface cracks or delaminations.

A knee simulator has been developed that places the tibial insert in an adverse environment: stair climbing with a tight PCL that places excessive posterior loading on the tibial plateaus at about 90° of flexion. This knee simulator was then used to test an insert that had undergone electron beam cross-linking with subsequent melting to reduce the concentration of residual free radicals. No subsurface cracks and delamination were detected at as many as 0.5 million cycles.

Although cross-linking polyethylene has been shown to reduce polyethylene volumetric wear rates, it also reduces its fracture toughness and elevates wear in abrasive conditions. With abrasive wear comes a greater percentage of particles smaller than 1 μm. Macrophages can phagocytose molecules of this size, leading to an osteolytic cascade reflected by an elevated tumor necrosis factor-α concentration found in patients with implants

containing cross-linked polyethylene compared with implants that are not cross-linked. Although less particle wear may occur, those particles produced may be more biologically active; however, the increase in biologic activity is likely offset by the decrease in particle number caused by decreased wear.

Summary

Periprosthetic osteolysis is a major cause of TKA failure, particularly in cementless systems. The primary initiator of osteolysis is polyethylene particulate debris. The major steps in the osteolytic cascade are generation of wear debris, access of that debris to bone, and the biologic reaction to the wear debris via osteoclasts. Patients are often clinically asymptomatic, but they may present with effusions. Radiographic diagnosis of osteolysis is difficult because of the geometry of the implant and the relative radiolucency of the cancellous bone surrounding the implant. Therefore, knowledge of the most common osteolytic lesion locations and patients at greatest risk for osteolysis is helpful in identifying TKAs with developing osteolysis. Early diagnosis may allow surgical treatment at a stage when necessary interventions are less complex. When planning a revision TKA, surgeons must be aware that radiographs often underestimate the extent of osteolysis. A variety of materials should therefore be readily available to address any unforeseen defects intraoperatively. There have been several advances in minimizing wear, particularly in the fields of polyethylene cross-linking, sterilization, and awareness of the adverse effects of a long shelf life.

Annotated Bibliography

Etiology

Akisue T, Yamaguchi M, Bauer TW, et al: "Backside" polyethylene deformation in total knee arthroplasty. *J Arthroplasty* 2003;18(6):784-791.

Using a semiquantitative scoring system to analyze 106 retrieved polyethylene tibial inserts, the authors found that the mean backside deformation score was 33% greater for implants from patients with osteolysis than for implants from patients without osteolysis.

Goodman S: Wear particulate and osteolysis. *Orthop Clin North Am* 2005;36(1):41-48.

This article reviews the causes of periprosthetic osteolysis.

Kovacik MW, Gradisar IA Jr, Haprian JJ, Alexander TS: Osteolytic indicators found in total knee arthroplasty synovial fluid aspirates. *Clin Orthop* 2000;379:186-194.

The authors of this study found elevated levels of IL-1β and tartrate-resistant acid phosphatase concentrations in TKA synovial fluid aspirates.

Mikulak SA, Mahoney OM, dela Rosa MA, Schmalzried TP: Loosening and osteolysis with the press-fit condylar posterior-cruciate-substituting total knee replacement. *J Bone Joint Surg Am* 2001;83-A(3): 398-403.

The authors of this study assessed press-fit condylar PCL-substituting implants and found that rotational forces were generated by impingement of the side walls of the intercondylar box on the polyethylene post and that rotational stresses are transmitted to the modular interfaces and to the metal-cement interfaces, resulting in loosening and osteolysis.

Muratoglu OK, Perinchief RS, Bragdon CR, O'Connor DO, Konrad R, Harris WH: Metrology to quantify wear and creep of polyethylene tibial knee inserts. *Clin Orthop Relat Res* 2003;410:155-164.

The authors present a metrologic method that uses a coordinate measuring machine to quantify the dimensions of the scar that forms on tibial insert articular surfaces.

Muratoglu OK, Vittetoe DA, Rubash HE: Damage of implant surfaces in total knee arthroplasty, in Callaghan JJ, Rosenberg AG, Rubash HE, Simonian PT, Wickiewicz TL (eds): *The Adult Knee.* Philadelphia, PA, Lippincott Williams & Wilkins, 2003, pp 297-313.

This chapter reviews TKA prosthesis wear mechanisms, including biologic and mechanical factors. Techniques to reduce articular surface damage are presented.

Puloski SK, McCalden RW, MacDonald SJ, Rorabeck CH, Bourne RB: Tibial post wear in posterior stabilized total knee arthroplasty: An unrecognized source of polyethylene debris. *J Bone Joint Surg Am* 2001;83-A(3):390-397.

The authors of this study show that the cam-post articulation in posterior-stabilized TKA implants can be an additional source of polyethylene wear debris. The variability in wear patterns observed among designs may be caused by differences in cam-post mechanics, post location, and post geometry.

Sethi RK, Neavyn MJ, Rubash HE, Shanbhag AS: Macrophage response to cross-linked and conventional UHMWPE. *Biomaterials* 2003;24(15):2561-2573.

The authors found that macrophages cultured on cross-linked and conventional polyethylene released levels of cytokines similar to levels on control tissue culture dishes. Macrophages cultured on titanium-alloy and cobalt-chromium alloy released levels of cytokines that were significantly higher than those cultured on polyethylene and from control tissue culture dishes.

Urban RM, Jacobs JJ, Tomlinson MJ, Gavrilovic J, Black J, Peoc'h M: Dissemination of wear particles to the liver, spleen, and abdominal lymph nodes of patients with hip or knee replacement. *J Bone Joint Surg Am* 2000;82(4): 457-476.

This study reported on the systemic distribution of metallic and polyethylene wear particles in patients with primary and revision joint prostheses. Systemic distribution of metallic and polyethylene wear particles was a common finding in patients with a previously failed implant and in those with a primary total joint prosthesis.

Incidence, Clinical Presentation, and Risk Factors

Berger RA, Rosenberg AG, Barden RM, Sheinkop MB, Jacobs JJ, Galante JO: Long-term followup of the Miller-Galante total knee replacement. *Clin Orthop* 2001;388:58-67.

The authors compared 172 patients with cemented MGI TKAs to 109 patients with cemented MGII TKAs at an average follow-up of 11 years and 9 years, respectively. The survivorship was 84.1% and 100%, respectively. No component had aseptic loosening or osteolysis. The MGI TKAs had a high prevalence of patellofemoral complications, whereas this was not a common problem in the patients with MGII TKAs.

Bozic KJ, Kinder J, Menegini M, Zurakowski D, Rosenberg AG, Galante JO: Implant survivorship and complication rates after total knee arthroplasty with a third-generation cemented system: 5 to 8 years followup. *Clin Orthop Relat Res* 2005;430:117-124.

The authors of this study assessed 334 patients who underwent primary TKA with a third-generation cemented prosthetic device using cruciate-retaining and posterior-stabilized designs at 5- to 8-year follow-up and found a survivorship of 95.9% and 99.5%, respectively. No significant difference in survivorship, reoperation rates, and complication rates was noted between the two groups.

Fehring TK, Murphy JA, Hayes TD, Roberts DW, Pomeroy DL, Griffin WL: Factors influencing wear and osteolysis in press-fit condylar modular total knee replacements. *Clin Orthop* 2004;428:40-50.

The authors of this study reported that at more than 5 year follow-up of 1,287 patients with PFC system TKAs, the prevalence of wear-related failure was 8.3%. The 13-year survivorship for all patients was 82.6%. Patient age, patient gender, polyethylene sheet vendor, polyethylene finishing method, and polyethylene shelf age were found to correlate with wear-related failure.

Goldberg VM, Kraay M: The outcome of the cementless tibial component: A minimum 14-year clinical evaluation. *Clin Orthop* 2004;428:214-220.

A prospective study of MGI cementless TKAs at a minimum 14-year follow-up showed osteolysis in 21% of the implants with tibial trays and 17% of the femoral components of the 113 knees studied. The overall knee survival rate was 87%.

Lachiewicz PF, Soileau ES: The rates of osteolysis and loosening associated with a modular posterior stabilized knee replacement: Results at five to fourteen years. *J Bone Joint Surg Am* 2004;86-A(3):525-530.

This prospective study of 193 knees implanted with the modular Insall-Burstein II posterior-stabilized total knee prosthesis showed excellent results in 112 patients, good results in 60, fair results in 15, and poor results in 6. Although eight patients had osteolytic lesions of the tibia, the authors found no clinical or radiographic evidence of loosening of the tibial component.

O'Rourke MR, Callaghan JJ, Goetz DD, Sullivan PM, Johnston RC: Osteolysis associated with a cemented modular posterior-cruciate-substituting total knee design: five to eight-year follow-up. *J Bone Joint Surg Am* 2002;84-A(8):1362-1371.

In a study of 128 Insall-Burstein II TKAs at an average 6.4-year follow-up, three knees had to undergo revision because of instability or infection, but none underwent revision because of loosening or osteolysis. Sixteen percent of the knees had radiographic evidence of osteolysis. Osteolysis was not found in any knee in which an all-polyethylene tibial component had been used.

Shanbhag AS, Bailey HO, Hwang DS, Cha CW, Eror NG, Rubash HE: Quantitative analysis of ultrahigh molecular weight polyethylene (UHMWPE) wear debris associated with total knee replacements. *J Biomed Mater Res* 2000;53(1):100-110.

The authors retrieved tissue from 18 failed TKAs to study the size and morphology of particulate wear debris. The mean wear debris size was 1.7 ± 0.7 μm, which was greater than three times larger than wear debris from failed THAs. The particles were predominantly spherical with occasional fibrillar attachments and flakes.

Radiographic Diagnosis

Berry DJ: Recognizing and identifying osteolysis around total knee arthroplasty. *Instr Course Lect* 2004;53:261-264.

The author of this article discusses the difficulty of identifying osteolysis radiographically, the common locations of osteolysis, and modalities that may make radiographic diagnosis of osteolysis more sensitive in the future.

Minoda Y, Kobayashi A, Iwaki H, et al: Polyethylene wear particles in synovial fluid after total knee arthroplasty. *Clin Orthop* 2003;410:165-172.

This study examined polyethylene particles in synovial fluid obtained 1 year after a TKA. The authors reported on the size, shape, and number of these particles.

Nadaud MC, Fehring TK, Fehring K: Underestimation of osteolysis in posterior stabilized total knee arthroplasty. *J Arthroplasty* 2004;19(1):110-115.

The authors of this study demonstrated the inaccuracy of radiographic diagnosis of osteolysis by obtaining standard AP and lateral radiographs of cadavers with simulated osteolytic lesions. They also demonstrated that these lesions can be more easily observed on oblique radiographs.

Intraoperative Assessment and Management of Osteolysis

Hockman DE, Ammeen D, Engh GA: Augments and allografts in revision total knee arthroplasty: Usage and outcome using one modular revision prosthesis. *J Arthroplasty* 2005;20(1):35-41.

The authors reported on the results of 65 Coordinate (DePuy, Warsaw, IN) revision TKAs at a minimum 5-year follow-up. Metallic augmentation was used in 89% of the revisions; large structural allografts were required in 48% of the revisions. Nine knees failed, requiring either revision or component removal. Eight others were clinical failures. At 8-year follow-up, survivorship was 79.4% ± 13.7%.

Hoeffel DP, Rubash HE: Revision total knee arthroplasty: Current rationale and techniques for femoral component revision. *Clin Orthop* 2000;380:116-132.

The authors of this article review currently used femoral revision techniques and their rationale and present a classification system of femoral deficiencies designed to guide the surgical decision-making process, particularly regarding the proper use of bone grafts, component augmentation, proper axial and rotational alignment, and femoral stems in revision TKA.

Rand JA, Ries MD, Landis GH, Rosenberg AG, Haas S: Intraoperative assessment in revision total knee arthroplasty. *J Bone Joint Surg Am* 2003;85-A(suppl 1):S26-S37.

This article proposes a guideline for treating contained and uncontained osteolytic defects with grafts.

Minimizing Osteolysis

Bhan S, Malhotra R: Results of rotating-platform, low-contact-stress knee prosthesis. *J Arthroplasty* 2003;18(8):1016-1022.

In this study, rotating-platform knee arthroplasties were assessed in 31 consecutive patients with 50 deformed knees. At a 4.5-year mean follow-up (range, 4 to 6 years), good results were reported in 72% of 22 osteoarthritic knees and 71.4% of 28 rheumatoid knees.

Buechel FF Sr: Long-term followup after mobile-bearing total knee replacement. *Clin Orthop Relat Res* 2002;404:40-50.

Clinical, radiographic, and survivorship analyses were conducted on a series of 309 cementless PCL-retaining meniscal-bearing and rotating-platform TKAs. At a mean follow-up of 12.4 years (range, 10 to 20 years), clinical results in patients surviving at least 10 years using a strict knee scoring scale were similar for patients with PCL-retaining and PCL-sacrificing prostheses. Good to excellent results were seen in

97.9% of patients with primary PCL-bearing prostheses and in 97.9% of those with primary rotating-platform prostheses.

Callaghan JJ, Squire MW, Goetz DD, Sullivan PM, Johnston RC: Cemented rotating-platform total knee replacement: A nine- to twelve-year follow-up study. *J Bone Joint Surg Am* 2000;82(5):705-711.

In this study, 119 consecutive TKAs (86 patients) with cemented rotating-platform femoral and tibial components and a Townley all-polyethylene dome patellar component were assessed. At 9- to 12-year follow-up, cemented LCS rotating-platform TKAs were reported to be performing well according to clinical and radiographic assessment.

Conditt MA, Stein JA, Noble PC: Factors affecting the severity of backside wear of modular tibial inserts. *J Bone Joint Surg Am* 2004;86-A(2):305-311.

This study examined the type and severity of backside wear in retrieved tibial inserts. Pitting, burnishing, and measurable polyethylene protrusions were observed on the backside of polyethylene inserts of implant designs with a variety of different capture mechanisms.

Fisher J, McEwen HM, Tipper JL, et al: Wear, debris, and biologic activity of cross-linked polyethylene in the knee: Benefits and potential concerns. *Clin Orthop* 2004; 428:114-119.

The authors reviewed the wear rates, wear debris, and biologic reactivity of various polyethylene inserts and concluded that the use of cross-linked polyethylene in the knee reduces the volumetric wear rate but also reduces fracture toughness, elevates wear in abrasive conditions, and elevates tumor necrosis factor-α release.

Harris WH, Muratoglu OK: A review of current cross-linked polyethylenes used in total joint arthroplasty. *Clin Orthop* 2005;430:46-52.

The authors discuss how differences in the polyethylene manufacturing processes may affect polyethylene wear, the rate of particle generation, oxidation, and mechanical properties.

Hopper RH Jr, Young AM, Orishimo KF, Engh CA Jr: Effect of terminal sterilization with gas plasma or gamma radiation on wear of polyethylene liners. *J Bone Joint Surg Am* 2003;85-A(3):464-468.

The authors conducted this study to test the hypothesis that conventional polyethylene liners that are cross-linked by sterilization with gamma radiation in air have better in vivo wear performance than non–cross-linked liners that are sterilized with gas plasma. The authors found that the in vivo wear of conventional polyethylene liners that had been sterilized with gamma radiation in air was, on average, 50% less than that of non–cross-linked liners sterilized with gas plasma.

Huang CH, Ma HM, Liau JJ, Ho FY, Cheng CK: Osteolysis in failed total knee arthroplasty: A comparison of mobile-bearing and fixed-bearing knees. *J Bone Joint Surg Am* 2002;84-A(12):2224-2229.

In this comparison of mobile-bearing and fixed-bearing TKA implants, the authors found that prevalence of osteolysis was higher in patients with a mobile-bearing prosthesis than in those with a fixed-bearing prosthesis. Radiographic analysis underestimated the degree of osteolysis, but found it to be predominantly on the femoral side, adjacent to the posterior aspect of the condyle.

Kilgus DJ: Polyethylene wear in mobile-bearing prostheses. *Orthopedics* 2002;25(2 suppl):S227-S233.

The author discusses the theoretic advantages of a mobile-bearing prosthesis in decreasing polyethylene wear via increased conformity.

Kuster MS, Horz S, Spalinger E, Stachowiak GW, Gachter A: The effects of conformity and load in total knee replacement. *Clin Orthop* 2000;375:302-312.

The authors studied the effects of conformity and load changes on TKA implant wear and found that surface and shear stress are more sensitive to changes in conformity than to changes in load.

Kuster MS, Stachowiak GW: Factors affecting polyethylene wear in total knee arthroplasty. *Orthopedics* 2002; 25(suppl 2):s235-s242.

The authors of this study assessed ways to minimize fatigue-type wear of TKAs and found that all stress parameters are more sensitive to conformity changes (design changes) than to load changes (activity restrictions). The effect of the mobile-bearing design on TKA implant wear is also discussed.

McGovern TF, Ammeen DJ, Collier JP, Currier BH, Engh GA: Rapid polyethylene failure of unicondylar tibial components sterilized with gamma irradiation in air and implanted after a long shelf life. *J Bone Joint Surg Am* 2002;84-A(6):901-906.

The authors of this study demonstrated that early, severe wear occurred in tibial polyethylene bearings that had been sterilized by gamma irradiation in air and stored for ≤ 4.4 years.

Muratoglu OK, Bragdon CR, Jasty M, O'Connor DO, Von Knoch RS, Harris WH: Knee-simulator testing of conventional and cross-linked polyethylene tibial inserts. *J Arthroplasty* 2004;19(7):887-897.

The authors used a knee simulator to compare the resistance to delamination and adhesive/abrasive wear of conventional and highly cross-linked polyethylene tibial inserts. They found that oxidation led to delamination, whereas increased cross-link density resulted in reduced adhesive/abrasive wear of tibial inserts.

Muratoglu OK, Bragdon CR, O'Connor DO, Jasty M, Harris WH: A novel method of cross-linking ultra-high-molecular-weight polyethylene to improve wear, reduce oxidation, and retain mechanical properties. *J Arthroplasty* 2001;16(2):149-160.

The authors present a novel method of increasing the cross-link density of polyethylene in which polyethylene is irradiated in air at an elevated temperature with a high-dose-rate electron beam and subsequently is melt-annealed. This treatment markedly improved the wear resistance of the polymer.

Muratoglu OK, Bragdon CR, O'Connor DO, Perinchief RS, Jasty M, Harris WH: Aggressive wear testing of a cross-linked polyethylene in total knee arthroplasty. *Clin Orthop Relat Res* 2002;404:89-95.

In this study, an aggressive in vitro knee wear and device fatigue model simulating a tight PCL balance during stair climbing was developed and used to assess the performance of three different polyethylene inserts. At 50,000 cycles, the authors found extensive delamination and cracking of the aged conventional polyethylene. At 0.5 million cycles, they did not find any subsurface cracking or delamination of the unaged conventional and highly cross-linked polyethylene inserts.

Rao AR, Engh GA, Collier MB, Lounici S: Tibial interface wear in retrieved total knee components and correlations with modular insert motion. *J Bone Joint Surg Am* 2002;84-A(10):1849-1855.

This study showed that backside wear correlated with the relative motion between the polyethylene insert and the metal base plate.

Wasielewski RC: The causes of insert backside wear in total knee arthroplasty. *Clin Orthop Relat Res* 2002;404:232-246.

The author of this article discusses the variables that increase the forces between the tibial polyethylene insert and the metal backing, thereby worsening backside relative micromotion and wear.

Classic Bibliography

Bohl JR, Bohl WR, Postak PD, Greenwald AS: The effects of shelf life on clinical outcome for gamma sterilized polyethylene tibial components. *Clin Orthop Relat Res* 1999;367:28-38.

Engh GA, Ammeen DJ: Classification and preoperative radiographic evaluation: Knee. *Orthop Clin North Am* 1998;29(2):205-217.

Hirakawa K, Bauer TW, Yamaguchi M, Stulberg BN, Wilde AH: Relationship between wear debris particles and polyethylene surface damage in primary total knee arthroplasty. *J Arthroplasty* 1999;14(2):165-171.

Peters PC Jr, Engh GA, Dwyer KA, Vinh TN: Osteolysis after total knee arthroplasty without cement. *J Bone Joint Surg Am* 1992;74(6):864-876.

Chapter 15

The Infected Total Knee Arthroplasty

David J. Jacofsky, MD

Arlen D. Hanssen, MD

Incidence

The incidence of deep infection following total knee arthroplasty is approximately 1% to 2.5%. One third of the deep infections occur within the first 3 months after surgery, and the remaining two thirds occur after 3 months. The risks of infection are increased in patients with rheumatoid arthritis, skin ulcerations, recurrent urinary tract infections, a history of prior knee joint infection, prior open surgical procedures, immunosuppressive therapy, poor nutrition, hypokalemia, diabetes mellitus, obesity, a history of smoking, and in patients with human immunodeficiency virus (HIV). Additional risk factors include revision procedures and surgical duration longer than 2.5 hours. There is no change in the infection rate when perioperative antibiotic prophylaxis is decreased from 48 to 24 hours after surgery. Many physicians advocate the use of antibiotic-impregnated bone cement for prophylaxis in primary and revision joint replacement surgery. Although some use this routinely, the risk of the development of drug-resistant organisms must be weighed against the potential benefit. Clearly, use in high-risk patients or procedures is worthwhile. The recommended use of prophylaxis with 2 g of amoxicillin 1 hour prior to dental procedures in patients with arthroplasties has helped decrease the incidence of late hematogenous joint infection. This recommendation is for patients who have one or more of the following: inflammatory arthropathy; immunosuppression because of disease, radiation, or medical therapy; type 1 diabetes mellitus; a prior septic joint replacement; malnourishment; hemophilia; or a joint replacement that is less than 2 years old. Despite the best prevention efforts, infection inevitably will occur following total knee arthroplasty in a certain number of patients.

Diagnosis

Early diagnosis of deep infection is imperative to salvage the prosthesis with débridement and retention; otherwise, prosthesis removal is required. Persistence of a moderately painful or stiff total knee arthroplasty implant should always alert the surgeon to the possibility of postoperative infection. Although the use of hematologic studies to determine erythrocyte sedimentation rate and C-reactive protein level are useful for screening, these tests should not be used for the definitive diagnosis of deep infection. Imaging studies, such as indium-labeled scans, are rarely indicated for the diagnosis of deep infection. Previous antibiotic use increases the risk of false-negative results with knee aspiration, and aspiration performed again at a later date can be expected to significantly improve results. As such, antibiotics should be discontinued for 7 to 10 days before aspiration. Some authors have reported that a longer time off antibiotics prior to aspiration may increase sensitivity, but the benefits of this must be weighed against the potential risks of a patient with an infected joint waiting a longer period for accurate diagnosis. Routine preoperative aspiration has a sensitivity of 75%, specificity of 96%, and accuracy of 90% and is strongly recommended as a routine test before virtually all total knee revisions. Aspiration also helps identify the antibiotic sensitivities of the offending organisms preoperatively to guide the use of specific antibiotics in the antibiotic-loaded cement spacers at surgery.

Persistent or copious wound drainage in the postoperative period should be aggressively treated with arthrotomy, débridement, and irrigation to prevent deep infection. Aggressive management of marginal skin edge necrosis or refractory wound healing by débridement of necrotic skin and primary wound closure is preferred to observation and oral antibiotic treatment because of a high likelihood of the subsequent development of deep infection with multidrug-resistant organisms. No clear consensus exists regarding the appropriate regimen of antibiotic treatment after débridement for drainage or wound complications in the absence of infection. Many physicians treat with intravenous antibiotics for a full 6 weeks, whereas others treat with oral or intravenous antibiotics until the wound is healed and dry. If the fascia is opened because of deep drainage, most physicians will exchange the polyethylene liner to maximally débride and irrigate the interface between the liner and the tib-

Table 1 | Treatment Options for Infected Total Knee Arthroplasty

Antibiotic suppression

Open débridement

Resection arthroplasty

Arthrodesis

Amputation

Single-stage or two-stage resection and reimplantation of another prosthesis

ial baseplate and to increase exposure for débridement of the posterior aspect of the knee.

Classification

Classification of periprosthetic infection is often related to the timing of onset from the initial index procedure, and the use of such a system is helpful in guiding appropriate management. A three-stage classification system was initially described based on the timing of presentation and the presumed mode of infection, and this system has been recently updated and modified. In this revised classification system, an infection in the immediate postoperative period is classified as type 2. Patients with a type 2 infection typically present during the first postoperative month, and a diagnosis is usually evident based on history and physical examination. These patients may report wound complications and/or superficial cellulitis around the time of their index procedure. The etiology of type 2 infections may include wound colonization at the time of surgery, infected hematomas, or the spread of superficial infection. Many of these infections are potentially preventable with appropriate preoperative antibiotics and careful surgical technique.

Type 3 infections are also believed to often originate during the index surgical procedure, but because they are often caused by a small inoculum or a low virulent organism, the onset of symptoms may be delayed. Patients with type 3 infections typically have a gradual deterioration in their function and an increase in pain. They may not have clear systemic or local findings consistent with definitive infection. In such patients, there may be a history of prolonged wound drainage at the time of the index procedure or perhaps a delay in discharge from the hospital. It is also worthwhile to ask patients with type 3 infections about previous prescriptions for ongoing courses of antibiotics, as well as whether these antibiotic treatment regimens transiently improved symptoms. Type 3 infections may be the most difficult periprosthetic infections to diagnose.

Type 4 infections are typically presumed to be secondary to hematogenous spread to a previously asymptomatic and aseptic joint replacement. There may be a history of associated febrile illness or acute infection, such as a urinary tract infection or pneumonia, followed by deterioration in joint function. Invasive or semi-invasive procedures such as colonoscopy, dental procedures, or local treatment of cutaneous infections may be reported. These infections are more common in patients who are immunocompromised, those who have recurrent episodes of bacteremia such as would be seen in intravenous drug abusers, those requiring repeated chronic urinary catheterization, or those who have had single episodes of bacteremia. Single episodes of bacteremia such as those that can occur with dental manipulations, respiratory infection, remote prosthetic infection, open skin lesions, endoscopy, or contaminated surgical procedures are often associated with type 4 prosthetic joint infections. Additionally, metallosis secondary to a failed arthroplasty may be an additional risk for the development of deep infection.

Many classification systems have expanded to include patients with positive intraoperative cultures (type 1). In a study of 106 infections, 31 patients initially thought to have aseptic failures were diagnosed with deep infection on the basis of positive intraoperative cultures. A minimum of two of five cultures were considered positive for infection. In this setting, culture results must be interpreted in conjunction with preoperative examination findings and laboratory study results, intraoperative culture results, frozen section histologic findings, and the overall clinical scenario. If positive culture results are deemed to be true positives, appropriate antibiotic therapy should be initiated.

Treatment

Once the diagnosis of deep infection has been established, several factors are important in determining the appropriate treatment, including the duration since index arthroplasty, consideration of the pathogen(s) and their antibiotic sensitivities, host factors that may adversely affect successful treatment, status of the soft-tissue envelope and extensor mechanism, whether the prosthesis is well fixed or loose, and assessment of the patient's expectations and functional demands. The six basic treatment options for an infected total knee arthroplasty are listed in Table 1.

Antibiotic Suppression

Antibiotic treatment alone will not eliminate deep infection in patients who have undergone total knee arthroplasty; therefore, it should rarely be selected as a treatment method. Unless the long-term goal is antibiotic suppression without eradication of infection in a patient with a known organism, the practice of prescribing antibiotics empirically for patients with a potentially infected arthroplasty is strongly discouraged and typically only complicates definitive treatment.

Débridement

The timing of the clinical presentation serves as a useful guide with regard to whether the prosthesis should be removed or whether an attempt at débridement with prosthesis retention should be considered. Although there are many prognostic variables associated with a successful outcome, timely débridement is important. Débridement attempts are not indicated when symptoms have been present longer than 4 weeks, and some evidence suggests a cutoff of only 2 weeks. The success of a débridement attempt is also likely affected by the microorganism. In a study of *Staphylococcus aureus* prosthetic joint infection treated with débridement and retention of the prosthesis, the probability of success was reported to be significantly higher when débridement was performed within 2 days of symptom onset. Acute hematogenous infection of a well-fixed and well-functioning prosthetic component can be successfully treated in 50% of patients when it is diagnosed 2 to 4 weeks from the onset of symptoms.

A relative contraindication for débridement with component retention may be the presence of other joint arthroplasties or indwelling prosthetic devices such as a heart valve. The literature does not support the use of débridement with prosthetic component retention in patients with late chronic infection. Furthermore, multiple attempts at débridement and component retention to salvage the joint are typically counterproductive, lead to extensive periarticular scarring, and make subsequent revision surgery more difficult.

Arthrotomy with open débridement has been shown to be the most successful treatment for patients with early deep infection after total knee arthroplasty. Arthroscopic débridement is less efficacious when compared with open débridement because most patients (68%) fail with arthroscopic treatment. Arthroscopic débridement prevents débridement of the polyethylene-prosthetic modular interface and provides access to the posterior aspect of the knee joint. Arthroscopic irrigation and débridement should be used only to treat medically unstable or anticoagulated patients or patients in whom the etiology of the infection is known to be within the last 72 hours (such as those who have recently undergone dental extraction).

Resection Arthroplasty

Although eradication of deep infection in patients after total knee arthroplasty has been well documented with this technique, with the exception of selected patients with limited ambulatory demands, this procedure is rarely used because of suboptimal functional results. The ideal candidate for this procedure is a patient with polyarticular rheumatoid arthritis with limited functional demands who is likely to have difficulty eradicating infection and/or tolerating more than one surgical procedure. Resection arthroplasty will allow the patient to sit more readily than will a knee arthrodesis. The primary disadvantage of resection arthroplasty is the frequent occurrence of knee instability and pain if the lower extremity is used for transfers or ambulation.

Arthrodesis

Arthrodesis has been historically considered the gold standard treatment option; however, this procedure adversely affects knee motion, making sitting and other associated activities more difficult. The most common indication for arthrodesis is the presence of extensor mechanism disruption in a patient with an infected total knee arthroplasty implant. Other indications for arthrodesis have been described, including young age, single joint disease, high functional demand, instability, unsalvageable soft tissues, poor host immune function, and highly-resistant infecting organisms. Relative contraindications to arthrodesis include significant ipsilateral hip or ankle arthritis, contralateral knee arthritis, contralateral upper extremity amputation, and severe segmental bone loss.

A variety of techniques are used for arthrodesis, including external fixators, plate fixation, and intramedullary nail fixation. Achieving union depends on the type of implant, extent of bony deficiency, successful control of infection, and type of arthrodesis fixation. Intramedullary devices have the highest union rates, but may have high reinfection rates if bacterial colonization is still present. External fixation is least likely to lead to septic failure, but it is technically demanding and has a higher nonunion rate in this setting. Although half pins may be used in conjunction with ring fixators, constructs using half pins only are far less stable and should be avoided. The most important factor in obtaining union is the apposition of the ends of the bone. Although most surgeons still use bone graft at the site of the arthrodesis, this has not been proved to have a significant difference in union rates, although study numbers are limited in most series. The use of soft-tissue flaps in patients with a poor-quality soft-tissue envelope should be considered to help minimize wound healing complications and the risk of reinfection and to provide healthy, well-vascularized tissue to the arthrodesis area.

Amputation

Amputation may be occasionally required for the treatment of an infected total knee arthroplasty implant in patients with life-threatening systemic sepsis, those who have undergone failed attempts at arthrodesis, those in whom the soft-tissue envelope cannot be predictably restored, or in patients who elect amputation over arthrodesis or the prospect of multiple surgical procedures. Amputation should be performed at a level that maximizes function, yet predictably eradicates infection. The

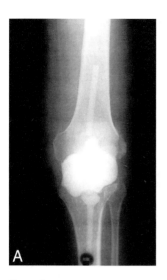
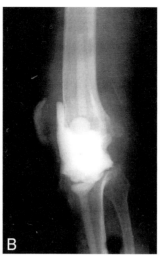
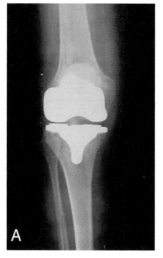
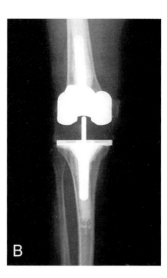

Figure 1 AP **(A)** and lateral **(B)** radiographs of a static interdigitated block spacer.

Figure 2 **A,** Preoperative AP radiograph of a patient with an infected TKA. **B,** AP radiograph of the same patient after a two-stage reimplantation was performed.

functional outcome after amputation performed above a total knee arthroplasty implant is poor because a substantial percentage of these patients are never fitted with prostheses; those who obtain prostheses seldom obtain functional independence.

Reimplantation

Most infected total knee arthroplasty implants require removal to eradicate the infection. The primary decision that must be made is whether a direct-exchange or a two-stage procedure should be performed. Although direct exchange has been advocated for this patient population, most authors recommend the two-stage approach because it appears to be more reliable and successful in that it avoids the difficulties encountered with the management of the soft-tissue envelope about the knee joint. Single-stage exchange is not commonly performed because of higher failure rates, but it may have a limited role in the treatment of patients who cannot tolerate two procedures and those who are infected with susceptible organisms and can be chronically suppressed after the exchange for extended periods or at times for life. Factors associated with the success of direct exchange include Gram-positive infections, absence of sinus formation, use of antibiotic-impregnated cement for the new prosthesis, and 12 weeks of antibiotic therapy. When using the two-stage reimplantation method, the surgical protocol includes removal of the prosthesis and all cement with thorough débridement of bone and soft tissues. Most authors recommend 4 to 6 weeks of parenteral antibiotics and then reimplantation of a new prosthesis when infection has proved to be eradicated.

In the interval between prosthesis removal and reimplantation, the use of a spacer is helpful for enhancing bone quality, providing local antibiotic delivery, provid-

ing greater patient comfort and mobility, improving soft-tissue healing, and maintaining collateral ligament tension; this is particularly true for patients who undergo treatment for bilateral infected total knee arthroplasty implants (Figures 1 and 2).

Mobile or articulating spacers allow continuous rehabilitation between stage one and stage two, maintain good alignment and stability of the knee, and provide reasonable range of motion before reimplantation (Figures 3 and 4). This range of motion helps maintain the soft-tissue planes, improves soft-tissue health, and eases the technical difficulties encountered at the second-stage procedure. Although some authors believe articulated spacers improve ultimate range of motion, others have found no significant difference in range of motion when comparing articulated spacers and mobile or static spacers. Most importantly, the antibiotic spacers provide the delivery of high-dose local antibiotic therapy.

Recently, one group of authors recommended that prerevision cultures be obtained in all patients 4 weeks after discontinuation of antibiotic treatment. This recommendation was made because it is believed that this technique helps identify continuing infection and that morbidity associated with recurrent infection is potentially avoided. Most have not found this approach to be beneficial and this protocol is not recommended. A recent study found no benefit and a 0% sensitivity in knee aspiration after resection for infection. The primary difficulty with obtaining prerevision cultures is determining whether an adequate sample has been obtained either by aspiration or via open biopsy. If culture samples are obtained via an open procedure, the additional morbidity and cost of the procedure when combined with the potential risk of introducing additional microorganisms seems to outweigh the benefits of this approach, but it is reasonable in the small group of pa-

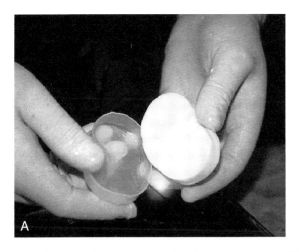
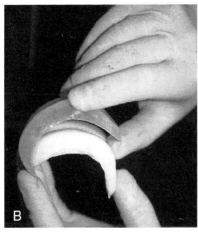
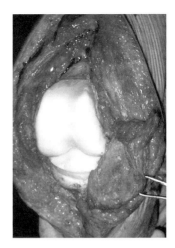

Figure 3 Photographs showing creation of tibial **(A)** and femoral **(B)** PROSTALAC-type articulating spacers.

Figure 4 Photograph of an implanted PROSTALAC-type articulating spacer.

tients with elevation of their serology tests (such as elevated C-reactive protein levels) or clinical recurrence of symptoms after discontinuation of antibiotics.

Summary

There are many variables that correlate with successful eradication of infection. There is currently general consensus that with careful patient selection, good débridement, and use of high-dose antibiotic-loaded cement spacers, a successful outcome can be obtained in 85% to 95% of patients with a two-stage reimplantation protocol. Although functional outcome after revision of septic total knee replacement is inferior to revision for aseptic reasons, patient satisfaction after revision and successful eradication of infection is equally high.

Annotated Bibliography

Incidence

Parvizi J, Sullivan TA, Pagnano MW, Trousdale RT, Bolander ME: Total joint arthroplasty in human immunodeficiency virus-positive patients: An alarming rate of early failure. *J Arthroplasty* 2003;18(3):259-264.

In this study, the authors reviewed the results of 21 total joint arthroplasties in 15 patients with HIV. At a mean follow-up of 10.2 years, 6 joints were infected, and 6 patients had died (all of complications of associated with acquired immunodeficiency disease).

Peersman G, Laskin R, Davis J, Peterson M: Infection in total knee replacement: A retrospective review of 6489 total knee replacements. *Clin Orthop Relat Res* 2001; 392:15-23.

In this study, 6,489 knee replacements were performed over a 6-year period in 6,120 patients at a single institution. Of these, infection was diagnosed in 116 knees. One third of the deep infections occurred within the first 3 months after sur-

gery, whereas the other two thirds occurred more than three months after surgery. Comorbidities that were reported to be statistically significant predictors of infection included prior open surgical procedures, immunosuppressive therapy, malnutrition, hypokalemia, obesity, smoking, and diabetes mellitus. Surgical times greater than 2.5 hours increased the risk of infection as well.

Diagnosis

Scher DM, Pak K, Lonner JH, Finkel JE, Zuckerman JD, Di Cesare PE: The predictive value of indium-111 leukocyte scans in the diagnosis of infected total hip, knee, or resection arthroplasties. *J Arthroplasty* 2000; 15(3):295-300.

The authors of this study evaluated the usefulness of indium-labeled bone scanning in the detection of infected joint replacement. In this study of 143 patients, the indium-labeled bone scan had a 77% sensitivity, 86% specificity, 54% and 95% positive and negative predictive values, respectively, and an 84% accuracy.

Tsukayama DT, Goldberg VM, Kyle R: Diagnosis and management of infection after total knee arthroplasty. *J Bone Joint Surg Am* 2003;85-A(suppl 1):S75-S80.

This review article helps classify the infection of a total joint for both descriptive and prognostic purposes and reviews the management of infected total knee replacement.

Treatment

Barrack RL, Engh G, Rorabeck C, Sawhney J, Woolfrey M: Patient satisfaction and outcome after septic versus aseptic revision total knee arthroplasty. *J Arthroplasty* 2000;15(8):990-993.

In this study, a consecutive series of 138 revision knees were prospectively assessed to compare the outcomes of those revised for septic versus aseptic etiology. Postoperatively, septic patients had a decreased range of motion and a markedly lower Knee Society clinical score (115 versus 135) than the aseptic group. However, patient satisfaction was equally high in both groups despite an inferior functional result.

Deirmengian C, Greenbaum J, Stern J, et al: Open debridement of acute gram-positive infections after total knee arthroplasty. *Clin Orthop Relat Res* 2003;416:129-134.

This study reviewed a series of 31 infected total knee arthroplasties treated with open débridement, component retention, and antibiotics. Seventy-eight percent were débrided within 10 days of symptom onset. At mean 4-year follow-up, 35% of patients retained their components, but only 1 in 13 (8%) were infected with *S aureus* compared with 56% of patients with *Staphylococcus epidermidis* or a streptococcal species.

Dixon P, Parish EN, Cross MJ: Arthroscopic debridement in the treatment of the infected total knee replacement. *J Bone Joint Surg Br* 2004;86(1):39-42.

This study showed that in a limited group of patients with acute infected total knee replacements, arthroscopic débridement with meticulous technique and focused, extended, antibiotic therapy can provide acceptable results.

Fehring TK, Odum S, Calton TF, Mason JB: Articulating versus static spacers in revision total knee arthroplasty for sepsis. *Clin Orthop Relat Res* 2000;380:9-16.

The authors of this study compared static versus articulating spacers for the treatment of infected total joint arthroplasty implants. Twenty-five patients were treated with static spacers and thirty were treated with articulating spacers before reimplantation. Although articulating spacers seemed to facilitate reimplantation, they offered no functional advantage nor increased risk of reinfection in this study group.

Kilgus DJ, Howe DJ, Strang A: Results of periprosthetic hip and knee infections caused by resistant bacteria. *Clin Orthop Relat Res* 2002;404:116-124.

The authors of this study of infected total hip and total knee arthroplasties compared the outcomes of patients infected with methicillin-sensitive versus methicillin-resistant strains of *S aureus*. In the knee groups, 89% of patients with sensitive organisms were successfully treated compared with only 18% of patients with resistant strains. Failure was defined as need for arthrodesis, amputation, or definitive resection arthroplasty because of recalcitrant infection.

Lee GC, Pagnano MW, Hanssen AD: Total knee arthroplasty after prior bone or joint sepsis about the knee. *Clin Orthop Relat Res* 2002;404:226-231.

The authors of this study assessed 20 total knee arthroplasty procedures performed in 19 patients who had a prior history of bone or joint sepsis. Careful preoperative screening for infection was performed and antibiotics were used in ce-

ment. Sixteen patients survived at greater than 2-year follow-up. One patient developed deep infection.

Meek RM, Masri BA, Dunlop D, et al: Patient satisfaction and functional status after treatment of infection at the site of a total knee arthroplasty with use of the PROSTALAC articulating spacer. *J Bone Joint Surg Am* 2003;85-A(10):1888-1892.

The authors of this study compared the results of revision for aseptic loosening with revision for septic failure. The infected group underwent a two-stage procedure with a prosthesis of antibiotic-loaded acrylic cement (PROSTALAC) articulating spacer. At 41-month follow-up, there was no statistical functional difference between the two groups, although a 4% reinfection rate was noted in the septic group.

Sierra RJ, Trousdale RT, Pagnano MW: Above-the-knee amputation after a total knee replacement: Prevalence, etiology, and functional outcome. *J Bone Joint Surg Am* 2003;85-A(6):1000-1004.

From 1970 to 2000, 18,443 primary total knee replacements were performed at one institution. A review of these procedures revealed an overall amputation rate of 0.36%. The rate of amputation for causes related to the knee replacement was 0.14%. Functional independence was rarely achieved after amputation above the knee in this group.

Silva M, Tharani R, Schmalzried TP: Results of direct exchange or debridement of the infected total knee arthroplasty. *Clin Orthop Relat Res* 2002;404:125-131.

In this literature review, 30 reports provided outcome data on 37 direct exchange arthroplasties, 530 open débridements, and 23 arthroscopic débridements. Factors associated with success of direct exchange included Gram-positive infections, absence of sinus formation, use of antibiotic-impregnated cement for the new prosthesis, and 12 weeks of antibiotic therapy. Factors associated with successful débridement included those done within 4 months of the index procedure, those done in patients with fewer than 4 weeks of symptoms, young healthy patients, and those with sensitive Gram-positive infections.

Trousdale RT, Hanssen AD: Infection after total knee arthroplasty. *Instr Course Lect* 2001;50:409-414.

This is a comprehensive review of the incidence, diagnosis, and management of infected total knee replacement.

Waldman BJ, Hostin E, Mont MA, Hungerford DS: Infected total knee arthroplasty treated by arthroscopic irrigation and debridement. *J Arthroplasty* 2000;15(4):430-436.

In this study, 16 patients with infected total knee arthroplasty implants were treated with arthroscopic irrigation and débridement. All had less than 8 days of knee symptoms. Arthroscopic débridement was found to be less efficacious than open treatment, and 62% of patients eventually required removal of components for treatment.

Wang CJ, Huang TW, Wang JW, Chen HS: The often poor clinical outcome of infected total knee arthroplasty. *J Arthroplasty* 2002;17(5):608-614.

The authors of this article compared the outcomes of various treatments of 26 infected total knee arthroplasties with successful eradication of infection. Arthrodesis was reported to achieve better pain relief, whereas reimplantation achieved better function. Half of the patients with reimplantations reported at least mild knee pain.

Wolff LH III, Parvizi J, Trousdale RT, et al: Results of treatment of infection in both knees after bilateral total knee arthroplasty. *J Bone Joint Surg Am* 2003;85-A(10): 1952-1955.

The authors of this study reviewed 21 patients treated for bilateral infected total knee arthroplasty implants and reported that the best rate of successful eradication of infection and functional outcome was achieved in patients who underwent bilateral resection arthroplasty with staged reimplantation. It is likely, however, that this retrospective study had a selection bias.

Classic Bibliography

Barrack RL, Jennings RW, Wolfe MW, Bertot AJ: The value of preoperative aspiration before total knee revision. *Clin Orthop Relat Res* 1997;345:8-16.

Section 2

Basic Science and General Knowledge

Section Editors:
Michael A. Mont, MD
Harry E. Rubash, MD

Chapter 16

Osteoarthritis and Inflammatory Arthritis

Joseph A. Buckwalter, MD

Gracia Etienne, MD, PhD

Osteoarthritis

Osteoarthritis, also referred to as degenerative joint disease, degenerative arthritis, osteoarthrosis, or hypertrophic arthritis, is among the most frequent and symptomatic medical problems for middle aged and older people. It affects people of all ethnic groups in all geographic locations, occurs in both men and women but more commonly in women, and it is the most common cause of long-term disability in patient populations older than 65 years. More than one third of people older than 45 years report joint symptoms that vary from a sensation of occasional joint stiffness and intermittent aching associated with activity to permanent loss of motion and constant deep pain. Those who are most severely affected have crippling joint deformity and instability. The joint degeneration that causes the clinical syndrome of osteoarthritis occurs most frequently in the hand, foot, knee, hip, and spine joints, but it can develop in any synovial joint; in all synovial joints the prevalence of degenerative changes increases with age.

Diagnosis

The clinical syndrome of osteoarthritis results from degeneration of a synovial joint: a generally progressive loss of articular cartilage accompanied by attempted repair of articular cartilage, remodeling and sclerosis of subchondral bone, and in many instances the formation of subchondral bone cysts and marginal osteophytes. In addition to the changes in the synovial joint, which are usually evident on plain radiographs, diagnosis of the clinical syndrome of osteoarthritis requires the presence of chronic joint pain. Many patients with osteoarthritis also have restriction of motion, crepitus with motion, and joint effusions. The most severely affected patients have joint deformities and subluxations.

Most patients with osteoarthritis seek medical attention because of joint pain. They often describe the pain as a deep, aching, poorly localized discomfort that has been present for years. The pain may increase with changes in the weather, especially storms or a drop in temperature, and increased activity. Activity-associated pain typically begins immediately or shortly after beginning joint use and may persist for hours after cessation of activity. Some patients first notice symptoms of degenerative joint disease after a minor joint injury or strenuous physical activity, even though radiographs may show evidence of changes consistent with long-standing joint degeneration. In the more advanced stages of the disease, the pain becomes constant and may awaken patients from sleep. As joint degeneration progresses, patients may notice loss of motion and feel grating, catching, and grinding sensations in the joint with motion. Joint enlargement caused by osteophyte formation and deformity occur later in the course of the disease.

The first signs of osteoarthritis include a decrease in the speed and freedom of active joint movement. Limitation of movement may result from incongruity or loss of articular cartilage, ligament and capsular contracture, muscle spasm and contracture, osteophytes, or intra-articular fragments of cartilage, bone, or menisci. Palpable crepitus, joint effusions, and joint tenderness also occur in many patients. Osteophytes can cause palpable and often visible bony prominences, and progressive loss of articular cartilage and subchondral bone will lead to joint subluxation and deformity. Muscle atrophy occurs with long-standing disease.

Physicians frequently diagnose osteoarthritis based on the patient's history and physical findings. Changes on plain radiographs typically confirm the diagnosis, but the correlation between the clinical presentation of the disease and radiographic changes varies considerably among patients. Some patients with radiographic evidence of advanced joint degeneration have minimal symptoms, whereas those with minimal radiographic changes may have severe symptoms. The radiographic changes associated with osteoarthritis include narrowing of the cartilage space, increased density of subchondral bone, and the presence of osteophytes. Although these three radiographic markers of joint degeneration often occur together, in some joints only one or two may be visible on standard radiographs. Subchondral cysts, or cavities, also develop in osteoarthritic joints. These cavi-

Table 1 | Known Causes of Joint Degeneration (Secondary Osteoarthritis)

Cause	Presumed Mechanism
Intra-articular fractures	Damage to articular cartilage and/or joint incongruity
High-intensity impact joint loading	Damage to articular cartilage and/or subchondral bone
Ligament injuries	Joint instability
Joint dysplasias (developmental and hereditary joint and cartilage dysplasias)	Abnormal joint shape and/or abnormal articular cartilage
Aseptic necrosis	Bone necrosis leads to collapse of the articular surface and joint incongruity
Acromegaly	Overgrowth of articular cartilage produces joint incongruity and/or abnormal cartilage
Paget's disease	Distortion or incongruity of joints caused by bone remodeling
Ehlers-Danlos syndrome	Joint instability
Gaucher's disease (hereditary deficiency of the enzyme glucocerebrosidase, leading to accumulation of glucocerebroside)	Bone necrosis or pathologic bone fracture leading to joint incongruity
Stickler's syndrome (progressive hereditary arthro-ophthalmopathy)	Abnormal joint and/or articular cartilage development
Joint infection (inflammation)	Destruction of articular cartilage
Hemophilia	Multiple joint hemorrhages
Hemochromatosis (excess iron deposition in multiple tissues)	Mechanism unknown
Ochronosis (hereditary deficiency of the enzyme homogentisic acid oxidase, leading to accumulation of homogentisic acid)	Deposition of homogentisic acid polymers in articular cartilage
Calcium pyrophosphate deposition disease	Accumulation of calcium pyrophosphate crystals in articular cartilage
Neuropathic arthropathy (Charcot's joints: syphilis, diabetes mellitus, syringomyelia, meningomyelocele, leprosy, congenital insensitivity to pain, amyloidosis)	Loss of proprioception and joint sensation results in increased impact loading and torsion, joint instability, and intra-articular fractures

(Reproduced with permission from Buckwalter JA, Mankin HJ: Articular cartilage: II. Degeneration and osteoarthrosis, repair, regeneration and transplantation. J Bone Joint Surg Am 1997;79: 612-632.)

ties vary in size and characteristically have dense bony borders. Osteochondral loose bodies, visible on radiographs as intra-articular bony fragments, occasionally develop from pieces of the joint surface. Joint subluxation, deformity, and malalignment develop with advanced disease. Bony ankylosis rarely occurs. Additional diagnostic imaging, including bone scanning, CT, and MRI, may be helpful in evaluating the early stages of degenerative joint disease, but they rarely are necessary for establishing the diagnosis.

Etiology

Osteoarthritis develops most commonly in the absence of a known cause, a condition referred to as primary or idiopathic osteoarthritis. Less frequently, it develops as a result of joint injuries, infections, or a variety of hereditary, developmental, metabolic, and neurologic disorders, a group of conditions referred to as secondary osteoarthritis (Table 1). The age of onset of secondary osteoarthritis depends on the underlying cause; thus, it may develop in young adults and even children as well as the elderly. In contrast, a strong association exists between primary osteoarthritis and age. The percentage of people with evidence of osteoarthritis in one or more joints increases from less than 5% of people between 15 and 44 years of age to 25% to 30% of people between 45 and 64 years of age. Moreover, evidence of osteoarthritis in one or more joints can appear in 60% to 90% of people older than 65 years. Despite this strong association and the widespread view that osteoarthritis results from normal wear and tear and eventually stiffens the joints of virtually everybody older than 65 years, the relationships between joint use, aging, and joint degeneration remain uncertain. Furthermore, normal lifelong joint use has not been shown to cause degeneration. Thus, osteoarthritis is not simply the result of mechanical wear from joint use.

Although the suffix "itis" implies that osteoarthritis is an inflammatory disease and some evidence of synovitis is frequently present, inflammation does not appear to be a major component of the disorder in most patients. Unlike the joint destruction caused by synovial inflammation, osteoarthritis consists of a retrogressive sequence of cell and matrix changes that result in loss of articular cartilage structure and function accompanied by cartilage repair and bone remodeling reactions. Because of the repair and remodeling reactions, the degeneration of the articular surface in osteoarthritis is not uniformly progressive, and the rate of joint degeneration varies among individuals and among joints. Occasionally, it occurs rapidly, but in most joints it progresses slowly over many years, although it may stabilize or even improve spontaneously with at least partial restoration of the articular surface and a decrease in symptoms.

Osteoarthritis usually involves all of the tissues that form the synovial joint, including articular cartilage, subchondral and metaphyseal bone, synovium, ligaments, joint capsules, and the muscles that act across the joint; however, the primary changes consist of loss of articular cartilage, remodeling of subchondral bone, and formation of osteophytes. The earliest articular cartilage structural changes seen in osteoarthritis are fraying or fibrillation of the superficial zone extending into the transitional zone and violation of the tidemark by blood vessels from subchondral bone. Some investigators have postulated that stiffening of subchondral bone precedes and causes articular cartilage degeneration and that progression of cartilage degeneration requires stiffening of subchondral bone, but others have argued that articular cartilage loss leads to increased peak stresses on subchondral bone that cause bone remodeling. It is not clear which of these views is correct or whether either is entirely correct, but in most instances articular cartilage degeneration and subchondral bone remodeling are both present when patients have symptoms, and it is the loss of articular cartilage that leads directly to loss of joint function.

Development and Progression

The earliest visible sign of osteoarthritis is fibrillation or disruption of the most superficial layers of the articular cartilage. As the disease progresses, the surface irregularities become clefts, more of the articular surface becomes roughened and irregular, and fibrillation extends deeper into the cartilage until the fissures reach subchondral bone. As the cartilage fissures grow deeper, the superficial tips of the fibrillated cartilage tear, releasing free fragments into the joint space and decreasing the cartilage thickness. At the same time, enzymatic degradation of the matrix further decreases the cartilage volume. The loss of cartilage matrix is accompanied by an increased rate of programmed cell death or apoptosis of chondrocytes in areas of articular cartilage degeneration. Eventually, the progressive loss of articular cartilage leaves only dense and often necrotic eburnated bone.

Articular Cartilage Changes

Many of the mechanisms responsible for progressive loss of cartilage in degenerative joint disease remain unknown, but the process can be divided into three overlapping stages (Table 2): cartilage matrix damage or al-

Table 2 | Stages in the Development and Progression of Osteoarthritis

Stage I Cartilage Matrix Disruption or Alteration

Disruption or alteration of the matrix macromolecular framework associated with an increase in water concentration may be caused by mechanical insults, degradation of matrix macromolecules, or alterations of chondrocyte metabolism. Initially, the type II collagen concentration remains unchanged, but the collagen meshwork may be damaged, and the concentration of aggrecan and the degree of proteoglycan aggregation decrease.

Stage II Chondrocyte Response to Matrix Disruption or Alteration

When chondrocytes detect a disruption or alteration of their matrix they can respond by increasing matrix synthesis and degradation and by proliferating. Their response may restore the tissue, maintain the tissue in an altered state, or increase cartilage volume. They may sustain an increased level of activity for years.

Stage III Decline in the Chondrocyte Response

Failure of the chondrocytic response to restore or maintain the tissue leads to loss of articular cartilage accompanied or preceded by a decline in the chondrocytic response. The causes for the decline in chondrocytic response remain poorly understood, but it may be partially the result of mechanical damage to the tissue, with injury to chondrocytes and a downregulation of the chondrocyte response to anabolic cytokines.

teration, chondrocyte response to tissue damage, and decline of the chondrocyte response.

In the first stage, either before or with the appearance of fibrillation, the matrix macromolecular framework is disrupted or altered at the molecular level and the water content increases. Early in this process, the chondrocytes increase their expression of enzymes that can degrade the matrix macromolecules. Although the concentration of type II collagen remains constant, decreases in proteoglycan aggregation and concentration and in the size of the glycosaminoglycan chains usually accompany the increase in water content. These changes increase the permeability (the ease with which water and other molecules move through the matrix) and decrease the stiffness of the matrix, alterations that may increase the vulnerability of the tissue to further damage. This first stage may occur as a result of a variety of mechanical insults, including high-intensity impact or torsional loading of a joint, accelerated degradation of matrix macromolecules caused by inflammation or similar insults, or metabolic changes in the tissue that interfere with the ability of chondrocytes to maintain the matrix.

The second stage begins when chondrocytes detect the tissue damage such as degradation of matrix macromolecules or alterations in osmolarity, charge density, or strain and release mediators that stimulate a cellular response that is often quite brisk. The response consists of both anabolic and catabolic activity as well as chondrocyte proliferation. Anabolic and mitogenic growth factors presumably have an important role in stimulating synthesis of matrix macromolecules and chondrocyte proliferation; clusters or clones of proliferating cells surrounded by newly synthesized matrix molecules constitute one of the histologic hallmarks of the chondrocytic response to cartilage degeneration. Recent studies have shown that intact fibronectin increases the anabolic activity of chondrocytes maintained in a spherical shape in culture and enhances their response to the anabolic cytokine insulin-dependent growth factor I. These observations suggest that intact fibronectin has a role in stimulating chondrocyte anabolic activity in vivo. Inflammatory cytokines such as interleukin (IL)-1 and tumor necrosis factor alpha (TNF-α) probably also influence chondrocyte activity because chondrocytes produce these molecules in response to a variety of mechanical and chemical stresses. IL-1 induces formation of nitric oxide, which diffuses rapidly and stimulates the activity of matrix metalloproteinases (MMPs), enzymes that degrade matrix macromolecules. Fibronectin fragments or other molecules present in damaged tissue may promote continued production of IL-1 and enhanced release of proteases. Degradation of type IX and type XI collagens and other molecules may destabilize the type II collagen fibril meshwork, leaving many of the type II fibrils intact initially, but allowing expansion of aggrecan and increased water content. Disruption of the superficial zone, a decline in aggregation, and an associated loss of aggrecan because of enzymatic degradation increase the stresses on the remaining collagen fibril network and chondrocytes with joint loading. Enzymatic degradation also clears damaged and intact matrix components and may release anabolic cytokines previously trapped in the matrix that stimulate synthesis of matrix macromolecules and chondrocyte proliferation.

During the second stage of osteoarthritis, enzymes that degrade articular cartilage matrix molecules have a critical role in causing progressive joint degeneration. MMPs destroy aggrecan and activate collagenase, which destroys collagen. The activity of these enzymes is controlled by molecules that increase MMP activity, including synovial and chondrocyte IL-1, tissue plasminogen activator, and matrix metalloproteinase activator, and molecules that suppress matrix degradation, including transforming growth factor-beta, tissue inhibitor of metalloproteinases, and to a lesser extent plasminogen activator inhibitor-1. The balance between MMP activators and suppressors influences the activity of MMPs, and the balance between degradative enzyme activity and matrix synthesis determines the rate of articular cartilage loss.

In this second stage of osteoarthritis, which may last for many years, the repair response (increased synthesis of matrix macromolecules and to a lesser extent cell proliferation) counters the catabolic effects of the proteases and may stabilize or, in some instances, restore the tissue. For example, findings on osteoarthritic hips and knees after osteotomy suggest that altering the joint mechanical environment may allow restoration of some form of articular surface.

Failure to stabilize or restore the articular cartilage leads to the third stage in the development of osteoarthritis, progressive loss of articular cartilage, and a decline in the chondrocytic anabolic and proliferative response. This decline could result from mechanical damage and death of chondrocytes no longer stabilized and protected by a functional matrix, but it also appears to be related to, or initiated by, a downregulation of chondrocyte response to anabolic cytokines. This may occur as a result of synthesis and accumulation of molecules in the matrix that binds anabolic cytokines including d*Eco*RIn, insulin-dependent growth factor binding proteins, and other molecules that can affect cytokine function.

Bone Changes

Alterations of the subchondral bone that accompany the degeneration of articular cartilage include increased subchondral bone density, formation of cyst-like bone cavities containing myxoid, fibrous, or cartilaginous tissue, and the appearance of regenerating cartilage within and on the subchondral bone surface. This response is usually most apparent on the periphery of the joint where bony and cartilaginous excrescences sometimes form sizable osteophytes. Increased bone density resulting from the formation of new layers of bone on existing trabeculae is generally the first sign of degenerative joint disease in subchondral bone, but in some joints subchondral cavities appear before a generalized increase in bone density. At the end stage of the disease, the articular cartilage has been completely lost, leaving thickened, dense subchondral bone articulating with a similar opposing denuded bony surface. The bone remodeling combined with the loss of articular cartilage changes joint shape and can lead to shortening of the involved limb, deformity, and instability.

In most synovial joints, growth of osteophytes accompanies the changes in articular cartilage and subchondral and metaphyseal bone. These fibrous, cartilaginous, and bony prominences usually appear around the periphery of the joint. Marginal osteophytes usually appear at the cartilage bone interface, but they may also appear along joint capsule insertions (capsular osteophytes). Intra-articular bony excrescences that protrude from degenerating joint surfaces are referred to as central osteophytes. Most marginal osteophytes have a cartilaginous surface that closely resembles normal articular cartilage and may appear to be an extension of the joint surface. In superficial joints, they usually are palpable and may be tender, and in all joints they can restrict motion and contribute to pain with motion. Each joint has a characteristic pattern of osteophyte formation. In the hip, they usually form rings around the rim of the acetabulum and the femoral articular cartilage. A prominent osteophyte along the inferior margin of the humeral articular surface commonly develops in patients with degenerative disease of the glenohumeral joint. Presumably, osteophytes represent a response to degeneration of articular cartilage and subchondral bone remodeling, including release of anabolic cytokines that stimulate cell proliferation and formation of bony and cartilaginous matrices.

Changes in Periarticular Tissues

Loss of articular cartilage leads to secondary changes in the synovium, ligaments, and capsules as well as in the muscles that move the involved joint. The synovial membrane often develops a mild to moderate inflammatory reaction and may contain fragments of articular cartilage. With time the ligaments, capsules, and muscles become contracted. Decreased use of the joint and decreased range of motion leads to muscle atrophy. These secondary changes often contribute to the stiffness and weakness associated with osteoarthritis.

Universal Risk Factors

In addition to the specific disorders responsible for the multiple forms of secondary osteoarthritis (Table 1), genetic predisposition and joint laxity have been identified as risk factors. Although these factors may increase the risk of osteoarthritis in selected populations, the most important risk factor in all populations is age. Mechanical loading that exceeds the ability of a joint to repair or maintain itself is another universal risk factor. Repetitive joint use over decades, joint injury, posttraumatic joint incongruity, instability, or malalignment and joint dysplasia all can create mechanical demands that damage articular surfaces.

Age

Recent studies suggest that age-related deterioration of chondrocyte function decreases the ability of the cells to maintain and restore articular cartilage. With increasing age, the cells synthesize smaller aggrecans and less functional link proteins, leading to the formation of smaller more irregular proteoglycan aggregates. Their mitotic and synthetic activities decline with age, and they become less responsive to anabolic cytokines and mechanical stimuli. Evidence that chondrocytes undergo age-related telomere erosion and increased expression of the senescence marker β-galactosidase suggests that cell senescence, possibly caused by oxidative damage, is responsible for the age-related loss of chondrocyte function.

Excessive Repetitive Joint Loading

Maintenance of normal synovial joint structure and function requires regular joint use. Lifelong normal daily activities and regular recreational running have not been shown to increase the risk of joint degeneration. There is evidence, however, that repetitive loading of normal joints can exceed the tolerance of a joint and cause degeneration. Surveys of individuals with physically demanding occupations (farmers, construction workers, metal workers, miners, and pneumatic drill operators) suggest that repetitive intense joint loading over a decade or more increases the risk of joint degeneration. Specific activities that have been associated with joint degeneration include repetitively lifting or carrying heavy objects, awkward work posture, vibration, continuously repeated movements, and working speed determined by a machine; other studies have suggested that participation in sports that repetitively expose joints to high levels of impact or torsional loading also increase the risk of joint degeneration. The contralateral knees of people with lower limb amputations have more degenerative changes than the knees of people without amputations, suggesting that the increased loading of the knees of their normal limbs caused degeneration of the knee. The degeneration of normal joints in people with joint fusions may have a similar explanation—that is, the loss of motion in the fused joint places increased mechanical demands on other joints.

Natural History

Although the view of osteoarthritis as a relentlessly progressive disease caused by steady wearing away of the articular surface is commonly accepted, the disease does not necessarily follow this course. Longitudinal studies of patients with hip and knee osteoarthritis show that over a decade or more the radiographic signs of joint degeneration do not progress in one third to two thirds of patients. Additionally, one longitudinal study of 63 patients showed that over 11 years 10% of patients had improvement in the radiographic signs of joint degeneration.

These studies also demonstrate that the correlation between the radiographic changes and the clinical course of osteoarthritis is not strong. The clinical syndrome of osteoarthritis may remain stationary, slowly progress over many years and even decades, improve temporarily, or occasionally progress rapidly to the point that the patient is completely disabled within a few years of the onset of the disease. Most patients with osteoarthritis have intervals of symptomatic improvement; in rare instances, the radiographic joint space spontaneously increases and symptoms decrease. The reasons for this variability in the natural history of the disease have not been discovered, although joint injuries, repetitive excessive joint torsion and impact loading, crystal deposition, and neuromuscular dysfunction have been associated with more rapid progression of joint degeneration.

Another factor that makes defining the natural history of osteoarthritis difficult is the limited correlation between the degree of joint degeneration and symptoms. Although the symptoms of osteoarthritis, primarily joint pain and stiffness, result from degeneration of the joint, the severity of articular cartilage loss is not necessarily closely related to the severity of symptoms. Patients with advanced joint degeneration may have relatively little pain and surprising mobility, whereas others with moderate joint degeneration may have severe symptoms and almost no joint motion. For this reason, it is important to distinguish the natural history of joint degeneration from the natural history of the clinical syndrome of osteoarthritis.

Inflammatory Arthritis

Although inflammation of the joint has various etiologies, the basic inflammatory process starts with migration of specific inflammatory cells incited by different triggers according to the specific disorder. The inflammatory cells then release molecules that mediate synovial proliferation and inflammation followed by soft-tissue and bone destruction.

Rheumatoid Arthritis

Rheumatoid arthritis is the most common type of inflammatory arthritis. Rheumatoid arthritis is usually manifested by the insidious onset of morning stiffness and polyarthralgia. The diagnosis is made according to the presence of specific criteria developed by the American College of Rheumatology, which include swelling, morning stiffness, nodules, positive laboratory findings, and positive radiographic analysis. A recent study found that testing of antibodies to cyclic citrullinated peptides in patients with undifferentiated arthritis can allow accurate prediction of those who will fulfill the American College of Rheumatology criteria. The inflammatory response is primarily mediated by mononuclear cells and is first directed against the periarticular soft tissues. Macrophage migratory inhibitory factors have been found to play an important role in the migration of inflammatory cells in the synovium of the joints of patients with rheumatoid arthritis via induction of IL-8. Macrophage migratory inhibitory factors regulate IL-8 and IL-1 β. Midkine (a heparin-binding growth factor) also appears to participate in the two distinct phases of rheumatoid arthritis: migration of leukocytes and osteoclast differentiation. Midkine is considered to be a key molecule in the pathogenesis of rheumatoid arthritis. Chondrolysis results later from the direct effect of lymphocytes on the cartilage. Characteristic radiographic evidence of periarticular bone resorption occurs much later in the destructive cascade. The positive laboratory test results include elevated erythrocyte sedimentation rate, elevated C-reactive protein level, and a positive rheumatoid factor titer. However, these findings are only encountered in approximately 80% of patients with rheumatoid arthritis. The characteristic radiographic findings include periarticular bone resorption, resulting into gross deviation and subluxation of small joints. In larger joints, there is generally a paucity of osteophytes for the degree of degeneration. In patients with advanced hip disease, there may be frank protrusio acetabuli.

The primary goals of the management of rheumatoid arthritis are to decrease soft-tissue inflammation, control pain, maintain joint function, and prevent deformity. These goals are achieved with the use of different modalities, including physiotherapy, medications, and surgery. The main therapeutic agents used in the treatment of rheumatoid arthritis are nonsteroidal anti-inflammatory drugs, antimalarial agents, remittive drugs, steroids, and cytotoxic agents. All of the specific treatment protocols are highly controversial and are constantly challenged by the introduction of new drugs. In a recent trial, adalimumab was shown to be effective in inhibiting the progression of structural joint damage, reducing symptoms, and improving physical function in patients with active rheumatoid arthritis who had demonstrated an incomplete response to treatment with methotrexate. Another study assessing the efficacy of the disease-modifying anti-rheumatic drugs (DMARDs) in patients with rheumatoid arthritis suggests that there are few consistent reliable predictors of treatment needs for this patient population. Surgical options for rheumatoid arthritis include synovectomy (through arthroscopy or arthrotomy), soft-tissue realignment, arthrodesis, and arthroplasty.

Systemic Lupus Erythematosus

Systemic lupus erythematosus (SLE) is the second most common inflammatory disease affecting the joint. It typically occurs in young women and is more prevalent among African Americans. The clinical symptoms include fever, rash, and polyarthralgia. In advanced stages of the disease, patients may have pancytopenia, pericarditis, and nephritis, which is usually the cause of mortality in patients with SLE. The inflammation is typically mediated by T-lymphocytes. The resulting destructive cascade starts with the soft tissue and then progresses to the cartilage and bone. The radiographic characteristics and the management of SLE are similar to those for rheumatoid arthritis.

Juvenile Rheumatoid Arthritis

Juvenile rheumatoid arthritis is a form of inflammatory disease that occurs in patients in the first two decades of life. The clinical symptoms include rash, morning stiffness, intermittent fever, and joint pain. The diagnostic workup may reveal inflammation of the pericardium, eye, and cervical spine. Ocular involvement in the form of iridocyclitis can lead to loss of vision if untreated. Therefore, frequent eye examination (twice a year) is critical to make an early diagnosis and initiate prompt treatment. Joint involvement caused by synovial proliferation can lead to chondrolysis, periarticular bone resorption, and contractures. Juvenile rheumatoid arthritis is also a major risk factor for protrusio acetabuli. Medical treatments include physiotherapy, high-dose salicylates, and remittive agents. Surgical options are synovectomy, realignment procedures, arthroplasty, and arthrodesis.

Crystal Deposition Disease

Three types of inflammatory arthritides are caused by crystal deposit in the joint: gout, chondrocalcinosis, and calcium hydroxyapatite crystal disease.

Gout is caused by the inflammation resulting from the production of monosodium urate crystal. The inflammation is mediated by proteases, prostaglandins, leukotrienes, interleukins, and free radicals. Gouty attacks may occur after any process that causes cellular death, such as chemotherapy, trauma, and surgery. The diagnosis is confirmed by the presence of monosodium urate crystals that are thin and strongly negatively birefringent. Medical treatments include indomethacin, colchicine, and allopurinol. Surgical options include débridement, arthrodesis, and arthroplasty.

Chondrocalcinosis is not a single entity but the clinical manifestation of different disorders such as ochronosis, hyperparathyroidism, pseudogout, hypothyroidism, and hemochromatosis. The inflammation is mediated by neutrophils. The classic radiographic finding is calcification of the cartilage (hyaline, meniscus, and fibrocartilage). The crystals are typically short, rhomboid-shaped, and weakly positively birefringent. Anti-inflammatory medications are used to control pain and inflammation. Intra-articular injections can be helpful on a short-term basis.

Calcium hydroxyapatite deposition disease is an inflammatory arthropathy associated with the precipitation of calcium salt crystals (calcium phosphate or calcium hydroxyapatite) in the joint. It leads to rapid degeneration of the involved joint and is most common in the knee and shoulder.

Spondyloarthropathies

The spondyloarthropathies are a cluster of often interrelated and overlapping chronic inflammatory rheumatic diseases characterized by a positive HLA-B27 and a negative rheumatoid factor titer. They classically include ankylosing spondylitis, reactive arthritis, psoriatic arthritis, and enteropathic arthritis. The primary patho-

logic sites are the bony insertions of ligaments and tendons, the axial skeleton, the limb joints. Extraskeletal tissues that may be involved include the intestines, skin, eye, lungs, and aortic valve. Although spondyloarthropathies are believed to be triggered by environmental factors in genetically predisposed patients, the cellular and molecular mechanisms of inflammation are not yet fully understood.

Ankylosing spondylitis is manifested by bilateral sacroiliitis and acute uveitis in HLA-B27 positive males. The disease has an insidious onset and progresses to spontaneous fusion of the spine. Hip involvement is always bilateral and is associated with protrusio acetabuli. Initial treatment consists of physiotherapy and nonsteroidal anti-inflammatory drugs. Extraskeletal involvement requires a multidisciplinary approach. Total hip arthroplasty has a poor prognosis in patients with ankylosing spondylitis because the acetabular protrusion makes the procedure technically difficult. In addition, patients with ankylosing spondylitis are at significant risk for heterotopic ossification.

Reiter syndrome is characterized by the classic triad of conjunctivitis, urethritis, and oligoarthritis. Skin involvement is also common. The arthritis typically presents with acute pain and effusion in the weight-bearing joints. Management typically consists of physiotherapy and nonsteroidal anti-inflammatory drugs.

Psoriatic arthritis is a chronic inflammatory disease characterized by progressive joint destruction associated with psoriasis. The disease runs a variable clinical course. The small joints are most often affected, although the disease often leads to degeneration of large joints. The treatment is largely empirical or anecdotal and is similar to that for rheumatoid arthritis. However, despite evidence of clinical improvement with current DMARDs treatment, psoriatic arthritis has been reported to result in radiographic damage in up to 47% of patients at a median follow-up of 2 years. Early diagnosis and treatment is critical for achieving satisfactory prognosis in the management of this disease.

Enteropathic arthritis is a form of inflammatory arthropathy associated with inflammatory bowel diseases. HLA-B27 plays an important role in enhancing the genetic susceptibility, but the underlying molecular mechanism is still unknown.

Polymyalgia Rheumatica

Polymyalgia rheumatica most commonly occurs in the geriatric population and is characterized by dull pain and stiffness of the hip and shoulder associated with headaches, malaise, and anorexia. In addition to an elevated erythrocyte sedimentation rate, laboratory abnormalities include anemia and elevated alkaline phosphatase levels. The treatment of polymyalgia rheumatica is largely supportive and symptomatic with physiotherapy, nonsteroidal anti-inflammatory drugs, and low-dose corticosteroids. High-dose corticosteroids are indicated only in patients with temporal arteritis.

Relapsing Polychondritis

Relapsing polychondritis is a rare inflammatory disorder affecting type II collagen. It leads to slow, progressive destruction of the articular cartilage. Extraskeletal involvement includes the ears, eyes, trachea, and heart. The management of relapsing polychondritis is mainly supportive.

Summary

Although in most patients the cause of osteoarthritis remains unknown and no cure has been identified, appropriate diagnosis and treatment, including patient education, can minimize symptoms and help patients maintain active and productive lives. Accomplishing this aim requires that physicians have an understanding of the pathophysiology of joint degeneration and the relationships between joint degeneration and the clinical syndrome of osteoarthritis. Even though much remains to be learned about the development and progression of the joint degeneration responsible for osteoarthritis, it is clear that the loss of articular cartilage results from disruption of the structural integrity of the articular cartilage coupled with or caused by an imbalance in the anabolic and catabolic activity of the tissue. The progression of joint degeneration varies considerably among patients; in some the joint degenerates rapidly, in some the degenerative changes progress slowly over decades, and in some the disease may remain stable. In rare instances, the joint degenerative changes spontaneously improve. Although joint degeneration is the underlying cause of the symptoms of osteoarthritis including joint pain and loss of joint function, not all patients with joint degeneration have symptoms of osteoarthritis. Future therapeutic approaches may include disease modifying drugs and surgical procedures that correct mechanical abnormalities, débride joints, and replace degenerated articular cartilage with implants that stimulate restoration of a cartilaginous joint surface. Development of methods to detect and monitor subtle changes in cartilage metabolism and identify the joint changes that precede loss of articular cartilage may make it possible to detect the earliest signs of osteoarthritis when therapeutic interventions have the greatest potential for preventing progression of the disease.

Inflammatory arthritis is typically bilateral. The laboratory findings vary significantly with the specific disorder in question. Initial treatment of inflammatory arthritis usually consists of physiotherapy and anti-inflammatory drugs. DMARDs play an important role in long-term management of these disorders. Ongoing studies continue to assess the efficacy of TNF-α blockers in the treatment protocol of joint inflammation; published data suggest that these agents are effective for the prevention of TNF-α–mediated destruction of bone because they act by reducing the number of osteoclasts in the inflammatory tissue.

Annotated Bibliography

Osteoarthritis

Buckwalter JA: Articular cartilage injuries. *Clin Orthop Relat Res* 2002;402:21-37.

The author discusses the mechanisms of articular cartilage injuries and the response of the tissues to these injuries.

Buckwalter JA: Sports, joint injury, and posttraumatic osteoarthritis. *J Orthop Sports Phys Ther* 2003;33:578-588.

This article reviews the relationship between sports participation, joint injury, and posttraumatic osteoarthritis.

Buckwalter JA, Heckman JD, Petrie DP: An AOA critical issue: Aging of the North American population. New challenges for orthopaedics. *J Bone Joint Surg Am* 2003;85-A:748-758.

This article outlines the impact of the aging of the North American population on needs for orthopaedic clinical care and future directions for the specialty of orthopaedics.

Coester LM, Saltzman CL, Leupold J, Pontarelli W: Long-term results following ankle arthrodesis for posttraumatic arthritis. *J Bone Joint Surg Am* 2001;83-A:219-228.

The authors of this article demonstrate that ankle arthrodesis is associated with osteoarthritis in the other joints of the foot and that this is a universal phenomena over time.

Martin JA, Buckwalter JA: Aging, articular cartilage chondrocyte senescence and osteoarthritis. *Biogerontology* 2002;3:257-264.

The authors of this article discuss the effect of aging on the function of articular cartilage chondrocytes and the role of loss of chondrocyte function in osteoarthritis.

Martin JA, Buckwalter JA: The role of chondrocyte senescence in the pathogenesis of osteoarthritis and in limiting cartilage repair. *J Bone Joint Surg Am* 2003;85-A(suppl 2):106-110.

This article examines how age-related changes in chondrocyte function may interfere with the ability of cartilage to maintain and repair itself.

Martin JA, Klingelhutz AJ, Moussavi-Harami F, Buckwalter JA: Effects of oxidative damage and telomerase activity on human articular cartilage chondrocyte senescence. *J Gerontol A Biol Sci Med Sci* 2004;59:324-337.

The authors of this article demonstrate the potential effects of oxidative damage on chondrocyte function and discuss the possible implications for the development of osteoarthritis.

Melzer I, Yekutiel M, Sukenik S: Comparative study of osteoarthritis of the contralateral knee joint of male amputees who do and do not play volleyball. *J Rheumatol* 2001;28:169-172.

This comparative study of osteoarthritis examines the possible relationship between increased loading and joint degeneration.

Inflammatory Arthritis

Chabaud M, Page G, Miossec P: Enhancing the effect of IL-1, IL-17, and TNF-alpha on macrophage inflammatory protein-3 alpha production in rheumatoid arthritis regulation by soluble receptors and Th2 cytokines. *J Immunol* 2001;167(10):6015-6020.

In this article, the authors examined the effects of the proinflammatory cytokines and chemokines on the production of macrophage inflammatory protein-3 alpha by rheumatoid arthritis synoviocytes. They found a direct enhancing effect and suggested a therapeutic application by inhibiting the cytokines and chemokines.

Conn DL: Resolved: Low-dose prednisone is indicated as a standard treatment in patients with rheumatoid arthritis. *Arthritis Rheum* 2001;45(5):462-467.

In this article, the author reviews the use of low-dose glucocorticoids in the treatment of rheumatoid arthritis. Glucocorticoids act by inhibiting the gene transcription of proinflammatory proteins and adhesion molecules. The author recommends low-dose glucocorticoids with adjuvant calcium and vitamin D as well as a regular surveillance program for patients with rheumatoid arthritis.

Ilowite NT: Current treatment of juvenile rheumatoid arthritis. *Pediatrics* 2002;109(1):109-115.

The author reviews the current treatment protocols used for juvenile rheumatoid arthritis and emphasizes the challenging aspects of managing patients with poor prognostic factors. Prompt diagnosis and treatment is crucial to improve the quality of life of patients with juvenile rheumatoid arthritis. The author suggests the use of nonsteroidal anti-inflammatory drugs as the first-line agent followed by methotrexate. One TNF inhibitor, etanercept, shows efficacy and safety in the treatment of juvenile rheumatoid arthritis; the more recently approved medications for rheumatoid arthritis have not been fully assessed for the treatment of juvenile rheumatoid arthritis.

Jenkins JK, Hardy KJ, McMurray RW: The pathogenesis of rheumatoid arthritis: A guide to therapy. *Am J Med Sci* 2002;323(4):171-180.

In this article, the authors discuss the immunopathogenesis of rheumatoid arthritis and report that the inflammatory cells secrete cytokines, such as IL-1 and TNF, which stimulate joint destruction by inducing prostaglandins, angiogenesis, chemokines, adhesion molecules, osteoclastogenesis, and matrix metalloproteinases.

Kane D, Stafford L, Bresnihan B, FitzGerald O: A prospective, clinical, and radiographic study of early psoriatic arthritis: An early synovitis clinical experience. *Rheumatology (Oxford)* 2003;42(12):1460-1468.

The authors conducted a prospective 2-year study to determine the clinical and radiographic outcomes of early psoriasic arthritis. They found that psoriatic arthritis is a chronic, progressive disease resulting in radiographic changes in up to 47% of patients.

Keystone EC, Kavanaugh AF, Sharp JT, et al: Radiographic, clinical, and functional outcomes of treatment with adalimumab (a human anti-tumor necrosis factor monoclonal antibody) in patients with active rheumatoid arthritis receiving concomitant methotrexate therapy: A randomized, placebo-controlled, 52-week trial. *Arthritis Rheum* 2004;50(5):1400-1411.

The authors investigated the ability of Adalimumab to suppress structural joint destruction, decrease the signs and symptoms, and improve physical function in patients with active rheumatoid arthritis who are receiving methotrexate. Adalimumad was found to be more effective than placebo in patients who did not respond to methotrexate therapy.

Khan MA: Update on spondyloarthropathies. *Ann Intern Med* 2002;136(12):896-907.

In this article, the author presents a comprehensive overview of the spondyloarthropathies and reviews the efficacy of the most recent therapeutic advances, including TNF-α.

Maruyama K, Muramatsu H, Ishiguro N, Muramatsu T: Midkine, a heparin-binding growth factor, is fundamentally involved in the pathogenesis of rheumatoid arthritis. *Arthritis Rheum* 2004;50(5):1420-1429.

Using immunoabsorbent assay, the authors found increased levels of midkine in serum and synovial fluid of patients with rheumatoid arthritis. In addition, the administration of midkine to genetically deficient mice raised the incidence of arthritis. Furthermore, midkine promoted the differentiation of macrophages to osteoclasts. They authors concluded that midkine participates in both phases of rheumatoid arthritis (migration of inflammatory cells and osteoclast differentiation).

Matsuno H, Yudoh K, Katayama R, et al: The role of TNF-alpha in the pathogenesis of inflammation and joint destruction in rheumatoid arthritis (RA): A study using a human RA/SCID mouse chimera. *Rheumatology* 2002;41(3):329-337.

The authors used mice engrafted with human rheumatoid arthritis tissue to investigate the roles of TNF-α and IL-6 in synovial inflammation. They perform histologic examinations of the synovium after treatment with anti-TNF-α monoclonal antibodies, TNF-α, and IL-6, respectively. The synovial inflammatory cells were significantly reduced by the administration of anti-TNF-α antibodies. There was a significant increase of inflammatory cells after treatment with TNF-α. The levels of TNF-α and IL-6 were also increased by the administration of TNF-α, whereas the treatment with IL-6 did not affect the levels of TNF-α. The authors concluded that TNF-α was a key molecule in the pathogenesis of inflammation of rheumatoid arthritis synovium. The study also suggests that TNF-α controlled IL-6 production.

Matteson EL, Weyand CM, Fulbright JW, et al: How aggressive should initial therapy for rheumatoid arthritis be? Factors associated with response to 'non-aggressive' DMARD treatment and perspective from a 2-year open label. *Rheumatology* 2004;43(5):619-625.

The authors of this study suggest that although there are few consistently reliable predictors of treatment for patients with rheumatoid arthritis, mild treatment with hydroxychloroquine can be greatly beneficial in patients in the early stages of the disease.

Pipitone N, Kingsley GH, Manzo A, et al: Current concepts and new developments in the treatment of psoriatic arthritis. *Rheumatology* 2003;42(10):1138-1148.

The authors performed a Medline search and present an overview of the management of psoriatic arthritis. The armamentarium should include nonsteroidal anti-inflammatory drugs, intra-articular glucocorticoid, DMARDs, and TNF-α blockers. They report that no treatment is curative, but prompt diagnosis and treatment is still paramount for a good prognosis.

Redlich K, Hayer S, Maier A, et al: Tumor necrosis factor alpha-mediated joint destruction is inhibited by targeting osteoclasts with osteoprotegerin. *Arthritis Rheum* 2002;46(3):785-792.

In this study, the authors found a significant decrease of joint inflammation in mice that were given osteoprotegerin and pamidronate. The findings suggest that osteoprotegerin alone or in combination with bisphosphonates may be an effective treatment option for TNF-mediated inflammation.

Reimold AM: New indications for treatment of chronic inflammation by TNF-alpha blockade. *Am J Med Sci* 2003;325(2):75-92.

The author discusses the effectiveness of two TNF-α blockers, etanercept and infliximab, in the treatment of various inflammatory arthritides.

Smith JB, Haynes MK: Rheumatoid arthritis: A molecular understanding. *Ann Intern Med* 2002;136(12):908-922.

The authors of this article present a comprehensive review of the molecular basis of rheumatoid arthritis with respect to potential for drug development.

van Gaalen FA, Linn-Rasker SP, van Venrooig WJ, et al: Autoantibodies to cyclic citrullinated peptides predict progression to rheumatoid arthritis in patients with undifferentiated arthritis: A prospective cohort study. *Arthritis Rheum* 2004;50(3):709-715.

The authors of this study concluded that testing for anti-cyclic citrullinated peptide antibodies in patients with undifferentiated arthritis allows accurate identification of a substantial number of patients who will fulfill American College of Rheumatology criteria for rheumatoid arthritis.

Classic Bibliography

Aigner T, Dietz U, Stoss H: Mark Kvd: Differential expression of collagen types I, II, III and X in human osteophytes. *Lab Invest* 1995;73:236-243.

Baici A, Lang A, Horler D, et al: Cathepsin B in osteoarthritis: Cytochemical and histochemical analysis of human femoral head cartilage. *Ann Rheum Dis* 1995;54: 289-297.

Buckwalter JA, Lane NE: Aging, sports and osteoarthritis. *Sports Med Arthritis Rev* 1996; 4:276-287.

Buckwalter JA, Lane NE, Gordon SL: Exercise as a cause of osteoarthritis, in Kuettner KE, Goldberg VM (eds): *Osteoarthritic Disorders.* Rosemont, IL, American Academy of Orthopaedic Surgeons, 1995, pp 405-417.

Buckwalter JA, Lohmander S: Operative treatment of osteoarthrosis: Current practice and future development. *J Bone Joint Surg Am* 1994;76:1405-1418.

Buckwalter JA, Mankin HJ: Articular cartilage: Tissue design and chondrocyte-matrix interactions. *Instr Course Lect* 1998;47:477-486.

Buckwalter JA, Martin JA: *Degenerative Joint Disease: Clinical Symposia.* Summit, NJ, Ciba Geigy, 1995, pp 2-32.

Buckwalter JA, Mow VC: Cartilage repair in osteoarthritis, in Moskowitz RW, Howell DS, Goldberg VM, Mankin HJ (eds): *Osteoarthritis: Diagnosis and Management,* ed 2. Philadephia, PA, WB Saunders, 1992, pp 71-107.

Callaghan JJ, Brand RA, Pedersen DR: Hip arthrodesis: A long-term follow-up. *J Bone Joint Surg Am* 1985;67: 1328-1335.

Chevalier X: Fibronectin, cartilage, and osteoarthritis. *Semin Arthritis Rheum* 1993;22:307-318.

Cooper C, Dennison E: The natural history and prognosis of osteoarthritis, in Brandt KD, Doherty M, Lohmander LS (eds): *Osteoarthritis*. Oxford, England, Oxford University Press, 1998, pp 237-249.

Cooper CR: Osteoarthritis and related disorders, in Klippel JH, Dieppe PA (eds): *Rheumatology*. London, England, Mosby, 1998, pp 8:2.1-8:2.8.

Szabo G, Roughley PJ, Plaas AH, Glant TT: Large and small proteoglycans of osteoarthritic and rheumatoid articular cartilage. *Arthritis Rheum* 1995;38:660-668.

Dieppe P: The classification and diagnosis of osteoarthritis, in Kuettner KE, Goldberg VM (eds): *Osteoarthritic Disorders*. Rosemont, IL, American Academy of Orthopaedic Surgeons, 1995, pp 5-12.

Ehrlich MG, Armstrong AL, Treadwell BV, Mankin HJ: The role of proteases in the pathogenesis of osteoarthritis. *J Rheumatol* 1987;14:30-32.

Felson DT: Epidemiology of osteoarthritis, in Brandt KD, Doherty M, Lohmander LS (eds): *Osteoarthritis*. Oxford, England, Oxford University Press, 1998, pp 12-22.

Felson DT: The epidemiology of osteoarthritis: Prevalence and risk factors, in Kuettner KE, Goldberg VM (eds): *Osteoarthritic Disorders*. Rosemont, IL, American Academy of Orthopaedic Surgeons, 1995, pp 13-24.

Gorman C: Relief for swollen joints. *Time.* October 28, 1996:86.

Hashimoto S, Ochs RL, Komiya S, Lotz M: Linkage of chondrocyte apoptosis and cartilage degeneration in human osteoarthritis. *Arthritis Rheum* 1998;41:1632-1638.

Hauselmann HJ, Oppliger L, Michel BA, et al: Nitric oxide and proteoglycan biosynthesis by human articular cartilage chondrocytes in alginate culture. *FEBS Lett* 1994;352:361-364.

Homandberg GA, Hui F: Arg-Gly-Asp-Ser peptide analogs suppress cartilage chondrolytic activities of integrin-binding and nonbinding fibronectin fragments. *Arch Biochem Biophys* 1994;310:40-48.

Homandberg GA, Meyers R, Williams JM: Intraarticular injection of fibronectin fragments causes severe depletion of cartilage proteoglycans in vivo. *J Rheumatol* 1993;20:1378-1382.

Lippiello L, Hall D, Mankin HJ: Collagen synthesis in normal and osteoarthritic human cartilage. *J Clin Invest* 1977;59:593-600.

Mankin HJ: The reaction of articular cartilage to injury and osteoarthritis: I. *N Engl J Med* 1974;291:1285-1295.

Mankin HJ: The reaction of articular cartilage to injury and osteoarthritis: II. *N Engl J Med* 1974;291:1335-1340.

Mankin HJ: The response of articular cartilage to mechanical injury. *J Bone Joint Surg Am* 1982;64:460-466.

Mankin HJ, Dorfman H, Lippiello L, Zarins A: Biochemical and metabolic abnormalities in articular cartilage from osteo-arthritic human hips: II. Correlation of morphology with biochemical and metabolic data. *J Bone Joint Surg Am* 1971;53:523-537.

Mankin HJ, Johnson ME, Lippiello L: Biochemical and metabolic abnormalities in articular cartilage from osteoarthritic human hips: III. Distribution and metabolism of amino sugar containing macromolecules. *J Bone Joint Surg Am* 1981;63:131-139.

Mankin HJ, Lippiello L: Biochemical and metabolic abnormalities in articular cartilage from osteo-arthritic human hips. *J Bone Joint Surg Am* 1970;52:424-434.

Mankin HJ, Thrasher AZ: Water content and binding in normal and osteoarthritic human cartilage. *J Bone Joint Surg Am* 1975;57:76-80.

Martel-Pelletier J, McCollum R, Fujimoto N, et al: Excess of metalloproteases over tissue inhibitor of metalloprotease may contribute to cartilage degradation in osteoarthritis and rheumatoid arthritis. *Lab Invest* 1994;70:807-815.

Martin JA, Buckwalter JA: Articular cartilage aging and degeneration. *Sports Med Arthritis Rev* 1996;4:263-275.

Martin JA, Buckwalter JA: Effects of fibronectin on articular cartilage chondrocyte proteoglycan synthesis and response to IGF-I. *J Orthop Res* 1998;16:752-757.

Middleton J, Arnott N, Walsh S, Beresford J: Osteoblasts and osteoclasts in adult human osteophyte tissue express the mRNAs for insulin-like growth factors I and II and the type 1 IGF receptor. *Bone* 1995;16:287-293.

Middleton JF, Tyler JA: Upregulation of insulin-like growth factor I gene expression in the lesions of osteoarthritic human articular cartilage. *Ann Rheum Dis* 1992;51:440-447.

Murrell GA, Jang D, Riley JW: Nitric oxide activates metalloprotease enzymes in articular cartilage. *Biochem Biophys Res Commun* 1995;206:15-21.

Myers SL, Flusser D, Brandt KD, Heck DA: Prevalence of cartilage shards in synovium and their association with synovitis in patients with early and endstage osteoarthritis. *J Rheumatol* 1992;19:1247-1251.

Poole AR, Rizkalla G, Ionescu M, et al: Osteoarthritis in the human knee: a dynamic process of cartilage matrix degradation, synthesis and reorganization. *Agents Actions Suppl* 1993;39:3-13.

Praemer AP, Furner S, Rice DP: *Musculoskeletal Conditions in the United States*. Park Ridge, Illinois, American Academy of Orthopaedic Surgeons, 1992.

Radin EL, Rose RM: Role of subchondral bone in the initiation and progression of cartilage damage. *Clin Orthop Relat Res* 1986;213:34-40.

Reimann I, Mankin HJ, Trahan C: Quantitative histologic analyses of articular cartilage and subchondral bone from osteoarthritic and normal human hips. *Acta Orthop Scand* 1977;48:63-73.

Spector TD, Dacre JE, Harris PA, Huskisson EC: Radiologic progression of osteoarthritis: An 11 year follow up study of the knee. *Ann Rheum Dis* 1992;51:1107-1110.

Testa V, Capasso G, Maffulli M, et al: Proteases and antiproteases in cartilage homeostasis: A brief review. *Clin Orthop Relat Res* 1994;308:79-84.

Trippel SB: Growth factor actions on articular cartilage. *J Rheumatol Suppl* 1995;43:129-132.

Tsuchiya K, Maloney WJ, Hoffman AR, et al: Osteoarthritis: Differential expression of matrix metalloprotease-9 nRNA in nonfibrillated and fibrillated cartilage. *J Orthop Res* 1997;15:94-100.

van Beuningen HM, van der Kraan PM, Arntz OJ, van den Berg WB: Transforming growth factor-beta 1 stimulates articular chondrocyte proteoglycan synthesis and induces osteophyte formation in the murine knee joint. *Lab Invest* 1994;71:279-290.

Varich L, Pathria M, Resnick D, et al: Patterns of central acetabular osteophytosis in osteoarthritis of the hip. *Invest Radiol* 1993;28:1120-1127.

Xie DL, Meyers R, Homandberg GA: Fibronectin fragments in osteoarthritis synovial fluid. *J Rheumatol* 1992;19:1448-1452.

Chapter 17

Conservative Management of Osteoarthritis of the Hip and Knee

David S. Hungerford, MD

Marc W. Hungerford, MD

Introduction

There have been significant changes in the conservative management of osteoarthritis of the hip and knee within the past 5 years, primarily because of the controversy surrounding the withdrawal of rofecoxib (Vioxx, Merck, Whitehouse Station, NJ) and valdecoxib (Bextra, Pfizer, New York, NY) from the market. Because of the publicity surrounding the complications associated with these two medications, patients are now openly resistant to the use of any nonsteroidal anti-inflammatory drug (NSAID). Patients with early osteoarthritis and even moderately advanced osteoarthritis are more open than ever to pursue conservative management. Therefore, it is important that physicians understand the effectiveness and safety of conservative management for osteoarthritis of both the hip and the knee. Many of the conservative treatment modalities that are in use today apply to both the hip and knee. However, there are some treatments that are specific to one joint or the other.

Many patients present to physicians having made the assumption that the pain that they are experiencing in the region of the hip or knee is the result of osteoarthritis. Because this is not always the case, the first step in conservative management is to establish the correct diagnosis. Osteoarthritis is commonly associated with painful limitation of motion, and radiographic changes show the typical signs of joint space narrowing, osteophyte formation, and sclerosis on either side of the joint. Although patients may be excused for making erroneous assumptions, physicians should never assume that symptoms arise from an osteoarthritic joint, but instead should positively establish the cause and effect relationship.

In every patient encounter involving a recommendation for treatment, a risk-benefit analysis should be conducted, and the results should be realistically discussed with the patient. Ultimately, physicians will recommend a specific form of treatment that patients will either accept or reject. This process cannot take place as it should unless patients and physicians thoroughly discuss risks and benefits. Patients are much more likely to be compliant with the proposed treatment if they understand how it works and why it is recommended. A discussion of the risks and benefits conveys to patients that physicians are cognizant of their rights and respect the role that they play as a partner in the treatment process. Physicians who circumvent this process do so at their own peril and are likely to have patients who are noncompliant and do not get well; worse yet, such patients may seek treatment elsewhere. Although most nonsurgical treatments are relatively low risk, some level of risk still exists, as has been recently shown with the problems associated with the cyclooxygenase (COX)-2 inhibitors. Explaining all aspects of treatment, even for low-risk nonsurgical recommendations, will build a relationship that will serve both patients and physicians well.

Education

Once patients understand the natural history of osteoarthritis and realize that simple modifications in their activities and lifestyle can positively impact their symptoms, they can participate in the management of their disease. Education includes helping the patient to understand the relationship between muscle strength, aerobic capacity, and body weight and their symptoms. The accelerated physical decline that is precipitated by the painful arthritic joint can be reversed. Weight reduction should be encouraged. A 1-lb weight loss results in a 3- to 4-lb force decrease across the affected joint. A patient who is 33 lb overweight is putting an additional 100 lb of force across the joint with each step, which, with a moderate level of activity, could translate to as much as 100 tons of extra force per day.

Physical Therapy

One of the characteristics of osteoarthritis is to lose range of motion and muscle strength around the affected joint. Physical therapy is aimed at improving range of motion through gentle active and active-assisted exercises and to increase strength to the muscles surrounding the joint. Additional methods for physical therapy include a variety of physical modalities (such as heat, cold, ultrasound, and electrical stimulation) as an adjunct to the exercise program. For the knee, exercise usually focuses on quadriceps strengthening. For the hip, exercises include all hip girdle muscles, but focus on the hip abductors. Increased strength improves functional stability around the arthritic knee and has been documented to decrease pain during walking. Strengthening exercises, particularly for muscles around the knee, must proceed with caution, and full range extension exercises against resistance are to be avoided. For both joints, functional exercises such as swimming, walking in waist-deep water, stair climbing on small steps, using an exercise cycle, and using a treadmill all have the potential to increase both functional capacity and muscle strength.

Aerobic Conditioning
One of the common reports of patients with osteoarthritis is that of decreased overall stamina. This results in decreasing ability to perform the activities of daily living. It has been documented that a supervised fitness walking program not only increases the functional capacity of participants but also decreases pain and the use of medication.

Assistive Devices
It has long been known that the use of a cane or crutch in the opposite hand can reduce the forces on the joint, hip, or knee by 50% to 60%. Because many patients with osteoarthritis of the lower extremity are also advanced in age and have balance problems that are made worse by the arthritic joint, the use of an assistive device may have the additional benefit of adding safety to activities. The difficulty has always been convincing the patient to comply with the use of such a device. Even so, patients need to be instructed in the benefits of assistive devices and the potential that exists for them to comfortably and significantly increase the extent of physical activities. Patients can often triple their walking distance with the use of a cane or crutch.

Nonsurgical Treatment Modalities
Because the knee is relatively superficial and the hip is covered by a thick layer of soft tissue, many of the treatment modalities used apply more to the knee than the hip. These include ultrasound, diathermy, interferential stimulation, local heat, local cold, and transcutaneous electrical neuromuscular stimulation. Many patients report short-term improvement in symptoms with the use of these modalities, but there is little convincing evidence of long-term improvement and no evidence of disease modification.

Acupuncture
Although acupuncture has been extensively used for relief of the pain of arthritis, there is no clear evidence of its value over placebo for treating pain in the hip or the knee.

Analgesics
Acetaminophen, over-the-counter NSAIDs, and aspirin have long been the mainstay for primary care physicians and rheumatologists for managing the symptoms of osteoarthritis. Patients are also likely to self-medicate with these drugs. Many patients with moderate level symptoms would do better if they took these medications on a regular basis rather than in response to elevating symptoms. All three have been demonstrated to be safe for intermittent and short-term self-medication. The only caveat with self-medication is that patients may be assuming that symptoms are the result of osteoarthritis, whereas they may actually be secondary to a more serious treatable condition for which the diagnosis is delayed. Patients with known chronic diseases and specifically gastrointestinal diseases should be discouraged from self-medicating.

Nonsteroidal Anti-inflammatory Drugs
The family of NSAIDs inhibits inflammation by blocking COX conversion of arachidonic acid to prostaglandin. Because prostaglandins are involved in many normal tissue processes, including mucosal defense and repair, the COX-1 inhibitors have been associated with significant adverse effects, particularly gastrointestinal symptoms. NSAIDs produce significant gastrointestinal morbidity and even mortality. Gastric disease secondary to NSAIDs has been called the second most deadly rheumatologic disease. As opposed to the COX-1 inhibitors, which are ubiquitous, the COX-2 enzyme is induced in areas of injury and inflammation. The class of COX-2 inhibitors was developed to avoid the adverse effects of the nonspecific COX inhibitors.

NSAIDs have been mass marketed and represent a multi-billion dollar industry. Until recently, patients demanded prescription strength NSAIDs for even mild disease. A survey of the practice patterns of general practitioners performed in the 1990s showed that 90% chose either sublevel anti-inflammatory or full anti-inflammatory doses of NSAIDs as the first line of treatment. Although most controlled and comparative studies show NSAIDs to be more effective than placebo, several studies have shown no substantive difference between therapeutic level NSAIDs, over-the-counter NSAIDs, and acetaminophen.

There is no compelling evidence that one NSAID is better than another. COX-1 inhibitors have more withdrawal symptoms secondary to adverse effects than COX-2 inhibitors, but neither has been found to be therapeutically more effective than the other.

Toxicity of NSAIDs

A 1998 publication estimated that 107,000 hospitalizations and 16,500 deaths annually in the United States were secondary to complications related to NSAID therapy. It was thought that the introduction of the COX-2 inhibitors would dramatically alter these statistics. However, the dominant story in the conservative management of osteoarthritis is the voluntary withdrawal of rofecoxib based on the increased risk of a cardiovascular event. Patients in this study received 25 mg of rofecoxib for 3 years to control recurrent colorectal polyps. Interim analysis of the patients who completed the 36-month study showed a statistically significant increase in cardiovascular events compared with placebo (7.2/1,000 compared with 5.3/1,000). Valdecoxib was also withdrawn voluntarily in April 2005 for similar concerns. Although many rheumatologists believe that the therapeutic advantages of the COX-2 inhibitors outweigh the adverse effects, and a US Food and Drug Administration panel recommended that both drugs be reapproved with a black box warning, both drugs currently remain off the market.

These highly publicized withdrawals, reinforced by advertising from trial lawyers seeking patients who can claim harm by virtue of taking these medications, have resulted in a significant shift in the public's attitude toward NSAIDs. In spite of the fact that its two competitors have been removed from the market, celecoxib (Celebrex, Pfizer) sales have decreased by 50%. Many patients refuse to even consider using an NSAID of any kind and are more open to conservative management of their symptoms or surgery.

Rational Use of NSAIDs

There is no evidence that chronic use of NSAIDs alters the natural history of osteoarthritis. Complications associated with NSAIDs are proportional to dose and duration. Complication rates also increase with patient age. Therefore, NSAIDs should be used sparingly, if at all, in the elderly patient population. Patients should begin on the lowest dose possible, and the medication should be discontinued as soon as possible. One long-term study compared naproxen (Naprosyn, Roche Pharmaceuticals, Basel, Switzerland) to acetaminophen. Only 35% of the patients completed the study. Withdrawal was higher in the acetaminophen group because of lack of efficacy and in the naproxen group because of adverse effects. The difference in efficacy between the two groups was not significant.

Hyaluronans

Hyaluronans are used for the treatment of osteoarthritis of the knee, and they are generally accepted as effective. Not all study findings agree that there is a significant difference between treated and control patients. Only three open label studies of hyaluronans used to treat osteoarthritis of the hip have reported findings, and all three showed positive results that justify a larger prospective randomized study.

Intra-articular Steroids

Although there are many reports on the effectiveness of intra-articular steroids for treatment of osteoarthritis of the knee, very few have been published on the hip. Injection of the knee can be done in a physician's office, whereas injection of the hip requires either ultrasound or fluoroscopic control. One controlled study of corticosteroid injection for the hip showed positive results, particularly for rest pain; improvement was maintained for the 12-week follow-up of the study. Although these findings suggest that intra-articular steroids may be more extensively used, there is also a disturbing report of four deep infections that occurred after total hip replacement in 40 patients (compared with no infections in 40 control subjects) who had received an intra-articular steroid injection before undergoing surgery.

Chondroprotective Agents

Glucosamine and chondroitin sulfate have enjoyed widespread acceptance among the lay public and considerable initial skepticism in the medical community. The medical literature and controlled studies on these two agents date back to the early 1980s. In vitro, in vivo, and clinical studies support glucosamine and chondroitin sulfate as having a positive effect on articular cartilage and the clinical symptoms of osteoarthritis. Glucosamine stimulates the production of glycosaminoglycans by chondrocytes and hyaluronic acid by synoviocytes, whereas chondroitin inhibits the enzymes that break down articular cartilage. At least five double-blind, single-joint, placebo-controlled studies using a validated outcome have been conducted to evaluate glucosamine, all of which have shown positive clinical results, and none of which have shown an adverse effect profile that is different from that of placebo. For chondroitin sulfate, two long-term studies have shown less progression of osteoarthritis of the knee in treated patients compared with control subjects, and one study showed a similar finding for osteoarthritis of the hand.

The most significant study has recently been conducted by the Glucosamine/Chondroitin Arthritis Intervention Trial study group funded by the US National Institutes of Health. This is a five-arm study that compared treatment with glucosamine alone, chondroitin sulfate alone, glucosamine and chondroitin sulfate together, NSAID (celecoxib), and placebo. Initial findings show that the combination of glucosamine and chondroitin sulfate resulted in a highly statistically significant improvement in patients with moderate and moderately severe osteoarthritis of the knee compared with placebo and celecoxib. This is an impeccably conducted, extensive trial that should put to rest any concerns about the efficacy of these two nutraceuticals in the treatment of osteoarthritis. Although only osteoarthritis of the knee was treated in the study, there is no reason to believe that the use of these agents for treatment of osteoarthritis of the hip would be any less effective.

This study used pharmaceutical grade glucosamine and chondroitin sulfate. A report from the University of Maryland Department of Pharmacology, which tested 32 commercially available products containing glucosamine, chondroitin sulfate, or both, noted that 7 products had no active ingredients and 9 had less than 50% of the active ingredients reported on their labels. Not all marketed products are the same. The Arthritis Foundation recommended that patients and physicians find out which products have been tested and use only those products.

Summary

There are many effective treatments that can be undertaken before considering surgery as a treatment for patients with almost any level of osteoarthritis. Even patients with severe pain can improve symptomatically with nonsurgical treatment. Even in patients in whom conservative therapy eventually fails, the period of nonsurgical treatment offers the opportunity for the surgeon to get to know the patient as a person, rather than to resort immediately to surgery.

Annotated Bibliography

Nonsurgical Treatment Modalities

Adebowale A, Cox DS, Zhongming L, Eddington ND: Analysis of glucosamine and chondroitin sulfate content in marketed products and the caco-2 permeability of chondroitin sulfate raw materials. *Am Nutraceutical Assoc* 2000;3(1):37-44.

This is an important article about the subject of nutraceuticals. The authors analyzed the contents of 32 marketed products containing glucosamine, chondroitin sulfate, or both. They found that seven of the products analyzed contained no active ingredients and additional nine contained less than 50% of the that claimed on the label.

Clegg DO, Reda DJ, Harris CL, Klein MA: The efficacy of glucosamine and chondroitin sulfate in patients with painful knee osteoarthritis (OA): The Glucosamine/chondroitin Arthritis Intervention Trial (GAIT). Available at: http://www.abstractsonline.com/viewer/browseOptions.asp?MKey={F5B9F43A-15A0-467D-8458-5DF32518B4E3}&AKey={AA45DD66-F113-4CDD-8E62-01A05F613C0D} [To view the abstract, copy the URL above into the browser and then type

"Chondroitin" into the search box and hit the enter button on your keyboard.]

This is the most important study of these two compounds to date. The study, which was funded by the US National Institutes of Health, included 1,583 patients with osteoarthritis of the knee who were randomly divided into five treatment arms: chondroitin sulfate, glucosamine, chondroitin sulfate and glucosamine, celecoxib, and placebo. The combination of chondroitin sulfate and glucosamine showed significant symptomatic improvement as measured by validated outcome measures in patients with moderate and severe osteoarthritis ($P = 0.002$). Patients with mild osteoarthritis did not show significant improvement, possibly because of a floor effect and the high placebo effect. The study continues to monitor subjects to determine whether there is a disease-modifying effect.

Fries JF, Bruce B: Rates of serious gastrointestinal events from low dose use of acetylsalicylic acid, acetaminophen, and ibuprofen in patients with osteoarthritis and rheumatoid arthritis. *J Rheumatol* 2003;30(10):2226-2233.

These authors studied 5,692 patients with rheumatoid arthritis and 3,124 patients with osteoarthritis from 12 databank centers (36,262 patient-years of observation) who had taken one of three study analgesics and examined the frequency of serious gastrointestinal events requiring hospitalization. None of the three analgesics had a gastrointestinal complication rate that was different from the background rate. If patients were also taking corticosteroids, the complication rates were higher. There was no difference between drugs. The authors concluded that these over the counter medications at low doses are safe in most patients.

Lippiello L, Woodward J, Karpman R, Hammad TA: In vivo chondroprotection and metabolic synergy of glucosamine and chondroitin sulfate. *Clin Orthop Relat Res* 2000;381:229-240.

This study tests glucosamine and chondroitin sulfate alone and in combination on a rabbit meniscectomy model of experimental arthritis. The results showed almost complete cartilage protection with combined treatment with glucosamine and chondroitin sulfate, whereas in the control specimen the cartilage was rapidly destroyed down to subchondral bone. These findings provide graphic and histologic evidence of the chondroprotective attributes of this glucosamine and chondroitin sulfate therapy.

McAlindon TE, LaValley MP, Gulin JP, Felson DT: Glucosamine and chondroitin for treatment of osteoarthritis: A systematic quality assessment and meta-analysis. *JAMA* 2000;283(11):1469-1475.

These authors reviewed studies using glucosamine or chondroitin sulfate for treating osteoarthritis of the knee that were controlled and used a validated outcome measure. They concluded that some degree of efficacy appears probable for this type of therapy.

Reginster JY: Long-term effects of glucosamine sulphate on osteoarthritis progression: A randomized, placebo-controlled clinical trial. *Lancet* 2001;357(9252):251-256.

This was a 3-year placebo-controlled randomized study of the effect of 1,500 mg of glucosamine on the progression of osteoarthritis of the knee. Two hundred twelve patients were enrolled. The control subjects averaged 0.3 mm of joint space narrowing, and there was no joint space narrowing in the treatment group. The authors reported that control subjects deteriorated clinically, whereas treated patients improved.

Roddy E, Zhang W, Doherty M, et al: Evidence-based recommendations for the role of exercise in the management of osteoarthritis of the hip or knee: The MOVE consensus. *Rheumatology (Oxford)* 2005;44(1):67-73.

This report reviews the entire literature on muscle strengthening, aerobic conditioning, and physical therapy in the treatment of osteoarthritis. Because use of these methods rests on a solid clinical and scientific foundation, orthopaedic surgeons should be aware of this literature and seek to use these tried, true, and safe methods in their practices.

Zhang W, Doherty M, Arden N, et al: EULAR evidence based recommendations for the management of hip osteoarthritis: Report of a task force of the EULAR Standing Committee for International Clinical Studies Including Therapeutics (ESCISIT). *Ann Rheum Dis* 2005;64(5):669-681.

This is a report of the whole spectrum of treatment of osteoarthritis of the hip. Ten recommendations are made that comprise evidenced-based treatment, the first eight of which fall under the category of conservative or nonsurgical management.

Classic Bibliography

Brand RA, Crowninshield RD: The effect of cane use on hip contact force. *Clin Orthop Relat Res* 1980;147:181-184.

Chapter 18

Perioperative Medical Management

Charles R. Clark, MD

Preoperative Evaluation

The purpose of the preoperative evaluation is to assess the current medical status of a patient and to determine the relative risk profile of the patient's medical condition. Although the medical management of patients undergoing total hip or knee arthroplasty is often conducted by an internist, it is very important for the orthopaedic surgeon to understand the principles and important factors involved.

The American Society of Anesthesiologists uses a stratification system to assess the risk of perioperative mortality based on the preoperative physical status of patients (Table 1). A comprehensive medical history and physical examination are the cornerstones of the preoperative assessment. Specific evidence of cardiovascular disease, cerebral vascular disease, pulmonary disease, neurologic conditions, uropathy, rheumatoid arthritis, obesity, and hematologic and endocrine disease can affect intraoperative and postoperative morbidity and mortality and must be carefully assessed. Judicious use of appropriate laboratory tests and radiographic imaging are necessary to provide optimal perioperative care.

Patients rarely die as a result of orthopaedic surgical procedures. In the United States, the rate of acute mortality after orthopaedic surgical procedures is approximately 0.5% for patients without hip fractures. One recent study identified the following five critical risk factors that are helpful in identifying which patients are at risk for death: chronic renal failure, congestive heart failure, chronic obstructive pulmonary disease, hip fracture, and age older than 70 years. It was reported that the mortality rate was 0.25% for patients with no critical risk factors and that a linear increase in the mortality rate was seen with an increasing number of critical risk factors ($P < 0.005$). Another recent study evaluated the 30-day mortality rate in a consecutive series of 30,000 patients who underwent elective total hip arthroplasty and found that the factors associated with an increased risk of mortality included older age, male gender, and history of cardiorespiratory disease. Additionally, a significant decline in the 30-day mortality rate

Table 1 | Preoperative Assessment Classification

American Society of Anesthesiologists Status	Examples of Preoperative Patients
Class 1: No disease	Healthy 25-year-old
Class 2: Mild to moderate systemic disease	65-year-old with well-controlled diabetes mellitus type 2
Class 3: Severe systemic disease	70-year-old with congestive heart failure and rest angina
Class 4: Life-threatening systemic disease	30-year-old with diabetes mellitus type 1 in ketoacidosis
Class 5: Morbidly ill	70-year-old with angina and mesenteric ischemia

E is added to each class if surgery is an emergency

(Reproduced with permission from Fiorillo AB, Solaro FX Jr: Preoperative medical evaluation, in Callaghan JJ (ed): The Adult Hip. Philadelphia, PA, Lippincott-Raven, 1998, pp 601-632; and Dripps RD: New classification of physical status. Anesthesiology 1963; 24:111.)

was identified in patients who underwent elective hip arthroplasty in the past decade (1990s) compared with those who underwent the same procedure in prior decades.

Specific Medical Conditions

The American College of Cardiology has established an algorithm regarding the perioperative cardiovascular evaluation of patients undergoing noncardiac surgeries (Figure 1). Total hip arthroplasty is typically categorized as elective surgery. The algorithm identifies major clinical predictors, including unstable coronary syndromes, decompensated congestive heart failure, significant arrhythmias, and severe valvular disease. Intermediate level predictors include mild angina pectoris, prior myocardial infarction, compensated or prior congestive heart failure, diabetes mellitus, and renal insufficiency. Minor clinical predictors include advanced age, an abnormal electrocardiogram, cardiac rhythm other than sinus, low functional capacity, prior stroke, and uncontrolled systemic hypertension. According to the guidelines established by the American College of Car-

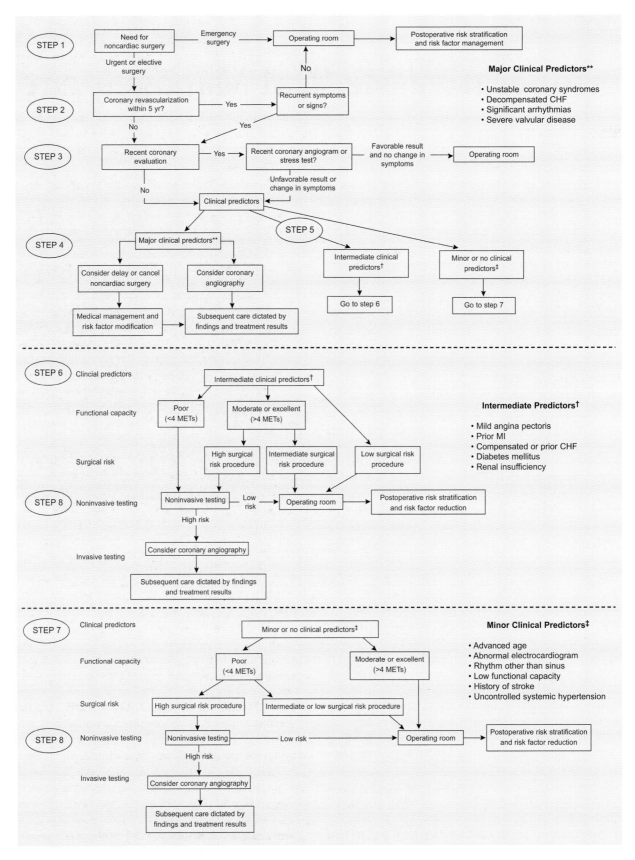

Figure 1 Stepwise approach to preoperative cardiac assessment. CHF = congestive heart failure, MET = metabolic equivalent, MI = myocardial infarction. (*Reproduced with permission from Eagle KA, Berger PB, Calkins H, et al: ACC/AHA guideline update for perioperative cardiovascular evaluation for noncardiac surgery: Executive summary. A report of the American College of Cardiology/American Heart Association Task Force on Practice Guidelines (Committee to Update the 1996 Guidelines on Perioperative Cardiovascular Evaluation for Noncardiac Surgery). J Am Coll Cardiol 2002;39(3):542-553.*)

diology, the overall cardiac risk for a patient with an intermediate clinical predictor who is undergoing orthopaedic surgery is generally less than 5%. This risk includes the combined incidence of cardiac death and nonfatal myocardial infarction.

Patients with mechanical heart valves are often maintained on warfarin; therefore, provisions need to be made to discontinue the warfarin preoperatively and place the patient on a "heparin window" in the interim. Low-molecular-weight heparins, as an alternative to unfractionated heparin, can be used on an outpatient basis to manage patients in the interim before surgery. After arthroplasty, the patient is treated with either heparin or low-molecular-weight heparin and warfarin therapy is resumed. The heparin compound is continued until the desired level of anticoagulation with warfarin is achieved based on the international normalized ratio.

Patients with significant cardiovascular disease should also be carefully examined for the presence of peripheral vascular disease. The examination should include an assessment of the vascular status of the extremity undergoing surgery. Careful documentation of pulses as well as assessment of skin temperature and hair distribution are important because patients with significant peripheral vascular disease may have substantial morbidity after arthroplasty.

Patients with a history of smoking and/or chronic obstructive pulmonary disease should be counseled regarding smoking cessation, and their pulmonary status needs to be optimized preoperatively. Epidural and/or spinal anesthesia is recommended for patients with significant pulmonary disease to obviate the effects of general anesthesia on their pulmonary status.

Patients undergoing total joint arthroplasty should be in good dental health before surgery and should be encouraged to seek professional dental care if necessary. Patients with diabetes mellitus deserve special consideration because the relative risk of perioperative morbidity, particularly infection, is increased in these patients. In a study of patients with diabetes mellitus who are undergoing total knee replacement, it was reported that all of the deep infections occurred in patients with type 1 diabetes mellitus. In addition, the revision rate, including revision for infection, was greater in patients with diabetes (3.6% versus 0.4%). The authors of this study recommended the routine use of cefuroxime-impregnated cement in this patient population.

Because patients with rheumatoid arthritis often have involvement of the hip and/or knee joints, there are several preoperative considerations for this patient population. First, the status of all multiple joints, particularly in the ipsilateral extremity, must be assessed. Second, because there is a high rate of cervical spine involvement in patients with rheumatoid arthritis (atlantoaxial subluxation is the most common abnormality) and because such involvement may often be rel-

atively asymptomatic, patients scheduled to receive a general anesthetic should undergo dynamic, lateral flexion-extension cervical spine radiography preoperatively to assess the status of the cervical spine. If significant instability is noted, alternative methods of anesthetic management should be considered, including awake intubation, fiberoptic intubation, and/or the use of spinal or epidural anesthesia. In addition, patients with rheumatoid arthritis who have been receiving long-term steroid therapy will likely require the use of stress doses of steroids during the perioperative period.

Obesity can have a significant impact on the outcome of patients undergoing total hip and total knee arthroplasty. One study reported that morbidly obese patients undergoing total knee arthroplasty can have successful results, but these results are associated with an increased risk of perioperative complications, including problems with wound healing, infection, and avulsion of the medial collateral ligament. The rate of perioperative complications was found to be significantly higher in the morbidly obese group; of the 55 total knee arthroplasties performed, 11 patients (22%) had wound complications, and 5 patients (10%) had an infection. Although it may be challenging to do so, it is important to counsel obese patients about weight reduction and its associated health benefits. A morbidly obese patient may also be a candidate for a gastric bypass procedure, and recommending consultation for such a procedure may be advisable, particularly in younger patients.

The knee is frequently involved in patients with hemophilic arthropathy. Total knee arthroplasty performed to treat hemophilic arthropathy has a high risk of failure as a result of infection. A recent study demonstrated a 90% survival rate at 5-year follow-up; however, the most common cause of failure in this series was infection. No significant difference in the CD4 lymphocyte counts was found between patients with infection and those without infection. Furthermore, it appeared that the human immunodeficiency virus status of the patient was not associated with infection. Thirteen of 38 patients died, and the most common cause of death was complications associated with the acquired immunodeficiency syndrome. The authors concluded, however, that the life expectancy of patients with hemophilia is lower than that of the general population who undergo total knee arthroplasty, and the improvement in the postoperative quality of life for patients with hemophiliac arthropathy may outweigh the risk of failure.

Social factors, such as the workers' compensation status of a patient, also appear to have an effect on surgical outcome. One study reviewed a series of patients receiving workers' compensation and who underwent total knee arthroplasty and concluded that surgeons should be aware that workers' compensation is one of several variables that can have an untoward influence on the perceived outcome of total knee arthroplasty.

Table 2 | Preoperative Testing: Incidence of Abnormalities Influencing Management and Indications*

Test	Incidence of Abnormalities Influencing Management	Indications
Hemoglobin[†]	0.1%	Anticipated major blood loss or symptoms of anemia
White blood cell count[†]	0.0%	Symptoms suggest infection, myeloproliferative disorder, or myelotoxic medications
Platelet count[†]	0.0%	History of bleeding diathesis, myeloproliferative disorder, or myelotoxic medications
Renal function (creatinine ± blood urea nitrogen)	2.6%	Older than 50 years, hypertension, cardiac disease, major surgery, medications that may affect renal function
Electrolytes	1.8%	Known renal insufficiency, congestive heart failure, medications that affect electrolytes
Glucose	0.5%	Obesity, known diabetes mellitus or risk for diabetes mellitus
Prothrombin time[‡]	0.0%	History of bleeding diathesis, chronic liver disease, malnutrition, recent or long-term antibiotic use
Activated partial thromboplastin time[‡]	0.1%	History of bleeding diathesis
Liver function tests[‡]	0.1%	No indication; consider albumin for major surgery or chronic illness
Urinalysis[‡]	1.4%	No indication (unless symptomatic)
Electrocardiogram	2.6%	Men older than 40 years, women older than 50 years, known coronary artery disease, diabetes mellitus, or hypertension
Chest radiograph	3.0%	Symptoms or examination suggest cardiac or pulmonary disease; consider if known cardiac or pulmonary disease

Preoperative testing should be directed at improving patient outcomes and avoiding excess costs; therefore, indications should be reviewed before ordering

[†]*All part of complete blood count (no differential needed unless indicated)*

[‡]*Rarely indicated*

Low-risk procedures rarely require preoperative testing (cataracts, endoscopy, biopsies)

For Medicare patients, electrocardiogram and chest radiograph require ICD-9 codes for the reason for the examination

(Adapted with permission from Smetana GW, Macpherson DS: The case against routine preoperative laboratory testing. Med Clin North Am 2003;87:7-40.)

Preoperative Radiographic Evaluation

Patients undergoing total hip arthroplasty typically require low AP pelvis, AP hip, and true lateral or Lowenstein radiographs as part of the preoperative evaluation. AP weight-bearing and lateral radiographs of the knee are particularly important in preoperative planning for patients undergoing total knee arthroplasty. A long leg weight-bearing radiograph that includes the hip, knee, and ankle joint as well as a Merchant or sunrise radiograph of the patellofemoral articulation may also be helpful.

Patients with significant deformity, particularly of the hip joint, may need additional radiographic evaluation. A patient with severe developmental dysplasia of the hip may require CT to assess not only the acetabular bone stock but also the rotational deformities of the proximal femur. A patient with posttraumatic arthritis of the hip or the knee may also require advanced imaging studies to assess bone stock status.

Patients with radiographic evidence of significant joint destruction (particularly of the knee) should be suspected for the possibility of neuropathic arthropathy.

Although many have considered neuropathic arthropathy to be a contraindication for total joint arthroplasty, one study reported the experience at the Mayo Clinic of total knee arthroplasty performed in patients with neuropathic (Charcot) joints and concluded that total knee arthroplasty may be offered to a select group of patients with end-stage neuropathic arthropathy. The basic principles of knee arthroplasty, which include restoring limb alignment, reinforcing bony defects by bone grafting or augmented prostheses, careful ligamentous balancing, and the appropriate selection of constrained prostheses, are important in these patients. Furthermore, this study reported that technical challenges were encountered in this patient population, particularly those with significant deformity, and hence required skilled implant placement and methods usually reserved for complex revision arthroplasty.

Preoperative Laboratory Studies

Preoperative testing should be directed toward improving patient outcomes and minimizing costs (Table 2). Because patients undergoing total hip or total knee arthroplasty are likely to experience major blood loss, obtaining prebaseline hemoglobin and hematocrit levels is important, as is obtaining a baseline white blood cell count. It is also important to assess renal function, particularly in patients with hypertension, cardiac disease, and those who take medications such as diuretics that may affect renal function. In addition, electrolyte levels should be determined for this patient population. A baseline glucose level should be obtained in obese patients and those with known diabetes mellitus. Baseline coagulation studies should also be performed in preparation for postoperative thromboprophylaxis. A preoperative urine analysis is often recommended in patients undergoing total joint arthroplasty. A patient with bacteria, even if symptomatic, is at risk for bacteremia, and an attempt should be made to sterilize the urine with antibiotic therapy preoperatively. Furthermore, antibiotic treatment is warranted before manipulation of the urinary tract, such as placement of an indwelling catheter for surgery.

The preoperative hemoglobin level has a significant impact on transfusion requirements after total joint arthroplasty. One study demonstrated that the preoperative hemoglobin level and weight of the patient predicted the need for blood transfusion after total hip and knee replacement. Patients with a preoperative hemoglobin level of less than 130 g/L were reported to have a 15.3 times greater risk of requiring a transfusion than those with a hemoglobin level of greater than 150 g/L. One group of authors conducted an analysis of blood management in 9,482 patients undergoing a total hip or total knee arthroplasty and found that the most important predictors of the transfusion of allogenic blood were a low baseline hemoglobin level and a lack of predonated autologous blood. A more recent study reported that clinical variables such as age, gender, hypertension, and body mass index have a synergistic effect on the risk of transfusion in patients undergoing total hip arthroplasty.

Perioperative/Postoperative Management
Analgesia

Postoperative pain management is a primary factor in the overall care of patients undergoing total hip and total knee arthroplasty. Although in many patients postoperative pain is jointly managed by an anesthesia/pain management service, orthopaedic surgeons should understand the basic principles involved.

Opioid analgesics comprise the cornerstone of pain management. Table 3 describes the basic opioid analgesic administration guidelines for patients who did not receive chronic opioid therapy before surgery. Doses must be based on individual patient needs and responses. Lower doses should be used initially and then titrated up to a level to achieve pain relief. Consider-

ation of the possibility of respiratory depression is important, particularly in older individuals. Respiratory depression can be reversed with naloxone injections (Table 4).

Patient-controlled intravenous opioid administration is often used for pain management in the postoperative period. Table 5 describes the typical loading doses and dosage ranges for patient-controlled analgesia. Note that the amount of opioid required to achieve comfort varies from patient to patient, and dosing should be adjusted to achieve patient comfort with minimum adverse effects. It is also important to appreciate the equivalent doses of various opioid analgesics; these are described in Table 6. (An example of opioid conversion is provided in Table 7.)

An important advance in perioperative pain management is preemptive analgesia. Findings on the use of preemptive analgesia in patients undergoing arthroscopic procedures as well as early experience using preemptive analgesia for those undergoing minimally invasive hip and knee procedures have been quite promising. Surgical procedures produce an initial afferent barrage of pain signals and generate a secondary inflammatory response, both of which contribute substantially to postoperative pain. Over the past decade, a greater understanding of pain mechanisms has led to this concept of analgesia. One study evaluated the efficacy of a cyclooxygenase (COX)-2 inhibitor coupled with regional anesthesia after total joint arthroplasty. Patients in the group that received epidural anesthesia and the COX-2 inhibitor had less pain than those in the other groups that did not, and the authors recommended the use of COX-2 inhibitors as an adjunctive analgesic after total hip arthroplasty.

Anesthesia and postoperative pain management protocols have been developed with the purpose of increasing the functional recovery of the patient by minimizing postoperative nausea and emesis and by increasing the patient's level of alertness during physical therapy. The basic tenet of such a program is to avoid epidural or intravenous narcotics. Typical protocols involve the use of a COX-2 anti-inflammatory medication along with an oral opioid such as oxycodone 1 hour before surgery. Intraoperative anesthesia is provided with an epidural catheter, and no general anesthetic agents are used. After arthroplasty, an additional dose of oxycodone is given orally, approximately 4 hours after the initial dose, and this is followed by the preemptive use of pain medication with oxycodone during the first 48 hours. In addition, a COX-2 anti-inflammatory drug is given every morning, and ketorolac can be used to treat breakthrough pain. Moreover, the use of an antiemetic agent such as ondansetron or metoclopramide administered near the end of the surgical procedure has also been reported to be useful in controlling postoperative nausea and emesis.

Table 3 | Opioid Analgesics*

Drug	Route	Starting Dose (Adults > 50 kg)	Onset	Peak	Duration
Codeine	PO	30 to 60 mg q 4 hr	30 min	1½ hr	6 hr
	IM	15 to 30 mg q 4 hr	15 to 30 min	30 to 60 min	4 to 6 hr
	SQ	15 to 30 mg q 4 hr	30 to 60 min	2 to 4 hr	4 to 8 hr
Fentanyl	IM	5 µg/kg q 1 to 2 hr	7 to 8 min	20 to 50 min	1 to 2 hr
(Sublimaze)	IV	0.25 to 1 µg/kg as needed	Immediate	1 to 5 min	30 to 60 min
					48 to 72 hr
(Duragesic)	Transdermal	25 µg/hr	12 to 24 hr	24 hr	
Hydrocodone with acetaminophen[†] (Lortab, Vicodin)	PO	5 to 10 mg hydrocodone q 4 to 6 hr	60 min	2 hr	4 to 6 hr
Hydromorphone	PO	2 to 4 mg q 4 to 6 hr	30 min	60 min	4 to 5 hr
(Dilaudid)	IM/SQ	2 mg q 4 to 6 hr	15 to 20 min	60 min	4 to 5 hr
	Slow IV	0.2 to 0.6 mg q 2 to 3 hr	15 to 20 min	60 min	4 to 5 hr
(Palladone)	PO-SR	12 mg daily	N/A	N/A	24 hr
Meperidine	IM/SQ	50 to 150 mg q 3-4 hr	10 to 45 min	30 to 60 min	2 hr
(Demerol)	IV	25 to 50 mg q 1-2 hr	2 to 5 min	20 min	2 hr
Methadone (Dolophine)	PO	2.5 mg 1 to 4 times daily	30 to 240 min	2 to 4 hr	4 to 24 hr
Morphine	PO/SL	10 to 15 mg q 3 to 4 hr	15 min	1½ to 2 hr	4 hr
	IM	4 to 10 mg q 3 to 4 hr	15 to 60 min	30 to 60 min	4 hr
	IV	2 to 4 mg q 2 to 4 hr	2 to 5 min	20 min	3 to 4 hr
	SQ	4 -10 mg q 3 to 4 hr	15 to 30 min	30 to 60 min	4 to 7 hr
(MS Contin)	PO-SR	MS Contin: 15 mg q 12 hr	N/A	N/A	8 -12 hr
(Avinza)	PO-SR	Avinza: 30 mg daily	N/A	N/A	24 hr
Oxycodone (Percocet)[‡]	PO/SL	5 -10 mg q 4 to 6 hr-alone or with acetaminophen	15 to 30 min	1 to 2 hr	4 to 6 hr
(OxyContin)	PO-SR	OxyContin: 10 mg q 12 hr	60 min	2 to 3 hr	12 hr

*These are general guidelines. Patient care requires individualization based on patient needs and responses. Lower doses should be used initially, then titrated up to achieve pain relief

[†]Analgesic duration of action does not correlate with half-life

[‡] Do not give more than 4 g of acetaminophen per day (from all sources)

PO = oral, IM = intramuscular, SQ = subcutaneous, IV = intravenous, SR = sustained-release product, UIHC = University of Iowa Hospitals and Clinics, N/A = not applicable

Antibiotics

The most effective means of preventing postoperative infection is the intravenous administration of a first-generation cephalosporin within 1 hour of the surgical incision. Intravenous cephalosporin is typically continued for a minimum of 24 hours. Alternative antibiotics must be used in patients who are allergic to cephalosporin and/or penicillin.

The American Academy of Orthopaedic Surgeons has published an advisory statement regarding the use of prophylactic antibiotics in orthopaedic medicine; it states that vancomycin should be reserved for the treatment of serious infection with β-lactam-resistant organisms, the treatment of infection in patients with life-threatening allergy to β-lactam-resistant organisms, or the treatment of infection in patients with life-threatening allergy to

Table 3 | Opioid Analgesics* (continued)

Metabolism	Half Life	Comments
Liver	2 to 4 hr	· IV use (even at low doses and when given very slowly) may cause marked decrease in blood pressure; IV use is not recommended. · IM or SQ routes are the preferred parenteral routes.
Liver	1 to 6 hr†	· Transdermal should NOT be used to treat acute pain. · Transdermal patch should be used only in opioid tolerant patients. Effects of patch last for 18 to 24 hours after the patch is removed. · Use of IV fentanyl is restricted to oncology, burn service, palliative care, intensive care units or based on recommendation by the Pain Service. Appropriate monitoring is required. Refer to Nursing Policies 8.021 and 8.025.
Liver	4 hr	Available at UIHC as: · Tablet with 5 mg hydrocodone and 500 mg acetaminophen. · Elixir with 2.5 mg hydrocodone and 167 mg acetaminophen per 5 mL.
Liver	2 to 3 hr 18.6 hr	· Chronic treatment may require q 3 to 4 hour dosing. · IV doses should be administered over at least 2-3 minutes. · Palladone is a long-acting dosage form and is restricted to Pain Service and Palliative Care. · Do not crush Palladone.
Liver	2 to 3 hr	· More than 72 hr of continuous use can cause accumulation of normeperidine which can lead to neuroexcitability (seizures). · Naloxone administration will increase neuroexcitability. · Use with caution in the elderly and patients with renal dysfunction. · Not for use in chronic pain. Do not exceed 600 mg/24 hours.
Liver	24 hr	· Used in chronic pain. · Continued dosing can result in accumulation and respiratory depression.
Liver	1.5 to 2 hr 2 to 4 hr 15 hr	· Oral liquid concentrate is available. · Active metabolite renally eliminated; use caution in elderly and patients with renal insufficiency. · Long-acting dosage forms should not be crushed. · Long-acting dosage forms should not be used to treat acute pain. · Avinza is not on the UIHC formulary, but is used by Medicaid.
Liver	4 hr	· Available at UIHC as an immediate-release tablet and oral liquid concentration. · Percocet contains oxycodone 5mg/acetaminophen 325 mg. · Other strengths of Percocet are available outside UIHC. · OxyContin is a sustained-release tablet. Do not crush. · OxyContin should not be used to treat acute pain.

β-lactam antimicrobial agents. As previously noted, antibiotics impregnated in cement should be considered for use in patients with diabetes mellitus who are undergoing cemented total knee arthroplasty.

Postoperative Laboratory Evaluation
A typical postoperative protocol for obtaining laboratory studies includes evaluating the hemoglobin status daily for the first few days until it is stable and monitoring the prothrombin time and/or international normalized ratio for patients receiving warfarin. A platelet count is recommended for patients receiving a low-molecular-weight heparin; electrolyte, blood urea nitrogen, and creatine levels must often be assessed in patients with chronic renal insufficiency, metabolic encephalopathy, diabetes, or in those taking medications that can al-

ter renal function (such as diuretics and angiotensin-converting enzyme inhibitors).

Patients with diabetes mellitus require special consideration. On the day before surgery, patients typically continue their usual medications; on the day of surgery, blood glucose level is monitored (target range on the morning of surgery, 100 to 180 mg/dL). Oral hypoglycemic agents are usually withheld on the morning of surgery, and then patients are managed with a basal dose of insulin followed by the use of short-acting insulin on a sliding scale.

Several studies have analyzed the efficacy of routine pathologic examination of surgical specimens obtained during primary total hip and knee arthroplasty. One such study concluded that benign conditions can be diagnosed accurately by an experienced surgeon. The pre-

Table 4 | Guidelines for Administering Naloxone for Reversal of Opioid-Induced Respiratory Depression

Opioid Overdose

0.4 mg to 0.8 mg IV/IM/SQ, titrated in accordance with the patient's response; repeat as needed. If given IV, each 0.4 mg should be given over 15 seconds.

Opioid-Induced Respiratory Depression

0.04 mg/mL (40 µg/mL) dilution in syringe (mix 0.4 mg/1 mL of naloxone and 9 mL of normal saline in a syringe for IV administration).

Administer 0.5 mL of diluted solution (0.02 mg or 20 µg) every 2 minutes until a change in alertness is observed.

Titrate naloxone until patient is responsive or a total of 0.8 mg (20 mL of diluted solution) has been given. Continue looking for other causes of sedation and respiratory depression.

Discontinue naloxone when patient is responsive to physical stimulation, respiratory rate is ≥ 8 breaths per minute and able to take deep breaths when told to do so.

Special Considerations

May need repeated doses or continuous infusion. Depending on amount and type of opioid given and time interval since last opioid administration, the duration of action of some opioids may exceed that of naloxone.

Titrate dose cautiously to avoid precipitation of profound withdrawal, seizures, and severe pain.

IV = intravenous, IM = intramuscular, SQ = subcutaneous

Table 6 | Equianalgesic Chart*

Analgesic	Dosage	
	Parenteral	Oral
Fentanyl (Sublimaze)	0.1 to 0.2 mg	N/A
Hydrocodone	N/A	30 mg
Hydromorphone (Dilaudid)	1.5 mg	7.5 mg
Meperidine (Demerol)	75 to 100 mg	300 mg[†] (N)
Morphine	10 mg	30 mg[‡]
Oxycodone	N/A	20 mg

Doses listed are equivalent to 10 mg of parenteral morphine. Doses should be titrated according to individual response. When converting to another opioid, the dose of the new agent should be reduced by 30% to 50% because of incomplete cross-tolerance between opioids.

[†]*Dosage in this range may lead to neuroexcitability*

[‡]*For a single dose, 10 mg intravenous morphine = 60 mg oral morphine. For chronic dosing, 10 mg intravenous morphine = 30 mg oral morphine*

N/A = not applicable, (N) = nonformulary drug at University of Iowa Hospitals and Clinics

Table 5 | Guidelines for Patient-Controlled Intravenous Opioid Administration for Adults With Acute Pain*

Drug[†]	Usual Loading Dose	Usual Patient-Controlled Analgesia Starting Dose for Demand Bolus	Usual Patient-Controlled Analgesia Dose Range	Usual Lockout Range	Usual Basal Rate
Morphine (1 mg/mL)	5 to 10 mg	1 mg	0.5 to 2.5 mg	5 to 10 min	None or 1 to 2 mg/hr
Hydromorphone (Dilaudid) (0.2 mg/mL)	0.5 to 1.5 mg	0.2 mg	0.05 to 0.4 mg	5 to 10 min	None or 0.1 mg/hr
Fentanyl (0.02 mg/mL)[‡]	0.015 to 0.05 mg	0.01 mg	0.01 to 0.025 mg	3 to 10 min	None or 0.02 to 0.1 mg/hr
Meperidine (Demerol) (10 mg/mL)[¶]	25 to 75 mg	10 mg	5 to 25 mg	5 to 10 mg	None or up to 25 mg/hr

The amount of opioid required to achieve comfort varies from patient to patient. Dosing should be adjusted to achieve patient comfort with minimal adverse effects.

[†]*Standard concentrations are listed in parentheses.*

[‡]*Fentanyl patient-controlled analgesia therapy is restricted to intensive care units, burn service, oncology, palliative care, or based on recommendation of the pain service. Appropriate respiratory monitoring is required.*

[¶]*Normeperidine, a metabolite of meperidine, is a central nervous system excitotoxin that produces anxiety, tremors, myoclonus, and generalized seizures when it accumulates with repetitive dosing. Patients with compromised renal function are at high risk. Naloxone does not reverse the effects of normeperidine and may exacerbate hyperexcitability. Meperidine should not be used for more than 48 to 72 hours for acute pain, even in patients without renal or central nervous system disease, or at doses greater than 600 mg/24 hours. Meperidine should not be prescribed for chronic pain.*

Table 7 | Example of Opioid Conversion

Patient is receiving a total of 5 mg of parenteral hydromorphone in a 24-hour period via a patient-controlled analgesia pump. The goal is to convert this to oral morphine for discharge. When converting from patient-controlled analgesia administration, add the total amount of opioid that the patient received in the last 24 hours, including
> Basal infusion
> Demand boluses administered by the patient
> Bolus doses administered by the medical/nursing staff.

The equianalgesic chart (Table 6) indicates that 1.5 mg of parenteral hydromorphone equals 7.5 mg of oral hydromorphone (a fivefold increase).

The patient's current dose of 5 mg per day of parenteral hydromorphone is equal to 25 mg per day of oral hydromorphone.

The next step is to convert 25 mg of oral hydromorphone to the daily oral morphine equivalent dose.

The equianalgesic chart indicates that 7.5 mg of oral hydromorphone is equal to 30 mg of oral morphine.

The patient's calculated dose of 25 mg of oral hydromorphone is equal to 100 mg of oral morphine.

The oral dose of morphine should be reduced by 30% to 50% to prevent any risk of overdose after the conversion because opioids do not have complete cross-tolerance. A 33% dose reduction from the calculated dose of 100 mg is equal to 67 mg of oral morphine per day.

The recommended dosing frequency of long-acting morphine (MS Contin) is every 12 hours (2 doses per day).

MS Contin is available in 15 mg, 30 mg, 100 mg, and 200 mg controlled-release tablets. The tablet strength closest to the calculated dose is 30 mg. The proper starting dose should therefore be 30 mg of sustained-release morphine every 12 hours.

Table 8 | Patients at Potential Increased Risk of Hematogenous Total Joint Infection

All patients during the first 2 years after prosthetic joint replacement

Immunocompromised/immunosuppressed patients
> Inflammatory arthropathies (rheumatoid arthritis, systemic lupus erythematosus)
> Drug-induced immunosuppression
> Radiation induced immunosuppression

Patients with comorbidities such as previous prosthetic joint infections, malnourishment, hemophilia, human immunodeficiency virus infection, insulin-dependent (type 1) diabetes, malignancy

Much of the current understanding about degenerative joint disease, osteonecrosis, and inflammatory arthropathies has been derived from careful but routine evaluation of specimens obtained during total joint arthroplasty. Therefore, the research and educational value of this process should not be overlooked. Nevertheless, it was concluded that although routine histologic evaluation of tissue excised from patients with uncomplicated osteoarthritis may not always be necessary, when careful gross examination of resected tissue suggests an unexpected finding or when the results of such analysis are used for undergoing quality assurance studies, histologic examination is warranted. Postoperative radiographs should be obtained in two planes to provide a baseline for additional follow-up as well as to ascertain whether any intraoperative complications including dislocation may have occurred.

Dental Prophylaxis
The American Academy of Orthopaedic Surgeons in conjunction with the American Dental Association published an advisory statement regarding antibiotic prophylaxis in patients with total joint arthroplasty. The advisory statement states that antibiotics are not routinely indicated for most dental patients with total joint arthroplasties. However, bacteremia may occur and lead to hematogenous seeding of a total joint arthroplasty, even years past arthroplasty; the period in which risk is greatest is apparently up to 2 years after undergoing total joint arthroplasty. Table 8 describes patients who are at potential increased risk of hematogenous total joint infection and Table 9 outlines the suggested antibiotic prophylaxis regimens for these patients.

Urologic Antibiotic Prophylaxis
The American Urologic Association in conjunction with the American Academy of Orthopaedic Surgeons has published an advisory statement on antibiotic prophylaxis for patients with urologic disorders and total joint arthroplasties. Although antibiotic prophylaxis is not

operative diagnosis should be determined on the basis of a careful history, a detailed physical examination, and a thorough examination of radiographs. To complete the clinical diagnosis, preoperative information should be combined with findings obtained through a careful intraoperative observation of resected specimens, which in hip arthroplasty includes inspection of the divided femoral head. In doing so, surgeons can usually exclude clinically the possibility of malignancy or another condition that may alter the management of the patient. It has been recommended that histologic analysis be reserved for situations in which the diagnosis is suspect or unexpected findings are noted intraoperatively.

A more recent study reported that routine pathologic examination of surgical specimens from patients undergoing primary total hip replacements because of the clinical diagnosis of osteoarthritis has limited cost-effectiveness because of the low prevalence of findings that alter patient management. Another recent article pointed out that whereas reducing cost is an important concern, histologic study of resected tissue still serves many purposes in addition to immediate patient care.

Table 9 | Suggested Antibiotic Prophylaxis Regimens*

Patient Status	Antibiotic	Dose
Not allergic to penicillin	Cephalexin, cephradine, or amoxicillin	2 g orally 1 hour before the procedure
Not allergic to penicillin and unable to take oral medications	Cefazolin or ampicillin	Cefazolin: 1 g; ampicillin: 2 g intramuscularly or intravenously 1 hour before the procedure
Allergic to penicillin	Clindamycin	600 mg orally 1 hour before the procedure
Allergic to penicillin and unable to take oral medications	Clindamycin	600 mg intravenously 1 hour before the procedure

No second doses are recommended for any of these dosing regimens

routinely indicated for most of these patients, it is recommended that premedication be considered in a small number of patients who may be at potential risk of hematogenous total joint infection. Patients who are at risk are the same as those described in Table 8; the only difference is that all patients with diabetes mellitus are considered at risk for urologic prophylaxis, not just diabetic patients who are insulin-dependent.

Stress Steroids

Patients receiving exogenous glucocorticoids such as prednisone may require supplemental (exogenous) glucocorticoids to meet the physiologic demands of surgery. One recent study found that patients undergoing total knee arthroplasty had a significant surgical stress response, whereas patients undergoing arthroscopy did not. It was concluded that the significantly increased cortisol production observed in nonsteroidal-dependent patients after total knee arthroplasty leaves open the possibility that steroid-dependent patients undergoing this procedure could benefit from perioperative glucocorticoid supplementation. This study, however, did not support the use of supplemental steroids for the less invasive knee arthroscopy procedure.

Summary

Although the perioperative management of patients undergoing total hip and total knee arthroplasty is often a team process, orthopaedic surgeons should have a good understanding of all the principles involved with such care. An exciting advance in perioperative management has been the introduction of preemptive analgesia, which includes the preoperative administration of anti-inflammatory and oral opioid agents. Such analgesic regimens combined with a comprehensive rehabilitation program have the potential to not only decrease the length of stay, but also facilitate the early rehabilitation of the patient. Although functional outcome studies are needed to determine the ultimate efficacy of such measures, they do appear to hold great promise for the future.

Annotated Bibliography

Preoperative Evaluation

Antibiotic Prophylaxis for Dental Patients With Total Joint Replacements: Advisory Statement. Rosemont, IL, American Academy of Orthopaedic Surgeons, 2003.

This advisory statement outlines recommendations for antibiotic prophylaxis for patients undergoing dental procedures who have total joint replacements.

Bhattacharyya T, Iorio R, Healy WL: Rate of and risk factors for acute inpatient mortality after orthopaedic surgery. *J Bone Joint Surg Am* 2002;84-A:562-572.

The authors used a predictive model to assess five critical risk factors for identifying patients at risk for death after orthopaedic surgery. They concluded that death is rare after orthopaedic surgery, with the overall mortality rate approaching 1% for all patients.

Eagle KA, Berger PB, Calkins H, et al: ACC/AHA guideline update for perioperative cardiovascular evaluation for noncardiac surgery: Executive summary. A report of the American College of Cardiology/American Heart Association Task Force on Practice Guidelines (Committee to Update the 1996 Guidelines on Perioperative Cardiovascular Evaluation for Noncardiac Surgery). *J Am Coll Cardiol* 2002;39:542-553.

This update of guidelines for perioperative cardiovascular risk assessment is a concise resource for the management of cardiovascular patients who are undergoing noncardiac procedures.

Meding JB, Reddleman K, Keating ME, et al: Total knee replacement in patients with diabetes mellitus. *Clin Orthop Relat Res* 2003;416:208-216.

The authors of this study routinely use cefuroxime-impregnated cement during total knee replacement in patients with diabetes mellitus. They reported a 1.2% infection rate in patients with diabetes mellitus compared with a 0.7% infection rate in those without diabetes mellitus. All deep infections occurred in patients with type I diabetes mellitus.

Norian JM, Ries MD, Karp S, Hambleton J: Total knee arthroplasty in hemophilic arthroplasty. *J Bone Joint Surg Am* 2002;84-A:1138-1141.

The authors of this study concluded that there is a high risk of failure as a result of infection in this patient population and that most infections occur late and are most often caused by *Staphylococcus epidermis*.

Parvizi J, Johnson BG, Rowland C, Ereth MH, Lewallen DG: Thirty-day mortality after elective total hip arthroplasty. *J Bone Joint Surg Am* 2001;83-A:1524-1528.

The authors found that factors associated with an increased risk of mortality within 30 days of elective total hip arthroplasty included older age, male gender, and a history of cardiorespiratory disease.

Parvizi J, Marrs J, Morrey BF: Total knee arthroplasty for neuropathic (Charcot) joints. *Clin Orthop Relat Res* 2003;416:145-150.

The authors suggest that total knee arthroplasty may be done in a selected group of patients with end-stage neuropathic arthropathy. Technical challenges are encountered in such patients, particularly in those with significant deformity, which may require skills, implant systems, and methods usually reserved for complex revision arthroplasty.

Pola E, Papaleo P, Santoliquido A, Gasparini G, Aulisa L, DeSantis E: Clinical factors associated with an increased risk of perioperative blood transfusion in nonanemic patients undergoing total hip arthroplasty. *J Bone Joint Surg Am* 2004;86-A:57-61.

The authors investigated several clinical parameters and found that clinical variables such as age, gender, hypertension, and body mass index may have a synergistic effect on the rate of transfusion in patients undergoing elective total hip arthroplasty.

Salido JA, Marin LA, Gomez LA, Zorrilla P, Martinez C: Preoperative hemoglobin levels and the need for transfusion after prosthetic hip and knee surgery. *J Bone Joint Surg Am* 2002;84-A:216-220.

The authors analyzed the relationship between preoperative hemoglobin levels, age, gender, weight, height, and type and duration of the total joint replacement surgery and the need for postoperative blood transfusion and concluded that the preoperative hemoglobin level ($P = 0.0001$) and weight of the patient ($P = 0.011$) predicted the need for blood transfusion after total hip and knee replacement.

Smetana GW, Macpherson DS: The case against routine preoperative laboratory testing. *Med Clin North Am* 2003;87:7-40.

The authors of this article suggest that almost all routine laboratory tests conducted before surgery have limited clinical value. They recommend that only a small number of routine tests should be ordered preoperatively based on age and that

selective use of other preoperative tests should be based on history and physical examination findings that identify subgroups of patients who are more likely to have abnormal results.

Perioperative/Postoperative Management

Antibiotic Prophylaxis for Urological Patients With Total Joint Replacements: Advisory Statement. Rosemont, IL, American Academy of Orthopaedic Surgeons, 2003.

This advisory statement details recommendations for the antibiotic prophylaxis of patients with urologic conditions who are undergoing total joint replacement.

Berry DJ, Berger RA, Callaghan JJ, et al: Minimally invasive total hip arthroplasty: Development, early results, and a critical analysis. *J Bone Joint Surg Am* 2003;85-A: 2235-2246.

The authors comprehensively discuss the topic of minimally invasive total hip arthroplasty.

Clark CR: Routine pathological examination of operative specimens from primary total hip and total knee replacement: Another look. *J Bone Joint Surg Am* 2000; 82-A:1529-1530.

The author suggests that although reducing cost is an important concern, the histologic study of resected tissue serves many purposes in addition to immediate patient care. Histologic examination is particularly warranted when a patient has another disorder that might complicate osteoarthritis, when careful examination of synovial tissue or a section of femoral head suggests an unexpected finding, or when the results of such analyses are used for ongoing quality assurance studies.

Kocher MS, Erens G, Thornhill TS, Ready J: Cost and effectiveness of routine pathological examination of operative specimens obtained during primary total hip and knee replacement in patients with osteoarthritis. *J Bone Joint Surg Am* 2000;82-A:1531-1535.

The authors concluded that routine pathologic examination of surgical specimens from patients undergoing primarily total hip or knee replacement because of a clinical diagnosis of osteoarthritis had limited cost-effectiveness because of the low prevalence of findings that altered patient management.

Leopold SS, Casnellie MT, Warme WJ, Dougherty PJ, Wingo ST, Shott S: Endogenous cortisol production in response to knee arthroplasty and total knee arthroplasty. *J Bone Joint Surg Am* 2003;85-A:2163-2167.

The authors found that patients undergoing total knee arthroplasty had a significant stress response, whereas patients undergoing arthroscopy did not.

Mallory TH, Lombard AV Jr, Fada RA, Dodds KL, Adams JB: Pain management for joint arthroplasty: Preemptive analgesia. *J Arthroplasty* 2002;17(4 suppl 1): 129-133.

The authors of this study retrospectively compared the results of a previously reported pain management protocol with two more recent groups of patients who were treated with modified pain protocols. In the earlier control protocol, epidural anesthesia was discontinued when patients arrived in the postanesthesia care unit, at which time administration of oral opioids and intravenous hydromorphone was initiated. The first group was given epidural anesthesia, and the second group was given spinal anesthesia.

Reuben SS, Sklar J: Pain management in patients who undergo outpatient arthroscopic surgery of the knee. *J Bone Joint Surg Am* 2000;82-A:1754-1766.

The authors of this article recommend that preemptive and multimodal analgesic techniques should be used in the management of patients undergoing anterior cruciate ligament reconstruction.

The Use of Prophylactic Antibiotics in Orthopaedic Medicine and the Emergence of Vancomycin-Resistant Bacteria: Advisory Statement. Rosemont, IL, American Academy of Orthopaedic Surgeons, 2003.

This advisory statement details recommendations for the antibiotic prophylaxis of patients with vancomycin-resistant bacterial infections.

Classic Bibliography

Bierbaum BE, Callaghan JJ, Galante JO, Rubash HE, Tooms RE, Welch RB: An analysis of blood management in patients having a total hip or knee arthroplasty. *J Bone Joint Surg Am* 1999;81:2-10.

Dripps RD: New classification of physical status. *Anesthesiology* 1963;24:111.

Fiorillo AB, Solaro FX Jr: Preoperative medical evaluation, in Callaghan JJ (ed): *The Adult Hip.* Philadelphia, PA, Lippincott-Raven, 1998, pp 601-632.

Lawrence T, Moskal JT, Diduch DR: Analysis of routine histological evaluation of tissues removed during primary hip and knee arthroplasty. *J Bone Joint Surg Am* 1999;81:926-931.

Mont MA, Mayerson JA, Krackow KA, Hungerford DS: Total knee arthroplasty in patients receiving workers' compensation. *J Bone Joint Surg Am* 1998;80:1285-1290.

Winiarsky R, Barth P, Lotke P: Total knee arthroplasty in morbidly obese patients. *J Bone Joint Surg Am* 1998;80:1770-1774.

Chapter 19

Blood Conservation for Total Joint Replacement

Steven T. Woolson, MD

Introduction

Despite continued improvements in the surgical techniques of total hip and knee replacement, perioperative blood loss from these procedures can represent a large amount of the patient's total blood volume. Because many patients undergoing total joint arthroplasty are elderly and have medical problems that can result in morbidity if significant blood loss occurs, preoperative planning for methods of safely replacing blood is imperative.

Cemented total knee replacement, which is routinely performed using tourniquet control, typically results in little intraoperative loss of blood; however, postoperative blood loss, if a drain is used, is usually between 500 and 1,000 mL. Studies that calculate the total hospital blood loss from formulas that use the patient's estimated blood volume and preoperative and postoperative hematocrit values have shown that unilateral knee replacement can result in an overall blood loss of between 1,500 to 1,900 mL (which is approximately 40% of the total blood volume of a 70 kg woman with a normal body habitus). This calculated total blood loss can be three to four times the volume of drainage from the surgical drain because a large portion of the blood that is lost is dispersed into the soft tissues or remains in the joint in the form of clot. Blood loss after cementless knee replacement is greater than that for cemented replacement because polymerized cement has a hemostatic effect on raw bone surfaces. Bilateral total knee replacement under one anesthetic or revision of a failed knee replacement result in a much higher risk of transfusion than a primary procedure.

Total hip replacement results in a blood loss of at least 1,000 mL for most primary procedures, with relatively equal amounts lost intraoperatively and postoperatively. Cementless fixation of hip components normally requires shorter surgical times and, thus, less intraoperative blood loss, but greater postoperative blood loss occurs with cemented fixation because of prolonged oozing from bone. As in total knee replacement, revision total hip replacement involves more surgical time, wider soft-tissue dissection, and often exposes a greater surface area of bleeding bone because of the need for trochanteric osteotomy and/or cup removal; the risk for transfusion is also high for patients who require replacement of both components.

Orthopaedic surgeons must plan for the possible need for blood replacement depending on individual patient characteristics, such as weight and preoperative hematocrit level and the type and complexity of the procedure. Because there are more risks of complications from allogeneic blood transfusion than autologous blood transfusion, it is important to attempt to eliminate the need for allogeneic blood. The use of autologous transfusion, red blood cell salvage, hemodilution, special surgical techniques, and treatment of preoperative anemia are all methods of blood loss management that can be used during surgical procedures. Appropriate and cost-effective use of these methods or combinations of each can result in a low complication rate from blood loss in most patients.

Allogeneic Blood Transfusion

Many patients have a preconceived fear of allogeneic blood transfusion that stems from the transmission of human immunodeficiency virus (HIV) and acquired immunodeficiency syndrome to bank blood and factor VIII cryoprecipitate recipients in the 1980s before stringent screening of blood donors was instituted. Although the risks of viral disease transmission from allogeneic transfusion have decreased dramatically over the years, the public is generally unaware that the risks of hepatitis and HIV are extremely low. The risks of allogeneic blood transfusion in order of decreasing prevalence are transfusion reactions such as fever caused by white blood cell antigens or late antibody development to red blood cell antigens, clerical error resulting in transfusion of the wrong type of blood, bacteremia from blood contamination, and transmission of viral or blood-borne infection.

The risk of the wrong type of blood being transfused may be fatal in some instances. Estimates for the risk of this iatrogenic error range from 1 in 400 units in Belgium to 1 in 36,000 units in Germany (where testing of blood type is done at the bedside before transfusion). One US study estimated that this error occurred in 1 of 19,000 units transfused. Because of the improved safety of transfusion from better donor selection and infectious disease testing, clerical error may be the most common serious transfusion-related risk.

Hepatitis is the most common transfusion-related illness. All blood units are now tested for the hepatitis B virus (HBV) and hepatitis C virus (HCV) using hepatitis B surface antigen, hepatitis B core antibody, HCV antibody, and a nucleic acid amplification test for HCV. HIV is screened for using HIV-1 and HIV-2 antibody tests and a nucleic acid amplification test for HIV-1. Human T cell leukemia viruses (HTLV-1 and HTLV-2) are tested for by detection of their antibodies. A serologic test for syphilis is routinely performed on each unit of blood, as is a nucleic acid amplification test for West Nile virus. These blood screening tests have resulted in a reduced risk of transmitting HBV via blood transfusion to 1 in 137,000 units of blood, HCV to 1 in 1 million units, and HIV to 1 in 1.9 million units. Other diseases that can be transmitted via blood transfusion include malaria, babesiosis, Chagas' disease, and Lyme disease, none of which can be detected by laboratory screening tests.

Directed donor blood donation is a form of allogeneic blood transfusion that may be chosen by some patients who are unable to or elect not to donate autologous blood. This form of transfusion is almost always chosen by patients who have a fear of contracting HIV from random blood bank units. Some studies have shown, however, that the incidences of markers for hepatitis and HTLV are higher in the population of directed donors than in the population of volunteer donors, making it possible that directed donor blood donation is less safe. Despite patient wishes that their own siblings, spouses, and friends are safer donors than the overall volunteer donor population, the use of directed donor blood donation should be discouraged. The increased cost of directing transfusions to certain recipients is not warranted unless the donor is a regular blood donor because of the possible slight increase in risk of transmission of infected units that have had false-negative test results.

Because of the risks involved with allogeneic transfusion, it is imperative that adequate informed consent be obtained from patients before ordering transfusions. A physician may be held negligent for ordering a transfusion that was not indicated because of a high hemoglobin level, for creating a situation in which transfusion is needed during a procedure that does not normally require transfusion, or for failing to use available autologous blood. Some states require surgeons to notify all patients undergoing elective surgery that autologous do-

nation is available to reduce the risks of allogeneic transfusion.

Studies have been conducted to determine the prevalence of allogeneic transfusion after total hip and knee replacement if only allogeneic blood is used for these procedures. One retrospective study of 161 total knee replacements and 209 total hip replacements in patients who had deep venous thrombosis prophylaxis with low-molecular-weight heparin showed an allogeneic transfusion rate of 29% and 39%, respectively, when a hemoglobin threshold of < 85 g/L was used and no autologous blood was transfused. Other studies have shown rates that vary between 35% and 70% for this patient population depending on the hemoglobin threshold. Using multivariate analysis, these transfusion rates have been shown to be statistically related to the patient's preoperative hemoglobin value ($P = 0.0001$) and weight ($P = 0.011$). If the preoperative hemoglobin level is between 130 and 150 g/L or < 130 g/L compared with > 150 g/L, then the prevalence of transfusion without autologous blood has been shown to be 4 or 15 times greater, respectively. The use of autologous blood has been shown to reduce the risk of allogeneic transfusion in almost all studies of patients undergoing total joint replacement, but cost-effective methods of using it are of concern.

In addition to the risks of clerical error and disease transmission, one study has shown a significantly higher risk of postoperative joint infection and fluid overload necessitating the use of diuretics when allogeneic blood is used after total joint arthroplasty ($P < 0.001$ for both postoperative joint infection and fluid overload). An association between allogeneic blood use and a longer hospital stay was also identified. These increased risks must be factored into any study assessing the efficacy and cost-effectiveness of autologous versus allogeneic blood transfusion.

Autologous Blood Transfusion

Three forms of autologous transfusion are available for patients undergoing total hip and knee replacement: predonated autologous blood, acute normovolemic hemodilution, and perioperative red blood cell salvage. Considerable controversy currently exists regarding the efficacy and cost-effectiveness of autologous transfusion, especially because the risk of viral disease transmission from allogeneic blood has been dramatically reduced over the past 10 years. However, although the cost of autologous transfusion in most instances is greater than that of allogeneic transfusion, a finite risk of transmission of hepatitis, HIV, or other infectious agents will always make allogeneic blood transfusion slightly more risky than autologous blood transfusion. Despite the unrealistic and probably unwarranted fears of contracting acquired immunodeficiency syndrome from a volunteer blood donor, autologous blood sources will likely continue to be used, and surgeons must continue to attempt to reduce allogeneic blood transfusion rates.

The oldest form of autologous transfusion uses predonated autologous blood; its use was first reported in 1968. Currently, predonated autologous blood is used in only 5% of all transfusions, and this percentage may be decreasing. Recommendations regarding the optimal use of predonated autologous blood require that it be used only when blood would be normally cross-matched before a surgical procedure, with the number of units requested being the same as would be cross-matched. In addition, predonated autologous blood should only be transfused if required. Patients may currently store blood safely for 42 days with an American Association of Blood Banks standard requirement of 70% viable erythrocytes (the same as for allogeneic blood). It is recommended that the interval between donations be at least 5 to 7 days and that a donation should not be made less than 3 days before the procedure. Patients must weigh at least 110 lb, have a hematocrit level of more than 33%, and have no recent history of infection or antibiotic use at the time of the donation. Patients who weigh less than 110 lb can donate partial units of blood with a reduction in the standard amount of anticoagulant in the collection bag. All patients are advised to take supplemental iron to prevent iatrogenic anemia, and it is useful to have them predonate blood as far in advance of the procedure as feasible to allow their hematocrit level to return to a normal range before surgery. Patients who require more than two units of autologous blood can donate blood over a longer preoperative interval by having some of the units frozen after the addition of glycerol. However, the use of frozen predonated autologous blood should be avoided whenever possible because the cost of freezing blood is high. Once thawed, there is only a 24-hour window in which frozen blood can be safely reinfused. Any patient who has significant cardiac conditions or uncontrolled hypertension must receive medical clearance to predonate blood, but advanced age is not a contraindication. Predonated autologous blood is screened for HIV and hepatitis, but it may still be reinfused to its recipient despite positive testing. Unused autologous and directed donor blood is discarded because these donors are not actual volunteers and may have a higher risk of disease transmission despite negative screening (false-negative test results).

The efficacy of the reduction in the risk of allogeneic blood exposure when predonated autologous blood is used has been reported in many studies. A study of 489 consecutive patients concluded that predonated autologous blood significantly reduced the requirements for allogeneic transfusion, with an allogeneic transfusion rate of 3% for predonated autologous blood donors versus 15% for nondonors ($P < 0.001$) in patients undergoing primary total hip and knee replacement. There was also a significant difference ($P < 0.001$) in allogeneic transfusion in patients undergoing revision or bilateral one-stage joint arthroplasty who had predonated autologous blood (19%) compared with patients who did not (49%). None of the patients undergoing primary total joint arthroplasty in this series who had a hemoglobin level of 150 g/L or more and none of the patients who had a preoperative hemoglobin of 130 to 150 g/L and were younger than 65 years required allogeneic blood. Of the 70 patients in these two categories, 83% of the predonated autologous blood that was collected was not used.

A multicenter study of transfusion requirements in patients undergoing total joint arthroplasty reported data from 9,482 consecutive patients. Fifty-seven percent of the 3,920 patients undergoing total hip replacement required transfusion compared with 39% of the 5,562 patients undergoing total knee replacement. Only 9% of the patients undergoing total hip replacement who predonated blood required allogeneic blood compared with 32% of the patients undergoing total hip replacement who were nondonors. The risk of allogeneic transfusion in 2,696 patients undergoing unilateral total knee arthroplasty who predonated blood was only 6% compared with 18% (347 of 1,946 patients) undergoing the same procedure who were nondonors. However, 45% of the predonated units were not used. The significant predictors of allogeneic transfusion included a low preoperative hemoglobin level and a lack of predonated blood.

In contrast to the previous two studies, a randomized, prospective study of patients undergoing primary total hip replacement demonstrated that 42 patients who predonated two units of predonated autologous blood had the same risk of allogeneic transfusion as 54 nondonors. No patients in either group received an allogeneic transfusion. However, the transfusion trigger in this study was lower than that reported in other studies for nondonors (< 70 g/L for healthy patients of any age and < 80 g/L for patients with a major medical comorbidity). Forty-one percent of the autologous blood was not used. However, in this study half of the nondonors had a hemoglobin of 90 g/L or less on postoperative day two and at discharge compared with 19% and 24% of predonated autologous blood donors, respectively, indicating that there was probably a study bias in favor of not transfusing the nondonors. This study demonstrates that a low hemoglobin trigger threshold for healthy, nonanemic patients undergoing total hip replacement will successfully eliminate the requirement for allogeneic transfusion, but these results would likely not have been found in a nonselected group of total joint arthroplasty patients, many of whom are anemic and have medical comorbidities.

There have been some retrospective reports of a large number of patients undergoing total joint replacement that showed a statistically significant decrease in the prevalence of postoperative deep venous thrombosis in those who have had both total hip and knee replacement when predonated autologous blood was obtained. However, because these studies were retrospective, the results may have been skewed by selection bias. Another study of blood management did not find an association between either autologous or allogeneic blood transfusion and postoperative thrombosis. The ability to carry out a prospective, randomized study on the effectiveness of autologous versus allogeneic blood transfusion is virtually impossible because few patients can be recruited to enter as a result of the continued public awareness of the risk, albeit small, of viral disease transmission from allogeneic blood transfusion.

Erythropoietin Therapy

Recombinant human erythropoietin was approved in 1995 for use in patients undergoing surgery in the United States. Erythropoietin is a glycoprotein produced by the kidney that stimulates red blood cell production from bone marrow. The US Food and Drug Administration has approved a preoperative dosing regimen of 600 U/kg of body weight (42,000 U for a 70-kg patient) given subcutaneously on a weekly basis starting 3 weeks before surgery, with the last dose given on the day of surgery (a total of 168,000 U/70-kg patient). Supplemental iron therapy is needed for these patients, with recommended doses of 325 mg of ferrous sulfate administered three times daily or 150 mg of polysaccharide-iron complex. Although concerns exist that a rapid increase in the hemoglobin level may be associated with thrombotic or vascular complications, no such association has been found in any study of orthopaedic patients.

Cost is a major consideration with erythropoietin therapy; at $0.01 per unit, the cost has been reported to be as high as $3,150 per patient in some published studies. A recent study of the efficacy of erythropoietin therapy reported that the cost of the high-dose regimen was $1,344 (Canadian); although this dose did not statistically decrease the allogeneic blood transfusion risk from the low-treatment dose, the authors believed that additional study of a larger number of patients would prove that the trend for better efficacy with a high dose is real. There is no question that erythropoietin therapy is more expensive than predonated autologous blood or red blood cell salvage methods and much more costly than using allogeneic blood.

Studies have shown that erythropoietin therapy can facilitate the predonation of autologous blood in orthopaedic patients by increasing erythropoiesis. Two randomized, prospective, double-blind multicenter studies have shown the efficacy of preoperative erythropoietin therapy in reducing the risk of exposure to allogeneic blood in patients who did not donate autologous blood for total joint replacement procedures. Each study included two treatment groups of high and low doses of erythropoietin (300 U/kg per day versus 100 U/kg per day given in 15 daily doses starting 10 days preoperatively in one study [a total of 315,000 U versus 105,000 U for a 70-kg patient] and 40,000 U versus 20,000 U given weekly for 4 weeks preoperatively [160,000 U versus 80,000 U] in the other study). Both studies showed a statistically significant reduction in the use of allogeneic blood in treated patients compared with those in the placebo groups (high dose, $P = 0.001$; low dose, $P = 0.003$), but neither showed a statistically significant difference in allogeneic blood transfusion risk between the high- and low-dose erythropoietin treatment groups ($P = 0.119$). There was no evidence in either study that the risk of deep venous thrombosis was greater in the treatment groups than in control groups.

If cost is not an issue, then erythropoietin therapy should be strongly considered for use in patients undergoing total joint replacement procedures who refuse to accept allogeneic blood transfusion, are too anemic to predonate blood, or are unable to predonate an adequate amount of their blood for a procedure that will usually require allogeneic blood transfusion, such as bilateral knee replacement or revision hip replacement.

Perioperative Red Blood Cell Salvage

Red blood cell salvage can be done intraoperatively during total hip replacement using devices that wash the suction drainage to remove fat, debris, and cement monomer and provide concentrated red blood cells with a hematocrit level of approximately 50%. Unwashed shed blood can be reinfused from the drainage tubes postoperatively after either total hip or knee replacement using one of several types of sterile collection devices that may or may not use an anticoagulant (Figure 1).

A recent retrospective study of 200 consecutive patients undergoing primary hip or knee replacement who did not predonate autologous blood and used only perioperative washed red blood cell salvage demonstrated a low rate of allogeneic blood transfusion (4%), with the same prevalence reported for patients undergoing hip and knee surgery. Other studies have corroborated these results and found that perioperative red blood cell salvage further reduces the allogeneic blood transfusion rate in patients who also had predonated autologous blood. Another randomized, prospective study of patients undergoing total knee replacement found that postoperative unwashed red blood cell salvage alone was equivalent to the use of one unit of predonated autologous blood in reducing the need for allogeneic blood transfusion. Because total knee replacement does not normally involve intraoperative blood loss when a tourniquet is used, postoperative salvage is an ideal method of autologous blood transfusion for that procedure. Studies on the composition of unwashed shed blood after total joint replacement have shown that this blood has a low hematocrit level (approximately 25%) and is defibrinated but probably poses no coagulopathy risk unless large volumes (> 1,000 mL) are reinfused.

Intraoperative washed red blood cell salvage should be standard for complex primary total hip replacement and revision total hip replacement when the femoral or both components are being replaced because these procedures may result in the salvage of three or more units of blood. This amount of autologous blood saving is definitely cost-effective, but the salvage of only one unit of blood (approximately 250 mL) is not cost-efficient. The use of postoperative unwashed or washed red blood cell salvage is cost-effective in patients undergoing unilateral primary total knee replacement who have not predonated autologous blood and in those undergoing bilateral knee replacement with or without predonated autologous blood. The cost of some sterile reinfusion drains is not prohibitive and, therefore, when predonated autologous blood is not available, this means of blood conservation is always warranted. However, for patients with an adequate amount of predonated autologous blood, perioperative red blood cell salvage may be excessive and unnecessary. The use of perioperative red blood cell salvage should be considered as an adjunctive blood conservation method in patients who have predonated adequate amounts of blood for their procedure, and it should be used routinely only for those who are at high risk to receive allogeneic blood for cost-saving reasons.

Acute Normovolemic Hemodilution

The technique of acute normovolemic hemodilution involves the collection of two to four units of blood (in standard transfusion blood bags with anticoagulant) from the patient immediately before surgery. Blood is collected until the hematocrit level reaches a low of 28%, and this blood is replaced on a 1:1 volume with hetastarch and lactated Ringer's solution. This autologous blood is reinfused intraoperatively when the hematocrit level drops below 24%. Contraindications to the use of this technique include a history of myocardial infarction, significant coronary artery disease, and/or uncontrolled hypertension. Randomized, prospective studies comparing acute normovolemic hemodilution to predonated autologous blood have been done in patients undergoing both total hip and total knee replacement at one institution. A study of 32 patients undergoing total knee replacement demonstrated no significant difference in the risk of allogeneic blood transfusion between acute normovolemic hemodilution and predo-

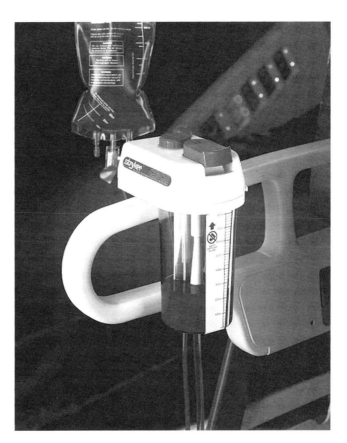

Figure 1 Photograph of a sterile closed-system blood salvage device that is used for unwashed red blood cell salvage and postoperative wound drainage.

nated autologous blood groups (25% versus 8%, respectively; $P = 0.5$). A study of 48 patients undergoing total hip replacement showed a significantly higher number of allogeneic blood units transfused in 23 patients in the acute normovolemic hemodilution group compared with 25 patients in the predonated autologous blood group (0.4 units versus 0, respectively, $P = 0.03$); the risk of allogeneic blood transfusion exposure was not statistically significantly different between the two groups (17% versus 0, respectively; $P = 0.3$). Additional studies of larger patient populations are needed (despite the claim that statistical significance was reached in these two studies) before the use of this hemodilution technique in patients undergoing total joint arthroplasty can be considered efficacious.

Surgical Considerations for Blood Conservation

Because the volume of intraoperative blood loss during total hip replacement represents a significant portion of the total hospital blood loss for this procedure (as opposed to total knee replacement when a tourniquet is used), the use of hypotensive regional anesthesia can lower blood loss significantly during total hip replacement. This technique should be considered for all patients undergoing revision hip surgery unless there is a medical contraindication. The effect of other surgical variables on blood loss and transfusion requirements such as the use of a tourniquet in total knee replacement and the use of a surgical drain have been debated for years. Whether to use a surgical drain remains controversial. Almost all studies assessing the efficacy of surgical drains have shown no differences in the blood loss, transfusion requirements, or early clinical results (knee or hip range of motion) when comparing patients who have had a drain to those who did not. One study of 136 patients undergoing total knee replacement showed that a significantly greater number of knees required dressing reinforcement as well as larger and more frequent ecchymoses when the surgical drain was not used, indicating that a surgical drain may be beneficial to the wound and soft tissues, even if it does not affect blood loss. Sealing the hole made in the femur for intramedullary instrumentation with either a bone or cement plug has proved to be helpful in reducing blood loss and the need for transfusion after total knee replacement. The use of a fibrin sealant on exposed bone and soft-tissue surfaces after total knee replacement has also been shown to be useful in reducing blood loss from surgical drains.

Summary

Planning for blood replacement after total joint arthroplasty should be based mainly on the type of procedure and secondarily on the blood volume and preoperative hemoglobin level of the patient. The goal should be to minimize exposure to allogeneic blood in a cost-effective manner. A low rate of allogeneic blood transfusion cannot be achieved unless surgeons are willing to use a lower hemoglobin threshold (< 8.5 g/L) than has been previously used (< 10 g/L [a hematocrit level of < 30%]). More importantly, surgeons must understand that blood transfusions should not be ordered unless patients become symptomatic regardless of the hemoglobin level. The exception to this, of course, is a medical comorbidity for which the prophylactic use of blood transfusion may be indicated solely on the basis of the hemoglobin level.

Patients undergoing unilateral primary or revision total knee replacement can have either postoperative red blood cell salvage alone or one unit of predonated autologous blood in most instances. Patients undergoing bilateral knee replacement will require at least two units of autologous blood and can also benefit from the reinfusion of postoperative salvage blood because of the high likelihood of losing more than 3,000 mL of blood perioperatively. Patients who have anemia preoperatively (hemoglobin level < 130 g/L) should be treated with oral iron or erythropoietin if the patient is opposed to receiving allogeneic blood. The use of red blood cell

salvage is cost-effective and does not delay the procedure or burden patients or surgeons with the added planning required for predonated autologous blood transfusions. The use of only one unit of predonated autologous blood will likely result in a low risk of unused blood and is usually a sufficient amount in uncomplicated total knee replacement procedures to prevent the need for allogeneic blood transfusion. Postoperative blood losses are greater when low-molecular-weight heparins are used, and procedures done with this type of prophylaxis may require the use of more predonated autologous blood units.

Primary unilateral total hip replacement may not require any predonated autologous blood or red blood cell salvage in young patients who have an adequate blood volume and who have a preoperative hemoglobin level greater than 150 g/L. Older patients undergoing total hip replacement who have medical comorbidities can be more safely treated with one or two units of predonated autologous blood or with perioperative washed red blood cell salvage techniques. Surgeons should not overorder predonated autologous blood, but have patients predonate the number of allogeneic units that are likely to be transfused if no autologous blood is used. The use of fewer units of predonated autologous blood combined with unwashed red blood cell salvage can reduce overall costs and be effective in eliminating the need for using bank blood. Patients with severe anemia must be treated with erythropoietin preoperatively to obviate the need for allogeneic blood transfusion.

Patients undergoing procedures that result in large amounts of blood loss may require multiple techniques, including hemoglobin enhancement, predonated autologous blood, and perioperative red blood cell salvage. It may not be possible for patients with anemia to avoid allogeneic blood transfusion after bilateral total knee replacement or revision total hip replacement procedures, but red blood cell salvage may reduce the amount of allogeneic blood needed.

A considerable reduction in the number of allogeneic blood transfusions can be accomplished by using hypovolemia (not the hemoglobin level) as the transfusion trigger and by avoiding the use of any one unit of allogeneic blood, which is often unnecessary. Most patients who receive one unit of allogeneic blood can be treated safely with observation alone.

Annotated Bibliography

Allogeneic Blood Transfusion

Salido JA, Marin LA, Gomez LA, Zorrilla P, Martinez C: Preoperative hemoglobin levels and the need for transfusion after prosthetic hip and knee surgery: Analysis of predictive factors. *J Bone Joint Surg Am* 2002;84-A(2):216-220.

This retrospective study of 296 patients (370 total joint replacements) in whom no autologous blood was used was done with a transfusion trigger of a hemoglobin level < 85 g/L. Analyses of multiple parameters showed that a higher preoperative hemoglobin level and greater patient weight were predictive for a lower risk of transfusion.

Autologous Blood Transfusion

Bae H, Westrich GH, Sculco TP, Salvati EA, Reich LM: The effect of preoperative donation of autologous blood on deep-vein thrombosis after total hip arthroplasty. *J Bone Joint Surg Br* 2001;83(5):676-679.

This retrospective study of patients who underwent total hip arthroplasty compared the prevalence of deep venous thrombosis in 1,037 patients who donated autologous blood preoperatively and 1,006 who did not predonate. The patients in the preoperative autologous blood donation group had a 9% incidence of venographically diagnosed deep venous thrombosis compared with a 13.5% incidence in the nondonor group ($P = 0.003$), but no increased risk for pulmonary embolism was reported.

Bierbaum BE, Callaghan JJ, Galante JO, Rubash HE, Tooms RE, Welch RB: An analysis of blood management in patients having a total hip or knee arthroplasty. *J Bone Joint Surg Am* 1999;81(1):2-10.

This multicenter study of blood management was done prospectively in 3,920 patients undergoing total hip replacement and 5,562 patients undergoing total knee replacement; 46% of the patients required a transfusion (66% of which received autologous blood). A low preoperative hemoglobin level and the lack of autologous blood were reported to be predictors for allogeneic transfusion. The authors also reported a high percentage (45%) of wasted autologous units.

Billote DB, Glisson SN, Green D, Wixson RL: A prospective, randomized study of preoperative autologous donation for hip replacement surgery. *J Bone Joint Surg Am* 2002;84-A(8):1299-1304.

This randomized, prospective study compared the requirement for allogeneic transfusion for patients undergoing total hip replacement, 42 of whom donated autologous blood preoperatively. Although no patients in either the donor or nondonor group received allogeneic transfusions, 49% of patients in the nondonor group were discharged with a hemoglobin level of 90 g/L or less versus 24% for those in the donor group.

Hatzidakis AM, Mendlick RM, McKillip T, Reddy RL, Garvin KL: Preoperative autologous donation for total joint arthroplasty: An analysis of risk factors for allogeneic transfusion. *J Bone Joint Surg Am* 2000;82(1):89-100.

The risk of receiving allogeneic blood was determined for 489 consecutive patients (347 total knee replacements and 271 total hip replacement). The authors found that autologous blood greatly reduced the risk of allogeneic transfusion ($P < 0.0001$). Revision one-stage bilateral total joint replacement and a lower

preoperative hemoglobin level were associated with a higher risk of allogeneic blood exposure.

Erythropoietin Therapy

Faris PM, Ritter MA, Abels RI: The effects of recombinant human erythropoietin on perioperative transfusion requirement in patients having a major orthopaedic operation. *J Bone Joint Surg Am* 1996;78(1):62-72.

This randomized, prospective, double-blind multicenter study of 185 orthopaedic patients (88% of whom underwent total joint replacement) compared two doses of erythropoietin with a placebo. The rate of exposure to allogeneic transfusion was 17% of patients in the high dosage group, 25% in the low dosage group, and 54% in the placebo group ($P < 0.001$ for both treatment groups).

Feagen BG, Wong CJ, Kirkley A, et al: Erythropoietin with iron supplementation to prevent allogeneic blood transfusion in total hip arthroplasty: A randomized, controlled trial. *Ann Intern Med* 2000;133:845-854.

This randomized, prospective, double-blind multicenter Canadian study assessed the preoperative use of erythropoietin in two dosage regimens in patients who underwent total hip replacement without preoperative autologous blood donation. Both treatment groups were found to be effective in reducing the risk of allogeneic transfusion compared with control subject (high dosage group, 11% allogeneic transfusion rate; low dosage group, 23%; control group [placebo], 45%).

Perioperative Red Blood Cell Salvage

Friederichs MG, Mariani EM, Bourne MH: Perioperative blood salvage as an alternative to predonating blood for primary total knee and hip arthroplasty. *J Arthroplasty* 2002;17:298-303.

The authors conducted this retrospective study of 200 consecutive total hip replacements (N = 68 patients) and total knee replacements (N = 132 patients) who received autologous transfusion with perioperative washed salvage blood only. The reported risk of allogeneic transfusion was only 4% for each procedure. Patients with a preoperative hematocrit level ≥ 37% were reported to have a 1.2% risk.

Woolson ST, Wall WW: Autologous blood transfusion after total knee arthroplasty: A randomized, prospective study comparing predonated and postoperative salvage blood. *J Arthroplasty* 2003;18:243-249.

This randomized, prospective study was conducted to determine the risk of allogeneic transfusion in patients who underwent total knee arthroplasty and had either autologous transfusion with one unit of preoperatively donated autologous blood alone or unwashed salvage blood. The allogeneic transfusion rate was 5% for 41 patients who preoperatively donated autologous blood versus 0 for 47 those in the unwashed salvage blood group ($P = 0.13$).

Acute Normovolemic Hemodilution

Goodnough LT, Despotis GJ, Merkel K, Monk TG: A randomized trial comparing acute normovolemic hemodilution and preoperative autologous blood donation in total hip arthroplasty. *Transfusion* 2000;40(9):1054-1057.

This randomized study of acute normovolemic hemodilution versus preoperative autologous donation in patients undergoing primary total hip replacement showed no significant difference in the exposure of patients to allogeneic blood from either technique. Four of 23 patients (15%) who had acute normovolemic hemodilution and none of 25 patients who had preoperative autologous donation received allogeneic blood ($P = 0.30$).

Surgical Considerations for Blood Conservation

Kumar N, Saleh J, Cardiner E, Devadoss VG, Howell FR: Plugging the intramedullary canal of the femur in total knee arthroplasty: Reduction in postoperative blood loss. *J Arthroplasty* 2000;15:947-949.

This was a randomized study of patients who underwent total knee replacement during which a bony plug was used to block the femoral intramedullary hole for the alignment rod. The authors found that a small but significant (17%) reduction in postoperative blood loss occurred when the bony plug was used compared to when it was not used.

Parker MJ, Roberts CP, Hay D: Closed suction drainage for hip and knee arthroplasty: A meta-analysis. *J Bone Joint Surg Am* 2004;86:1146-1152.

The authors conducted a meta-analysis of 18 randomized, prospective studies that compared the use of a drain or no drain for total hip and knee arthroplasty. They found no difference in the risk of wound infection, hematoma, or other wound complications requiring reoperation in the two groups. Use of a drain was not only related to a higher transfusion rate, but also to a greater amount of wound drainage requiring dressing changes.

Classic Bibliography

Ayers D, Murray D, Duerr D: Blood salvage after total hip arthroplasty. *J Bone Joint Surg Am* 1995;77:1347-1351.

Cushner FD, Friedman RJ: Blood loss in total knee arthroplasty. *Clin Orthop Relat Res* 1991;269:98-101.

Etchason J, Petz L, Calhoun L, et al: The cost effectiveness of preoperative autologous blood donations. *N Engl J Med* 1995;332:719-724.

Faris PM, Ritter MA, Keating EM, et al: Unwashed filtered shed blood collected after knee and hip arthroplasties: A source of autologous red blood cells. *J Bone Joint Surg Am* 1991;73:1169-1178.

Goodnough LT, Rudnick S, Price TH, et al: Increased preoperative collection of autologous blood with recombinant human erythropoietin therapy. *N Engl J Med* 1989;321(17):1163-1168.

Mallory TH, Kennedy M: The use of banked autologous blood in total hip replacement surgery. *Clin Orthop* 1976;117:254-257.

Nelson CL, Stewart JG: Primary and revision total hip replacement in patients who are Jehovah's Witnesses. *Clin Orthop* 1999;369:251-261.

Stevens CE, Aach RD, Hollinger FB, et al: Hepatitis B virus antibody in blood donors and the occurrence of non-A, non-B hepatitis in transfusion recipients: An analysis of the transfusion-transmitted viruses study. *Ann Intern Med* 1984;101:733-738.

Woolson ST, Watt JM: Use of autologous blood in total hip replacement: A comprehensive program. *J Bone Joint Surg Am* 1991;73(1):76-80.

Chapter 20

Anesthesia

Nigel E. Sharrock, MB, ChB

Introduction

Approximately 500,000 hip and knee replacements are performed annually in the United States. The success and safety of these procedures depends in large part on anesthetic and perioperative care, which has evolved significantly over the years. This has contributed to a reduction in perioperative in-hospital morbidity for hip surgery from 1% to 2% of patients in the 1960s to about 0.3% of patients today. Mortality rates in high-volume centers range from 0.01% to 0.15% of patients. As a result of improved care, patients currently recover more quickly and the duration of hospital stays has declined from weeks to days.

Preoperative Care

Assessment

The medical condition of any patient undergoing major surgery needs to be defined to ensure that the patient's medical conditions are optimally characterized and stabilized before surgery. Medical conditions, which are associated with a higher incidence of perioperative complications, include cirrhosis, renal insufficiency, pulmonary hypertension, congestive heart failure, diabetes, ischemic heart disease, cardiac arrhythmias, severe pulmonary disease, and dementia. Patients with these conditions should be stabilized medically before surgery and carefully monitored during surgery.

The medical workup is usually individualized based on physician, patient, and local practice. The workup also depends on the degree of surgical injury. For example, complex revision surgery or one-stage bilateral joint arthroplasty is a high-risk procedure, justifying extensive medical workup. By contrast, a primary total joint arthroplasty is a moderate risk procedure, especially when performed in less than 2 hours with the patient under regional anesthesia and receiving effective pain management. In moderate-risk surgical procedures, evidence to date does not seem to justify conducting an exhaustive preoperative assessment to identify ischemic heart disease.

Medication

As a general rule, it is preferable to maintain each patient's preoperative medications up to and including the morning of surgery and restart them as soon as possible following surgery. Anticoagulation should be discontinued preoperatively. For other medications, such as insulin, the dosage may need to be adjusted. Routine perioperative administration of beta-blockers has been advocated in higher-risk patients, but whether this has a measurable effect in patients undergoing joint arthroplasty is unclear. Nevertheless, perioperative control of heart rate, especially in higher-risk patients, is warranted to reduce the risk of perioperative myocardial ischemia.

Surgical Issues

The status of patients with severe rheumatoid arthritis and ankylosing spondylitis should be carefully assessed because patients may have unstable or fused cervical spines, necessitating bronchoscopic intubation if general anesthesia is required. Positioning these patients in the lateral decubitus position requires input from both surgical and anesthetic personnel.

If the surgical procedure is likely to be complex, the anesthesiology staff should be informed. Factors that may influence intraoperative anesthetic planning include severe protrusio of the hip (which can result in vascular injury to the iliac vessels), valgus deformity of the knee (which can lead to peroneal nerve injury or compartment syndrome), arterial disease of the iliac or femoral vessels (which can lead to arterial thrombosis and therefore may require intraoperative anticoagulation or avoiding the use of a tourniquet), and the implantation of long-stem cemented femoral components.

Intraoperative Care

Reaming the medullary canal and inserting cemented components into the femur and the tibia results in showers of emboli (fat, bone marrow, and associated thrombi), which enter the pulmonary circulation. The thrombi can be small (especially during knee replacement) or large, and its generation is typically accompanied by an acute activation of thrombogenesis. Although small thrombi do not result in any measurable change in a patient's cardiopulmonary status, larger thrombi can lead to pulmonary hypertension, a reduction in cardiac output, hypotension and even cardiac arrest, which can occur with the first-time implantation of long-stem cemented components. Resuscitation is best performed with epinephrine administration via a central line as soon as any sign of hypotension ensues. Circulatory collapse is uncommon after routine primary total hip replacement with modern cement restricters or when using noncemented components.

Cardiac arrest during total hip replacement is a catastrophic event, but it is fairly uncommon. It occurs primarily with the insertion of long-stem cemented total hip replacement components and is caused by massive fat thromboembolism. Cardiac arrest may also occur during spinal and epidural anesthesia, especially when patients become volume depleted or when no beta agonists, such as ephedrine or epinephrine, are used to preserve cardiac output.

Intraoperative fat emboli may lead to an increase in pulmonary artery pressure after total joint arthroplasty resulting from the mechanical occlusion of the pulmonary vasculature or subsequent endothelial injury. Studies have demonstrated that the emboli may enter the systemic circulation via a patent foramen ovale or, more commonly, via the pulmonary circulation. Emboli have been detected in the middle cerebral artery intraoperatively in 40% of patients during total hip and total knee replacement. It is unknown whether the presence of emboli contributes to cognitive changes in patients after total joint arthroplasty.

Tourniquet Use

Inflation of a tourniquet around the thigh leads to a variety of physiologic effects. Tissue ischemia and venous stasis can contribute to deep vein thrombosis formation during total knee replacement. The pressure beneath the tourniquet likely injures the thigh muscle, adversely affecting early rehabilitation. Prolonged tourniquet inflation may predispose patients to nerve injury. Although tourniquet pressures of 300 mm Hg usually are sufficient unless a patient's arterial pressure exceeds 200 mm Hg, hypotensive anesthesia enables reduced tourniquet pressure to be applied. Inflation of the tourniquet increases arterial and central venous pressures. Inflation of the tourniquet on both legs at once is usually well tolerated, but deflation must be performed sequentially to avoid profound hypotension. After the release of the tourniquet, several physiologic changes occur (most notably hypotension) resulting from acute blood loss, vasodilatation of the ischemic leg, and circulatory effects secondary to the ischemic metabolites.

Performing total knee replacement without a tourniquet offers several possible advantages, including enhanced rehabilitation and a reduced risk of deep vein thrombosis. However, studies suggest that the rate of deep vein thrombosis is not reduced without the use of a tourniquet during total knee replacement and that perioperative blood loss is similar with or without tourniquet use.

Vascular Obstruction During Total Hip Replacement

During total hip replacement, the femoral vessels can become twisted, kinked, and obstructed during preparation of the femoral canal. A slight increase in arterial pressure occurs when the artery is obstructed and a reduction in pressure when the leg is straightened. Occlusion of the femoral vein leads to venous stasis of the lower extremity, which predisposes patients to deep vein thrombosis. After relocation of the hip, a reduction in central venous oxygenation can be detected using an SVo^2 monitor to reflect periods of femoral venous and/or arterial occlusion. Intraoperative intravenous administration of heparin during femur surgery when the vessels are obstructed reduces the likelihood of deep vein (and possibly arterial) thrombosis following total hip replacement.

Thrombogenesis During Joint Arthroplasty

Deep vein thrombosis and subsequent pulmonary embolism are major complications after total joint arthroplasty and may account for up to 50% of perioperative deaths. It is now recognized that the thrombi form initially during surgery, although they may extend or reform in a dynamic process after surgery. Thus, anesthesiologists and surgeons should give careful consideration to the intraoperative factors that affect deep vein thrombosis formation.

Evidence for the intraoperative genesis of deep vein thrombosis is derived from several sources. First, measurement of markers of deep vein thrombosis demonstrates an initiation of thrombosis intraoperatively. During total hip replacement, thrombogenesis begins during surgery on the femur, but not during reaming the acetabulum or insertion of the cup. This action coincides with obstruction of the femoral vein and the release of bone marrow contents into an obstructed femoral vein. During total knee replacement, thrombogenesis occurs throughout surgery.

Anesthetic practice can influence the rates of deep vein thrombosis and pulmonary embolism. Regional anesthesia (epidural, spinal, and possibly nerve blockade) result in a 30% to 50% reduction in deep vein thrombosis rate after total hip replacement and a 20% reduction in deep vein thrombosis after total knee replacement (proximal deep vein thrombosis is reportedly reduced by at least 50% with epidural anesthesia after total knee re-

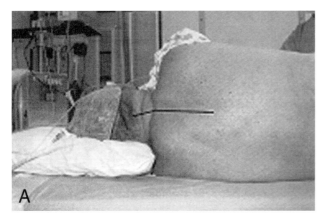

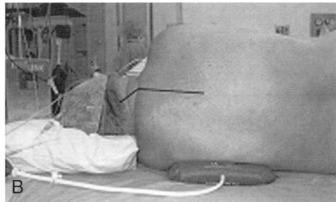

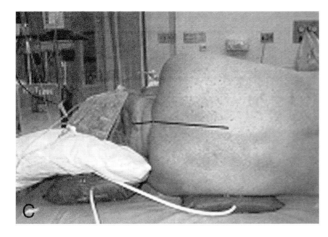

Figure 1 **A** through **C,** Photographs showing how inflation of a shoulder pillow decompresses the dependent shoulder and the inflation of another shoulder pillow beneath the head eliminates angulation of the neck for patients placed in the lateral position for total hip replacement.

placement). The mechanism for this effect is unknown, but it may relate to an enhancement of lower extremity blood flow during or immediately after surgery or a reduction in blood loss. In patients who receive hypotensive epidural anesthesia, the reported rate of deep vein thrombosis is 11% and the rate of proximal deep vein thrombosis 3%, which is far below rates normally observed with normotensive epidural anesthesia. Hypotensive epidural anesthesia is associated with an increase in skeletal muscle blood flow and low blood loss (100 to 200 mL).

Other intraoperative factors that decrease the deep vein thrombosis rate when combined with regional anesthesia include pneumatic compression during or immediately after surgery and the administration of intravenous unfractionated heparin (15 U/kg) before surgery. Intraoperative unfractionated heparin has been reported to result in a deep vein thrombosis rate of 7% to 8% of patients and a pulmonary embolism rate of 0.5% of patients at 3-month follow-up.

Regional Versus General Anesthesia

Total joint arthroplasties can be performed using general or regional anesthesia. However, studies demonstrate that regional anesthesia provides better outcome. When regional anesthesia is used during total hip replacement, the amount of blood loss and rates of deep vein thrombosis,

pulmonary embolism, and mortality are reportedly reduced. When regional anesthesia is used during total knee replacement, the rates of deep vein thrombosis and mortality are reportedly reduced. Furthermore, rehabilitation is facilitated by the use of epidural and/or femoral nerve blockades.

Patient Positioning

Although relatively few positioning problems occur when patients undergoing total knee replacement are placed in the supine position, ulnar nerve pressure must be minimized at the elbow and airway obstruction during sedation should be avoided.

By contrast, total hip replacement performed with patients in the lateral position poses several problems. First, compression over the dependent femoral triangle can lead to femoral nerve injury and/or ischemia of the dependent limb during prolonged surgery. More commonly, inadequate bolsters (or axillary rolls) lead to dependent shoulder pain, patient movement during surgery, and the possibility of compression of the dependent brachial plexus. By using inflatable pillows, adequate decompression of the brachial plexus and dependent shoulder can be obtained. By also using an additional adjustable pillow beneath the head, the cervical spine can be correctly aligned (Figure 1).

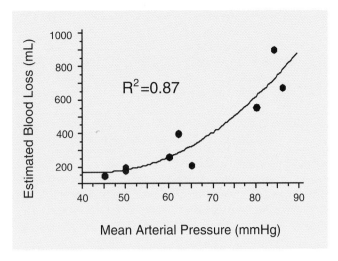

Figure 2 Diagram showing the mean intraoperative blood loss during primary unilateral total hip replacement; data were compiled from published studies in which mean arterial pressure during surgery was reported.

Blood Loss

Blood loss during and following total joint arthroplasty is a common complication. Between 30% and 50% of patients undergoing primary total hip replacement require homologous blood transfusion. Rates of transfusion are higher for patients undergoing complex revision and one-stage bilateral surgery. Anesthetic practice can affect blood loss. During total hip replacement, blood loss can be reduced by the use of epidural, spinal, or lumbar plexus blocks. Blood loss can also be affected by induced hypotension (Figure 2). With hypotensive epidural anesthesia, only 6% of patients require homologous blood transfusions following total hip replacement. Hypotensive epidural anesthesia not only reduces transfusion requirements, but it also provides a clearer surgical field and improved fixation of cemented components. Additionally, hypotensive epidural anesthesia can reduce blood loss after total knee replacement, but this requires that blood pressure to be kept low postoperatively.

Other factors that can reduce perioperative transfusion include the use of autologous blood, preoperative erythropoietin, intraoperative cell salvage, and the use of antifibrinolytic agents including aprotinin and tranexamic acid.

Postoperative Care

Pain

Pain following total hip replacement is usually well managed with a combination of narcotics, acetaminophen, and nonsteroidal anti-inflammatory drugs or cyclooxygenase (COX)-II inhibitors. However, superior postoperative analgesia can be provided using epidural analgesia or a lumbar plexus block. Femoral nerve blocks provide ineffective pain relief after total hip replacement. Whether optimal pain relief results in enhanced outcome or improved rehabilitation after total hip replacement is unknown.

Pain after total knee replacement is a major problem. Narcotics frequently are inadequate. Epidural analgesia, a femoral nerve block, or a combination of both result in superior pain relief and enhanced rehabilitation (improved range of motion of the knee and the achievement of other rehabilitation milestones).

The benefits of continuous regional anesthesia pain control techniques after surgery include a reduction in narcotic usage. This results in fewer adverse gastrointestinal effects and a reduction in light-headedness with early ambulation. Continuous peripheral nerve blockade (femoral, lumbar plexus, and sciatic blocks) may, if proved to be safe, become the preferred mode of pain relief in the future.

COX-2 inhibitors also improve pain relief, leading to reduced narcotic usage and fewer complications, such as itching, nausea, and adverse cognitive effects. These agents appear to be better tolerated after surgery than nonteroidal anti-inflammatory drugs, but they may be contraindicated when noncemented compounds are used.

Use of Regional Anesthesia and Perioperative Anticoagulants

A significant number of instances of epidural hematoma were reported with the introduction of low-molecular-weight heparin (LMWH), necessitating a review of the safety of epidural and spinal anesthesia when LMWH and other anticoagulants were used. As a result, consensus statements from the American Society of Anesthesiologists have been published, the latest in 2004, that conclude that the use of regional anesthesia in patients receiving anticoagulants increases the risk of epidural hematoma. The consensus statements also suggest that the risk associated with withdrawing epidural catheters, especially in patients receiving warfarin, has probably been overstated.

Monitoring and Fluid Management

Patients undergoing primary total joint arthroplasty require careful monitoring. Continuous arterial monitoring is preferable when induced hypotension is to be used and for monitoring rapid changes in hemodynamic status resulting from blood loss during or immediately following surgery. Central venous monitoring is useful to assess filling pressure when induced hypotension is used. For major surgical procedures (revision surgery, periprosthetic fracture, and one-stage bilateral surgery), both arterial and central venous monitoring are recommended. For one-stage bilateral cemented total hip replacement and long-stem cemented total hip replacement, pulmonary artery catheters are useful. Although transesophageal echocardiography is a useful diagnostic tool, it is difficult to use in patients receiving regional anesthesia.

Fluid management is very important after total joint arthroplasty. There is a tendency to administer excessive fluids, which is likely to result in pulmonary edema, hypoxia, and confusion for several days after surgery. It is possible that pulmonary endothelial injury secondary to intraoperative embolism predisposes patients to fluid accumulation in the lungs. Because the risk of renal failure is uncommon for patients who have undergone total joint arthroplasty, it is advisable to restrict rather than overload fluids. Blood is transfused to maintain a hematocrit level of 30% in high-risk patients, but it can be maintained in the 20% to 24% range in healthier patients if those patients remain stable hemodynamically.

Urinary catheters should be inserted perioperatively when regional anesthesia is used. Evidence suggests that the use of catheters does not appear to increase the risk of urinary sepsis or infection of the total hip prosthesis. The temperature of patients should be maintained by warming blankets and/or fluids.

Summary

Optimal anesthesia care has been shown to improve perioperative care and outcome for patients who undergo orthopaedic procedures. An understanding of these factors by orthopaedic surgeons should help integrate these modalities into routine practice.

Annotated Bibliography

Preoperative Care

Buvanendran A, Kroin JS, Tuman KJ, et al: Effects of perioperative administration of a selective cyclooxygenase 2 inhibitor on pain management and recovery of function after knee replacement: A randomized controlled trial. *JAMA* 2003;290(18):2411-2418.

In this randomized, double-blind, drug company–sponsored study, 70 patients received either rofecoxib or placebo daily for 2 weeks after total knee replacement. Pain scores, narcotic consumption, nausea, vomiting, and sleep disturbances were lower for the rofecoxib than the group receiving placebo. The rofecoxib group also had an improved range of motion after surgery with no demonstrable difference in bleeding. All patients also received epidural analgesia.

Eagle KA, Berger PB, Calkins H, et al: ACC/AHA guideline update for perioperative cardiovascular evaluation for noncardiac surgery: Executive summary. A report of the American College of Cardiology/American Heart Association Task Force on Practice Guidelines (Committee to Update the 1996 Guidelines on Perioperative Cardiovascular Evaluation for Noncardiac Surgery). *Circulation* 2002;105(10):1257-1267.

This in-depth discussion of preoperative assessment of patients undergoing noncardiac surgery focuses on cardiac workup. The authors attempt to classify surgery into high-, medium-, and low-risk categories and allocate workup accordingly. The indications for preoperative beta-blocker therapy and the usefulness of perioperative monitoring are discussed.

Holte K, Sharrock NE, Kehlet H: Pathophysiology and clinical implications of perioperative fluid excess. *Br J Anaesth* 2002;89(4):622-632.

The authors of this article outline the pathophysiology of excessive perioperative fluid administration and cite a tendency to administer excessive fluid for a variety of reasons, including efforts to counter circulatory depression from anesthesia, prevent renal dysfunction, and avoid blood transfusion. The limitations of relying on urine output as a marker of hydration and approaches to limit fluid administration are also discussed.

Rodgers A, Walker N, Schug S, et al: Reduction of postoperative mortality and morbidity with epidural or spinal anaesthesia: Results from overview of randomised trials. *BMJ* 2000;321(7275):1493.

The authors conducted a meta-analysis of spinal or epidural anesthesia compared with general anesthesia and found that patients receiving regional anesthesia for hip surgery had a reduced rate of mortality (30%), deep vein thrombosis (40%), pulmonary embolism (55%), pneumonia (39%), and transfusion (55%). Whether postoperative epidural analgesia contributes to this benefit is unknown.

Rosencher N, Kerkkamp HE, Macheras G, et al: Orthopedic Surgery Transfusion Hemoglobin European Overview (OSTHEO) study: Blood management in elective knee and hip replacement in Europe. *Transfusion* 2003; 43(4):459-469.

In a multicenter prospective study of 3,996 patients in Europe, allogenic blood was transfused in 48% of patients undergoing primary unilateral total hip replacement and 46% of those undergoing primary unilateral total knee replacement. The risk of transfusion was reported to be related to the preoperative hemoglobin level. Patients receiving allogenic blood had a higher incidence of postoperative infection (4%) compared with patients receiving autologous blood (1%).

Veien M, Sorensen JV, Madsen F, Juelsgaard P: Tranexamic acid given intraoperatively reduces blood loss after total knee replacement: A randomized, controlled study. *Acta Anaesthesiol Scand* 2002;46(10):1206-1211.

In this study, 30 patients were randomized to receive 10 mg/kg of intravenous tranexamic acid as the tourniquet was deflated and 10 mg/kg 3 hours later. The authors found that blood loss was reduced from 760 to 409 mL with the use of tranexamic acid.

Intraoperative Care

DiGiovanni CW, Restrepo A, Gonzalez Della Valle AG, et al: The safety and efficacy of intraoperative heparin in total hip arthroplasty. *Clin Orthop Relat Res* 2000;379: 178-185.

In this study, 989 patients undergoing primary total hip replacement under hypotensive epidural anesthesia received a single injection of 15 U/kg of unfractionated heparin preoperatively. At 3-month follow-up, five patients developed clinical pulmonary emboli, but none died. One patient developed major bleeding. Six percent of patients received allogenic blood; 87% received aspirin and 13% received warfarin postoperatively. The authors concluded that intraoperative heparin is a safe and effective form of thromboprophylaxis when used in combination with hypotensive epidural anesthesia.

Edmonds CR, Barbut D, Hager D, Sharrock NE: Intraoperative cerebral arterial embolization during total hip arthroplasty. *Anesthesiology* 2000;93(2):315-318.

In this study, 20 patients undergoing total hip replacement were assessed using transcranial Doppler imaging; echogenic showers were observed in the middle cerebral artery of 8 patients during impaction of the cemented femoral component or after relocation of the hip. The authors suggested that these emboli traverse the pulmonary circulation and may influence postoperative cognitive function.

Gonzalez Della Valle A, Salonia-Ruzo P, Peterson MG, Salvati EA, Sharrock NE: Inflatable pillows as axillary support devices during surgery performed in the lateral decubitus position under epidural anesthesia. *Anesth Analg* 2001;93(5):1338-1343.

In this crossover study, an inflatable axillary roll was reported to provide less pressure on the shoulder and chest wall and better alignment of the cervical spine than a 1-L saline bag. The authors reported that the inflatable pillow resulted in excellent comfort during surgery performed with the patient under epidural anesthesia.

Pitto RP, Hamer H, Fabiani R, Radespiel-Troeger M, Koessler M: Prophylaxis against fat and bone-marrow embolism during total hip replacement reduces the incidence of postoperative deep-vein thrombosis: A controlled, randomized clinical trial. *J Bone Joint Surg Am* 2002;84-A(1):39-48.

Transesophageal echocardiography was performed to detect intraoperative echogenic material in the right heart on 131 patients undergoing primary total hip replacement with a cemented femoral component. Evidence of small emboli was observed after insertion of the cup and with reaming of the femur. Evidence of large emboli (> 5 mm) was observed after relocation of the hip in patients who did not have venting of the femur. The rate of deep vein thrombosis (using ultrasonography) was lower in the group that had venting of the femur.

Salvati EA, Pellegrini VD Jr, Sharrock NE: Recent advances in venous thromboembolic prophylaxis during

and after total hip replacement. *J Bone Joint Surg Am* 2000;82(2):252-270.

This extensive review discusses the perioperative factors involved in thrombogenesis during total hip replacement. It outlines the mechanisms for intraoperative genesis of deep vein thrombosis and outlines a multimodal approach to deep vein thrombosis prevention in the immediate perioperative period enabling the use of less powerful anticoagulants thereafter.

Williams-Russo P, Sharrock NE, Mattis S: Randomized trial of hypotensive epidural anesthesia in older adults. *Anesthesiology* 1999;91(4):926-935.

The authors of this study reported that hypotensive epidural anesthesia to a mean arterial pressure of 50 ± 5 mm Hg did not result in any significant impairment of cognitive function in elderly or high-risk patients undergoing total hip replacement. No adverse effects were noted in renal or cardiac functions of this group of patients when compared a control group with a mean arterial pressure of 60 ± 5 mm Hg. The authors concluded that hypotensive epidural anesthesia is safe to use in high-risk patients.

Postoperative Care

Capdevila X, Barthelet Y, Biboulet P, Ryckwaert Y, Rubenovitch J, d'Athis F: Effects of perioperative analgesic technique on the surgical outcome and duration of rehabilitation after major knee surgery. *Anesthesiology* 1999;91(1):8-15.

In this randomized prospective study of 56 patients who underwent total knee replacement, the authors reported that epidural analgesia and continuous femoral nerve blockade provided better pain control with enhanced rehabilitation as assessed by range of motion of the knee than intravenous patient-controlled morphine. Patients who received epidural analgesia and continuous femoral nerve blockade were discharged from the rehabilitation center earlier than patients who received intravenous patient-controlled morphine.

Juelsgaard P, Larsen UT, Sorensen JV, Madsen F, Soballe K: Hypotensive epidural anesthesia in total knee replacement without tourniquet: Reduced blood loss and transfusion. *Reg Anesth Pain Med* 2001;26(2):105-110.

In this study, 30 patients undergoing total knee replacement were randomly assigned to receive spinal anesthesia with a tourniquet or hypotensive epidural anesthesia without a tourniquet. The authors found a statistically significant reduction in blood loss and transfusion with hypotensive epidural anesthesia.

Stevens RD, Van Gessel E, Flory N, Fournier R, Gamulin Z: Lumbar plexus block reduces pain and blood loss associated with total hip replacement. *Anesthesiology* 2000;93(1):115-121.

Sixty patients undergoing primary total hip replacement under general anesthesia were randomly assigned to receive a lumbar plexus block with 0.5% bupivacaine or no block before surgery. It was reported that narcotic requirements, postoperative pain scores for 6 hours, and blood loss (both during and following surgery) were significantly lower in the patients receiving a lumbar plexus block.

Wu CL, Anderson GF, Herbert R, Lietman SA, Fleisher LA: Effect of postoperative epidural analgesia on morbidity and mortality after total hip replacement surgery in Medicare patients. *Reg Anesth Pain Med* 2003;28(4): 271-278.

The authors conducted a review of 5% of Medicare patients undergoing total hip replacement between 1994 and 1999 and found that the 7-day mortality rate was 0.3%. The authors were unable to demonstrate a reduction in mortality rate using epidural analgesia and provided an extensive discussion about the limitation of this methodology.

Classic Bibliography

Bierbaum BE, Callaghan JJ, Galante JO, Rubash HE, Tooms RE, Welch RB: An analysis of blood management in patients having a total hip or knee arthroplasty. *J Bone Joint Surg Am* 1999;81(1):2-10.

Byrick RJ, Mullen JB, Mazer CD, Guest CB: Transpulmonary systemic fat embolism: Studies in mongrel dogs after cemented arthroplasty. *Am J Respir Crit Care Med* 1994;150(5 Pt 1):1416-1422.

Christie J, Burnett R, Potts HR, Pell AC: Echocardiography of transatrial embolism during cemented and uncemented hemiarthroplasty of the hip. *J Bone Joint Surg Br* 1994;76(3):409-412.

Liguori GA, Sharrock NE: Asystole and severe bradycardia during epidural anesthesia in orthopedic patients. *Anesthesiology* 1997;86(1):250-257.

Patterson BM, Healy JH, Cornell CN, Sharrock NE: Cardiac arrest during hip arthroplasty with a cemented long-stem component: A report of seven cases. *J Bone Joint Surg Am* 1991;73:271-277.

Sharrock NE, Cazan MG, Hargett MJ, Williams-Russo P, Wilson PD Jr: Changes in mortality after total hip and knee arthroplasty over a ten-year period. *Anesth Analg* 1995;80(2):242-248.

Sharrock NE, Go G, Harpel PC, Ranawat CS, Sculco TP, Salvati EA: Thrombogenesis during total hip arthroplasty. *Clin Orthop Relat Res* 1995;319:16-27.

Sharrock NE, Go G, Williams-Russo P, Haas SB, Harpel PC: Comparison of extradural and general anaesthesia on the fibrinolytic response to total knee arthroplasty. *Br J Anaesth* 1997;79(1):29-34.

Sharrock NE, Go G, Sculco TP, Salvati EA, Westrich GH, Harpel PC: Dose response of intravenous heparin on markers of thrombosis during primary total hip replacement. *Anesthesiology* 1999;90(4):981-987.

Sharrock NE, Haas SB, Hargett MJ, Urquhart B, Insall JN, Scuderi G: Effects of epidural anesthesia on the incidence of deep-vein thrombosis after total knee arthroplasty. *J Bone Joint Surg Am* 1991; 73(4):502-506.

Sharrock NE, Salvati EA: Hypotensive epidural anesthesia for total hip arthroplasty: A review. *Acta Orthop Scand* 1996;67(1):91-107.

Singelyn FJ, Deyaert M, Joris D, Pendeville E, Gouverneur JM: Effects of intravenous patient-controlled analgesia with morphine, continuous epidural analgesia, and continuous three-in-one block on postoperative pain and knee rehabilitation after unilateral total knee arthroplasty. *Anesth Analg* 1998;87(1):88-92.

Sulek CA, Davies LK, Enneking FK, Gearen PA, Lobato EB: Cerebral microembolism diagnosed by transcranial Doppler during total knee arthroplasty: Correlation with transesophageal echocardiography. *Anesthesiology* 1999;91(3):672-676.

Westrich GH, Farrell C, Bono JV, Ranawat CS, Salvati EA, Sculco TP: The incidence of venous thromboembolism after total hip arthroplasty: A specific hypotensive epidural anesthesia protocol. *J Arthroplasty* 1999;14(4): 456-463.

Williams-Russo P, Sharrock NE, Mattis S: Randomized trial of hypotensive epidural anesthesia in older adults. *Anesthesiology* 1999;91(4):926-935.

Chapter 21

Venous Thromboembolic Disease and Prophylaxis in Total Joint Arthroplasty

Clifford W. Colwell, Jr, MD

Mary E. Hardwick, MSN, RN

Introduction

Hemostasis is a balance between clotting and bleeding in the circulatory system. By stopping blood loss from damaged vessels, hemostasis allows the body to control the flow of blood after vascular injury. In addition to being the process the body uses to stop blood flow when the vascular system is damaged, hemostasis also maintains blood flow under normal conditions.

Primary hemostasis is the first phase of coagulation, consisting of the initial vessel reaction and formation of a platelet plug at the site of the injury. Primary hemostasis occurs rapidly (within seconds) to stop blood loss. Hemostasis is a complex process involving the blood vessels, blood cells, and plasma, with the initial deposit of platelets and the activation of coagulation factors creating a fibrin clot. Three mechanisms combine to begin primary hemostasis: vascular spasms, platelet plug formation, and activation of the normal coagulation or clotting process.

The blood vessels and the components within the blood are involved in primary hemostasis and coagulation. Components in the blood include red blood cells, white blood cells, platelets, proteins carried in the plasma (zymogens and cofactors), and nonprotein cofactors (calcium and phospholipids). These components are inactive in the blood until vessel damage or stagnation occurs. Each component plays a role in stopping bleeding at the site of an injury.

Coagulation begins as soon as the body recognizes that damage to a blood vessel has occurred. The normal clotting process takes place through a chain of events initially stemming from vessel damage and subsequently the body's reaction to correct the damage. Tissue thromboplastin is released from the damaged cells, initiating a complex chemical cascade in which a prothrombin activator converts prothrombin to thrombin. Thrombin acts to convert fibrinogen to fibrin, which forms filamentous strands that weave together in a mesh that traps platelets, blood cells, and plasma to form a semisolid clot. Fibrin, the product of chemical reactions known as the coagulation cascade, is important in clot formation because it acts as a "glue," binding platelets to each other and firmly attaching the clot to the blood vessel surface (Figure 1). Fibrin provides stability to the clot.

Virchow first described conditions leading to thrombus formation in 1856. Virchow's triad describes three conditions that are required for clotting: blood stasis (slow or nonflowing blood), direct injury to the vessel, and hypercoagulability (Figure 2). All of these conditions exist when a patient undergoes lower extremity joint arthroplasty or has experienced trauma such as fractured hip.

Stasis occurs with decreased blood flow, immobility, partial immobility, reduced blood pressure, swelling, or tourniquet use. Patients undergoing joint arthroplasty or hip fracture repair typically receive regional or general anesthesia and are therefore immobile during surgery. Patients with hip fractures may be partially immobile because of pain and/or splinting after injury, both of which decrease blood flow. Additionally, blood pressure may be lowered by the body as a protective measure or during surgery by anesthesia to prevent excess bleeding, both of which decrease blood flow and can contribute to stasis. Tourniquet use during knee arthroplasty decreases blood loss at the surgical site and can also contribute to stasis. Postoperatively, pain with movement and swelling can result in immobility and contribute to stasis.

Vessel injury occurs during lower extremity surgery because some vessels (usually small vessels) are interrupted. Large vessels can also be injured perioperatively. For example, when the hip is dislocated during hip arthroplasty, the leg is usually internally or externally rotated depending on the approach, which contorts large vessels and can cause vessel endothelium cells to rupture, thereby initiating hemostasis and the coagulation cascade. Similarly, retractors and instruments used during surgery can damage vessel wall cells and initiate the formation of a blood clot.

Hypercoagulability occurs during surgery because of an increase of tissue factor, the presence of fat particles, the presence of other activated factors, and a decrease in coagulation inhibitors. During lower extremity sur-

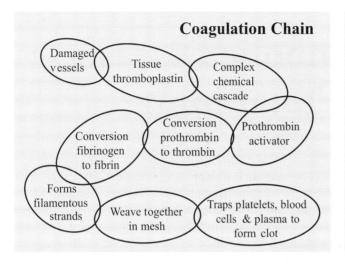

Figure 1 Graphic representation of the coagulation chain from vessel damage to clot formation.

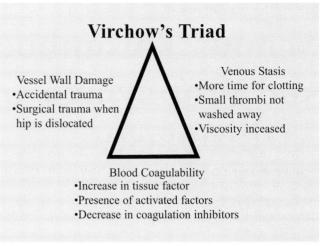

Figure 2 Graphic representation of Virchow's triad illustrates the three aspects of blood clotting.

gery, reaming to prepare bone for a prosthesis can release antigens that stimulate clot formation into the bloodstream.

Venous Thromboembolic Disease

Venous thromboembolic disease is the third most common vascular disease after heart attack and stroke, and one of the most common causes of death in hospitalized patients. Each year, 600,000 patients will experience venous thromboembolism. At least 50,000 and as many as 200,000 patients may die from a pulmonary embolism (a blood clot that obstructs blood flow to the lungs). Routine autopsy data have led researchers to estimate that 10% to 25% of all hospital deaths involve pulmonary embolism, many of which are extensive enough to be considered the cause of death.

Without prophylaxis, venous thromboembolism occurs in 40% to 84% of patients who undergo knee arthroplasty, 45% to 57% of patients who undergo hip arthroplasty, and 36% to 60% of patients who undergo hip fracture repair. Because 90% of instances of pulmonary embolism are thought to originate in the proximal (popliteal and higher) vessels, prevention of proximal thrombi is important. The incidence of proximal deep venous thrombosis without prophylaxis is 9% to 20% for patients undergoing knee arthroplasty, 23% to 36% for those undergoing hip arthroplasty, and 17% to 36% for those undergoing hip fracture surgery. In the general population, blood clots occur in one of every 2,000 people (0.05%).

The prevalence of pulmonary embolism without prophylaxis in patients undergoing knee arthroplasty is 1.8% to 7%; fatal pulmonary embolism occurs in 0.2% to 0.7%. In patients undergoing hip arthroplasty without prophylaxis, pulmonary embolism and fatal pulmonary embolism occur in 0.7% to 30% and 0.1% to 0.4% of

patients, respectively. In patients undergoing hip fracture surgery without prophylaxis, pulmonary embolism occurs in 4.3% to 24% of patients and fatal pulmonary embolism occurs in 3.6% to 12.9%. Approximately 1 in every 100 people (1%) with venous thromboembolism dies; 80% of patients with pulmonary embolism die without any symptoms and two thirds of these deaths occur within 30 minutes of the pulmonary embolism. Some patients who have died suddenly at home are thought to have experienced massive, unforeseen pulmonary embolism.

As mentioned previously, major orthopaedic surgery of the lower extremities poses unique risks for venous thromboembolism, including slowed blood flow, vein damage, and debris from bone cuts. Other underlying risk factors may also be present in individual patients that increase the risk for venous thromboembolism.

A previous history of thromboembolic disease increases the risk for another thromboembolic event after surgery approximately eightfold, and is one of the most serious risk factors for venous thromboembolism after surgery. A history of ischemic stroke also increases the risk of venous thromboembolism.

A hypercoagulable state in which genetics plays a factor, such as activated protein C resistance, increases the risk for venous thromboembolism after major lower extremity surgery. In addition, the presence of a lupus anticoagulant or deficiencies in protein S and antithrombin III reduce the fibrinolytic activity and increase the risk of venous thromboembolism.

A history of cancer also increases the risk of venous thromboembolism because both increased procoagulation activity and reduction of fibrinolytic activity are typically present in this patient population. Additionally, chemotherapy has a toxic effect on the endothelium and may produce an additional risk. Because cancer increases the risk of venous thromboembolism without surgery, it greatly increases risk of venous thromboembolism after surgery.

Age is also a risk factor for many patients undergoing lower extremity surgery. Although age 40 years has traditionally been used as a threshold for increased risk, the risk of venous thromboembolism increases exponentially between the ages of 20 and 80 years: for each decade over 40 years, the risk of venous thromboembolism doubles. Age is also a risk factor for venous thromboembolism in patients undergoing total joint arthroplasty or hip fracture surgery.

Obesity has been reported to increase the risk of venous thromboembolism. Use of oral contraceptives also has been reported to increase the risk of venous thromboembolism; however, whether the use of hormone replacement therapy poses an increased risk is a controversial topic. Tobacco use has also been reported to increase the risk of venous thromboembolism, especially in conjunction with other risk factors. Many patients undergoing lower extremity surgery have these additional risk factors beyond those posed by the surgical procedure itself. All specific risk factors must be evaluated when selecting the type and duration of prophylaxis.

Classic signs and symptoms of deep venous thrombosis include swelling of the leg, change in color of the leg, pain, and a positive Homan's sign. Approximately 50% to 80% of the instances of deep venous thrombosis are clinically silent (exhibit no signs or symptoms). Therefore, clinical signs and symptoms are an inaccurate method of diagnosing venous thromboembolism.

Signs and symptoms of pulmonary embolism include shortness of breath, difficulty breathing, chest pain, tachycardia, cyanosis, hemoptysis, hypotension, and anxiety. Patients diagnosed with pulmonary embolism or fatal pulmonary embolism, however, may exhibit none of these symptoms. Patients who are at high risk and have any symptoms of pulmonary embolism should undergo clinical examination to rule out the presence of pulmonary embolism.

Contrast venography is still considered to be the gold standard for the diagnosis of deep venous thrombosis. Venography, an invasive procedure performed by injecting radiopaque medium into a vein in the foot and obtaining a series of radiographs as the contrast medium travels through the vessels of the leg, is diagnostic of deep venous thrombosis when veins do not fill adequately, thereby indicating a clot blocking the vein. However, the use of venography is limited because it is difficult to obtain a clear view of the veins behind the knee and the large vessels in the groin. The radiopaque medium used contains iodine and can cause an allergic anaphylactic reaction in some patients. The radiopaque medium that is currently used has been reported to cause deep venous thrombosis in fewer than 0.1% of patients; the incidence of deep vein thrombosis was significantly higher with previous media. If the radiopaque medium is injected into the tissue instead of the vein, it can cause necrosis and sloughing of the tissue.

Venous ultrasound of the lower extremities is generally preferred by surgeons and patients because it is noninvasive. Ultrasound uses sound waves to help visualize the vessels in the lower extremities. In most institutions, ultrasound has a high rate of predictive accuracy; it is also highly sensitive and specific when used to assess vessels in the thigh. The accuracy, sensitivity, and specificity of ultrasound, however, are reduced when used to assess vessels in the calf. Ultrasound is not universally used in hospitals, and the procedure must be performed by a skilled technician. If the technician is not proficient at performing the test, ultrasound can be inaccurate. An additional issue with ultrasound in patients who undergo lower extremity surgery is the occasional difficulty viewing the veins adequately because of swelling, particularly in the calf. Ultrasound also cannot clearly visualize the large vessels after entry into the trunk of the body. Contrast MRI can be used to visualize pelvic veins.

If a patient has symptoms that suggest the presence of a pulmonary embolism, tests are done to attempt to rule it out. The first tests that are usually done for such patients include chest radiography and electrocardiography, neither of which will definitively show a pulmonary embolism, but can reveal other causes for the symptoms. After chest radiography and electrocardiography, a ventilation/perfusion scan usually is performed. This test requires that a patient breathe in a radiopaque medium. A picture of the lungs is then obtained that differentiates between ventilation and perfusion of the lung to help identify any potential defect. The result of a ventilation/perfusion scan is negative, low probability, or high probability. If the result is negative, the patient is diagnosed as not having a pulmonary embolism. If the result is low probability, no definitive diagnosis is obtained. If the result is high probability, treatment for a pulmonary embolism is typically initiated.

Pulmonary angiography may be performed if a diagnosis of pulmonary embolism is still possible or in question. As with venography, pulmonary angiography is an invasive examination that requires the use of a radiopaque medium. The medium is injected into a vein, usually in the arm, and radiographs are obtained as it travels through the veins of the lungs. If an area shows no medium in a specific area of the lung, the diagnosis of pulmonary embolism is made.

A relatively new examination for venous thromboembolism is the use of CT pulmonary angiography or venography. CT pulmonary angiography appears to be highly accurate in the diagnosis of pulmonary embolism, but it is an expensive procedure and not available at all institutions. Examination using CT pulmonary angiography can help diagnose patients with questionable ventilation/perfusion scan results, possibly in place of invasive pulmonary angiography.

Prophylaxis

The ideal prophylaxis should be effective, practical, and cost-effective and have a low risk of adverse effects. Prophylaxis for venous thromboembolism can be nonpharmacologic or pharmacologic. The results of randomized clinical trials can be examined and compared to identify the prevalence of venous thromboembolism with placebo or no prophylaxis. One way to compare prophylactic methods is to assess relative risk reduction, which is determined by comparing the results of the method tested with those of a comparator and arriving at the percent decrease gained by using the prophylactic method being studied. The selection of a prophylactic tool depends on patient risk factors and medical condition. Determination of the venous thromboembolism risk of each patient is important in deciding which type of prophylaxis to use. Prophylaxis is even more important in patients with multiple risk factors. Intraoperative factors that can decrease the risk of venous thromboembolism include decrease in surgical time; decrease in the duration that the leg is maximally flexed, internally rotated, or abducted; and the use of regional anesthesia. Early mobilization and heightened awareness of venous thromboembolism signs and symptoms also can be beneficial. None of these factors, however, will decrease the incidence of venous thromboembolism as effectively as pharmacologic prophylaxis.

Nonpharmacologic

One of the most common and oldest nonpharmacologic methods of prophylaxis is early ambulation, which involves mobilizing the patient as soon as possible after surgery. Although early ambulation continues to be practiced, the effects of venous thromboembolism using early mobilization alone have been shown to be similar to those of placebo. A second type of nonpharmacologic prophylaxis involves the use of active ankle pumps (flexing and extending the foot to tense and relax the calf muscles, which, by simulating walking, increases the pressure in the veins of the leg). Although active ankle pumps have been shown to increase venous velocity up to 175%, these devices used alone do not significantly decrease the incidence of venous thromboembolism in patients who have undergone lower extremity surgery. Elastic stockings are another type of nonpharmacologic prophylaxis, but this type of therapy has not been proved to be effective in this patient population. One study reported that the use of elastic stockings alone for 6 months in a cohort of 1,162 patients who underwent hip arthroplasty resulted in a 3.4% incidence of venous

thromboembolism, with a 1.6% incidence of pulmonary embolism (0.3% of which were fatal).

Knee-high or thigh-high intermittent pneumatic compression of the legs has also been used as nonpharmacologic prophylaxis in patients who have undergone lower extremity surgery and in trauma patients. Although intermittent pneumatic compression is often selected for initial prophylaxis in trauma patients because it can be applied preoperatively and does not increase the risk of bleeding, studies have not shown that intermittent pneumatic compression alone is adequately effective in this patient population. In one study of 110 patients who underwent total knee arthroplasty and 423 patients who underwent total hip arthroplasty, intermittent pneumatic compression was shown to be moderately effective. In patients who underwent total knee arthroplasty, the incidence of deep venous thrombosis was reduced to 28.2% and the incidence of proximal deep venous thrombosis was reduced to 73% (relative risk reduction, 56%). In patients who underwent total hip arthroplasty, the incidence of deep venous thrombosis was reduced to 20.3% and the incidence of proximal deep venous thrombosis was reduced to 13.7% (relative risk reduction, 63%.)

Venous foot pumps, in which a bladder is attached to the bottom of the foot to provide intermittent pressure to the arch, have also been used as a type of nonpharmacologic prophylaxis. One study reported on the use of venous foot pumps in 172 patients who underwent total knee arthroplasty and showed a 40.7% incidence of total deep venous thrombosis and a 2.3% incidence of proximal deep venous thrombosis (relative risk reduction, 37%). No known randomized, controlled studies on the use of venous foot pumps have been reported to date. Although both intermittent pneumatic compression and venous foot pumps appear to decrease the incidence of venous thromboembolism, the limited number of patients in the studies assessing these two types of nonpharmacologic prophylaxis, the difficulty of using either device on an outpatient basis, and poor patient compliance combined with decreased hospital stay limit their use as an adjunctive treatment to pharmacologic prophylaxis.

Pharmacologic

Warfarin is currently the only commercially available oral anticoagulant. Warfarin is a vitamin K antagonist that produces its anticoagulant effect by interfering with the cyclic interconversion of vitamin K. Warfarin has a high bioavailability, is rapidly absorbed from the gastrointestinal tract, and affects coagulation factors within 24 hours; however, it can take 72 to 96 hours to reach a therapeutic level in the blood. The half-life of warfarin is 36 to 42 hours. Warfarin circulates in the blood by binding to plasma proteins, and it accumulates in the liver, where it is metabolically transformed and excreted. The terminal half-life (the time to elimination from the body) of warfarin after a single dose is approximately 1 week. The effect of warfarin can be counteracted by vitamin K, either administered therapeutically or ingested in food.

The dose response relationship of warfarin is influenced by genetic and environmental factors. In addition to known and unknown genetic factors, various disease states, drugs, and dietary factors can interfere with a patient's response to warfarin. Other drugs may influence the pharmacokinetics of warfarin by reducing its absorption from the gastrointestinal tract or by disrupting its metabolic clearance through the liver. Variability in the anticoagulant response may also occur because of inaccurate laboratory testing, patient noncompliance, and poor patient-physician communication.

Hereditary resistance to warfarin can occur; patients with this type of resistance may require doses that are 5 to 20 times higher than average to achieve the anticoagulant effect. Dietary intake of foods high in vitamin K can potentiate the anticoagulant effect of warfarin. Disease states involving fever or hyperthyroidism can also increase warfarin responsiveness. Additionally, hepatic disease increases the anticoagulant effect of warfarin because of the impaired synthesis of coagulation factors. Warfarin, therefore, should be used with caution in patients with these medical conditions.

Approximately 50% of the orthopaedic surgeons surveyed in the United States reported that they use warfarin as the prophylaxis of choice after orthopaedic surgery of the lower extremity. Dosing may begin the day before surgery, a few hours before surgery, or after surgery, with a loading dose of 5 to 10 mg, followed daily by a single dose adjusted to maintain the international normalized ratio within the therapeutic range of 2 to 3. Warfarin therapy requires monitoring, initially on a daily basis until a satisfactory international normalized ratio is achieved, then once or twice weekly depending on the patient. The dose is adjusted according to the prothrombin time results to maintain a stable international normalized ratio within the therapeutic range. The usual dose of warfarin ranges from 2 to 10 mg during maintenance therapy. Warfarin therapy may continue from 10 days to 6 weeks after surgery.

Warfarin, as with other types of pharmacologic prophylaxis, is associated with many adverse effects, the most serious of which is bleeding (particularly bleeding into various tissues and organs of the body). Less frequently (in < 0.01% of patients), necrosis and/or gangrene of the skin and other tissues occur. Other adverse effects may include nausea, vomiting, loss of appetite, diarrhea, and abdominal cramping.

Twelve clinical trials were conducted to assess the use of warfarin in patients who underwent total knee arthroplasty. Overall, a 37.0% incidence of deep venous thrombosis and a 6.6% incidence of proximal deep venous thrombosis were reported, with a relative risk reduction of 43% compared with placebo. Twelve clinical trials were also conducted to assess the use of warfarin in patients who underwent total hip arthroplasty. Overall, a 22.3% incidence of deep venous thrombosis and a 5.2% incidence of proximal deep venous thrombosis were reported, with a relative risk reduction of 59% compared with placebo. A study of 126 patients who underwent hip fracture surgery and received warfarin therapy reported an overall 20% incidence of deep venous thrombosis and a 9% incidence of proximal deep venous thrombosis, with a relative risk reduction of 60%.

Low-molecular-weight heparins are derived from heparin by chemical or enzymatic depolymerization, which yields molecule fragments that are approximately one third the size of those of unfractionated heparin. Because the method of preparation is different in each type of low-molecular-weight heparin, the pharmacokinetic properties and anticoagulant profiles may not be clinically interchangeable. Low-molecular-weight heparins vary in weight from 1,000 to 10,000 daltons, with a mean molecular weight of 4,500 to 5,000 daltons.

Low-molecular-weight heparins, as with unfractionated heparin, produce their major anticoagulant effects by activating antithrombin and inhibiting both factors Xa and IIa (thrombin). Low-molecular-weight heparins have a longer plasma half-life (4.5 hours), better bioavailability at low doses, and a more predictable dose response than unfractionated heparin. Low-molecular-weight heparins are eliminated through the kidneys. The results of laboratory tests such as partial thromboplastin time or prothrombin time change very little with use of low-molecular-weight heparins and are therefore not monitoring tools for low-molecular-weight heparin therapy. Blood cell counts, particularly platelets, should be assessed because instances of thrombocytopenia and heparin-induced thrombocytopenia have been reported, although the incidence with low-molecular-weight heparin therapy is extremely low.

Uses for low-molecular-weight heparins include venous thromboembolism prophylaxis, venous thromboembolism treatment, treatment of unstable angina, and coronary angioplasty. The principal adverse effect with low-molecular-weight heparins, as with unfractionated heparin, is bleeding into soft tissue or into a wound site from surgery or trauma. Protamine sulfate has been recommended to neutralize low-molecular-weight heparins; however, antifactor Xa activity is not completely neutralized with protamine sulfate because protamine manifests reduced binding to low-molecular-weight components.

Although several low-molecular-weight heparins are commercially available, only two have been approved for use in the United States by the US Food and Drug

Administration: enoxaparin and dalteparin. All low-molecular-weight heparins are administered by subcutaneous injection. Doses vary, but all are administered in a fixed dose once or twice daily. For prophylactic treatment after major lower extremity surgery, low-molecular-weight heparins are recommended for at least 10 days, but in patients who have undergone total hip arthroplasty or hip fracture surgery, prophylaxis may be extended from 28 to 35 days after surgery. With hospital stays decreasing to 4 days or less, patient must learn to self administer low-molecular-weight heparin, have home health care workers administer the injections, or go to a rehabilitation or skilled nursing facility for the remainder of the treatment.

In 19 clinical trials using low-molecular-weight heparin prophylaxis for patients who underwent total knee arthroplasty, the overall reported prevalence of deep venous thrombosis and proximal deep venous thrombosis was 35.1% and 5.6%, respectively (relative risk reduction against placebo, 46%). In 33 clinical trials using low-molecular-weight heparin prophylaxis for patients who underwent total hip arthroplasty, the overall reported prevalence of deep venous thrombosis and proximal deep venous thrombosis was 14.8% and 4.7%, respectively (relative risk reduction, 73%). For 887 patients who underwent hip fracture surgery, the overall reported prevalence of deep venous thrombosis and proximal deep venous thrombosis was 18% and 6%, respectively (relative risk reduction, 64%).

Fondaparinux, a factor Xa inhibitor for venous thromboembolism prophylaxis in total joint arthroplasty and hip fracture surgery, is a chemically synthesized pentasaccharide that has a half-life of 17 to 21 hours and affects the coagulation cascade only at the level of factor Xa. Fondaparinux is eliminated through the kidneys and should be used with caution in patients with decreased kidney function. The major adverse effect of fondaparinux is bleeding, particularly in soft tissue or into the wound.

Administered by subcutaneous injection once daily in a static dose of 2.5 mg, this factor Xa inhibitor has been shown to be more efficacious than the low-molecular-weight heparin enoxaparin in clinical trials of patients who underwent total knee arthroplasty, total hip arthroplasty, or hip fracture surgery. Fondaparinux is currently approved for use in total knee arthroplasty, total hip arthroplasty, and hip fracture surgery, and clinical trials are underway for other uses.

In a clinical trial of 361 patients who underwent total knee arthroplasty, the overall reported prevalence of deep venous thrombosis and proximal deep venous thrombosis was 12.5% and 2.4%, respectively (relative risk reduction, 81%). In two clinical trials comparing fondaparinux and enoxaparin in 1,695 patients who underwent total hip arthroplasty, the overall reported prevalence of deep venous thrombosis and proximal

deep venous thrombosis was 4.7% and 1.2%, respectively (relative risk reduction, 91%). In a clinical trial of 626 patients who underwent hip fracture surgery, the reported prevalence of deep venous thrombosis and proximal deep venous thrombosis was 8.0% and 0.9%, respectively (relative risk reduction, 84%).

The results of early phase III trials of a direct thrombin inhibitor, ximelagatran, in patients who underwent total knee arthroplasty are currently before the US Food and Drug Administration for approval. After oral administration, ximelagatran is rapidly absorbed, inhibits both free and clot-bound thrombin, and has predictable pharmacokinetics, with no clinically relevant interactions with food and a low potential for drug interactions. Excreted through the renal system, ximelagatran should be used with caution in patients with decreased renal function. It is administered orally twice daily with no need for routine monitoring to adjust doses. In addition to bleeding, transient elevation of liver function levels may be caused by ximelagatran.

In a study comparing warfarin and ximelagatran (36 mg twice daily administered orally) in patients who underwent total knee arthroplasty, the overall reported incidence of deep venous thrombosis and proximal deep venous thrombosis was 20.3% and 2.5%, respectively (relative risk reduction against placebo, 68.4%). Ximelagatran is effective in the prevention of deep venous thrombosis and does not require monitoring in patients who have undergone total knee arthroplasty. Other types of direct thrombin inhibitors that can be administered orally are also currently under investigation in clinical trials.

Although aspirin is frequently used for prophylaxis, sufficient randomized controlled trials have not been conducted to indicate whether it is effective as a single prophylactic agent in patients undergoing total joint arthroplasty and hip fracture surgery. In five clinical trials of patients undergoing total knee arthroplasty, the overall incidence of deep venous thrombosis and proximal deep venous thrombosis was 54.6% and 8.9%, respectively (relative risk reduction compared with placebo, 15%). In five clinical trials of patients undergoing total hip arthroplasty, the overall incidence of deep venous thrombosis and proximal deep venous thrombosis was 41.7% and 11.4%, respectively (relative risk reduction, 35%). Three trials of patients undergoing hip fracture surgery reported an overall incidence of deep venous thrombosis and proximal deep venous thrombosis of 39% and 13%, respectively (relative risk reduction, 39%).

Summary

Both nonpharmacologic and pharmacologic types of prophylaxis are available for use after major lower extremity surgery. The American College of Chest Physicians Consensus Conference has published guidelines based on randomized prospective trials with clear end points for prophylaxis after major lower extremity surgery. These evidence-based guidelines assert that many established prophylactic protocols are effective and safe for use. Recent controlled trials indicate that prophylaxis for patients who have undergone total knee or hip arthroplasty and hip fracture surgery can be achieved with warfarin at an international normalized ratio of 2 to 3; low-molecular-weight heparins administered either twice or once daily, depending on the agent; or 2.5 mg of fondaparinux administered 6 to 8 hours after surgery and then once daily.

The recommended duration of prophylaxis for patients who have undergone total knee arthroplasty is reasonably well established as 7 to 10 days postoperatively. Patients who have undergone total hip arthroplasty or hip fracture surgery may also receive prophylaxis for 7 to 10 days, but venographic evidence has indicated that 28 to 35 days may add efficacy to the shorter course of prophylaxis without significant risk of adverse effects.

Pharmacologic agents should be used with caution when combined with spinal or epidural anesthesia and analgesia. If a patient has multiple or traumatic punctures, nonpharmacologic prophylaxis should be used initially and then replaced with pharmacologic prophylaxis when the risk of bleeding diminishes. If pharmacologic prophylaxis is used after neuraxial anesthesia or analgesia, the removal of the catheter should be coordinated with the half-life of the agent and the timing of the next dose. For low-molecular-weight heparins, the catheter should not be removed sooner than 2 hours before the next dose. If using warfarin, the catheter should be removed on the morning of the second day before the international normalized ratio reaches 1.5. Because of the prolonged half-life of fondaparinux, it is recommended for use after removal of the catheter.

Because venous thromboembolism is a common and potentially lethal condition, especially in patients who undergo major lower extremity surgery, the use of thromboprophylaxis is essential. The choice of prophylaxis should be determined on an individual patient basis by carefully assessing each patient's risk factors and the type of prophylaxis to be used.

Annotated Bibliography

Venous Thromboembolic Disease

Heit JA: Risk factors for venous thromboembolism. *Clin Chest Med* 2003;24:1-12.

The author discusses the risk factors for venous thromboembolism, acknowledges the multifactoral aspects of the disease (which has both genetic and environmental components), and offers suggestions for improved identification of persons at risk.

Westrich GH, Rana AJ: Prevention and treatment of thromboembolic disease: An overview. *Tech Orthop* 2001;16:279-290.

The authors provide information on risk factors associated with venous thromboembolism and discuss current diagnostic methods. Treatment and prophylactic regimens are reviewed.

White RH: The epidemiology of venous thromboembolism. *Circulation* 2003;107:I4-I8.

The author provides an overview of venous thromboembolism incidence and risks and discusses recurrence and mortality rates.

Prophylaxis

Anderson FA Jr, Hirsh J, White K, Fitzgerald RH Jr: Temporal trends in prevention of venous thromboembolism following primary total hip or knee arthroplasty 1996-2001: Findings from the Hip and Knee Registry. *Chest* 2003;124:349S-356S.

The authors used an outcomes database to provide data regarding the incidence of venous thromboembolism and practice changes in total joint arthroplasty.

Colwell CW Jr: *Practice Patterns in DVT Prophylaxis.* Rosemont, IL, Orthopaedic Research Foundation, 2003. Available at http://www.oref.org/DVT/DVTPromofor Website.doc. Accessed June 13, 2005.

This article discusses the practice patterns of orthopaedic surgeons who perform total joint arthroplasty; data were obtained from a survey of orthopaedic surgeons.

Geerts WH, Heit JA, Clagett GP, et al: Prevention of venous thromboembolism. *Chest* 2001;119(suppl 1): 132S-175S.

This article provides consensus guidelines for the management of prophylaxis that were derived from a meta-analysis of studies of venous thromboembolism after major surgery of the lower extremity.

Mesko JW, Brand RA, Iorio R, et al: Venous thromboembolic disease management patterns in total hip arthroplasty and total knee arthroplasty patients: A survey of the AAHKS membership. *J Arthroplasty* 2001;16:679-688.

The practice patterns of orthopaedic surgeons practicing total joint arthroplasty are described; data were obtained from a survey of members of the American Association of Hip and Knee Surgeons.

Turpie AG, Bauer KA, Eriksson BI, Lassen MR: Fondaparinux vs enoxaparin for the prevention of venous thromboembolism in major orthopedic surgery: A meta-analysis of 4 randomized double-blind studies. *Arch Intern Med* 2002;162:1833-1840.

The authors of this study conducted a meta-analysis of four trials of patients who underwent total knee arthroplasty, total hip arthroplasty, or hip fracture surgery and received fondaparinux prophylaxis.

Classic Bibliography

Charnley J: Prophylaxis of postoperative thromboembolism. *Lancet* 1972;2:134-135.

Geerts WH, Pineo GH, Heit JA, et al: Prevention of venous thromboembolism: The Seventh ACCP Conference on Antithrombotic and Thrombolytic Therapy. *Chest* 2004;126:338S-400S.

Prevention of venous thrombosis and pulmonary embolism: NIH Consensus Development. *JAMA* 1986; 256:744-749.

Chapter 22

Bone Grafts and Bone Graft Substitutes

Jean F. Welter, MD, PhD

Victor M. Goldberg, MD

Introduction

More than 500,000 bone graft procedures are performed each year in the United States, making this one of the most commonly performed orthopaedic procedures. More than half of these bone grafts are used during spinal arthrodeses, with the rest being used during other general orthopaedic and maxillofacial applications. Indications for bone grafting are listed in Table 1.

Bone grafting is a fairly mature technology. The last major breakthrough was the introduction of free vascularized bone transplants in 1975, and relatively little has changed in bone grafting techniques and indications since then. In contrast, considerable effort is being put into developing bone graft substitutes based on diverse natural and synthetic structural materials, bioactive compounds, and combinations of these substances. Bone graft substitutes represent approximately 10% of the bone graft market, but their share is increasing. They have the potential to expand the range of clinical conditions that can be treated. Experimental approaches, including gene therapy and tissue engineering, may someday make bone grafts obsolete. Nevertheless, currently no single type of implant or graft is ideally suited for all circumstances. Thus, the choice of the proper method remains the responsibility of the surgeon.

Bone Grafts

General Considerations and Terminology

The term "bone graft" refers to transplanted bone, and can thus apply to autografts (tissue transferred from one anatomic site to another in the same individual), allografts (a graft between genetically dissimilar individuals of the same species), or xenografts (tissue transplanted across species barriers). Some authors prefer the use of the term "graft" to describe living tissue and the term "implant" for all others. The term "bone graft substitute" generally refers to manmade or processed, naturally occurring substances.

Bone can be repaired or regenerated by three processes: osteogenesis, osteoconduction, and osteoinduction (Table 2).

Osteogenesis is the formation of new bone by viable cells in the graft or by invading cells from the surrounding host tissue. Approximately 10% of the graft cells in cancellous bone survive to participate in bone formation. Thus, except in the instance of vascularized grafts, the surrounding host tissue (the graft bed) contributes all the blood vessels and most of the cells required to incorporate the graft.

Osteoconduction is a largely passive function of the graft. In osteoconduction, new bone formation occurs along the graft, which serves as a passive scaffold, trellis, or template for the host vascular and cellular responses. The graft stimulates the attachment and migration of vascular and osteogenic cells within the graft material. The physical characteristics of the graft (porosity, pore size, pore connectivity, and three-dimensional architecture) affect its osteoconductive activity. Interactions between graft matrix proteins and cell surface receptors also influence the response of the host to the graft material.

Osteoinduction is the process whereby bone formation is stimulated by an implant or transplant. New bone formation occurs because residual cells and/or signaling molecules in the graft stimulate, recruit, and direct the proliferation and differentiation of pluripotent mesenchymal stem cells. Substances that participate in osteoinduction include growth factors, cytokines, enzymes, enzyme inhibitors, and matrix components.

Bone grafts can be further classified according to their composition (cortical, corticocancellous, or cancellous), anatomic site of origin, or blood supply (nonvascularized or revascularized). Allografts are described based on preservation method (fresh or freeze-dried) or other processing steps (demineralized or irradiated). Because these factors affect the properties of the material, they influence the proper choice of material for a particular clinical situation.

Bone Graft Biology

It has been noted that when a defect in the course of a long bone is filled by a transplant, nature must perform

Table 1 | Indications for Bone Grafting

Enhancing or promoting healing in patients with delayed union, nonunion, osteotomies, arthrodesis, poor or limited healing potential, and in some instances infection

Bridging fracture defects and providing bony continuity and structural support

Replacing cortical segments in patients with complete bone loss resulting from severe fractures or tumor excision

Filling cavities from cyst, sequestrum, tumor removal, or in revision arthroplasty

Reconstructing deficient bone stock for revision arthroplasty

three tasks: (1) preserve nutrition and reestablish circulation of the transplant, (2) unite the ends of the transplant with the ends of the fragments, and (3) transform the transplant into a duplicate of the normal bone whose place it fills.

Although some of the cell and molecular details have been further defined since these tasks were noted by Phemister in 1914, the understanding of the basics of bone graft incorporation has not changed significantly. Incorporation of all grafts occurs in predictable stages, although there are variations in the sequence and intensity of these stages depending on the type of graft (autologous, allogeneic, or revascularized). Immediately after implantation, the graft is surrounded by a hematoma. Entrapped platelets degranulate, releasing growth factors such as platelet-derived growth factor (PDGF) and transforming growth factor-beta 1 (TGF-β 1). Because their vascular supply has been interrupted, most cells within the graft die within the first days, and an inflammatory/wound-healing response is initiated. Host-derived osteoclasts begin focal resorption of the graft material, often along existing haversian and Volkmann's canals. This provides an ingress path for endothelial cells and for osteoblast precursors, which arise from proliferating mesenchymal stem cells. These cells then deposit osteoid on the fresh resorption surfaces. During the subsequent weeks and months, the sequence of local osteoclastic resorption and revascularization, recruitment and ingress of mesenchymal precursor cells and their differentiation, and new bone formation is repeated throughout the graft. For a large graft, the incorporation process can take years to complete. These events transiently weaken the graft below its initial strength; in addition to the reduction in mass resulting from osteoclastic resorption, the initial new bone is frequently woven bone. Woven bone is highly cellular and disorganized, with limited mechanical strength. The woven bone gradually undergoes remodeling to lamellar bone. With the exception of vascularized grafts, most grafts take years to become fully mechanically supportive.

It is well recognized that bone is a mechanosensitive tissue (it adapts to its mechanical environment). Bone grafts share this property, albeit it occurs differently at different stages of incorporation. Dead implants, such as allografts and most cortical grafts, are initially not responsive to loads. However, if the graft is mechanically unstable, excessive resorption and fibrosis will likely prevent incorporation. Conversely, once the graft becomes at least partially integrated and remodeled, mechanical loading without excessive movement will promote further graft remodeling and integration. In vascularized grafts in particular, weight bearing can have a profound effect on graft integration and hypertrophy.

Table 2 | Overview of Osteogenic, Osteoinductive, Osteoconductive, and Mechanical Properties of Commonly Used Bone Grafts and Bone Graft Substitutes*

Type of Graft		Osteogenesis	Osteoinduction	Osteoconduction	Mechanical Support
Autograft	Cancellous	++	+++	+++	–
	Cortical	+	++	++	+++
	Vascularized	+++	++	++	+++
Allograft	Cancellous	–	+++	+++	–
	Cortical/Frozen	–	+	+	+++
	Cortical/Freeze-dried	–	+	+	–
Substitute	Osteoconductive	–	–	+++	+
	Osteoinductive	–	+++	+	+
	Nonbiologic	–	+	+	+++
Gene therapy		++	+++	–	–
Tissue engineering		+++	++	++	++

*For each property, +, ++, and +++ are qualitative degrees of positive; – indicates negative

Bone Grafting Complications

In addition to donor site morbidity, bone grafting procedures are affected by three major complications: fractures, nonunions, and infections. Fractures primarily affect cortical grafts and may occur because the graft was inadequately sized for the host bone. The remodeling process described previously weakens cortical grafts, predisposing them to late fracturing. Nonunions may be caused by inadequate stabilization, or in the instance of allografts, by immunologic rejection. Graft infections, although they can often be treated or prevented with antibiotics, may require graft removal.

Autografts

General Considerations

Autogenous bone remains the material of choice when it can be harvested without risk to the patient. Cancellous or corticocancellous iliac crest grafts are the most frequently used, but other sources are useful as well (corticocancellous rib grafts or the cortical fibular diaphysis). Disadvantages of autogenous bone include that the available amount, shape, or size of autologous bone graft may be inadequate, and donor site morbidity is a serious and frequent concern.

Cancellous Autografts

Cancellous grafts are composed of porous, highly cellular trabecular bone and are used to stimulate and enhance bone healing. In terms of clinical outcome, cancellous autografts remain the gold standard against which all other grafting procedures are judged. Cancellous autografts are the only commonly used grafts that provide osteogenesis; they provide osteoconduction and osteoinduction as well. Because of their open structure and large surface area, the incorporation of these grafts is the quickest; complete turnover and integration with the host site can be completed as early as 6 to 12 months postoperatively. Donor site complications can include hematomas, seromas, infection, fracture, herniations, postoperative pain, and sensory loss.

Cortical Autografts

Cortical autografts are composed of relatively nonporous, lamellar bone. They are used primarily to provide immediate mechanical support for a major bony defect. They incorporate much the same as cancellous grafts, but at a much slower pace. A relative drawback of large cortical grafts is the necrosis that affects most of the graft because of the loss of its blood supply. Compared with cancellous grafts, the balance between resorption and new bone formation is shifted in favor of resorption at early time points. The resulting relative osteopenia, which can last for 6 to 18 months, can make partial weight bearing necessary as a precaution during this period. Vas-

cularized cortical grafts can help overcome this complication.

Vascularized Autografts

Bone grafts can be transferred as vascularized grafts, either on a vascular pedicle or as a free graft with a microsurgically reanastomosed blood supply. Free grafts were first introduced in the mid 1970s. Although experimental work has been done on vascularized allografts, in clinical practice the procedure is generally reserved for autogenous tissue, primarily for cortical grafts such as the fibula. Because the blood supply is preserved, these grafts undergo much less cell necrosis, and thus bypass much of the lengthy repair process involved in conventional (avascular) bone graft incorporation. Vascularized bone graft healing is conceptually analogous to fracture repair. In particular, the transient structural weakening that can occur during conventional graft incorporation is eliminated. Vascularized grafts have only 40% of the stress fracture rate of nonvascularized grafts that are more than 12 cm in length.

Vascularized autografts are ideal for repairing large, critical-sized defects or grafting into poorly vascularized, scarred, or irradiated beds. Persistent nonunions and osteonecrosis of the hip are other indications. A further advantage is that the bone graft can be part of a composite free transplant, including soft tissue and skin, for major reconstructive surgery. Drawbacks are the even more limited supply of suitable donor sites, an increase in donor site morbidity because of the extensive dissection of the vascular pedicle and muscle cuff, and the increased technical difficulty of the microvascular anastomosis.

Allografts

General Considerations

In patients in whom suitable amounts or types of autologous material are not available, allograft can be used. The attractive feature of allografts is that essentially unlimited amounts are available for use, and donor site morbidity is not a consideration. Most revision arthroplasties require the use of some form of allograft. Allografts are available as cancellous, corticocancellous, or purely cortical material. The incorporation of allografts is similar to that of autografts, but it occurs much more slowly. It also tends to be a surface phenomenon, in which new bone encases the graft, which remains histologically distinguishable from host bone for years. The incorporation is also invariably accompanied by inflammation, likely related to an immune response to the graft. The potential for disease transmission or immunologic complications is similar to that associated with any allotransplantation. Processing and packaging of the material (by freezing or freeze-drying) can degrade its osteoinductive and mechanical properties. Cultural or religious biases against allotransplantation (and xenotransplantation) in general may also apply to bone grafting.

Cancellous Allografts

Cancellous allografts do not provide live cells for osteogenesis, but are osteoconductive and osteoinductive. Long-term results using cancellous allograft are similar to those using autograft. The bone can be obtained from many anatomic sites, such as the proximal and distal femur, tibial plateau, calcaneus, and talus. It is generally processed into blocks or chips and packaged either frozen or freeze-dried.

Cortical Allografts

Cortical allografts are the most commonly used cortical graft because sufficient autologous cortical bone is often not available and morbidity at the donor site is a concern. The grafts are usually frozen or freeze-dried and therefore are obviously not viable; however, cortical autografts are not viable either, so this is not a major disadvantage. Processing the grafts by freezing is convenient for storage, reduces immunogenicity, and may reduce the risk of disease transmission. Healing and incorporation of these grafts can be enhanced by adding fresh, autogenous cancellous bone or marrow to the graft-host junctions.

Fresh-Frozen Cortical Allografts Fresh-frozen cortical allografts are the most commonly used cortical graft. They function primarily as structural supports and contribute osteoconduction and osteoinduction, but no osteogenesis. A major advantage is that they can be matched anatomically and structurally to the bone being replaced.

Freeze-Dried Cortical Allografts Freeze-drying cortical bone significantly reduces immunogenicity, allows room-temperature storage, and can substantially increase the shelf life of the product. Osteoconduction and osteoinduction are preserved, but freeze-drying drastically reduces the mechanical properties of the graft.

Vascularized Allografts

The need for long-term immunosuppression and the risk of graft-versus-host disease are difficult to justify, given the limited potential advantages of this graft type. Thus, although experimental work has been conducted on vascularized allografts, they are not used clinically. Possible exceptions may include patients already undergoing immunosuppression for other reasons (for example, renal transplant recipients) or bone transplanted in the context of whole-limb transplantation.

Xenografts

Bone xenografts are not used fresh or fresh-frozen. Heavily processed (organic extraction, high temperature calcinations) bovine bone is commercialized as Bio-Oss or OrthOss (Geistlich, Biomaterials, Wolhusen, Switzerland) or EndoBon (Biomet Europe, Dordrecht, The Netherlands). Bovine bone is also available in a sintered bone formulation. Coral exoskeletons are also arguably xenografts. All of these materials retain their microstructure and are osteoconductive.

Bone Graft Substitutes

General Considerations

Except for solid metal implants such as those used in arthroplasty, bone graft substitutes can be subdivided into osteoconductive and osteoinductive materials. Bone graft substitutes have the advantages of unlimited supply and easy sterilization and storage over autografts and allografts. Disadvantages can include poor handling properties, variable resorption rates, poor mechanical properties, and potentially adverse effects on normal bone remodeling. In many patients, bone graft substitutes may be better used as bone graft extenders in concert with autogenous or allogeneic bone.

Osteoconductive bone graft substitutes are generally porous structures, which, when implanted into bone, serve as a structural template for host-derived new bone formation. Some types may provide some structural support (at least transiently). Conversely, osteoinductive bone graft substitutes are generally cytokines or growth factors, which stimulate the recruitment and differentiation of undifferentiated, host-derived stem cells to the osteogenic lineage. As such, they generally provide no initial mechanical support and must be used in conjunction with rigid fixation. The prototypical osteoinductive agents are bone morphogenetic proteins (BMPs) pioneered by Marshall Urist. Other compounds with osteogenic potential are TGF-ß, fibroblast growth factors (FGFs), insulin-like growth factors (IGFs), and PDGFs. Although some of these products may be approved for specific applications, it is nevertheless the responsibility of the surgeon to decide (and of the manufacturer to prove) whether it is the best available product for that application.

Osteoconductive Materials

Osteoconductive materials serve as a passive scaffold for the host vascular and cellular responses. The implant stimulates the attachment and migration of vascular and osteogenic cells within the graft material. Osteoconductive materials increase the probability that the entire gap or void space will become filled with host bone. They also serve as a placeholder or spacer that blocks the ingress of soft tissues into the gap. The porosity, pore size, pore connectivity, and three-dimensional architecture, as well as the chemical composition and surface structure of the implant all affect osteoconduction. Pore sizes of 100 to 500 μm with lateral interconnections of 100 μm or greater seem to be ideal.

Calcium Sulfate (Plaster of Paris)

Calcium sulfate was first used as a resorbable bone graft substitute in the 19th century and remains in use today. Calcium sulfate is used as pellets (for example, Osteo-Set, Wright Medical Technology, Arlington, TN) or in injectable form (for example, MIIG, Wright Medical Technology; BonePlast, Interpore Cross, Irvine, CA). It is useful in antibiotic-laden form for the treatment of infected defect sites. It offers little mechanical support and dissolves relatively rapidly (in 30 to 60 days) in vivo.

Ceramics

Calcium phosphate-based bone graft substitutes are the hydroxyapatite-based (coral-based or synthetic) and β-tricalcium phosphate-based ceramics. Their primary use is as void fillers and as coatings on metallic implants. Ceramics are osteoconductive. Ceramics are composed of hydroxyapatite or tricalcium phosphate or a combination of the two.

Hydroxyapatite, the major constituent of the inorganic component of bone, is biocompatible and nonimmunogenic. Various forms of injectable or moldable apatite-based cements have been developed for use in metaphyseal fractures. For example, Norian Skeletal Repair Systems (Norian SRS, Norian Core, Cupertino, CA) is an injectable, fast-setting carbonated apatite cement used to fill defects in cancellous bone from cysts or metaphyseal fractures. It offers some mechanical integrity.

Beta-tricalcium phosphate granules can be mixed with patient-derived bone marrow and used as a void-filler (for example, Cellplex TCP, Wright Medical; Conduit, DePuy, Warsaw, IN). Beta-tricalcium phosphate ceramics are biocompatible and resorbable.

Another calcium phosphate-based product, alpha-Bone Substitute Material (α-BSM, ETEX, Cambridge, MA), is also used for the treatment of bone voids. It is a low-crystallinity, high-porosity calcium phosphate cement with good resorption characteristics; it is hydrated before use and hardens rapidly at body temperature.

Coral

The microstructure of some coral (*Porites* and Goniopora species) exoskeletons is grossly similar to bone, with interconnecting porosity. Coral of the genus *Porites* has an average void volume of 66%; parallel channels are 230 μm in diameter, with interconnecting fenestrations between these channels.

In Europe, coral exoskeletons are used in the native calcium carbonate form (Biocoral, Inoteb, Saint-Gonnery, France). In North America, porous hydroxy-

apatite (Pro-osteon, Interpore 200, or 500, Interpore Cross International, Irvine, CA) is derived from marine coral, processed through the replamineform process. This converts the coral calcium bicarbonate exoskeleton into hydroxyapatite through a hydrothermal reaction. This hydroxyapatite matrix is osteoconductive; it is used for cyst and void repair and, in conjunction with rigid fixation, for fracture repair.

Extracellular Matrix Scaffolds

Extracellular matrix proteins, including collagen, laminin, fibronectin, and glycosaminoglycans, can be fabricated into porous scaffolds. These scaffolds are readily resorbable and osteoconductive. Type I collagen-based scaffolds are the most frequently used. Type I collagen is the major collagen of bone and the most abundant protein in bone extracellular matrix. By itself, type I collagen offers little mechanical stability, but it is used to augment and enhance other bone graft substitutes. Several commercial products are available. One such product (Collagraft, Zimmer, Warsaw, IN) is made from purified type I bovine dermal fibrillar collagen, combined with hydroxyapatite granules and beta-tricalcium phosphate. It is approved for use in patients with acute long bone fractures and traumatic bone defects, and for those with voids or gaps that are not intrinsic to the stability of the bony structure. The material is resorbable and can be combined with autogenous bone graft as a bone graft extender. Another product (Healos, Orquest, Mountain View, CA) is also resorbable; it is based on a porous, open cell matrix formed from cross-linked collagen fibers coated with resorbable hydroxyapatite.

Osteoinductive Materials

When used as bone graft substitutes, osteoinductive agents are intended to induce and promote differentiation of undifferentiated mesenchymal stem cells to osteogenic cells. Compounds with known osteoinductive properties include bone marrow, TGF-β, BMPs, FGFs, IGFs, and PDGFs.

Bone Marrow

Bone marrow has been used to directly stimulate bone formation in bone defects and nonunions. Autogenous bone marrow can be harvested through a minute incision using a large-bore cannula with minimal morbidity. For nonunions, the marrow can be injected percutaneously to the site. Its efficacy is based on the presence of pluripotent mesenchymal stem cells in the marrow. These cells, however, are quite rare (0.001% or less of the nucleated cells) and become significantly rarer among the debilitated or elderly patient populations most likely to require such adjuvant therapy. Thus, it may be advantageous to attempt to enrich or culture-expand these cells before reimplantation. Bone marrow can also be used as an adjuvant to augmentation, bone grafts, or bone graft substitutes.

Demineralized Bone Matrix

Demineralized bone matrix (DBM) is prepared from pulverized cortical bone by extracting the mineral phase with a 0.5 N hydrochloric acid solution. The demineralization unmasks acid-resistant BMPs and other growth factors that remain in the matrix. BMPs promote bone formation by inducing the differentiation of mesenchymal cells to chondroblasts, which deposit a chondroid extracellular matrix. This subsequently undergoes endochondral ossification. Since the initial studies by Urist, the osteoinductive capacity of DBM has been well established; however, although animal studies have demonstrated that DBM can promote spinal fusion, clinical studies of DBM for inducing spinal fusion have yielded disappointing results compared with autografts. Limitations of DBM include batch-to-batch variability and the potential for infectious disease transmission. DBM is resorbable and provides no structural strength. It may be more useful as an extender by adding autograft, allograft, or bone marrow cells. An injectable putty containing DBM (Allomatrix, Wright Medical) is commercially available. Because BMPs are the primary active agent in DBM, it is probable that recombinant BMPs will replace DBM.

Bone Morphogenetic Proteins

The BMPs (BMP 1 through 7) are members of the expanding TGF-β superfamily of growth factors. BMPs have been cloned and sequenced and are available as highly purified recombinant proteins. The most extensively studied BMPs are osteogenic protein-1 (OP-1)/BMP-7 and BMP-2.

OP-1 Implant (Stryker Corporation, Kalamazoo, MI) contains rhOP-1 and a bovine collagen carrier which has US Food and Drug Administration (FDA) approval. It is intended to be used as an autograft alternative to treat patients with refractory nonunions. It is reconstituted from a lyophilized powder, and then implanted as a paste.

A new material containing rhBMP-2 collagen sponge carrier has been approved for spine fusions (In-Fuse, Medtronic-Somafor-Danek, Minneapolis, MN). In clinical studies, rhBMP-2 bone graft substitutes along with titanium interbody fusion cages for lumbar spinal fusion demonstrated osteoinduction capabilities.

Growth Factors

Growth factors can be enriched from the blood of patients at the time of surgery, or they can be obtained as highly purified or recombinant proteins. In the future, gene therapy may allow the delivery of genetically modified cells as growth factor factories to the graft site. In addition to the BMPs discussed previously, numerous other growth factors have osteoinductive capacity. Some of these are still in the experimental stages; some are commercial products. For example, PDGF has been shown to have a stimulatory effect on fracture healing in a rabbit osteotomy model, and basic FGF is produced in bone during the early phase of fracture healing and has been shown to have an anabolic and mitogenic effect on osteoblasts and their precursors.

Mixtures of bone-derived growth factors are also undergoing clinical trials, either alone or as adjuvants with DBM or ceramics. One such product (Ossigel, Orquest, Mountain View, CA) is an injectable matrix that combines hyaluronic acid and basic FGF. It is intended to promote fracture union and is currently under clinical evaluation in Europe. In the Autologous Growth Factors (AGF, Interpore Cross International, Irvine, CA) approach, a proprietary gel is enriched by the buffy coat of the patient's blood and is placed at the fracture site. The gel is thus enriched with growth factors, especially TGF-β and PDGF.

Nonbiologic Materials

Nonbiologic bone graft substitutes have an advantage over biologic materials in that the physical properties (mechanics, surface chemistry, porosity and connectivity) can be controlled during manufacture. Drugs, growth factors, or cytokines can be incorporated during manufacture for subsequent delayed release. Synthetic biodegradable polymers and metals are the most commonly used.

Polymers

Polylactic- and polyglycolic-acid-based polymers have a long history of use as resorbable surgical suture materials. They have also been used as resorbable fracture fixation implants. One such product (PolyGraft BGS, Osteobiologics, San Antonio, TX) is a porous polylactide-coglycolide, calcium sulfate, and polyglycolide fiber composite that has been approved by the FDA to fill bony voids or gaps caused by trauma or surgery that are not intrinsic to the stability of the bony structure. The PolyGraft product family includes granules, preformed cubes, blocks, and cylinders. The material is resorbable.

Metals

Metal implants are most commonly used as solid implants for arthroplasty. No bone ingrowth occurs into the metal implants directly, but a variety of porous metal coatings has been used as bone ingrowth surfaces to interlock the implants and the host bone. The technologies include sintered beads and fibers and plasma-sprayed surfaces. These are generally low-porosity surfaces, but more exotic coatings with much higher porosities are becoming available. Highly interconnected porous tantalum meshes are made by chemical vapor deposition of tantalum onto a vitreous carbon substrate. These meshes (with 75% to 80% porosity and an average pore size of approximately 400 to 500 μm) are in use in total hip arthroplasty components (Zimmer). They appear to be exceptionally biocompatible and support impressive bone ingrowth. Their use in segmental bone reconstruction and spinal fusion is currently being investigated. Hydroxyapatite or other ceramic coatings can be applied to metal implants to improve integration, usually by plasma-spraying, alone, or in combination with other coatings.

The Future of Bone Grafts and Bone Graft Substitutes

As tools for reconstructing or replacing deficits of the skeleton, bone grafts represent a fairly mature technology. The last major advance was the introduction of free vascularized transplants in 1975, which was brought on by the development of microvascular surgery techniques. Relatively little has changed in bone grafting techniques and indications since that time. The comparatively recent addition of bone graft substitutes, including synthetic structural materials, bioactive compounds, and combinations of these, has greatly expanded the range of clinical conditions that can be treated. Nevertheless, no single type of implant or graft is currently ideally suited for all circumstances. Two experimental approaches, gene therapy and tissue engineering, have the potential to change this in the not-too-distant future, and they may someday make the harvesting of bone grafts obsolete.

Gene Therapy

Findings from animal studies suggest that gene therapy will eventually become clinically useful. In gene therapy, genetic information in the form of DNA (or occasionally RNA) is transferred to cells to alter their gene expression patterns for therapeutic purposes. The alteration can be positive—the cell expresses or overexpresses the protein encoded by the gene (for example, cytokines or growth factors that are beneficial to the repair process). The alteration can also be negative—the genetic information is designed to inhibit or downregulate the expression of endogenous genes.

An advantage to this approach is that it can easily be used in conjunction with most of the bone grafts or bone graft substitutes discussed previously. The genetic material can be injected directly at the site of interest, as naked DNA, as a complex designed to facilitate entry into the cells, or in a viral (adenoviral or retroviral) vector. It is possible to target the expression of the gene product by using, for example, regulatory sequences that function only in selected cell types. Alternately, a patient's own cells can be harvested, culture expanded, genetically modified, and then reimplanted.

One challenge with this approach is controlling the duration of the expression of the gene product at the target site. In most instances, a short-term, reversible, localized therapeutic effect is desired and is usually achieved. However, the possibility of creating stable transformants with long-term expression of the gene product exists, as does the possibility of inadvertent malignant transformation of the modified cells.

Tissue Engineering

Tissue engineering is the result of the confluence of biologic, physical, and engineering sciences. The goal of tissue engineering is to create living biologic analogs of tissues in vitro for subsequent implantation. This can be as simple as culture-expanding progenitor cells from various sources (bone marrow, fat, peripheral blood) for reimplantation, or it can involve extensive in vitro bioreactor culture in combination with specialized scaffolds and cytokines or growth factors. Although currently the subject of much academic and industry research, no actual products of this type are commercially available for use as bone graft substitutes at this time. Limited clinical trials are underway in The Netherlands for a cell-scaffold composite product as an adjunct in hip revision surgery (VivescOs, IsoTis, Bilthoven, The Netherlands). A major tissue-engineering–related problem is that bone is a vascular tissue. Thus, the successful tissue engineering of large bone implants is dependent on the formation of a built-in microvascular system in vitro, which is still a major challenge.

Annotated Bibliography

Bone Grafts

Bodde EW, de Visser E, Duysens JE, Hartman EH: Donor-site morbidity after free vascularized autogenous fibular transfer: Subjective and quantitative analyses. *Plast Reconstr Surg* 2003;111(7):2237-2242.

Ten patients who underwent free vascularized autogenous fibular transfer and six age-matched, healthy control subjects were included in this donor-site morbidity study. Reported complications included pain (60% of patients), dysesthesia (50%), ankle instability (30%), and inability to run (20%). Gait analyses revealed objective changes in gait patterns, particularly at a high velocity.

Goldberg VM: Selection of bone grafts for revision total hip arthroplasty. *Clin Orthop* 2000;381:68-76.

This article provides a review of the selection criteria for bone graft materials in revision total hip arthroplasty based on bone graft biology.

Bone Graft Substitutes

Bucholz RW: Nonallograft osteoconductive bone graft substitutes. *Clin Orthop* 2002;395:44-52.

This is an in-depth review of synthetic bone graft substitutes that are currently approved for orthopaedic use in the United States. The author discusses the composition and histologic features of these bone graft substitutes and highlights the current lack of well-designed clinical trials on which to base clinical indications for their use.

Greenwald AS, Boden SD, Goldberg VM, Khan Y, Laurencin CT, Rosier RN: Bone-graft substitutes: Facts, fictions, and applications. *J Bone Joint Surg Am* 2001; 83(suppl 2):98-103.

The authors of this article discuss the clinical use of bone graft substitutes, with emphasis on the need to critically evaluate the claims made regarding commercial materials.

Nelson CL, McLaren SG, Skinner RA, Smeltzer MS, Thomas JR, Olsen KM: The treatment of experimental osteomyelitis by surgical debridement and the implantation of calcium sulfate tobramycin pellets. *J Orthop Res* 2002;20(4):643-647.

In this placebo-controlled study, calcium sulfate was used to deliver antibiotics in an osteomyelitis model to New Zealand white rabbits that were infected with *Staphylococcus aureus*. Rabbits treated with 10% tobramycin sulfate pellets showed a significantly higher eradication of infection (85%) than those treated with débridement only (42%), placebo pellets and systemic tobramycin (36%), or placebo pellets alone (23%).

The Future of Bone Grafts and Bone Graft Substitutes

Gamradt SC, Lieberman JR: Genetic modification of stem cells to enhance bone repair. *Ann Biomed Eng* 2004;32(1):136-147.

The authors of this article examine the potential and limitations of genetic modification of mesenchymal stem cells to produce and respond to osteogenic growth factors with the goal of developing a tissue engineering strategy for bone repair.

Mauney JR, Blumberg J, Pirun M, Volloch V, Vunjak-Novakovic G, Kaplan DL: Osteogenic differentiation of human bone marrow stromal cells on partially demineralized bone scaffolds in vitro. *Tissue Eng* 2004;10(1-2): 81-92.

Three-dimensional, partially demineralized bone scaffolds were investigated for their ability to support osteogenic differentiation of human bone marrow stromal cells in vitro. Seeded scaffolds were cultured for 7 and 14 days in the presence of dexamethasone. Analysis supports the osteoblastic differentiation of the marrow cells.

Classic Bibliography

Bobyn JD, Stackpool GJ, Hacking SA, Tanzer M, Krygier JJ: Characteristics of bone ingrowth and interface mechanics of a new porous tantalum biomaterial. *J Bone Joint Surg Br* 1999;81(5):907-914.

Brown KL, Cruess RL: Bone and cartilage transplantation in orthopaedic surgery: A review. *J Bone Joint Surg Am* 1982;64:270-279.

Chase SW, Herndon CH: The fate of autogenous and homogenous bone grafts: A historical review. *J Bone Joint Surg Am* 1955;37:809-841.

Ludwig SC, Boden SD: Osteoinductive bone graft substitutes for spinal fusion: A basic science summary. *Orthop Clin North Am* 1999;30(4):635-645.

Phemister D: The fate of transplanted bone and regenerative power of its various constituents. *Surg Gynecol Obstet* 1914;19(3):303-333.

Scaduto AA, Lieberman JR: Gene therapy for osteoinduction. *Orthop Clin North Am* 1999;30(4):625-633.

Taylor GI, Miller GD, Ham FJ: The free vascularized bone graft. A clinical extension of microvascular techniques. *Plast Reconstr Surg* 1975;55(5):533-544.

Younger EM, Chapman MW: Morbidity at bone graft donor sites. *J Orthop Trauma* 1989;3(3):192-195.

Chapter 23

Polymethylmethacrylate Bone Cement and Polyethylene

Stuart B. Goodman, MD, PhD, FRCSC, FACS

Orhun K. Muratoglu, PhD

Polymethylmethacrylate Bone Cement
Constituents and Physical Properties

Polymethylmethacrylate (PMMA) bone cement, which is still commonly used in joint arthroplasty surgery of the lower extremity, consists of a liquid and a powder in a ratio of about 1:2. The liquid contains monomeric methylmethacrylate, an activator (dimethyl paratoluidine), and a stabilizer (hydroquinone). The powder contains spherical balls of PMMA alone or added PMMA/methacrylate or PMMA-styrene copolymer, an initiator (benzoyl peroxide), and a radio-opacifier (usually barium sulfate or zirconium oxide). Additionally, bone cement may contain antibiotics (with the powder) or dye (usually chlorophyll).

The curing of PMMA is exothermic. In vitro tests yield maximum curing temperatures of 60°C to 80°C; however, maximum in vivo temperatures are much lower (40°C to 46°C), primarily because of heat dissipation to the prosthesis, surrounding tissues, and blood. The time for curing of PMMA depends on numerous factors, including the ambient and local temperature, relative amounts of liquid and powder, type and amounts of additives and inclusions, method of preparation and handling, and cement thickness. These factors also affect the physical properties of PMMA. When bone cement cures, volume shrinkage of approximately 2% to 7% occurs; the more air bubbles present in the cement, the less the volume shrinkage. Thus, mixing technique directly affects the degree of shrinkage (for example, vacuum-mixed cement shrinks more than hand-mixed cement, which contains many entrapped air bubbles associated with mixing in an open bowl). During the weeks after it has cured, PMMA slowly expands because of the uptake of water, which negates to a great degree the previous volume shrinkage. Because polymerization is incomplete, residual monomer of approximately 2% to 6% remains. During the first few weeks after surgery, most of the remaining monomer is either polymerized or metabolized. Although bone cement hardens in approximately 10 to 20 minutes, the physical properties of cement improve for about 24 hours after polymerization.

The molecular weight of PMMA is approximately 200,000; this is determined by the cement constituents, length of the chains resulting from polymerization, and form of sterilization. Gamma sterilization generally lowers the molecular weight, whereas ethylene oxide sterilization has little effect.

The mechanical properties of bone cement must be sufficient to withstand loads that are multiples of the patient's body weight. According to standards established by the International Organization for Standardization, the static mechanical properties of cement must exceed compressive strength of 70 MPa, bending strength of 50 MPa, and bending modulus of 1,800 MPa. PMMA is much weaker than cortical bone (25% weaker in tension and 50% weaker in compression and shear). For this reason, when used in load-bearing applications, bone cement should be supported by bone to avoid fracture of the cement.

Surgeons and manufacturers generally refer to cement as being of low or high viscosity. Low-viscosity cement flows easily, whereas high-viscosity cement is doughy and less fluid. The viscosity of cement is determined by the chemical composition of the cement, ratio of powder to monomer, and cement temperature. Prechilling of the monomer slows the polymerization process and produces lower viscosity cement, whereas warming the monomer has the opposite effect.

Originally, PMMA was radiolucent; however, this made it difficult to visualize the cement mantle and identify deficiencies, cracks, or other abnormalities. The two additives that are currently used by manufacturers to make PMMA radiopaque are barium sulfate and zirconium oxide. Barium sulfate constitutes about 10% of the cement weight, whereas zirconium oxide constitutes almost 15%. These compounds are found in the powder and constitute small micron-sized particles that are dispersed throughout the cement during polymerization; however, they do not take part in the polymerization process. When the cement cracks or otherwise degrades, these particles are released and can be abrasive, causing third-body wear of the implant. There is some controversy as to whether these small particles exacerbate periprosthetic osteolysis because of the small particle size and their composition. Furthermore, barium ions can be released into the surrounding tissue and result in toxicity.

Antibiotics and Bone Cement

Antibiotics are frequently added to bone cement to reduce the occurrence of infection during joint arthroplasty. The addition of antibiotics also functions as a mechanism of delivery of high-dose antibiotics to areas of previous infection. The use of antibiotics in cement during joint arthroplasty has both a theoretical and practical basis: the Norwegian Hip Registry has documented a lower risk of infection if antibiotic-laden cement is used in addition to systemic antibiotics. In general, the antibiotics added to bone cement should be bactericidal, broad-spectrum antibiotics that are particularly effective against gram-positive cocci and gram-negative rods. The antibiotics should also have a low rate of developing resistant pathogens and have a low allergic potential. In addition, the antibiotics should be thermostable (so as not to degrade during the exothermic polymerization reaction) and water soluble (to elute from the cement and diffuse into the local tissues). The antibiotic should be delivered in fine powder form and thoroughly mixed with the powder component before addition of the monomer. It should be noted that when surgeons create their own antibiotic-laden cement, the mechanical properties of the cured cement may be impaired because of clumping and suboptimal dispersion of the antibiotic powder. These properties are affected differently by the addition of various types and amounts of cements in different physical forms. During prosthesis fixation, antibiotics are generally used in a ratio of approximately 1 g of antibiotic to 40 to 80 g of bone cement. This combination usually has less than a 10% detrimental effect on the static properties of cement. If the cement is also centrifuged or vacuum mixed, the mechanical properties are less affected by the addition of antibiotics.

The addition of antibiotics also affects the fatigue life of bone cement. One study reported that compared with hand-mixed cement, vacuum-mixed Simplex P bone cement (Stryker Howmedica Osteonics, Allendale, NJ) improved the fatigue life in diametral tension from approximately 10,000 cycles to failure to 230,000 cycles in a testing apparatus. Vacuum-mixed Simplex P with tobramycin cement decreased the fatigue life to approximately 160,000 cycles, but this was not significantly different from that of vacuum-mixed Simplex P without tobramycin. However, hand-blending of 1.2 g of tobramycin crystals in a simulated operating room environment resulted in significantly weaker cement (approximately 40,000 cycles to failure), even when vacuum mixing was used. These findings indicate that hand-

blending of antibiotic into bone cement should be avoided.

Several antibiotic containing cements are currently available commercially in the United States, including Palacos R with gentamicin (Biomet, Warsaw, IN) and Simplex P with tobramycin. Palacos R has 0.835 g of gentamicin sulfate (equivalent to 0.5 g of gentamicin) in 40.8 g of powder. Simplex P with tobramycin contains 1 g of the antibiotic per 40 g of powder. Manufacturers are currently seeking approval for other antibiotic-loaded cements. A unique hip implant called the Prosthesis of Antibiotic-Loaded Acrylic Cement (PROSTALAC, DePuy, Warsaw, IN) has humanitarian device approval with the US Food and Drug Administration. This device is a temporary hip prosthesis containing vancomycin and tobramycin, and it is used for two-stage hip replacement in patients with confirmed infection with susceptible organisms.

Clinical Use of Bone Cement

The use of bone cement for implant fixation has undergone four generations of surgical technique. First-generation cement technique included mixing the cement with a spatula in an open bowl and then finger packing the cement within bone. Second-generation methods consisted of delivering the cement distally to proximally into an occluded femoral canal using a cement gun. Third-generation techniques added the use of pulsatile lavage to clean the bone more thoroughly, centrifugation or vacuum mixing of the cement to improve the mechanical properties, and a pressurization device to intrude the cement into the cleaned interstices. The implant was often precoated with PMMA to create a chemical bond with the cement, or the femoral component was macrotextured to improve the cement-prosthesis interlock. Fourth-generation techniques include measures to centralize the implant proximally and distally within the femoral canal to ensure a more uniform cement mantle thickness.

The use of bone cement is both an art and a science. The mixing and handling of bone cement must be meticulously performed so as to maximize the interlock of the cement with the surrounding bone. In this respect, bone cement is a grout without adhesive properties to bone. Because research showed that many cement cracks originated at the cement-implant interface, some prostheses were precoated with a thin layer of bone cement to enhance the bonding of the newly applied cement to the precoated implant. However, clinicians found debonding occurring at the interface; therefore, precoating of implants is less common now.

Centrifugation and vacuum mixing of bone cement are techniques that help rid the cement of large bubbles, which are areas of stress concentration. Although the former technique has generally been abandoned because it is cumbersome, vacuum mixing is a mainstay of modern cementing technique. Centrifugation and vacuum mixing have been shown to decrease cement porosity and improve the ultimate compressive strength and strain, improve flexural strength, increase the flexural modulus of elasticity, increase the resistance to creep, and improve fatigue performance. However, the enhancements of the physical properties of cement with centrifugation and vacuum mixing are different for different formulations of cement, the type of device, and mixing technique used. Vacuum mixing of bone cement has been associated with enhanced long-term clinical results according to the Swedish Hip Registry. In addition, potentially harmful methacrylate fumes are contained and evacuated in a closed system.

Meticulous cleaning of the bone with pulsatile lavage together with careful drying, use of cement containment devices, a cement gun, and instrumentation to centralize the prosthesis in bone has become routine (fourth-generation cement technique). The use of systemic or regional hypotension and local vasoconstriction also diminish blood intrusion into the cancellous bone. Enhancing cement penetration into the cancellous interstices by increasing bone porosity and cement pressure has been shown to improve fracture toughness at the bone-cement interface.

New Nonbiodegradable Acrylic Cements

PMMA bone cements have excellent long-term material properties and biocompatibility. Unfortunately, some have tried to improve upon PMMA bone cement with disastrous results; for example, Boneloc bone cement (Biomet) was associated with high rates of early aseptic loosening. Researchers have attempted to alter the monomer, polymer, activator, and other components, as well as vary the more traditional molar concentrations of the constituents to improve the mechanical properties (strength and fatigue toughness) and minimize toxic residuals. Incorporating a toughening or reinforcing agent such as polybutylmethacrylate particles or reinforcement with fibers of titanium, polymethylmethacrylate, carbon, or polyethylene terephthalate in the powder has led to increased fatigue life or strength in vitro. However, these additives are not currently used commercially.

Polyethylene

Ultra-high molecular-weight polyethylene (UHMWPE) has been the material of choice for load-bearing, articular surfaces in total joint arthroplasty since the 1960s. Total joint arthroplasty has a good survivorship rate during the first postoperative decade. In the second postoperative decade, total joint arthroplasty is commonly compromised, primarily because of adhesive and abrasive wear and fatigue damage of polyethylene com-

ponents. Adhesive and abrasive wear of polyethylene generates particulate debris that eventually can result in periprosthetic osteolysis, which is a major problem in patients who have undergone total hip arthroplasty and a growing concern in patients who have undergone total knee arthroplasty. Fatigue damage of polyethylene components in the form of delamination is more of an issue in patients who have undergone total knee arthroplasty. This type of damage is often accelerated by oxidative embrittlement secondary to the oxygen exposure of the residual free radicals generated by gamma sterilization.

Significant Changes to Polyethylene in the Past Decade

Oxidation of polyethylene is initiated when the residual free radicals generated by the gamma sterilization react with oxygen. A complex cascade of events leads to the formation of peroxy free radicals, hydroperoxides, and ultimately carbonyl species (primarily ketones, esters, and acids). The formation of the carbonyl species can be accompanied by chain scission, thereby reducing the molecular weight of the polymer. This eventually leads to recrystallization, increase in stiffness, and embrittlement of the polyethylene. During the mid 1990s an industry-wide substitution of gamma sterilization in air with gamma sterilization an inert gas occurred to eliminate the exposure of polyethylene implants to oxygen during storage. This change was instituted in an effort to reduce the oxidative embrittlement and fatigue damage of polyethylene components.

Since the late 1990s, a more far-reaching, widely recognized development led to the clinical introduction of radiation cross-linked and thermally treated polyethylenes. This technology is expected to decrease adhesive and abrasive wear and increase the oxidative stability of polyethylene components compared with the traditional (gamma sterilized in air) and more conventional (gamma sterilized in nitrogen) polyethylenes.

Polyethylene Microstructure and Cross-Linking

Polyethylene is a hydrocarbon with a repeat unit of $-(C_2H_4)-_n$ and a molecular weight of more than 1 million g/mol. At room temperature, polyethylene molecules form two distinct phases: the amorphous phase and the crystalline phase (Figure 1). The amorphous matrix consists of randomly oriented chain segments. The crystalline domains, also called lamellae, are typically 10 to 50 nm in thickness and 10 to 50 μm in length. The chains in the crystals are packed in a long-range order.

Ionizing radiation induces cross-links in polyethylene. During irradiation, carbon-hydrogen bonds are cleaved to form free radicals (Figure 2). Cross-linking results from the recombination of two free radicals to form an interchain covalent bond. Cross-linking takes place mainly in the amorphous phase of the polymer,

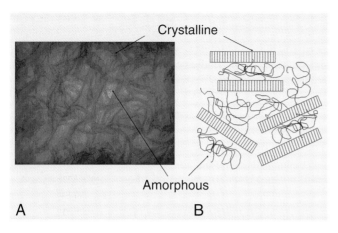

Figure 1 A transmission electron micrograph **(A)** and a schematic representation **(B)** of UHMWPE shows the lamellae embedded in an amorphous matrix. The long-chain polyethylene molecules assume a random orientation in the amorphous regions. In the crystalline lamellae, the molecules are oriented in a long-range order. *(Reproduced with permission from Muratoglu OK, Vittetoe DA, Rubash HE: Damage of implant surfaces in total knee arthroplasty, in Callaghan JJ, Rosenberg AG, Rubash HE, et al (eds): The Adult Knee. Philadelphia, PA, Lippincott Williams & Wilkins, 2003, pp 297-313.)*

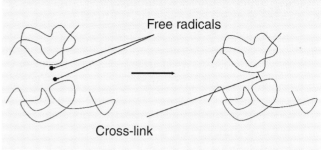

Figure 2 Schematic representation of carbon-hydrogen bonds that are broken during irradiation to form free radicals along the backbone of the polyethylene molecule. The reaction of two free radicals in two separate molecules results in the formation of a cross-link. *(Reproduced with permission from Muratoglu OK, Kurtz SM: Alternative bearing surfaces in hip replacement, in Sinha RK (ed): Hip Replacement: Current Trends and Controversies. New York, NY, Marcel Dekker, 2002, pp 1-46.)*

when the molecules are in close enough proximity to allow the recombination. In the crystalline phase, because of the increased distance between the molecules, cross-linking is not favored. As a result, the free radicals generated in the crystalline regions become trapped. These residual free radicals are the known precursors of the oxidation-induced embrittlement secondary to gamma sterilization. Therefore, thermal treatment is done after radiation cross-linking to reduce or eliminate the residual free radicals so as not to compromise long-term performance of components through oxidative embrittlement.

The thermal treatment after irradiation includes either melting or annealing. Melting is more effective in eliminating residual free radicals. This is achieved by heating the polyethylene to above its melting point (> 137°C), which converts all crystalline matter to amorphous matter and allows the residual free radicals to recombine with each other. Annealing (or heating below the melting point) is much less effective and results in only partial reduction of residual free radicals.

Contemporary Cross-Linked Polyethylenes

Several highly cross-linked polyethylenes are available for clinical use in both total hip and total knee implants (Table 1). Either gamma or electron-beam irradiation is used at dose levels ranging from 50 to 105 kGy. Thermal treatment after irradiation is either melting or annealing. The irradiated and melted polyethylenes are gas-sterilized using either ethylene oxide gas or gas plasma. Unlike gamma sterilization, the gas sterilization techniques do not have adverse effects on the oxidative stability of polyethylene. Because there are residual free

radicals in the irradiated and annealed polyethylenes, these components need to be stored in nitrogen until implantation. Gas sterilization techniques require the implant packaging to be gas permeable; therefore, the manufacturers must package components fabricated from irradiated and annealed polyethylene in nitrogen and use gamma sterilization. This final gamma sterilization step inherently increases the concentration of the residual free radicals in the irradiated and annealed polyethylene to above that of conventional polyethylene, which is a potential concern for long-term performance.

In Vitro Testing of Cross-Linked Polyethylenes (Total Hip Implants)

The adhesive and abrasive wear rate of polyethylene decreases with increasing radiation dose (increasing cross-link density) (Figures 3 and 4). The greatest reduction in wear occurs at the radiation dose level of 100 kGy, beyond which the benefit of cross-linking is minimal. All cross-linked polyethylenes that are currently in use are cross-linked with a radiation dose level of approximately 100 kGy or less. Hip simulator studies showed that the wear rate of highly cross-linked polyethylene is markedly lower than that of conventional polyethylene even in the presence of clinically relevant third-body particles. An added benefit of cross-linked polyethylenes is that larger femoral head sizes can be used. There is clinical evidence of increased volumetric wear and increased risk for osteolysis associated with larger femoral head diameters and conventional polyethylene. A recent in vitro study showed that the wear rate of 100-kGy electron-beam irradiated and melted polyethylene was independent of the femoral head size between 22 and 46 mm. Currently, 36-, 38-, and 44-mm femoral head sizes are available with electron-beam cross-linked and melted polyethylene acetabular liners.

Table 1 | Contemporary Uses of Highly Cross-Linked Polyethylenes

	Manufacturer	Irradiation Temperature	Radiation Dose (kGy)	Radiation Type	Thermal Treatment After Irradiation	Sterilization Method	Total Radiation Dose Level (kGy)	Residual Free Radicals Present?	Comments
Longevity	Zimmer, (Warsaw, IN)	~40°C	100	Electron beam	Melted	Gas plasma	100	No	Total hip implants only; also used with large femoral heads
Prolong	Zimmer	~125°C	65	Electron beam	Melted	Gas plasma	65	No	Total knee implants only with cruciate-retaining design
Durasul	Zimmer	~125°C	95	Electron beam	Melted	Ethylene oxide gas	95	No	Total hip implants and cruciate-retaining knee implants; also used with large femoral heads in total hip implants
Marathon	DePuy	Room temperature	50	Gamma	Melted	Gas plasma	50	No	Total hip implants only
XLPE	Smith & Nephew (Memphis, TN)	Room temperature	100	Gamma	Melted	Ethylene oxide gas	100	No	Total hip implants only
Crossfire	Stryker Howmedica Osteonics	Room temperature	75	Gamma	Annealed	Gamma in nitrogen	105	Yes	Total hip implants only

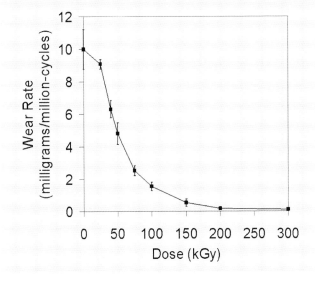

Figure 3 Graph illustrating the average wear rate of cylindrical pins as a function of radiation dose level. The pins were machined from GUR 1050 UHMWPE blocks that were first irradiated to the indicated radiation dose level and subsequently melted. The wear rate decreases with increasing radiation dose level. *(Reproduced with permission from Muratoglu OK, Bragdon CR, O'Connor DO, et al: Unified wear model for highly crosslinked ultra-high molecular weight polyethylenes (UHMWPE). Biomaterials 1999; 20:1463-1470.)*

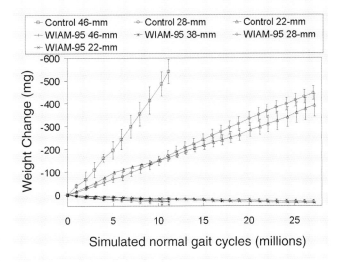

Figure 4 Graph illustrating the average weight change of acetabular liners as a function of simulated gait cycles. Control liners were machined from GUR 1050 resin and gamma sterilized in nitrogen. Warm-irradiated with adiabatic melting (WIAM)-95 liners were machined from GUR 1050 resin with electron-beam at a dose level of 95 kGy and subsequently melted. The WIAM-95 liners were sterilized using ethylene oxide. The key lists the femoral head sizes used during the hip simulator testing. Note that the wear rate (slope of weight change versus cycles) of the control polyethylene increases with increasing femoral head size, whereas the wear rate of the highly cross-linked polyethylene remains unchanged with increasing femoral head size. *(Reproduced with permission from Muratoglu OK, Bragdon CR, O'Connor D, et al: Larger diameter femoral heads used in conjunction with a highly cross-linked ultra-high molecular weight polyethylene: A new concept. J Arthroplasty 2001;16(suppl 1):24-30.)*

In Vitro Testing of Cross-Linked Polyethylenes (Total Knee Implants)

The effect of radiation cross-linking and melting was also studied with cruciate-retaining tibial knee inserts using knee simulators. Simulated normal gait or simulated stair climbing with a simulated tight posterior cruciate ligament resulted in delamination type fatigue damage on the articular surfaces of accelerated-aged, conventional polyethylene inserts. Under the same test conditions, the accelerated-aged, 100-kGy electron-beam cross-linked and melted polyethylene showed no delamination type damage. The in vitro adhesive wear rate of electron-beam irradiated and melted polyethylene was significantly lower than that of conventional polyethylene with two different types of cruciate-retaining tibial insert designs. The abrasive wear rate of cross-linked polyethylene was lower than that of conventional polyethylene when tested with surgically explanted femoral components that had been roughened in vivo through third-body damage. Overall, the in vitro knee simulator studies showed improved adhesive and abrasive wear resistance and delamination resistance with highly cross-linked polyethylenes. It is important to note that the in vitro testing of cross-linked polyethylenes in total knee implants has been limited to cruciate-retaining, fixed-bearing designs. Additional analysis is needed for implant designs that are more demanding in terms of stresses, such as posterior-stabilized knee implants.

Summary

PMMA bone cement is a material with excellent physicochemical properties and long-term biocompatibility in vivo. Newer products now contain specific antibiotics and have been shown to decrease the risk of revision because of infection. Meticulous surgical techniques in preparing bone and proficient handling of cement, including vacuum mixing, have been shown to improve the clinical longevity of cemented implants.

The technology of radiation cross-linking and melting is expected to reduce the incidence of revision surgery. Because patients undergoing total hip and total knee replacement include not only elderly patients (older than 75 years), but also younger and more active patients, the demand for polyethylene components with low wear is increasing. The significance of the development of new highly cross-linked polyethylenes will likely be identified in a decrease in mortality and morbidity rates, better patient outcomes, long-term successful surgical treatment of young and active patients, and a decrease in health-care costs.

Highly cross-linked polyethylenes have been in use since 1998 in total hip implants and since 2000 in total knee implants. Several short-term (up to 3-year follow-up) in vivo radiographic studies have shown a marked reduction in the femoral head penetration with highly cross-linked polyethylenes compared with conventional polyethylenes. In addition, analysis of explanted acetabular liners has shown improved wear resistance with cross-linking. These in vivo observations corroborate findings from in vitro hip simulator tests. A few instances of rim fracture with highly cross-linked acetabular liners have been reported. In all of these instances, the acetabular placement was in excess of 45° of abduction, resulting in subluxation and adverse component placement. Five-year follow-up studies have shown that the performance of highly cross-linked UHMWPE liners has not been compromised.

Preliminary in vitro testing of cross-linked polyethylenes in total knee implants is encouraging in that it has been shown to significantly reduce adhesive and abrasive wear and delamination. Although these in vitro analyses were rigorous, all of the physiologic variables were not replicated. Therefore, continued long-term analysis of in vivo performance of highly cross-linked polyethylene tibial inserts is needed.

Annotated Bibliography

Polymethylmethacrylate Bone Cement

Graham J, Ries M, Pruitt L: Effect of bone porosity on the mechanical integrity of the bone-cement interface. *J Bone Joint Surg Am* 2003;85-A(10):1901-1908.

This in vitro study demonstrated that the fracture resistance of the cement-bone interface is greatly improved when the ability of the cement to flow into the intertrabecular spaces is enhanced.

Joseph TN, Chen AL, Di Cesare PE: Use of antibiotic-impregnated cement in total joint arthroplasty. *J Am Acad Orthop Surg* 2003;11(1):38-47.

This is a comprehensive article on the use of antibiotic-impregnated cement in primary and revision joint arthroplasty; the authors assess in vivo and in vitro studies.

Kuhn KD: *Bone Cements: Up-to-Date Comparison of Physical and Chemical Properties of Commercial Materials.* New York, NY, Springer Verlag Telos, 2000.

This is a comprehensive book that outlines the material properties of bone cements.

Lewis G: Fatigue testing and performance of acrylic bone-cement materials: State-of-the-art review. *J Biomed Mater Res B Appl Biomater* 2003;66(1):457-486.

This article documents the fatigue properties of many different bone cements; the author discusses the testing conditions and factors that alter fatigue life.

The Norwegian Arthroplasty Register. Bergen, Norway, Haukeland University Hospital. Available at http://www.haukeland.no/nrl/. Accessed July 15, 2005.

This Web site documents the demographics and outcomes of hip and knee arthroplasties performed by Norwegian surgeons in a national registry.

The Swedish National Hip Register. Göteborg, Sweden, Göteborg University. Available at http://www.jru.orthop.gu.se/. Accessed July 15, 2005.

This Web site documents the demographics and outcomes of hip arthroplasties performed by Swedish surgeons in a national registry.

Polyethylene

Bragdon CR, Jasty M, et al: Third-body wear of highly cross-linked polyethylene in a hip simulator. *J Arthroplasty* 2003;18(5):553-561.

The authors of this article used a hip simulator to demonstrate that the wear rate of electron-beam cross-linked and melted UHMWPE is lower than that of gamma in nitrogen and conventional UHMWPE under third-body abrasive conditions.

Collier J, Currier B, Kennedy FE, et al: Comparison of cross-linked polyethylene materials for orthopaedic applications. *Clin Orthop* 2003;414:289-304.

The authors conducted this study to evaluate the effect of the various cross-linking processes on physical and mechanical properties of UHMWPE; commercially available cross-linked polyethylenes from six orthopaedic manufacturers were tested. Cross-linked materials were evaluated as they were received and after an accelerated aging protocol. The authors report the free radical identity and concentration, oxidation, crystallinity, melt temperature, ultimate tensile strength, elongation at break, tensile stress at yield, and toughness of each material.

Digas G, Karrholm J: RSA evaluation of wear of conventional versus cross-linked polyethylene acetabular components in vivo, in *Proceedings of the 49th Annual Meeting of the Orthopaedic Research Society*. Rosemont, IL, Orthopaedic Research Society, 2003, p 1430.

The authors report that electron-beam cross-linked UHMWPE acetabular liners have lower femoral head penetration in vivo than conventional UHMWPE acetabular liners.

Engh GA, Koralewicz LM, Pereles TR: Clinical results of modular polyethylene insert exchange with retention of total knee arthroplasty components. *J Bone Joint Surg Am* 2000;82(4):516-523.

The authors of this article report that patient outcomes can be compromised when a UHMWPE tibial insert is exchanged because of severe damage to the component.

Johnson TS, Laurent M, Yao JQ, Blanchard CR: Comparison of wear of mobile and fixed bearing knees tested in a knee simulator. *Wear* 2003;255(7):1107-1112.

The authors of this study found that the in vitro wear rates of the knee implants tested were comparable to those of conventional UHMWPE implants. They also found that highly cross-linked UHMWPE can substantially reduce the wear of cruciate-retaining implants.

Martell JM, Incavo SJ: Clinical performance of a highly cross-linked polyethylene at two years in total hip arthroplasty: A randomized prospective trial, in *Proceedings of the 49th Annual Meeting of the Orthopaedic Research Society*. Rosemont, IL, Orthopaedic Research Society, 2003, p 1431.

The authors report that femoral head penetration is lower in patients with highly cross-linked UHWMPE acetabular liners than in those with conventional acetabular liners.

McKellop H, Shen FW, Lu B, Campbell P, Salovey R: Effect of sterilization method and other modifications on the wear resistance of acetabular cups made of ultra-high molecular weight polyethylene: A hip-simulator study. *J Bone Joint Surg* 2000;82A:1708-1725.

The authors report improvement in wear resistance of UHMWPE with cross-linking and discuss the increased wear rate in conventional UHWMPE sterilized with ethylene oxide compare with conventional UHMWPE sterilized with gamma radiation.

Muratoglu OK, Bragdon CR, O'Connor DO, Jasty M, Harris WH: A novel method of crosslinking UHMWPE to improve wear, reduce oxidation and retain mechanical properties. *J Arthroplasty* 2001;16(2):149-160.

Using a simulated tight posterior cruciate ligament, the authors found that accelerated aged highly cross-linked UHMWPE tibial inserts can withstand stair climbing loading better than conventional UHMWPE.

Muratoglu O, Deluzio KJ: The use of high-dose irradiation and melt treated ultra-high molecular weight polyethylene in total knee replacement to decrease the incidence of delamination and wear debris generation. *Semin Arthroplasty* 2002;13(4):338-343.

The authors of this article report that cross-linking reduces the adhesive wear of tibial inserts. They also report that postirradiation melting avoids oxidation and delamination in these components.

Muratoglu OK, Merrill EW, Bragdon CR, et al: Effect of radiation, heat, and aging on in vitro wear resistance of polyethylene. *Clin Orthop* 2003;417:253-262.

The authors found that wear resistance of UHMWPE can decrease when residual free radicals are present and when components are subjected to accelerated aging.

Nivbrant B, Roerhl S: In vivo wear and migration of high cross-linked poly cups: A RSA study, in *Proceedings of the 49th Annual Meeting of the Orthopaedic Research Society*. Rosemont, IL, Orthopaedic Research Society, 2003, p 358.

The authors report that the wear rate in patients with highly cross-linked acetabular liners was lower than in those with conventional liners.

Saikko V, Calonius O, Keranen J: Wear of conventional and cross-linked ultra-high-molecular-weight polyethylene acetabular cups against polished and roughened CoCr femoral heads in a biaxial hip simulator. *J Biomed Mater Res* 2002;63(6):848-853.

The authors report that highly cross-linked UHMWPE acetabular liners, when articulating against either polished or roughened cobalt-chromium femoral heads, have improved wear resistance compared with conventional UHMWPE acetabular liners.

Classic Bibliography

Cadambi A, Engh GA, Dwyer KA, Vinh TN: Osteolysis of the distal femur after total knee arthroplasty. *J Arthroplasty* 1994;9(6):579-594.

Collier JP, Sperling DK, Currier JH, Sutula LC, Saum KA, Mayor MB: Impact of gamma sterilization on clinical performance of polyethylene in the knee. *J Arthroplasty* 1996;11(4):377-389.

Dole M: Cross-linking and crystallinity in irradiated polyethylene. *Polym Plast Technol Eng* 1979;13(1):41-64.

Frankel A, Balderston RA, Booth RE Jr, Rothman RH: Radiographic demarcation of the acetabular bone-cement interface: The effect of femoral head size. *J Arthroplasty* 1990;5(suppl):S1-S3.

Harris WH: The problem is osteolysis. *Clin Orthop* 1995; 311:46-53.

Jahan MS, Wang C, Schwartz G, Davidson JA: Combined chemical and mechanical effects on free radicals in UHMWPE joints during implantation. *J Biomed Mater Res* 1991;25(8):1005-1017.

Kashiwabara H, Shimada S: Free radicals and crosslinking in irradiated polyethylene. *Radiat Phys Chem* 1991; 37(1):43-46.

Kurtz SM, Muratoglu OK, Evans M, Edidin AA: Advances in the processing, sterilization, and crosslinking of ultra-high molecular weight polyethylene for total joint arthroplasty. *Biomaterials* 1999;20(18):1659-1688.

Lewis G: Properties of acrylic bone cement: State of the art review. *J Biomed Mater Res* 1997;38:155-182.

Livermore J, Ilstrup D, et al: Effect of femoral head size on wear of the polyethylene acetabular component. *J Bone Joint Surg Am* 1990;72-A:518-528.

McGinniss V: Crosslinking with radiation, in Bandrup J, Immergut EH (eds): *Polymer Handbook*. New York, NY, John Wiley & Sons, 1989, vol 4, pp 418-449.

McKellop H, Shen F-W, et al: Wear of gamma-crosslinked polyethylene acetabular cups against roughened femoral balls. *Clin Orthop Relat Res.* 1999;369:73-82.

McKellop H, Shen FW, Lu B, Campbell P, Salovey R: Development of an extremely wear resistant ultra-high molecular weight polyethylene for total hip replacements. *J Orthop Res* 1999;17(2):157-167.

Muratoglu OK, Bragdon CR, O'Connor DO, et al: Unified wear model for highly crosslinked ultra-high molecular weight polyethylenes (UHMWPE). *Biomaterials* 1999;20(16):1463-1470.

Randall JC, Zoepfl FJ, Silverman J: A 13C NMR study of radiation-induced long-chain branching in polyethylene. *RMacromol Chem Rapid Commun* 1983;4:149-157.

Sutula LC, Collier JP, Saum KA, et al: Impact of gamma sterilization on clinical performance of polyethylene in the hip. *Clin Orthop* 1995;319:28-40.

Chapter 24

Imaging

Thomas A. Gruen, MS

Introduction

Since the discovery of x-rays in 1895, significant technological advancements have been made in diagnostic imaging for patients undergoing total joint arthroplasty procedures as well as those who have already undergone reconstructive procedures. The challenges using any of the diagnostic imaging modalities are related to the complex four-dimensional nature (three-dimensional structural geometry and time [temporal feature of biology and biomechanics]) of the reconstructed hip and knee joint in heterogeneous patient populations.

Plain Radiography

Plain radiography is the conventional imaging method for preoperative planning and serial postoperative assessment in patients who undergo hip or knee reconstruction. No consensus currently exists, however, regarding which radiographic views reliably and reproducibly predict outcomes. Moreover, few data have been reported on the use of true lateral projections, which can provide a more realistic overall spatial assessment of the reconstructed hip joint.

Serial radiographic follow-up assessments rely on a properly performed baseline examination that permits comparison of subsequent postoperative radiographs with those obtained during the initial postoperative examination. Baseline radiographs document the initial component position and orientation as well as interface features associated with initial skeletal fixation.

The key parameters in the postoperative examination, particularly in patients with concurrent symptoms of pain, include progressive changes in component alignment or position, evidence of new interface radiolucencies suggestive of aseptic loosening, and changes in the structural integrity of the implant components (wear of the polyethylene-bearing insert, fracture, deformation, and liner/insert dissociation) and supporting bone. With improved primary and secondary implant fixation techniques, the diagnosis of irregular radiolucencies associated with periprosthetic osteolysis caused by wear particles also requires serial radiographic follow-up, particularly when supportive structural bone loss is symptomatic; if undiagnosed, it could lead to complex periprosthetic bone fractures with resultant severe instability of the reconstructed joint. The assessment of radiolucencies or osteolytic lesions requires zonal analysis of each component to monitor its location and progression of radiographic signs. When assessing total hip implants radiographically, the femoral zones are designated as 1 through 7 for the AP view and 8 through 14 for the lateral view; the zones for the acetabular component are designated as I through III for the AP view.

Total Hip Arthroplasty

During the radiographic assessment of patients who have undergone total hip arthroplasty, the recommendations for optimal orientation of the acetabular component include 45° ± 10° socket inclination as measured on the AP view of the pelvis and 15° ± 10° cup anteversion as measured on a lateral cross-table (shoot-through) view. Accurate assessment of patients with femoral stem-type components requires the Lauenstein (table-down) lateral view of the proximal femoral shaft, for which positioning during interval examinations is more easily reproducible. Accurate assessment of patients with resurfacing components requires the Johnson axiolateral view of the femoral neck. The need for good lateral views has been emphasized in recent reports on computerized software used to quantify polyethylene wear in three-dimensional and two-dimensional radiographic studies of patients after total hip arthroplasty.

Total Knee Arthroplasty

When obtaining a long leg weight-bearing AP radiograph of the entire lower extremity in patients who have undergone total knee arthroplasty, the optimal placement of the knee joint for classical alignment schemes is 7° of anatomic valgus, as measured between the mechanical axis (defined by a line drawn from the center of the femoral head to the middle of the talus) and the femoral anatomic axis (defined by a line drawn along the shaft of the femur to the middle of the knee joint and then from the middle of the knee joint to the ankle joint). For standard (short) films of the knee, the tibiofemoral angle is calculated from the intersection of the femoral anatomic axis with the tibial anatomic axis. Other radiologic alignment angles include the femoral flexion angle (which is subtended by a line parallel to the femoral condyles and the distal femoral axis delineated by two femoral shaft midpoints) and the tibial angle (which is subtended by a line drawn parallel to the plateau of the tibial component and the proximal tibial axis delineated by two tibial shaft midpoints). Using the base plate undersurface as a reference line, the tibial component should be perpendicular to the tibial shaft for classical alignment conditions.

On the lateral view of the knee joint, the femoral component should be approximately parallel to the long axis of the femur and nearly perpendicular to the central femoral cut surface; hence, the defined femoral flexion angle should be 90°. The tibial component's position should be central or slightly posterior relative to the central line of the tibial shaft; the tibial angle (which is subtended by a line along the base plate subsurface and the tibial shaft axis) should be slightly posteriorly tilted (< 90°) to match the normal anatomic posterior slope of the patient.

Implant Fixation and Stability

Diligent attention to imaging technique and patient positioning is important in detecting interface radiolucencies. The x-ray beam should be as perpendicular as possible to the component to increase the conspicuity of possible thin radiolucent lines.

At the cement- or implant-bone interface, a thin (< 2 mm wide) radiolucency suggests a stable fibrous fixation (evidence of a fibrous layer that forms after arthroplasty). This radiolucency becomes stable by 2 years postoperatively and is often demarcated from the adjacent bone by a thin (radiodense) line of sclerosis. Radiographic signs of aseptic loosening (unstable fibrous fixation) for cemented or cementless components include progression beyond the normal thin (1 to 2 mm) radiolucent zone at the cement- or implant-bone interface. A contiguous lucency completely around the components, particularly with progression over time, delineates complete loosening. Continued progressive widening of the interface radiolucency generally precedes formation of a granulomatous membrane, which is associated with unstable fixation and/or reaction to particulate debris. There appears to be a consensus that minimal (< 5 mm) subsidence of the femoral hip component without progression over time does not necessarily imply loosening, particularly for cemented collarless, polished tapered stems. The reported signs of greater reliability for cementless component loosening include progressive sub-

sidence or migration of the component, particularly when accompanied by pain.

A recent meta-analysis found that subtraction arthrography may be more sensitive than contrast arthrography in the assessment of aseptic loosening of total hip prostheses, particularly for the femoral component.

Periprosthetic Sepsis

Although no plain radiographic signs are reliably diagnostic of infection, aggressive patterns of periosteal elevation, rapid progression of osteolysis, progressive interface radiolucency, and evidence of endosteal scalloping resorption in combination with clinical symptoms heralding joint infection suggest infection. Some studies report that concurrent radionuclide arthrography and/or aspiration arthrography may enhance sensitivity for diagnosing septic loosening. It is important to understand the relative usefulness of preoperative and intraoperative tests for diagnosing periprosthetic sepsis, particularly when more patients have an increased incidence of resistant organisms and severe resorptive bone loss, which makes treatment difficult.

Quantitative CT

Recent improvements in CT technology, such as more rapid data acquisition using helical (spiral) scanning techniques, improved image processing, and better analytical measurement methods have been shown to help detect periprosthetic bone loss associated with particle-mediated osteolysis. Quantitative CT substantially adds three-dimensional data sets from the transverse sectional images to the routine CT coronal and sagittal images. Specialized software eliminates streaking artifacts associated with metallic implants and allows for three-dimensional segmentation of the CT image and reconstruction of the segmented image, which provides a more accurate visualization and volumetric size measurement of osteolytic lesions than is possible with plain radiography (Figure 1). Quantitative CT, therefore, can be helpful in preoperatively detecting the extent of bone loss and determining whether patients may require bone grafting during revision arthroplasty.

Computer-Assisted Imaging

The most recent advance in diagnostic imaging involves the use of CT- and MRI-based images in computer-assisted orthopaedic surgery of the hip and knee. Preoperative and intraoperative applications during arthroplasty procedures are typically implemented via navigation, robotic, or image-guided systems. Computer-assisted imaging is a fertile field of research, and its successful integration into daily clinical practice depends, as with plain radiography, on accurate measurements, precision, and error variability. The current and future research directions for CT- and MRI-based diagnostic im-

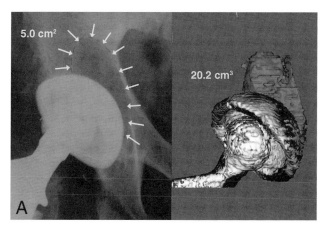

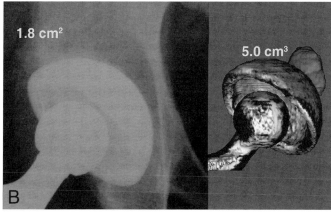

Figure 1 Two-dimensional lesion area as measured using plain radiography and three-dimensional volume-based CT. **A,** A large osteolytic lesion is evident in both images. **B,** A smaller lesion was identified using CT but it was not conspicuously evident using conventional radiography. (Courtesy of Charles A. Engh Sr, MD.)

aging advances include improved region-based point identification and requisition (registration, statistical shape modeling, and bone morphing) and kinematic analysis of hip and knee arthroplasties (range of motion and implant-related factors).

Noninvasive Bone Density Measurement

It has been established that a decrease in bone mass of at least 30% is necessary to be detected on plain radiographs. Despite this limitation, plain radiography is still useful in the initial clinical evaluation of patients with osteopenia. Noninvasive bone density measurement, however, provides more detailed information about the mineral density of bone at a specific site being assessed, such as the proximal femur. Bone mineral density is now routinely measured using dual-energy x-ray absorptiometry (DEXA), not only for screening for osteopenia and osteoporosis, but also for the longitudinal monitoring of pharmacologic treatment options for patients with osteoporosis. DEXA is the current gold standard for diagnosing osteoporosis, which is defined by the World Health Organization on the basis of bone mineral density that is 2.5 standard deviations below established values (T-score).

DEXA allows for measurement of bone mineral density by accounting for the attenuation of a second x-ray signal by the surrounding soft tissues. Bone mineral density (in g/cm^2) is determined by the measured bone mineral content (in grams) divided by the corresponding areal size of the bone within the specified region of interest. DEXA can determine the bone mineral density of specific bones, such as the proximal femur, as well as the lumbar spine, total body, and other skeletal sites. DEXA obtains a planar image of bone, and its two-dimensional nature compromises the potential efficacy of its methodology because some simple assumptions must be made regarding the geometry and structure of the bone being assessed. Numerous studies have

demonstrated that DEXA is a precise measurement method for small changes in bone mineral density. DEXA has also been shown to be sensitive to rotation of the femur; hence, correct and careful positioning of patients is essential for reliable and reproducible results.

As with good-quality serial radiographs, highly skilled DEXA operators are essential for obtaining high-quality longitudinal (four-dimensional) studies, particularly in patients in who small changes in bone characteristics are expected. Several studies have shown that inaccuracies can occur beyond precision errors related to the use of DEXA. These inaccuracies have been attributed to intraosseous and extraosseous fat content, which may compromise patient-specific evaluations of fracture risk and, in prospective studies, overestimate or underestimate clinically significant true changes in bone mineral density.

Other recent applications of DEXA in orthopaedics include the serial assessment of periprosthetic implant-related bone changes associated with stable hip and knee components (stress shielding). Most studies have demonstrated net bone loss localized in the most proximal regions of the femur (zones 1 and 7) and the greater trochanter. These findings corroborate the findings of previous radiographic studies that reported localized decreased density as evidenced by radiographic signs of corticocancellization within the intact cortex of the medial femoral neck. A recent meta-analysis of studies of the effects of bisphosphonates (clinically proven inhibitors of bone resorption) on periprosthetic bone quality examined the findings of six randomized controlled trials (four of which included patients who underwent total hip replacement and two of which included patients who underwent total knee replacement) with small patient populations (range, 13 to 54 patients). The meta-analysis demonstrated that bisphosphonate treatment up to 1 year had significant beneficial effects with regard to maintaining more periprosthetic bone mineral density in patients who underwent total hip or knee replacement than in control subjects. Patients who underwent total knee arthroplasty were noted to derive more benefit from bisphosphonate treatment than those who underwent total hip arthroplasty. These findings, however, were interpreted with caution by the authors because of the lack of analyses of clinically relevant outcome measures among the included studies.

Over the past decade, orthopaedic researchers have come to a greater awareness that the quantity of bone mineral density is not the only factor that determines fracture risk. Clinicians have observed that some bones of poor quality do not fracture, whereas apparently healthy bones do. Bone mineral density, therefore, cannot statistically account for all of the reduction in fracture risk. Among the other parameters for bone quality currently being studied is the relative contribution to the overall mechanical strength of cortical bone and cancellous bone. High-resolution imaging with DEXA, CT, and MRI is beginning to reveal the geometry and internal architecture of bones. Newer generation DEXA systems have improved spatial resolution to permit morphometric measurements of other geometric features (hip axis length, femoral neck length, and relative cortical thickness) that may account for bone quality, many of which may be determined from clinical radiographs.

Summary

The current evolution of imaging modalities, from digital or computed radiography, 3-T MRI units, and 64-slice helical CT systems to the latest generation of newer DEXA, hybrid positron emission tomography and single photon emission CT technologies, is rapidly generating a daily volume of images that may soon overload the capacity of radiologists and orthopaedic surgeons to interpret them. Nevertheless, with the growing acceptance of evidence-based orthopaedics, it is important to know the indications for each imaging modality, understand the standards for obtaining the appropriate radiographic image for diagnosis, be able to reliably and reproducibly interpret imaging results, and be familiar with recommended methods for reporting of imaging results including appropriate terminologies.

Annotated Bibliography

Plain Radiography

Bossuyt PM, Reitsma JB, Brusn DE, et al: Standards for Reporting of Diagnostic Accuracy: The STARD statement for reporting studies of diagnostic accuracy: Explanation and elaboration. *Ann Intern Med* 2003;138(1): W1-W12.

In response to the suboptimal quality of reporting of studies of diagnostic accuracy, a group of scientists and editors developed a checklist of 25 items and a flow diagram to facilitate the inclusion of all relevant information and better decision making in health care.

Claus AM, Anderson CA Jr, Sychterz CJ, Xenos JS, Orishmo KF, Engh CA Sr: Radiographic definition of pelvic osteolysis following total hip arthroplasty. *J Bone Joint Surg Am* 2003;85-A(8):1519-1526.

The authors evaluated eight cadaveric hips after implantation of hip components and obtained four radiographs of each hip from different views. Defects were created to simulate osteolytic lesions for interobserver and intraobserver agreement studies of films after reimplantation of the hip components. The percentage of lesions that were correctly identified ranged from 11.4% for small lesions to 95% for large lesions. The overall sensitivity according to radiographic view varied from 37.7% for the AP pelvic view to 73.6% when all four views were examined. Two significant observations were made as a result of these findings: (1) the actual lesion volume was typically more than two times greater than the lesion size as measured radiographically and (2) the limitations of using plain radiographs assess (simulated) periacetabular osteolytic lesions were quantified.

Dumbleton JH, Manley MT, Edidin AA: A literature review of the association between wear rate and osteolysis in total hip arthroplasty. *J Arthroplasty* 2002;17(5):649-661.

In an attempt to define a wear rate threshold for polyethylene debris for the development of periprosthetic osteolysis after hip arthroplasty, the authors of this study conducted an extensive review of the literature and found that the incidence of osteolysis increased as the wear rate increased. However, a closer review of the tabulation from the literature review showed evidential variation in the reporting of osteolytic lesions by location, shape, and size.

Engh CA Jr, Sychterz CJ, Young AM, Pollock DC, Tommey SD, Engh CA Sr: Interobserver and intraobserver variability in radiographic assessment of osteolysis. *J Arthroplasty* 2002;17(6):752-759.

Interobserver and intraobserver agreement studies, using kappa coefficients, were performed using AP pelvic radiographs from 60 randomly selected patients. The authors concluded that consistent comparisons could not be made with osteolysis rates reported by different observers and that it was more accurate to analyze a series of radiographs than the most recent radiograph.

Goergen TG, Dalinka MK, Alazraki N, et al: Evaluation of the patient with painful hip or knee arthroplasty: American College of Radiology. ACR Appropriateness Criteria. *Radiology* 2000;215(suppl):295-298.

Guidelines prepared by an expert panel on musculoskeletal imaging based on a literature review of imaging studies are discussed. The authors recommended use of these guidelines for appropriate diagnosis of component loosening in patients with painful hip or knee arthroplasty.

Kundel HL, Polansky M: Measurement of observer agreement. *Radiology* 2003;228(2):303-308.

The authors discuss measures of observer agreement, including the statistical application of chance-corrected indices, such as kappa, weighted-kappa, and multiobserver kappa.

Miura H, Mitsuda S, Mawatari T, et al: The oblique posterior femoral condylar radiographic review following total knee arthroplasty. *J Bone Joint Surg Am* 2004;86-A(1):47-50.

Three observers analyzed 55 sets of radiographs, including true lateral and oblique posterior condylar views, for detecting posterior radiolucencies and found better detection with the latter using interobserver and intraobserver agreement analysis.

Nadaud MC, Fehring TK, Fehring K: Underestimation of osteolysis in posterior stabilized total knee arthroplasty. *J Arthroplasty* 2004;19(1):110-115.

The authors found that large simulated lesions of 36 mm (prepared in two cadaveric femurs) were easily recognized on oblique films when such simulated lesions were not recognized on standard AP and lateral views.

Saleh KJ, Holtzman J, Gafni A, et al: Development, test reliability and validation of a classification for revision hip arthroplasty. *J Orthop Res* 2001;19(1):50-56.

The authors demonstrated the concise stepwise methodologic details involved in the development of a valid and reliable classification system for the severity measure of radiographic assessment of femoral bone defects before revision arthroplasty.

Teeny SM, York SC, Mesko JW, Rea RE: Long-term follow-up care recommendations after total hip and knee arthroplasty: Results of the American Association of Hip and Knee Surgeons' member survey. *J Arthroplasty* 2003;18(8):954-962.

With a response rate of 66% (447 of 682) from the members of the American Association of Hip and Knee Surgeons, 80% of the respondents recommended annual or biennial follow-up examinations for patients who have undergone total hip or total knee arthroplasty, with more frequent follow-ups recommended for patients clinical or radiographic signs of (impending) implant failure.

Quantitative CT

Stulberg SD, Wixson RL, Adams AD, Hendrix RW, Bernfield JB: Monitoring pelvic osteolysis following total hip replacement surgery: An algorithm for surveillance. *J Bone Joint Surg Am* 2002;84-A(suppl 2):116-122.

In a follow-up of 80 patients from an initial study, each with a unique cohort of hip implants, the authors evaluated the feasibility of using CT to detect pelvic osteolysis in clinically silent lesions. They found that the prevalence of such lesions was 48% using CT and 24% using radiography. From this experience, an algorithm was developed to guide medical and surgical treatment in this patient population.

Computer-Assisted Imaging

Potter HG, Nestor BJ, Sofka CM, Ho ST, Peters LE, Salvati EA: Magnetic resonance imaging after total hip arthroplasty: Evaluation of periprosthetic soft tissue. *J Bone Joint Surg Am* 2004;86-A(9):1947-1954.

The authors of this study correlated modified MRI techniques in 28 hips (27 patients) with radiographic and intraoperative findings and found that MRI more reliably estimated the extent and location of acetabular lytic lesions than the corresponding radiographs; MRI also allowed visualization of hypertrophic intracapsular synovial deposits that accompanied the bone resorption in 89% of patients.

Noninvasive Bone Density Measurement

Watts NB: Fundamentals and pitfalls of bone densitometry using dual-energy x-ray absorptiometry (DXA). *Osteoporos Int* 2004;15(11):847-854.

The author discusses the errors in patient positioning, incorrect DEXA scan analysis, mistakes in DEXA interpretation, and errors in patient demographic data that lead to erroneous results and can result in incorrect clinical decisions or actions.

Classic Bibliography

Bland JH, Soule AB, Van Buskirk FW, Brown E, Clayton RV: A study to inter- and intra-observer error in reading plain roentgenograms of the hands: "To err is human". *Am J Roentgenol Radium Ther Nucl Med* 1969;105(4):853-859.

Bobyn JD, Mortimer ES, Glassman AH, Engh CA, Miller JE, Brooks CE: Producing and avoiding stress-shielding: Laboratory and clinical observations of noncemented total hip arthroplasty. *Clin Orthop* 1992;274:79-96.

Brand RA, Yoder SA, Pedersen DR: Interobserver variability in interpreting radiographic radiolucencies about total hip reconstructions. *Clin Orthop* 1985;192:237-239.

Caterrall RC: Ex umbris erudito: "The study of radiographs is, and will always remain, a practical art." *J Bone Joint Surg Br* 1968;50-B(3):455.

DeLee JG, Charnley J: Radiologic demarcation of cemented sockets in total hip replacement. *Clin Orthop* 1976;121:20-32.

Engh CA, Massin P, Suthers KE: Roentgenographic assessment of the biologic fixation of porous-surfaced femoral components. *Clin Orthop* 1990;257:107-128.

Ewald FC: The Knee Society total knee arthroplasty roentgenographic evaluation and scoring system. *Clin Orthop* 1989;248:9-12.

Gruen TA, McNeice GM, Amstutz HC: "Modes of failure" of cemented stem-type femoral components. *Clin Orthop* 1979;141:17-27.

Gruen T: A simple assessment of bone quality prior to hip arthroplasty: Cortical index revisited. *Acta Orthop Belg* 1997;63(suppl 1):20-27.

Hodgkinson JP, Shelley P, Wroblewski BM: The correlation between the roentgenographic appearance and operative finding at the bone-cement junction of the socket in Charnley low friction arthroplasties. *Clin Orthop* 1988;228:105-109.

Johnston RC, Fitzgerald RH Jr, Harris WH, Poss R, Muller ME, Sledge CB: Clinical and radiographic evaluation of total hip replacement: A standard system of terminology for reporting results. *J Bone Joint Surg Am* 1990;72(2):161-168.

Kramhoft M, Gehrchen PM, Bodtker S, Wagner A, Jensen F: Inter- and intraobserver study of radiographic assessment of cemented total hip arthroplasties. *J Arthroplasty* 1996;11(3):272-276.

Robinson PJ: Radiology's Achilles' heel: Error and variation in the interpretation of the Roentgen image. *Br J Radiol* 1997;70(839):1085-1098.

Smith MJ: *Error and Variation in Diagnostic Radiology*. Springfield, IL, Charles C. Thomas, 1967.

West JD, Mayor MB, Collier JP: Potential errors inherent in quantitative densitometric analysis of orthopaedic radiographs: A study after total hip arthroplasty. *J Bone Joint Surg Am* 1987;69(1):58-64.

Chapter 25

Information Management in Reconstructive Orthopaedic Practices

Ira H. Kirschenbaum, MD

Introduction

Optimizing the continuum of care for patients undergoing hip and knee reconstruction requires a global understanding of a wide range of issues. Surgical techniques, issues related to preoperative and postoperative care as well as long-term follow-up results remain the foundation of care. All of these aspects of the management of patients who have undergone hip and knee reconstruction generate multiple levels of information. Successful management of this information affects clinical outcomes, direct patient care, surgeon time management, financial decisions, and communication concerns.

Management of information concerning patients who have undergone joint reconstruction is best handled in the electronic setting. The basic principles that serve as a road map for the reconstructive surgeon in the development and use of any information management system are listed in Table 1.

The world of information technology has expanded from back-office operational support to the management of all information that enters the clinical arena. What is the nature of the information? All information that flows into a clinical practice can be divided into three general categories: (1) information generated from the clinical encounter (electronic medical record [EMR]), (2) information received from outside of the office (document management/EMR), and (3) practice management-scheduling and financial information (practice management program). Expanding these general categories provides additional detail regarding the nature of information in the medical office (Tables 2 through 4).

In general, this information has three key elements: it is collected from varying sources, it is collected at different periods of time, and the type of information varies (it can be numerical, subjective, templated, and relational; part of the information is permanent, but part of it can change).

When the types of information with these generalized key elements are combined, the complexity and dependency of the information that eventually constitutes the entirety of the medical chart of each patient is apparent. Additional complication of medical information technology occurs when the attempt is made to combine the information in one patient's chart with data sets from other patient charts to obtain information about a practice, procedures, or trends.

Medical information effectively exists as an individual record of the moment, a record that is part of a larger set of records from an individual and part of a larger set of records from other patients. This makes for one extremely complex universe of information that is nearly impossible to manage without a meticulously planned and consistently applied information management strategy.

Developing an Information Management Strategy

The foundation of any information management strategy must be electronic in nature. It is tempting to believe that one strategy and/or one computer program or family of programs can help organize an entire practice and its medical records. Reviewing the basic parameters previously discussed makes it clear that the search for a single, unified information management solution would be futile and fraught with expense, error, and failure.

Table 1	Basic Principles for the Development and Use of an Information Management System
What type of information flows into the reconstructive practice?
What are the ways of technically managing this information?
What are the methods of logistically managing this information flow?
How can key information be communicated and shared?
What are some key techniques to use information from the reconstructive clinical experience to maximize an individual patient's care?
What are some strategies to use information from the reconstructive clinical practice to add to the global information database of reconstructive patients?
What are some of the methods to leverage information technology to clinically and financially improve operations in the office?

Table 2 | Information From the Clinical Encounter

Patient intake data
  Registration form
    Personal demographics
    Financial information
    Referral doctor (communications profile)
  Medical/surgical history form
    Basic past medical history
    Injury specific information
  Outcomes measures (optional)
Interview communications
  Confirmation of intake information
  Subjective history
  Templated history
  Physical examination
    Assistant input
      Vital signs
      Basic examinations of normal areas
    Attending physician input
      Confirmation of assistant
      Disease specific
      General physical examinations and provocative testing
      Office actions
  Radiographs
  Testing
    Electromyography/nerve conduction velocity testing
    Gait analysis
    Bone density
  Injections
  Bracing/durable medical equipment
  Casting
  Suture removals
Exit actions (referrals/tests/prescriptions)
  Imaging
    MRI, nuclear medicine
  Surgical booking
  Prescriptions
  Treatment referrals
    Epidural steroids
    Rheumatologist second opinion
    Orthopaedic consultant referrals
  Communications
  Work/disability assessment and note
  School note
  Handicap permit
  Exit information for staff
  Return visit (dates and instructions)

Table 3 | Information From Outside of the Office

At time of visit
  Imaging studies
    Actual films for review
    Reports
  Previous notes of treatment
  Injury/accident information
After visit
  Imaging
    Reports
    Actual films
  Laboratory tests
  Legal letters
  Reports from consultants
  Insurance information
  Surgical information
    Surgical reports
    Discharge summaries
    Consultant reports

Table 4 | Information From Practice Management/Financial

Billing demographics
  Insurance
  Eligibility status
  Benefits coverage (itemized)
Financial response
  Claims posting
  Receivables posting
  Reporting of outstanding information
Schedule
  Patient panels
  Physician (academic)
  Physician (vacation)
  Resource services
    Technicians
    Key staff

It must be determined whether it is reasonable to expect that one software program can be developed to process all three types of medical information that flow into a clinical practice. Currently, such software is not practical primarily because the tools needed to acquire, analyze, and use various forms of medical information change at dramatic rates. Arguably, any single software program can only effectively process two of the three types of medical information.

Complicating this further is the fact that generational changes in practice management software occur at a different rate than those of EMR and document management software. After many years of use, practice manage-

Table 5 | General Features of an Electronic Office

Staff training is a priority. The concepts will be new to any staff and errors are more easily exposed.

Information can be entered from multiple sites at different times. This means that while the physician is seeing a patient, the medical assistant can enter general medical information, the fellow can perform a follow-up study, and the physician can be analyzing a radiograph. When all of these tasks are completed, the EMR collects the information into one cohesive note.

The transfer of electronic information is more rapid, comprehensive, and secure than paper.

Everyone can view a record simultaneously. No more lost charts or asking who has a chart.

All levels of information can be stored in one electronic chart, whether that is a medical narrative, a hip or knee score, or images.

---

ment software offers solid and predictable function. As a result, major upgrades occur infrequently, usually years apart. EMR and document management software, conversely, is relatively new and major upgrades occur one to three times a year. Practice management software must have stability and long-term reliability, whereas EMR and document management software must be flexible to respond to the changing demands of the type of information it processes. The solution to this problem is actually quite simple. As long as the software programs that manage each of the three aspects of the information can "talk" to each other, then both types of software can be used to develop a customized information technology solution for an orthopaedic reconstruction practice.

The Modern Electronic Office

The general features of any electronic office are listed in Table 5. The modern orthopaedic reconstruction practice has several important needs that can be met by shifting to electronic documentation and digital imaging. Electronic technology can make producing the medical record, appropriate referrals and prescriptions more efficient (Figure 1). Preoperative planning can also be more efficient in that electronic technology can help streamline requests for surgical equipment and ancillary services. Data in the form of standardized scoring or outcomes measures can also be collected and organized more efficiently using electronic technology. Additionally, electronic technology now has tools to help analyze radiographs in a consistent manner.

The modern electronic office should be EMR-centric (the office should be run off of the EMR). This is not a trivial point. Many offices are run according to the practice management schedule. This may make it easier to schedule appointments and improve staffing issues at the front desk, but it does not allow physicians to harness the power of managing clinical information and revenue generated from the EMR (the actual clinical encounter).

PATIENT: SAMPLE, BOB   DOB (AGE): 10/10/1950 (54 year(s) old)   EXAM DATE: 02/21/05

CC/HPI: []
MEDICAL HX: Alzheimer's Disease; Arthritis; Asthma
SURGICAL HX: Aortic Valve Replacement; Arthroplasty; UNI KNEE
ALLERGIES: Penicillins; Animals; Antibiotics; Antidepressants; Anti-Inflammatories
MEDICATIONS: a. Abutrol Vioxx (Dosage: 25 mg SIG: 1 tab po q daily prn Dispense: 30 Refills: 0)
SOCIAL HX: Alcohol – Never; Alcohol – Occasionally; Drug Use – Pos. Hx Marijuana; Employment: Disabled; Marital Status: Married; STD – Denies Hx; Tobacco: Chew; Tobacco: Cigar; Tobacco: Cigarettes <1PPD; Tobacco: Cigarettes >3 PPD; Tobacco Cigarettes 2-3 PPD; Tobacco: Never Smoked
FAMILY HX: Cataracts
REVIEW OF SYSTEMS: General: health excellent
Eyes: denies vision loss, blurry vision, eye pain
ENT: no loss of vision, pain
CV: denies chest pains, palpitations
Resp: no wheezing, shortness of breath
GI: denies nausea, vomiting, diarrhea, constipation, change in bowel habits, abdominal pain
GU: denies urinary symptoms
MSK: excluding current complaint, denies back pain, joint pain, joint swelling, muscle cramps, muscle weakness, stiffness, arthritis
Skin: no rashes
Neuro: no headaches, numbness, weakness
Endo: no weight change Heme: no abnormal bruising, bleeding
ASA GRADE: ( ) No chronic conditions ( ) Mild chronic problems ( ) Severe chronic problems ( ) Incapacitating chronic problems ( ) Moribund patient
PRIMARY DIAGNOSIS: ( ) Osteoarthritis ( ) Rheumatoid Arthritis ( ) Osteocrosis ( ) Post-traumatic ( ) Other
OTHER DISABLING DISEASES: ( ) None ( ) Contralateral Hip ( ) Back ( ) Ipsilateral knee ( ) Contralateral knee ( ) Upper extremity ( ) Foot/ankle ( ) Other []
HIP SCORE:
    Pain: ( ) None(44) ( ) Slight(40) ( ) Mild(30) ( ) Moderate(20) ( ) Marked(10) ( ) Totally disabled(0)
    Limp: ( ) None(11) ( ) Slight(8) ( ) Moderate(5) ( ) Severe(0)
    Support: ( ) None(7) ( ) Cane, long walks(5) ( ) Cane, mostly(3) ( ) 1 crutch(3) ( ) 2 canes(2) ( ) crutch/unable(0)
    Distance: ( ) Unlimited(11) ( ) 6 blocks(8) ( ) 2-3 blocks(5) ( ) Bed and chair(0)
    Stairs: ( ) Normally without railing(4) ( ) Normally with railing (2) ( ) In any manner(1) ( ) Unable(0)
    Shoes: ( ) With ease(4) ( ) With difficulty(2) ( ) Unable (0)
    Sitting: ( ) 1 hour(5) ( ) 30'(3) ( ) Unable(0)
    Transport: ( ) Able(1) ( ) Unable(0)
PHYSICAL EXAM:

Vital Signs: Pulse, respiratory rate- WNL
General: Well nourished, well hydrated, no acute distress
Cardiovascular: No peripheral edema, pulses 2+
Lymphatic: No adenopathy
Head and Neck: Inspection/Palpitation: normal alignment and mobility; Range of motion: full flexion, extension, rotation, and side to side bending; Stability: normal; Strength and tone: normal; Sin: no rashes or lesions
Spine, ribs, pelvis: Inspection/Palpitation: normal alignment and mobility, no deformity; Range of motion: flexion, extension, lateral bending and rotational ROM is normal; Stability: normal; Strength and tone: normal
Right upper extremity: elbow, wrist, and hand is normal; Stability: no laxity; Strength and tone: normal throughout; Skin: no rashes or suspicious lesions
Left upper extremity: Inspection/Palpitation: no joint enlargement or tenderness; Range of motion: shoulder, elbow, wrist, and hand ROM is normal; Stability: no laxity; Strength and tone: normal throughout; Skin: no rashes or suspicious lesions
Right lower extremity: [] Trendelenburg.
Tenderness: [].
Pain on testing []
Strength: Hip: Flexion-[], Abduction-[]. Quadriceps-[]. Hamstrings-[].

HIP SCORE:
Range of motion: Flexion[], Abduction [], Adduction []. External rotation [], Internal rotation [] = Total []
( ) 210-300(5) ( ) 160-209(4) ( ) 100-159(3) ( ) 60-99(2) ( ) 30-59(1)
Flexion contracture: ( ) >=30(-1) ( ) <30(0)
LLD: ( ) >3.2cm(-1) ( ) <3.2 cm(0) Actual: []
Left lower extremity: [] Trendelenburg.
Tenderness: [].
Pain on testing []
Strength: Hip: Flexion-[], Abduction-[]. Quadriceps-[]. Hamstrings-[].

HIP SCORE:
Range of motion: Flexion[], Abduction [], Adduction []. External rotation [], Internal rotation [] = Total []
( ) 210-300(5) ( ) 160-209(4) ( ) 100-159(3) ( ) 60-99(2) ( ) 30-59(1)
Flexion contracture: ( ) >=30(-1) ( ) <30(0)
LLD: ( ) >3.2cm(-1) ( ) <3.2 cm(0) Actual: []
Skin: No rashes or suspicious lesions
Neuro: Reflexes. Bilaterally: biceps- 2+, patella- 2+, plantar- 2+, (-) Babinski, (-) clonus. Sensation. intact, no hypesthesias, paresthesias
DIAGNOSIS: No data for Diagnosis
TREATMENT AND ORDERS: No data for CPT
COMMENTS: []
PLAN: []

Figure 1 This screen capture provides an example of a template that combines regular medical notes with an embedded Harris Hip score. The sections signified by a "[]" are areas where voice recognition or prescripted text (SmartText, which is software that uses XML to allow complex use of well-defined and discreet objects in what otherwise appears as free text) can be entered. The *International Classification of Diseases, 9th Edition* and *Current Procedural Terminology* codes are entered on another screen.

Table 6 | Characteristics of a Full-Featured Information Management System

The Practice Management Program

Capture all necessary demographic and insurance data

Have many options for data entry

Staff typing

Web kiosk

Office kiosk

Ability to automatically flag patient charts with customized and specific practice management issues such as:

Copayment required

Owes a balance

Study patient

The program cannot be proprietary to the point where the data cannot be easily exported to another program. Once business information is entered in the practice management program, a simple keystroke should enable physicians to transfer that information to another program, such as a digital imaging program or an EMR program (often referred to as data catch or data scraping programs). This prevents the need to reenter data and more importantly allows physicians to choose different vendors for different services if they determine there is a better solution in part of the technology mix

Electronic billing

Full practice scheduling of all providers. Ideally, this schedule should be able to synchronize with a physician's personal schedule or a handheld device.

Multiple levels of security features.

The Electronic Medical Record

Import data from any practice management program

Have an intuitive, easy to understand interface

Have multiple templates that are easily customizable

Templates can be transferable not only to users in a physician's practice but nationally to forum and discussion groups

Multiple options in data entry

Voice recognition: high-level voice recognition programs are currently so sophisticated that an EMR without a voice entry option should immediately be discarded as a choice

Data entry can be done by allied staff simultaneously while physicians are working on their portion of the chart (for example, while physicians are entering the subjective history, the medical assistant is entering all past medical history data)

Option for checkboxes

Ability to develop what is referred to as SmartText or Autotext for data entry. For example, if physicians have a five paragraph, standard informed consent discussion dictation, this can be entered simply by saying "INSERT consent total hip." This can be expanded to unlimited amounts of SmartText (such as "INSERT hip score," in which the framework of a hip score would appear on the screen and physicians can then click on the checkboxes)

Import an image into the body of the note

Referrals, prescriptions and other actions must first come off of the note physicians are working on

Physicians should be able to send a message to anyone in the office and track that message throughout its entire life in the office

Some practices have advanced digital imaging systems coupled with rudimentary EMR systems. Although this allows for elegant radiograph reviews, it fails to take into account the fact that diagnostic imaging represents a relatively small component of the clinical encounter, work flow, and revenue generation. It is therefore recommended that an orthopaedic reconstruction practice should optimize EMR technology by making the EMR the "command center" of the practice.

Requirements for an Information Management System for Reconstructive Orthopaedics

In developing the framework of an information management system for any surgical practice it is critical to understand that the needs of practices vary from community to community and even within communities. What is important to an academic faculty-based practice may be less so to a busy private practice and vice versa.

It is essential, therefore, to assess the needs of the practice in an honest, straightforward manner. One of the simplest paradigms is to attempt to understand the behavior and motivation patterns of a group. Technology decisions are often easier to make after this assessment. Six distinct factors typically motivate surgeon behavior: (1) doing the right thing, (2) making money, (3) defensive medicine, (4) marketing the practice, (5) power and glory, and (6) going home. In this equation, no single factor represents more than 50% of a physician's motivation, nor is any single factor eliminated entirely. These six motivating factors are relative to each other in general and specific ways:

Table 6 | Characteristics of a Full-Featured Information Management System (cont)

ICD and CPT codes could be entered by anyone in the office at any time. For example, when a patient is sent to the radiography suite, when the technician obtains a knee radiograph, the person obtaining the radiograph enters the CPT code 73560 into the chart. This prevents dropout of procedures in the office. It is recommended that the key nonsurgeon in the office be responsible for CPT entry. For example, when the medical assistant draws up a cortisone injection, that data should be entered into the developing note for the day, which saves time for the surgeon and prevents errors.

Any referral or prescription from the EMR should be able to be printed in the office or automatically transmitted via fax using an electronic fax server.

Physicians should have complete design control over the final look of the note. Notes that are too technical are often tedious and cumbersome, not to mention difficult to read

Scoring systems should have the ability to seamlessly be incorporated into the note so physicians do not have to have separate records for patient notes and study notes. The example in Figure 2 combines a high-level evaluation and management code with a scoring system (hip score) that can be reported on at any future time. The reporting part of the program culls out the hip score from clinical data so physicians do not have to do it. The note looks more like a consultation note that physicians can send to a referring physician

Physicians need to be able to easily transmit the final note via fax to the referring physician with a customized message

Full reporting functions and data analysis through open architecture programs are a requirement. If data can be analyzed by any third-party software, then physicians are not dependent on the EMR company for all of their reporting needs

The ability to quickly list any unfinished and notes or messages

  A full-featured EMR will be able to show physicians the list of patients seen on any range of days and show either finished examinations or unfinished examinations. This would allow physicians to easily see which notes are pending and simply finish them from this screen. The same can be done for messages.

The ability to transmit the note via fax to anyone, especially the referring physician, directly from the note through a computer-based fax server

Integrated document management system

  Document management means handling data that is sent to physicians from elsewhere. Although it may be desirable to have documents sent electronically, it is unlikely that all outside sources are electronically capable. In general, patients bring forms to the office or forms are transmitted via fax to the office

  Currently, one of the simplest methods of getting documents into the EMR is to use some form of scanning.

  Scanning paradigm

    The office should have an automated multiple document scanner and each workstation should have an individual sheet scanner. In this way, responsibility for document scanning is spread throughout the office, with each person scanning their own documents

    An alternate paradigm would be a central scanning group, but this may be expensive

  The scanned documents should have the following features:

    The images should be highly compressed

    The images should be saved in a standard format like Adobe PDF files or TIF images

    The images should be linked to the chart easily

    You should be able to annotate the images

    You should be able to print and transmit the images via fax

Integrated digital imaging

  Seamless integration attached to each patient chart

  Ability to manipulate images for various views such as zoom, edge definition, etc

  Ability to overlay templates or measuring systems that can be collated and reported on

---

marketing an orthopaedic reconstruction practice may result in increased revenues, and it may also contribute to a physician's power and glory in the academic and regional communities; doing the right thing most often is the best form of defensive medicine and is a surefire way to market a practice.

Once a profile of the individual surgeons in a group is developed and then the group is averaged as a whole, what at first seemed to be a business decision is now a total practice decision. An information management system should include EMR, digital imaging, a practice management program, and other features to maximize both individual and practice goals. In other words, the most appropriate information management system for any given practice will optimize each of the factors that motivate physicians. With this in mind, any full-featured

information management system should have the characteristics listed in Table 6.

EMR systems should be evaluated as to whether they have all of these characteristics. It is also important to cross-reference the features of an EMR software program with the actual practice goals. Does a particular EMR software program optimize all six of the motivational factors discussed previously?

Logistical Application of an EMR

The modern electronic office includes a variety of software packages to manage scheduling and billing, development of a clinical note, and the production of clinical actions from the notes (such as prescriptions, referrals, messages, letters to referred doctors that include findings, and internal communications including surgical

Table 7 | Logistical Application of an EMR

Clinical Event	Use of the EMR
The patient registers basic demographic information at the front desk through a paper intake form, at a kiosk in the office, or on a web-based form that the patient completes.	Information is keyed into or automatically transferred (web-based) to a practice management software program. The demographic information is then transferred electronically to the EMR/document management program and a digital radiography system.
The patient completes a comprehensive "past medical history" form (paper, kiosk, or web-based).	A medical assistant, nurse, or physician's assistant then enters or checks the information and transfers it to the patient's EMR. This can be done at any time, using any computer in the office.
The patient arrives with important paper-based information from previous medical encounters.	The surgeon or an assistant enters this information using a variety of methods. An effective method is a combination of voice recognition and preassembled templates. Figure 1 shows a sample template that can be used for a hip replacement patient.
The patient goes to the radiology department and has a digital radiograph taken.	The patient's demographic information was already transferred to the radiology department so reentry is unnecessary. The digital radiograph is taken and automatically transferred to a screen in the patient's room or to another location for viewing by the surgeon.
The surgeon discusses the radiographic findings with the patient and either performs an office treatment (such as a joint injection), or orders a test (such as a MRI), or prescribes medication.	The surgeon enters notes on the treatment, ordered test, or prescription using the EMR. The treatment is automatically coded in the office. The requested test or prescription is printed at the office exit window and cataloged in the EMR.
The patient prepares to exit the office.	The information on all office treatments (such as radiographs or injections), referrals, and prescriptions has been sent electronically to the exit staff. They properly counsel the patient and collect all necessary copayments (such as for the office visit or radiograph) and discharge the patient.
The final note is completed.	The surgeon then enters the impression or other comments (using voice recognition or templates). The case is then coded. The information from the past medical history that had been entered and all of the treatments entered by the staff (injection, radiographs) are brought into the note completing a comprehensive record.
The referral doctor receives a communication.	After the note is completed and reviewed, the EMR automatically faxes the completed note with a customized cover letter to the referral doctor. This action occurs through a computerized fax server.
Coding/billing information transmittal	The front desk gets an instantaneous "superbill" for collection. The EMR can then send this information directly to the billing department for review and billing.
After the patient leaves the office, the staff needs to precertify referrals (such as for MRI scans)	The staff runs a report on all the patients seen that day and prints a list of all referrals that require staff intervention. This list is displayed on the screen for the staff to work with. When the precertification number is obtained, it is entered in the EMR chart.
The patient calls the next day for the (MRI) precertification number.	The staff obtains the record from any computer screen in the office and gives the number to the patient.
The patient has the test and the MRI facility faxes the report to the surgeon's office.	The faxed report is scanned into the patients EMR in the document management section.
The patient calls for the MRI results.	A message is placed in the patient's EMR that he/she called for the MRI results. That message becomes a permanent part of the EMR and the surgeon receives the message in his/her message box.
The patient discusses the case with the surgeon.	The surgeon, either in the office or remotely (from any internet connection) views the clinical note, the MRI report, or the MRI radiographs on the computer screen. The results are discussed with the patient and details of the discussion, further action (referrals to specialist, surgical bookings, and/or prescriptions) are entered on the EMR.

booking forms and letters of medical necessity). An example of the practical application of an EMR system is shown in Table 7, which presents the basic logistics of a simple patient encounter. This example can be used to extrapolate the endless connections of messages, prescription renewals, and future office visits that can all be connected together in a web of information. It is important to recognize that, unlike with a paper record, an EMR allows all encounters to be linked to each other, and allows simultaneous viewing of charts and records by all staff members. An accurate chronological patient record also is maintained.

Summary

The world of information management is changing rapidly. Current medical practices would achieve great benefits in adopting the features of EMR, document management, and digital imaging. The specifics of each type of software have importance, but the logistics of the application of the EMR in the office is of equal or more importance. This includes staff training, development of the proper application of the EMR to a specific flow of patients, and an understanding of the specific ways in which an information management system can help achieve practice goals.

Annotated Bibliography

Using information technology, in *Crossing the Quality Chasm: A New Health System for the 21st Century*. Washington, DC, Committee on Quality of Healthcare in America, Institute of Medicine, National Academies Press, 2001. Available at: http://www.nap.edu/catalog/10027.html. Accessed October 14, 2005.

This is a thorough review of a wide range of issues in electronic health records and their implications for the quality of medial care. Topics such as consumer health, clinical care, administrative issues, public health concerns, clinical outcomes research, and privacy issues are covered. This chapter also provides an overview from a national as well as practitioner level and includes a comprehensive bibliography

Kirschenbaum I, Mabrey J, Wood G III, Alexander H: *Instructional Course Lecture Series: The Electronic Medical Office. Optimizing Solutions.* [Audiotape Series.] Rosemont, IL, American Academy of Orthopaedic Surgeons, 2003.

This is a comprehensive 3-hour symposium discussing the basis of a paperless office, digital imaging, electronic medical records, and the use of personal digital assistants.

Chapter 26

Outcomes Assessment in Hip and Knee Arthroplasty

Kevin J. Mulhall, MD, MCh, FRCSI (Tr & Orth)

Khaled J. Saleh, MD, MSc (Epid), FRCSC, FACS

Introduction

Total joint arthroplasty of the hip and knee is widely acknowledged to be a successful and cost-effective procedure from the perspective of patients and third-party payers. Many long-term studies attest to the significant improvement in the quality of life after total joint arthroplasty procedures, which has been propelled by recent technologic advancements in prosthetic design, instrumentation, surgical techniques, and rehabilitation. These results, when combined with an aging population, explain the dramatic rise in the number of total joint arthroplasty procedures seen in the United States and internationally.

Most total joint arthroplasty studies reported findings retrospectively on a small number of subjects with varying severity of disease and short follow-up periods. Furthermore, total joint arthroplasty results are reported in a nonstandardized fashion and frequently use nonvalidated outcome measures. This creates difficulty in formulating predictive models that can enhance patient selection, rationalize geographic variation, or allow researchers to arrive at universally accepted treatment guidelines. These observations are not new, and various commentaries within the field have called these shortcomings to be addressed.

Quality of life measurement has become an increasingly important medical activity as people live longer and incur more chronic illnesses. The specific measurement of health-related quality of life is important both in patient care and in clinical research, helping to determine such issues as prognosis, compensation, placement, and estimating health care requirements and the nature, timing, and results of any medical or surgical interventions.

The ideal hip or knee arthroplasty outcome system should be applicable to all patients so that genuine comparisons can be made for an individual at different time points or among individuals. Unfortunately, such a system does not currently exist, despite the desirability of a universal tool for assessing outcome after total joint arthroplasty being identified as long ago as 1975. Several systems have been proposed to quantify the outcomes of different medical and surgical interventions. Unfortunately, the validity of many of these instruments has not been established.

In a systematic study of rating scales for total knee arthroplasty (TKA), 34 different rating systems in the published literature were identified between 1972 and 1992. This study highlighted the wide variations in characteristics recorded and the emphasis placed on each by the differing scoring systems. It has also been found that patients report that their most bothersome symptoms are not covered by most outcome questionnaires. The challenge for any rating system of total joint arthroplasty is to objectively assess the function of the hip or knee, independent of the overall function of the patient, which may be limited by something entirely different. The problem becomes more complex as instruments designed for primary procedures are applied to revision procedures for which domains such as bone loss, ligament attenuation, component removal, and extensor or abductor mechanism integrity need to be factored in.

Health-Related Quality of Life in Total Joint Arthroplasty

The concept of health itself can be complex. Health was defined by the World Health Organization more than 40 years ago as "a state of complete physical, mental, and social well-being." Health, however, is only one aspect of quality of life. Other factors such as income, freedom, and quality of the environment are also determinants of the quality of life. It was because of this that the term health-related quality of life has been recommended as more specific and applicable.

Some health-related quality of life measures consist of a single question, such as, "how is your quality of life?" More commonly, health-related quality of life instruments are questionnaires made up of several items or questions. These items are added up in several dimensions or domains, which refer to the outcome of interest that is being measured. Domains include such things as mobility, self-care, and well-being.

Administration of health-related quality of life questionnaires can be performed by trained interviewers or can be self-administered. Response rates are typically maximized when an interviewer administers a health-related quality of life survey by limiting missing items and ensuring patient comprehension of the item or questionnaire. However, this is an extremely costly and time-consuming method of survey administration because of the need to train the interviewer and the time required to perform interviews.

Although self-administered health-related quality of life instruments are more cost-efficient, they may have a greater likelihood of a lower response rate, missing items, or misunderstood questions. One compromise between the two approaches is to have an instrument completed by the subject under supervision. Cost-effective supervision can be best achieved electronically in the form of software that will not allow the subject to move on to the next question without appropriately completing the preceding question.

The goals of a health-related quality of life instrument may be either (1) differentiating factors that have a higher measure of health-related quality of life than those that have a worse measure (a discriminative instrument) or (2) measuring how much a health-related quality of life changes over time after an intervention (an evaluative instrument).

For either a discriminative or evaluative instrument, two fundamental properties are required: reproducibility (the ability of a test to reproduce the same results when repeated under the same conditions) and accuracy (the instrument really measures what it is intended to measure). Reproducibility in discriminative instruments is termed reliability; in evaluative instruments, it is termed responsiveness.

Like all psychometric instruments, health-related quality of life instruments must meet two general standards: reliability (the ability of the instrument to consistently discriminate among patients with a great deal or a little of the characteristic of interest; a reliable instrument is one in which patients score consistently high or low across different observers [interrater] and different situations [test-retest]) and validity (the ability of the instrument to demonstrate that it is actually assessing the characteristic of interest).

Validity may depend on whether a gold standard exists. Although no gold standards for health-related quality of life exist, scenarios may arise in which a specific target for a health-related quality of life measure exists that can be treated as a criterion. In such circumstances, a health-related quality of life instrument is determined to be measuring what it is intended to measure if its results correspond to those of the criterion standards. Alternatively, when no gold standard or criterion standard exists, clinical research relies on techniques used by experimental psychologists to deal with this problem, such

Table 1 | Techniques Used to Determine Validity of Health-Related Quality of Life Instruments	
Face and content validity	Judgment by a criterion group of experts, patients, or caregivers that the questions asked appear to tap into the relevant domain and cover all the important content areas
Concurrent validity	The instrument correlates with other measures of the same underlying characteristic
Construct validity	The absence of a gold standard of the characteristic, construct validity amounts to the demonstration that the instrument changes in the anticipated direction when administered to groups who differ on other characteristics thought to be related to the characteristic of interest; the construct is the hypothesis relating the two characteristics

as face and content, concurrent, and construct validity (Table 1). The most reported type of validity is construct validity, which involves comparisons among measures. This method of instrument validation examines whether correlations exist (and to what degree) between the new instrument and a more established and perhaps better understood instrument. An example of such validation would be the evaluation of a new arthroplasty instrument against the Medical Outcomes Study 36-Item Short Form Health Survey (SF-36).

A key property of a health-related quality of life is ease of interpretability. For discriminative instruments, this can be defined as whether an instrument score signifies the degree to which that state exists. For example, the degree of impairment experienced with osteoarthritis or rheumatoid arthritis can be classified as mild, moderate, or severe. Interpretability of an evaluative instrument refers to the differences in patients during a time period and can be signified as trivial, small, moderate, or large. It has also been stated that practicality is another critical facet of any health-related quality of life instrument. The essence of this belief is that even in the best context, greater efforts should be made to facilitate the ease of application of health-related quality of life instruments into medical decision making.

Specific and Generic Measures of Health Status

The two basic approaches to health-related quality of life instruments that already exist are generic and specific. The strength of the generic instruments such as the Nottingham Health Profile and the SF-36 is that these are single instruments that can detect differential effects on different aspects of health status. (The Medical Outcomes Study 12-Item Short Form Health Survey is validated for arthroplasty and is essentially just a shortened version of SF-36.) Generic instruments have the ability to compare various interventions in various conditions at various times and discriminate well among individuals with varying levels of self-reported general health status and comorbidities. However, the biggest weakness of generic instruments is that they can lack responsiveness as a result of not adequately focusing on the area of interest or study. Specific instruments such as the Western Ontario and McMaster University Osteoarthritis Index (WOMAC), Harris Hip Score, the Oxford questionnaires, and the Hospital for Special Surgery Score are disease-specific or population-specific instruments. Although specific instruments are more responsive than generic instruments, comparability across differing conditions may be difficult.

Generic Measures of Health Status

The SF-36 is a generic instrument that measures health status and is probably one of the most widely used tools globally. It includes eight subscales, with 35 items among them (1 additional item is not used in the scores). The developers of the SF-36 have proposed two summary scores: the physical component score (more heavily weighted toward pain and physical function) and the mental component score (more heavily weighted toward mental health and vitality). Although the physical component score more closely correlates with the status of patients who have undergone total hip or knee replacement, the mental component score has also been shown to improve with total joint arthroplasty.

For example, using the SF-36, highly significant improvement at 2 years after total joint arthroplasty has been demonstrated for physical function, social function, physical role function, emotional role function, mental health, energy, and pain. However, regression analysis failed to indicate a predictive relationship between preoperative and postoperative scores for any scale. Using the SF-36, it has also been shown that total joint arthroplasty dramatically improves the quality of life and function of patients with arthritis. However, because the SF-36 cannot reliably predict postoperative improvement on an individual basis, it cannot be used alone to determine treatment selection. These findings support the inclusion of both a generic and a disease-specific health-related quality of life instrument to assess patient outcomes fully.

Specific Measures of Health Status

The WOMAC Index is a self-administered health questionnaire that was specifically designed for patients with osteoarthritis of the hip or knee, and it is one of the most widely used instruments used to report outcomes after total joint arthroplasty. It consists of 24 multiple-choice items grouped into three categories: pain, stiffness, and physical function. The questions are ranked on a five-point Likert scale (1 point = best result and 5 points = worst result), and the scores are added for each category.

A major component of the joint-specific scoring systems is range of motion. This measure is widely used because it is an easily understood, direct measure of the joint's condition. Despite the intuitive connection between joint flexibility and surgical success, it remains to be shown how range of motion influences the most important outcome: a patient's ability to use the prosthetic joint in activities of daily living.

In a study of knee range of motion and outcome of TKA, only modest correlations were found between knee range of motion and WOMAC function. At 12-month follow-up, significantly worse WOMAC function scores were found in patients with less than 95° of flexion compared with patients with greater than 95° of flexion. In linear regression models, WOMAC pain and function scores at 12-month follow-up were both correlates of patient satisfaction and perceived improvement in quality of life, but knee flexion was not. These findings suggest that knee range of motion is difficult to predict from self-administered surveys of a patient's functional status. In addition, the authors of this study recommended use of the WOMAC questionnaire rather than collecting range of motion data by self-administration.

The choice of the ideal outcome instrument to assess total joint arthroplasty remains a complex issue. The most appropriate method is likely a combination of an acceptable hip or knee scoring system, a generic instrument (such as the SF-36), and a specific instrument (such as the WOMAC). Both physician-oriented and patient-oriented methodologies should be used routinely.

Factors Affecting Outcomes
Domain Variability

In an assessment of 34 knee rating systems, it was noted that variability exists among the instruments with regards to key domains such as pain and function. More specifically, including an assessment of pain as part of the overall global score results in a broad range of variability, with weights (coefficients assigned to parts of a frequency distribution to represent the relative importance of those parts) ranging from as little as 7% to as high as 60%. Functional assessment includes multiple factors that are not consistently included from one instrument to the next. Important attributes such as the ability to ascend or descend stairs, to walk, to transfer, to rise from a chair, to squat or kneel, to sit for a period of time, extremity weakness, spinal pathology, and other comorbidities as they impact the knee are not consistently assessed in all outcome instruments.

Instrument Psychometric Properties

There is a paucity of psychometric testing (validation and reliability testing) in the literature on the various outcome instruments. For example, poor correlation has been found among the items that comprise the Knee Society Clinical Rating System, which may indicate that the instrument is not focused on the outcome of interest. A review of six outcome instruments used to assess patients who underwent knee arthroplasty (Knee Society Clinical Rating System, WOMAC, SF-36, 6-minute walk, 30-second stair climb, and quality of life/time tradeoff) demonstrated that each of the outcome instruments offered a slightly different perspective. However, the WOMAC and Knee Society Clinical Rating System were found to be the most responsive outcome instruments. A comparison of the reliability and validity of three scoring systems (the Knee Society score, the British Orthopaedic Association score, and the Oxford 12-item questionnaire) demonstrated that the Oxford 12-item questionnaire was the most reliable outcome instrument because of the elimination of interobserver variation. This indicated that patient self-assessment was more reliable and reproducible than the objective components of the other two investigator-dependent instruments.

Outcome instruments used to assess patients who have undergone hip replacement have also been compared. Good correlation has been found among commonly used instruments, including the Harris Hip Score, a modified Harris Hip Score, the Merle D'Aubigne score, and the Hospital for Special Surgery Hip Rating. However, scores from these outcome instruments may decline over the course of a 10- to 20-year follow-up period because of changes in a patient's age and/or medical condition rather than any factor relating to the hip arthroplasty, which is a shortcoming in the reliability of these instruments.

Patient (and Physician) Expectations

The expectations of patients have been shown to strongly influence the postoperative outcome of total joint arthroplasty. Moreover, because these procedures are performed for pain relief and restoration of joint function, the goals for individual patients will differ with respect to postoperative function and activity. Nonetheless, to a considerable extent these goals will determine whether the total joint arthroplasty is successful and whether the patient believes that significant residual disability is present.

In terms of functional outcomes, poor correlation has been found between the use of objective (physician-assessed) knee scores and subjective (patient-assessed) visual analog scale scores. It has been demonstrated that surgeons usually focus on range of motion, alignment, and stability, whereas patients focus on the functionality of the knee as a whole. Several studies have also demonstrated that surgeons tend to expect better symptomatic relief than is expected from the patients undergoing total hip arthroplasty (THA) and TKA. Evaluations

tend to be comparable when patients have little or no pain and are satisfied with the results, but diverge when patients' ratings for pain increase. This discrepancy increases when the patient is not satisfied with the outcome. These findings indicate that the use of self-administered patient questionnaires as well as physician-generated assessments may provide a more complete evaluation of the results of total joint arthroplasty. Because it has also been shown that patient expectations are important independent predictors of improved functional outcomes and satisfaction following total joint arthroplasty and do not correlate with preoperative functional health status, a greater understanding of exactly how expectations affect outcomes and whether it is possible to modify these factors is needed.

Range of Motion

Preoperative range of motion has been shown to be an important factor affecting postoperative outcomes for total joint arthroplasty. In one study, it was demonstrated that patients who underwent TKA and had a high range of motion preoperatively will lose motion, whereas those with poor preoperative motion will gain motion, and those in the midrange will stay in the midrange. The statistical model was able to predict 50% to 60% of the preoperative change by simply assessing the preoperative scores. It has also been demonstrated that functional components of both the WOMAC and Harris Hip Scores correlate well with physician-measured range of motion 1 year after THA. Range of motion, therefore, seems to be a reasonably predictable outcome factor that should be discussed with patients before surgery, thus helping to avoid the unrealistic goals or expectations of some patients.

Age

Whether patient age and the number and type of comorbidities have an effect on the outcomes of total joint arthroplasty remains controversial. In a community-based cohort of patients who underwent primary THA or TKA, preoperative and postoperative WOMAC and SF-36 scores showed no age-related differences in joint pain, function, or quality of life. Although patients in the older and younger groups had a comparable number of comorbid conditions and complications, those in the older group were more likely to be transferred to a rehabilitation facility.

Preoperative Functional Status

Over the past decade, the importance of functional assessment after total joint arthroplasty has been recognized and has led to the creation of standard instruments to assess the outcome of these operations. The association of preoperative functional status with the outcome of total joint arthroplasty has been analyzed. Studies using the SF-36 and WOMAC have shown that patients with lower preoperative physical function and pain do not improve after total joint arthroplasty to the level achieved by those with higher preoperative function (especially those who undergo TKA). This indicates that surgery performed later in the natural history of functional decline secondary to osteoarthritis of the knee and possibly osteoarthritis of the hip results in poorer postoperative functional status. However, other studies have demonstrated that patients with the poorest health-related quality of life preoperatively gained most from surgery. Furthermore, it has also been found that patient satisfaction correlates significantly with general health and disease-specific outcome measures, with the highest correlation occurring with the domains relating to pain and function; therefore, patients who underwent later surgery were more satisfied with their outcomes.

Activity

Activity measurements have also been used to assess patients who undergo total joint arthroplasty. This patient population has been shown to be reliable in the self-evaluation of activity levels, with studies confirming the accuracy of self-administered questionnaires in assessing the frequency and level of activity (using pedometry, for example). Because activity may ultimately influence the relative longevity of certain implants or of an implant in different patient populations, activity may prove to be an important indicator of survivorship outcomes.

Radiographic Parameters

Several studies have analyzed the relationship between preoperative and postoperative radiographs and clinical outcomes. The uniform reporting of the radiographic results of TKA has enabled investigators to compare different implants. Domains assessed in this manner have included component position, extremity and knee alignment, as well as the prosthesis-bone interface as assessed on AP, lateral, and patella skyline or Merchant view radiographs. One study measured the width of radiolucent lines in all zones around each of the three implant components in millimeters. The sum of these measurements for each component resulted in a numerical score, with a high value or presence of radiolucencies in 10 or more zones signifying possible or impending implant failure.

The relationship between the extent of the radiographic evidence of preoperative osteoarthritis and the clinical results of THA has also been analyzed. Greater degrees of cartilage space loss have been found to correlate with lower hip scores preoperatively, but not with preoperative pain scores. Furthermore, patients who underwent THA also had less pain at 1 and 3 years postoperatively; pain was independent of preoperative radiographic evidence of osteoarthritis. In addition, hip scores at any stage of follow-up were independent of the degree of osteoarthritis observed on preoperative radiographs.

A retrospective gait analysis was done on patients with cemented THAs, all of whom had excellent clinical results on the basis of a Harris Hip Score of 95 or better; it was determined that varus positioning of the stem resulted in abnormal gait characteristics in the range of hip motion, the flexion-extension moments at the hip, and stride length. Because a large percentage of patients with varus eventually experience mechanical failure, such changes in gait may be significant.

Arthroplasty Registries and Databases

To address the numerous problems regarding the nature of total joint arthroplasty studies, such as retrospective studies conducted on a small number of subjects with varying severity of disease, short follow-up periods, results reported in a nonstandardized fashion, and the use of nonvalidated outcome instruments, the international orthopaedic community has initiated large-scale data collection projects, with varying degrees of success.

Data registries in general have contributed much to the field of orthopaedics, and particularly to hip and knee surgery. Accurate databases can be used to characterize practice patterns, identify and investigate prostheses failure, establish benchmarks, develop guidelines, and to quantify present and future health care resource utilization. Such data should inevitably lead to improvements in patient outcomes, such as that evidenced by the drop in revision THAs observed in Sweden after implementation of the national registry there. However, troublesome issues still need to be resolved in establishing effective, inclusive databases. The arguments regarding such issues as individual institution and surgeon profiling, case mix stratification as it relates to outcomes, confidentiality, legal discoverability, and use of data for public accountability are far from resolved. Clinicians need to feel confident that these databases will accomplish the desired mutual objective of ensuring the best outcomes for their patients, and the potential uses of resultant data need to be clearly outlined at the outset. The public too needs to feel that the process is appropriately transparent and must be educated in the process and objectives of these databases. The general requirements of successful health data registries are listed in Table 2. It is important to reduce the cost and data collection burden of this process, and it stands to reason that data collected should coincide with what is already collected both clinically and administratively. Although a complex process, uniform databases and related software, incorporating outcomes instruments, should ideally be established to interact efficiently with electronic medical records.

Table 2 | General Guidelines for a Successful Health Data Registry

Clear objectives

A valid protocol design

Clear inclusion and exclusion criteria

A study sample that is representative of the universal population

A comprehensive collection of variables necessary to answer the project objective(s)

Mechanisms implemented to track patients

Mechanisms implemented to ensure a high level of data integrity

Blinding of data collection personnel

A method to rectify methodologic problems

Although industry, government, and the consumer stand to gain from the decreased revision rates anticipated with the establishment of effective registries, the issue of who should pay for what in an initially expensive process remains to be fully resolved.

The AAOS MODEMS Experience

In 1994, the American Academy of Orthopaedic Surgeons (AAOS) established an outcomes initiative following a 3-year planning and development process: the Musculoskeletal Outcomes Data Evaluation and Management System (MODEMS). This project had two goals: (1) to create validated patient-based functional health questionnaires that would become the gold standard for musculoskeletal research, and (2) to collect data from practicing orthopaedists using these instruments.

In 1998, Version 2.0 of the MODEMS questionnaire was released and database elements included demographic and clinical information and health and well-being scales. The MODEMS initiative began in 1997 with a target of 1,000 surgeons enrolled in the project and 50,000 records to be completed by 1999. The project was terminated in 2000 after failing to meet this target goal. Although the AAOS Lower Limb Outcomes Questionnaire comprised the largest subset of data in the database, many of the data regarding patients who underwent THA and TKA could not be used because of various data integrity issues and lack of follow-up.

Future Directions

Problems encountered with the MODEMS data collection project are instructive if the objective of a useful, large-scale arthroplasty database is to be achieved. Factors identified as critical to the process include clear design, specific processes to recruit and follow-up patients, and clear inclusion and exclusion criteria.

Careful design of data collection forms is required to capture pertinent patient, procedure, surgeon, institution, and outcome variables (describe the population concerned), and allow for analyses that will be both de-

scriptive as well as more formal (posit testing of specific hypothesis). Deriving a conceptual model with the variables for which data must be collected to answer the objectives and delineating the interactions between these variables not only averts important variable omissions, but also helps in developing aims and forming an analytic plan. Forms must also be streamlined to minimize respondent (patient as well as physician) burden to minimize dropout. Data collection management must be able to quickly identify errors and remedy them. Because of its slow and laborious nature, paper-based data collection is associated with weak corrective feedback. More recently developed automated data collection systems will hopefully circumvent the issues associated with paper-based data collection and protect against entering conflicting or missing data elements. It seems critical, therefore, that a data operation center should be established and charged with collecting the information from patients and surgeons; ensuring accurate and timely form completion and data entry; maintaining the database; data analyses; and maintaining patient and surgeon confidentiality.

Structured postoperative follow-up schedules are a requirement, and accurate completion of follow-up questionnaires is essential to enable any data analysis to take place. When a patient is no longer available for follow-up, there must be mechanisms in place to track the patient.

Feedback loops are necessary to affect not only the data collection process, but the consumers of this information, who would include patients, surgeons, hospitals, and third-party payers. These feedback loops would serve to improve quality of care, identify issues, and streamline health care expenditures.

Summary

It is widely accepted now that effective outcomes analysis is critical to the future development of quality care in total knee and hip arthroplasty. Surgeons need to remain at the forefront of this effort to ensure that appropriate systems are established according to the principles outlined previously. It will be important for physicians to maintain a degree of control over the system because surgeons are best positioned to act as patient advocates in this process by directing the development of total joint arthroplasty in a responsible and progressive fashion. This will only be possible through the successful establishment of comprehensive and universally accepted total joint arthroplasty outcome assessment instruments.

Annotated Bibliography

Health-Related Quality of Life in Total Joint Arthroplasty

Davies AP: Rating systems for total knee replacement. *Knee* 2002;9(4):261-266.

The author summarizes many of the scoring systems available for the assessment of patients undergoing TKA. It was concluded that the WOMAC, SF-36, and Oxford 12-Item Knee Questionnaire have undergone the most thorough assessment of reliability and validity and are therefore appropriate for the assessment of outcome after TKA.

Holtzman J, Saleh K, Kane R: Effect of baseline functional status and pain on outcomes of total hip arthroplasty. *J Bone Joint Surg Am* 2002;84-A(11):1942-1948.

This study assessed 1,120 patients who underwent THA regarding activity level, pain, need for assistance for walking, the distance that the patient could walk, and ability to perform instrumental activities of daily living. The findings suggested that the poorer the preoperative status, the more patients may benefit from THA. Findings also showed that patients with a poor preoperative status may not have as good an outcome as those with a better preoperative status.

Holtzman J, Saleh K, Kane R: Gender differences in functional status and pain in a Medicare population undergoing elective total hip arthroplasty. *Med Care* 2002; 40(6):461-470.

This study of 1,120 Medicare patients undergoing THA demonstrated that women reported more severe pain and functional deficits preoperatively (independent of comorbidities and age) than men. Functional discrepancies persisted at 1 year postoperatively. The authors also reported that women covered by Medicare are more disabled at the time of THA and do not do as well 1 year postoperatively.

Kiebzak GM, Campbell M, Mauerhan DR: The SF-36 general health status survey documents the burden of osteoarthritis and the benefits of total joint arthroplasty: But why should we use it? *Am J Manag Care* 2002;8(5): 463-474.

In a prospective study of 622 patients who underwent THA or TKA, the SF-36 was administered over 2 years postoperatively. The SF-36 was found to have the sensitivity to document improvement in health-related quality of life and to reveal differences between THA and TKA and between men and women. However, the authors concluded that routine use of outcome assessment instruments to monitor these patients is costly and unjustified.

Mahomed NN, Liang MH, Cook EF, et al: The importance of patient expectations in predicting functional outcomes after total joint arthroplasty. *J Rheumatol* 2002;29(6):1273-1279.

The authors prospectively evaluated a cohort of 191 patients who underwent THA or TKA with self-reported SF-36 WOMAC scores as well as a satisfaction scale before and 6 months after surgery. Patient expectations regarding surgery were not associated with their age, gender, index joint of surgery, or correlated with preoperative functional health status, but were important independent predictors of improved functional outcomes and satisfaction.

Robertsson O, Dunbar MJ: Patient satisfaction compared with general health and disease-specific questionnaires in knee arthroplasty patients. *J Arthroplasty* 2001; 16(4):476-482.

The results of two self-administered postal surveys of the same group of patients who underwent TKA were compared in this study. The first simple questionnaire regarding patient satisfaction had a much greater response than the second, which contained the same simple satisfaction questionnaire along with several general health (Nottingham Health Profile, SF-36, SF-12) and disease/site-specific (Oxford 12-Item Knee Questionnaire, WOMAC) questionnaires. The authors found that patient satisfaction correlated significantly with general health and disease-specific outcome measures, and that patients who did not respond were more often dissatisfied.

Specific and Generic Measures of Health Status
Bach CM, Feizelmeier H, Kaufmann G, Sununu T, Gobel G, Krismer M: Categorization diminishes the reliability of hip scores. *Clin Orthop* 2003;411:166-173.

Scoring systems related to outcomes of THA may generate results as a numeric system (score) or as a category system (excellent, good, fair, and poor). This study analyzed 83 THAs that were followed up at an average of 6.2 years and scored using five different hip scores. Higher interobserver reliability (correlation coefficient, 0.71 to 0.81) and interscore correlation (correlation coefficient, 0.81 to 0.92) were found for the numeric systems.

Boardman DL, Dorey F, Thomas BJ, Lieberman JR: The accuracy of assessing total hip arthroplasty outcomes: A prospective correlation study of walking ability and 2 validated measurement devices. *J Arthroplasty* 2000; 15(2):200-204.

This study of 30 patients who underwent THA and were evaluated preoperatively and 1 year postoperatively with the WOMAC and SF-36 and objectively evaluated at the same interval with basic stride analysis and the 6-minute walk test established a correlation between walking ability and the functional aspects of the WOMAC and the SF-36, thereby supporting the use of these instruments in assessing functional outcome after THA.

Hunsaker FG, Cioffi DA, Amadio PC, Wright JG, Caughlin B: The American Academy of Orthopaedic Surgeons outcomes instruments: Normative values from the general population. *J Bone Joint Surg Am* 2002;84-A(2):208-215.

The standardization of 11 AAOS musculoskeletal outcomes measures is described based on an overall panel response rate of 67.4%. All 11 scales exhibited high internal reliability as well as discriminant and convergent validity, thus meeting the objective of providing reliable and valid normative data for use in clinical and research settings.

Lingard EA, Katz JN, Wright RJ, Wright EA, Sledge CB: Kinemax Outcomes Group: Validity and responsiveness of the Knee Society Clinical Rating System in comparison with the SF-36 and WOMAC. *J Bone Joint Surg Am* 2001;83-A(12):1856-1864.

This is a prospective observational study of the outcomes of primary TKA designed to validate the Knee Society Clinical Rating System (knee and function scores) and to compare its responsiveness with that of the WOMAC and the SF-36 in 697 patients with a mean age of 70 years. The WOMAC, SF-36, patient satisfaction, and demographic data were obtained with self-administered questionnaires. The WOMAC and SF-36 were found to be more responsive measures of the outcome of TKA, and were less labor-intensive in removing observer bias compared with the Knee Society Clinical Rating System.

Nilsdotter AK, Roos EM, Westerlund JP, Roos HP, Lohmander LS: Comparative responsiveness of measures of pain and function after total hip replacement. *Arthritis Rheum* 2001;45(3):258-262.

In this study the Functional Assessment System, WOMAC, and SF-36 were used to assess 20 patients who underwent THA (mean age, 72.6 years) preoperatively and up to 1 year postoperatively. The pain and function scores of the WOMAC and SF-36 showed greater responsiveness than the Functional Assessment System. Self-administered questionnaires such as the WOMAC and SF-36 are more responsive measures of pain and function than range of motion, performance tests, and observer-administered questions (as in the Functional Assessment System).

Ragab AA: Validity of self-assessment outcome questionnaires: Patient-physician discrepancy in outcome interpretation. *Biomed Sci Instrum* 2003;39:579-584.

Patient assessment outcome index questionnaires were reviewed for 103 patients who underwent cementless THA. A modified Harris Hip Score was compared with the clinical Harris Hip Score obtained at the last office visit at mean follow-up of 4 years. Although there was a low correlation between the scores, particularly in patients with a pain score of less than 30 points, it was found that the etiology of perceived hip pain was actually the hip in only 5 of 26 patients. The validity of self-administered outcome questionnaires may therefore be impacted by patients' misinterpretation of apparently straightforward questions.

Saleh KJ, Macaulay A, Radosevich DM, et al: The Knee Society Index of Severity for failed total knee arthroplasty: Development and validation. *Clin Orthop* 2001; 392:153-165.

This article describes the development and validation of an Index of Severity for Failed Total Knee Arthroplasty by the Knee Society.

Saleh KJ, Radosevich DM, Kassim RA, et al: Comparison of commonly used orthopaedic outcome measures using palm-top computers and paper surveys. *J Orthop Res* 2002;20(6):1146-1151.

The collection of health-related quality of life data (SF-36 and WOMAC) from patients who underwent hip and/or knee arthroplasty was compared using handheld computers and self-administered (paper) questionnaires. Although the handheld computers and self-administered (paper) questionnaires provided comparable results, there was a lack of reliability across modes of administration, which indicates that additional study is needed before implementing newer data-capture technologies.

Arthroplasty Registries and Databases

The Norwegian Arthroplasty Register. Bergen, Norway, Haukeland University Hospital. Available at http://www.haukeland.no/nrl/. Accessed July 15, 2005.

This Web site documents the demographics and outcomes of hip and knee arthroplasties performed by Norwegian surgeons in a national registry.

The Swedish National Hip Register. Göteborg, Sweden, Göteborg University. Available at http://www.jru.orthop.gu.se/. Accessed July 15, 2005.

This Web site documents the demographics and outcomes of hip arthroplasties performed by Swedish surgeons in a national registry.

Classic Bibliography

Bellamy N, Buchanan WW, Goldsmith CH, Campbell J, Stitt LW: Validation study of WOMAC: A health status instrument for measuring clinically important, patient-relevant outcomes following total hip or knee arthroplasty in osteoarthritis. *J Rheumatol* 1988;15:1833-1840.

Brinker MR, Lund PJ, Cox DD, Barrack RL: Demographic biases found in scoring instruments of total hip arthroplasty. *J Arthroplasty* 1996;11(7):820-830.

Fortin PR, Clarke AE, Joseph L, et al: Outcomes of total hip and knee replacement: preoperative functional status predicts outcomes at six months after surgery. *Arthritis Rheum* 1999;42:1722-1728.

Insall JN, Dorr LD, Scott RD, Scott WN: Rationale of the Knee Society Clinical Rating system. *Clin Orthop* 1989;248:13-14.

Lieberman JR, Dorey F, Shekelle P, et al: Differences between patients' and physicians' evaluations of outcome after total hip arthroplasty. *J Bone Joint Surg Am* 1996;78(6):835-838.

Lieberman JR, Dorey F, Shekelle P, et al: Outcome after total hip arthroplasty: Comparison of a traditional disease-specific and a quality-of-life measurement of outcome. *J Arthroplasty* 1997;12(6):639-645.

McGuigan FX, Hozack WJ, Moriarty L, Eng K, Rothman RH: Predicting quality-of-life outcomes following total joint arthroplasty: Limitations of the SF-36 Health Status Questionnaire. *J Arthroplasty* 1995;10:742-747.

Schmalzried TP: Quantitative assessment of walking activity after total hip or knee replacement. *J Bone Joint Surg Am* 1998;80(1):54-59.

Ware JE, Kosinski M: *SF-36 Physical and Mental Health Summary Scales: A Manual for Users of Version 1.* Lincoln, RI, Quality Metric Incorporated, 2001.

Wolf AM: Reproducibility and validity of a self-administered physical activity questionnaire. *Int J Epidemiol* 1994;23(5):991-999.

Zahiri CA, Schmalzried TP, Szuszczewicz ES, Amstutz HC: Assessing activity in joint replacement patients. *J Arthroplasty* 1998;13(8):890-895.

Chapter 27

Arthrodesis of the Hip and Knee

John J. Callaghan, MD

Francis W. Cooke, PhD

David A. McQueen, MD

John R. Schurman II, MD

Arthrodesis of the Hip

With the proven ability of total hip arthroplasty to obtain durable long-term fixation with cementless implants and possibly reduce bearing surface wear with the use of newer polyethylenes and hard-on-hard bearings, hip arthrodesis is no longer the treatment of choice for patients with incapacitating unilateral end-stage hip arthritis. Nonetheless, no long-term total hip arthroplasty outcomes studies have yet been published for active patients younger than 25 years with unilateral arthritis of the hip.

Indications and Contraindications

Hip arthrodesis should be considered as a treatment option for young active patients with unilateral arthritis of the hip, especially if these patients have no potential for employment other than hard manual labor. Hip arthrodesis has also recently been reported as a treatment for patients with pelvic tumors and proximal femoral focal deficiency.

Before performing hip arthrodesis, an extensive preoperative history and physical examination are necessary to ensure that patients have no other lower extremity musculoskeletal conditions or symptoms, such as back, ipsilateral knee, or contralateral hip pain. Education and counseling of patients and their families is also necessary to ensure that they understand the limitations associated with the procedure, such as inconvenience in sitting, as well as the only indications for takedown of the fusion (markedly limiting back, contralateral hip, or ipsilateral knee pain).

The long-term benefits as well as the optimal position of the fusion have been well documented in 35-year follow-up studies. Although ipsilateral knee, contralateral hip, and low back pain develop in most patients over time, only 15% to 20% require conversion to total hip replacement, usually later than 20 years after the procedure. The position of the fusion to prevent late-onset symptoms involves flexion of 20° to 35°, rotation of neutral to 5° external, and adduction of 0° to 5°. Abduction and internal rotation should be avoided to prevent long-term lower extremity symptoms and abnormal gait.

Various methods of fusion have been described, with a cobra plate technique being the most commonly used in the past. Success with double plating, dynamic compression screws, and external fixation has recently been reported, with fusion rates of 80% to 100%.

Conversion of the hip arthrodesis to total hip replacement should be considered only for patients with severe back, ipsilateral knee, and contralateral hip pain. Ipsilateral knee replacement and contralateral hip replacement without fusion takedown can be considered, but should be limited to inactive patients. A recent long-term follow-up study of 208 patients who underwent hip arthrodesis conversion to total hip replacement and were followed for an average of 9.2 years found that 79% of patients reported minimal if any pain, 83% reported good or excellent function, and 79% reported good or excellent range of motion. Only 12 patients required revision. The 10- and 26-year implant survival rates were 96% and 73%, respectively. Fifty percent of the patients required ambulatory supports. Another study demonstrated better postoperative gait if the hip was reconstructed to the original anatomic hip center.

Arthrodesis of the Knee

Arthrodesis of the knee has long been considered a demanding procedure that is subject to a variety of postoperative complications and often results in marginal or unacceptable outcomes. For these reasons, arthrodesis has typically been held in reserve as a final salvage procedure for patients with irretrievably failed total knee arthroplasties and other comparable conditions. Initially, the indications for arthrodesis were poliomyelitis, tuberculosis, and sepsis. The pioneering surgeons who first treated these conditions with arthrodesis were quick to recognize the necessity for rigid fixation and firm compressional apposition of the femoral and tibial osteotomies. With the proliferation of total knee replacement surgery in the last quarter of the 20th century, failed total knee arthroplasty became the primary indication for

Table 1 | Success Rate of Early Attempts to Salvage Failed Total Knee Arthroplasties by Arthrodesis

Study	Predisposing (Failed) Arthroplasty Type	Success Rate (%)
Vlasak et al (1995)	Resurfacing	75
Hagemann et al (1978)	Resurfacing	71
	Hinged	57
Brodersen et al (1979)	Resurfacing	81
	Hinged	56
Vahvanen (1979)	Resurfacing	50
Knutson et al (1984)	Resurfacing	68
	Constrained	39

knee arthrodesis. Failed total knee arthroplasty introduced additional arthrodesis problems associated with shortened limbs and reduced periarticular soft tissue and bone stock. Initially, arthrodesis salvage of irretrievably failed total knee arthroplasty resulted in relatively high rates of nonunion (Table 1). More recently, advances in technique and instrumentation have simplified the procedure and improved the success rate.

Indications and Contraindications

Currently, the primary indication for surgical arthrodesis of the knee is an irretrievably failed total knee arthroplasty resulting from persistent infection and involving such extensive destruction of soft and hard tissue that exchange arthroplasty is not a reasonable option. Other indications include total knee arthroplasties that are subject to recurring aseptic loosening, knees with a grossly deficient extensor mechanism, and knees that have undergone tumor resection. In addition, some patients with intractable pain or persistent instability associated with total knee arthroplasty may also be candidates for arthrodesis. When these primary indications are present, certain secondary factors may support the choice of arthrodesis as the most appropriate treatment. These secondary indications include young patient age, high functional demands, and the absence of complicating comorbidities.

Contraindications for arthrodesis include significant disability because of age or multiple joint disease, especially ipsilateral hip or ankle arthropathy, or contralateral amputation or knee fusion. Persistent nonunion of a periarticular fracture or massive periarticular bone loss may also militate against successful arthrodesis. Finally, patient reluctance may be an important factor in patients with a long history of repeated failed surgeries.

Alternatives to Arthrodesis

In patients for whom primary or revision arthroplasty of the knee is contraindicated, the only alternatives to ar-

throdesis are resection arthroplasty and amputation. Although both of these procedures generally result in poor functional outcomes, they may be appropriate in patients with persistent life-threatening infection, extreme disability (especially in those who are already nonambulatory), and bone loss or soft-tissue deficiency that is so extensive as to obviate arthrodesis as an option. Some patients with a resection arthroplasty may be capable of limited ambulation, usually with the aid of assistive devices. Above-knee amputees are capable of considerable mobility with a prosthesis if other comorbid factors are limited, but such patients are also likely to be good candidates for arthrodesis. Although amputation or resection arthroplasty may be appropriate for selected patients, for most severely compromised knee patients, successful arthrodesis provides a sound sensate limb that facilitates ambulation and the performance of daily activities at a higher level of efficiency and cost-effectiveness than either of these alternatives.

Procedures

In patients with infection, especially those with established persistent infection and those in whom the causative organism is particularly virulent, every effort must be made to ensure that the infection is fully resolved before an attempt is made to perform arthrodesis with implanted fixation hardware. Anti-infective therapy should be based on a proven protocol equivalent to the first step of the two-stage revision of infected total knee arthroplasty. Such protocols will generally recommend removal of all previous implants and materials, including bone cement and soft tissue, hard tissue débridement if necessary, aggressive antibiotic therapy, and a thorough assessment of treatment effectiveness.

In current practice, two arthrodesis techniques, external fixation and intramedullary nailing, provide the highest rates of fusion and the shortest fusion times. Because of the limited amount of subcutaneous hardware associated with external fixation, this method has been recommended by some for patients in whom the complete elimination of infection cannot be ensured. Ring type external fixation devices, such as the Ilizarov system, that rely on relatively thin wires for transcutaneous skeletal engagement can provide adequate intraoperative compression, but not dynamic compression, while minimizing the amount of subcutaneous hardware required. These systems are tedious to apply, however, and are so bulky that they may not be well accepted by the patient. Nonring external fixation devices, such as the Hoffman and the Wagner systems, are better tolerated, but may yield somewhat lower fusion rates because adequate intraoperative compression is more difficult to achieve.

Intramedullary rod fixation is becoming a relatively routine arthrodesis procedure that provides a high level

Table 2 | Outcomes for Arthrodesis Procedures

Study	Fixation Method	No. of Patients	Success Rate (%)	Mean Fusion (weeks)	Mean Complication Rate* (%)
Garberina et al (2001)	Ring external fixation	19	68	20.0	84
David et al (2001)	Ring external fixation	12	100	27.6	58
Manzotti et al (2001)	Ring external fixation	5	100	29.5	N/A
Oostenbroek et al (2001)	Ring external fixation	15	93	28.0	80
Hak et al (1995)	One- and two-column external fixation	36	61	N/A	59
Domingo et al (2003)	One- and two-column external fixation	15	100	26.9	47
	Short intramedullary rod	11	91	19.5	36
Waldman et al (1999)	Long intramedullary rod	21	95	27.3	38
Lai et al (1998)	Short intramedullary rod	33	94	22.5	33
Arroyo et al (1997)	Long intramedullary rod	21†	90	36.4	38
Ellingsen et al (1994)	Long intramedullary rod	18	89	23.8	55

*Rate of complication among patients who achieved prompt fusion
†Includes 16 patients who underwent previous tumor resection

of success and good patient acceptance. Both long rod and short rod systems are available. The long rods extend through most or all of the femur and tibia. Some are unitary and some are bicomponent devices requiring a connecting fitting at the level of the knee. Cross-locking screws provide excellent intraoperative compression and rotational stability. Some long rods require incisions at the hip as well as at the knee and may be impossible to insert in patients with femoral deformity or in those with an ipsilateral hip prosthesis. Distal and proximal dissemination of knee sepsis is also a possibility with long rods in patients in whom complete resolution of a preexisting infection has not been achieved. Some early long rod designs did not provide for cross-locking screws, and these devices were less successful in providing compression and rotational control.

Several designs that rely on short femoral and tibial intramedullary rods are now available. These devices are inserted (retrograde in the femur and antegrade in the tibia) through a single incision at the knee. Cross-locking screws are typically installed percutaneously with a drill guide, and no fluoroscopy is required. A coupling fixture between the two rods provides effective intraoperative compression and at least one design (the Wichita fusion nail, Stryker Howmedica Osteonics, Allendale, NJ) includes a dynamic compression capability as well. The short rod systems offer several advantages. They are compatible with an ipsilateral hip prosthesis, a tourniquet can be used to minimize blood loss, and up to 10° of (permanent) flexion can be accommodated where desirable because of the shortness of the rods. Furthermore, in patients who experience reinfection of an established arthrodesis, the short rods are much easier to remove without disrupting the fusion. In patients

with a periarticular fracture, however, the short rods have proved to be inadequate as a combined fracture fixation and arthrodesis stabilization system.

Assessment of Fusion Status

The evaluation of fusion status relies on radiographic evidence, preferably from two orthogonal views of trabecular bridging of the osteotomy gap. This is combined with clinical assessment of fusion stiffness and pain, which is evaluated by subjecting the limb of the patient to a manually applied bending moment. Both these assessment methods involve a degree of subjectivity and uncertainty. The assessment of trabecular bridging is difficult to perform unambiguously unless the plane of the osteotomy is precisely parallel with the x-ray beam. Likewise, the determination of fusion stiffness is somewhat compromised by the contribution that the fixation device makes to the overall stiffness of the construct. For these reasons, it is advisable to implement both methods of assessment during the early postoperative period so that changes, or the lack thereof, can be more readily appreciated.

Postoperative Management

The principal objective of arthrodesis fixation is to provide firm bony apposition and a high degree of rigidity and stability at the fusion site. Consequently, little biomechanical advantage is derived from restricting limb loading, and patients are generally allowed to begin ambulation on the first postoperative day.

Outcomes

The rate of successful arthrodesis generally falls in the range of 90% to 100% for both external fixation devices and intramedullary rods (Table 2). The mean time required to achieve fusion is also similar for the two methods, falling in the range of 20 to 30 weeks for external fixation devices and 20 to 36 weeks for intramedullary rods. A variety of postoperative complications, both minor and serious, are common with these systems. The complication rate for external fixation devices falls in the range of 55% to 85%, whereas that for intramedullary rodding is somewhat lower at 33% to 60%. It should be noted, however, that the higher complication rate encountered with the external devices is largely a result of pin tract infections that are generally controllable.

Once fusion has been confirmed, most patients are able to walk and perform the activities of daily living at an acceptable level, although as many as half may have to rely on some type of assistive device for ambulation. Patients are likely to express some degree of dissatisfaction with their stiff knees, but most are generally accepting of the rationale that this is preferable to a flail knee or an amputation.

An additional element of concern is the limb-length discrepancy that may result from arthrodesis procedures in which significant bone loss has occurred as a result of trauma, tumor surgery, or repeated revision of an infected total knee arthroplasty. If the discrepancy is minimal (< 2 cm), the knee can be fused in 5° to 10° of flexion to provide for ground clearance during the swing phase of gate. This amount of flexion can be obtained with either an external fixation device or a short intramedullary rod system. However, attempts at providing a flexion allowance have not generally been successful when long intramedullary rods are used.

For fused limbs that are short by 2 to 4 cm, it is advisable to fuse the knee in full extension to reduce gait abnormalities because ground clearance is no longer a problem. For limb-length discrepancies greater than 4 cm, bone grafting or prosthetic spacers should be considered to reduce the difference.

For patients who have endured a large number of surgical procedures for failed total knee arthroplasty, it is instructive to compare outcomes for an additional attempt at revision arthroplasty with the results for arthrodesis. Under these conditions, the success rate for revision total knee arthroplasty is typically lower than that for arthrodesis. Patients who undergo successful revised total knee arthroplasty are likely to have higher functional scores (Knee Society scoring system), but less pain relief.

Complications

The two most serious clinical complications of arthrodesis are failure to achieve fusion and sepsis (not including minor wound or pin tract infections). Nonunions usually respond to corrective surgery with revised osteotomies, renewed compression, and occasionally bone grafting.

Deep infection, especially reinfection, usually requires removal of all implanted components followed by aggressive antibiotic therapy. A small percentage of compromised arthrodesis attempts may fail to respond to revision, in which instance amputation or a flail knee may be the only treatment option.

Additional arthrodesis complications associated with intramedullary rod stabilization include rod fracture, ipsilateral limb fracture, peroneal nerve palsy, and rod migration in patients without cross-locking screws. With external fixation, complications include pin tract infections, neurovascular injury resulting from pin insertion, and pin site fractures.

Annotated Bibliography

Arthrodesis of the Hip

Joshi AB, Markovic L, Hardinge K, Murphy JC: Conversion of a fused hip to total hip arthroplasty. *J Bone Joint Surg Am* 2002;84:1335-1341.

In this study, 208 conversion total hip arthroplasties from hip arthrodesis were followed at an average of 9.2 years after total hip replacement. The authors reported that 15 nerve palsies occurred and there were only 12 revisions. The implant survival rate was 96% at 10-year and 73% at 26-year follow-up.

Stover MD, Beaule PE, Matta JM, Mast JW: Hip arthrodesis: A procedure for the new millennium? *Clin Orthop Relat Res* 2004;418:126-133.

The authors discuss abductor sparing techniques used for hip arthrodesis and detail the need for preoperative education. They also highlight the appropriate position of fusion and describe the conversion to total hip replacement procedure.

Arthrodesis of the Knee

Christie MJ, DeBoer DK, McQueen DA, Cooke FW, Hahn DL: Salvage procedures for failed total knee arthroplasty. *J Bone Joint Surg Am* 2003;85(suppl 1):S558-S562.

New alternatives for treating patients with infected total knee arthroplasties after multiple revisions and severe bone loss are discussed. Treatment options include (1) exchange arthroplasty with new or custom-made prostheses, (2) structural allograft composites, (3) reconstruction of osseous defects with porous implants, and (4) arthrodesis with a short intramedullary rod system that provides excellent compression, good rotational and alignment control, and dynamic compression.

David R, Shtarker DR, Horesh Z, Tsur A, Soudry M: Arthrodesis with the Ilizarov device after failed knee arthroplasty. *Orthopedics* 2001;24(1):33-36.

In this study, patients with failed total knee arthroplasty because of infection (12 patients) or aseptic loosening (1 patient) underwent arthrodesis using the Ilizarov external fixator. Solid fusion was achieved in all patients; average healing time was 27.6 weeks.

Domingo LJ, Caballero MJ, Cuenca J, Herrera A, Sola A, Herrero L: Knee arthrodesis with the Wichita fusion nail. *Int Orthop* 2003;28(1):25-27.

In this article, arthrodesis experience with external fixators and other fixation systems is compared with the results obtained with a new short intramedullary rod system.

Garberina MJ, Fitch RD, Hoffman ED, Hardaker WT, Vail TP, Scully SP: Knee arthrodesis with circular external fixation. *Clin Orthop Relat Res* 2001;382:168-178.

In this retrospective study, 19 patients who underwent knee arthrodesis with circular external fixation were assessed. Postoperative radiographs were evaluated for evidence of bony fusion (defined as trabecular bridging between the femur and tibia), and fusion was successful in 13 of 19 patients (68%).

Incavo SJ, Lilly JW, Bartlett CS, Churchill DL: Arthrodesis of the knee. *J Arthroplasty* 2000;15(7):871-876.

The authors discuss arthrodesis using a variety of long and short intramedullary rods in 22 patients with infected total knee arthroplasties. Successful fusion occurred in all patients, but four patients required additional surgery.

Manzotti A, Pullen C, Deromedis B, Catagni MA: Knee arthrodesis after infected total knee arthroplasty using the Ilizarov method. *Clin Orthop Relat Res* 2001;389: 143-149.

Of five patients who underwent knee arthrodesis using the Ilizarov method after infected total knee arthroplasty, all were reported to have a stable knee arthrodesis after a mean external fixation time of 6.8 months without additional surgery or bracing. All patients were satisfied with the outcomes.

Oostenbroek HJ, van Roermund PM: Arthrodesis of the knee after an infected arthroplasty using the Ilizarov method. *J Bone Joint Surg Br* 2001;83(1):50-54.

The authors discuss their experience with 15 infected total knee arthroplasties that were treated with external fixation to achieve arthrodesis.

VanRyn JS, Verebelyi DM: One-stage debridement and knee fusion for infected total knee arthroplasty using the hybrid frame. *J Arthroplasty* 2002;17(1):129-134.

The authors present only two instances of arthrodesis with a ring-type external fixation device, but this is accompanied by a review of 10 related studies (394 patients) from the literature.

Wang CJ, Huang TW, Wang JW, Chen HS: The often poor clinical outcome of infected total knee arthroplasty. *J Arthroplasty* 2002;17(5):608-614.

The authors of this study compared treatment of infected total knee arthroplasties by arthrodesis and total knee arthroplasty reimplantation on the basis of knee scores. They reported that the infected total knee arthroplasties had significantly better outcomes when compared with noninfected total knee arthroplasties. No significant difference in knee scores was noted when comparing the two groups.

Wiedel JD: Salvage of infected total knee fusion: The last option. *Clin Orthop Relat Res* 2002;404:139-142.

The author discusses the relative merits of external fixation and intramedullary rodding for arthrodesis of infected total knee arthroplasties.

Classic Bibliography

Arroyo JS, Garvin KL, Neff JR: Arthrodesis of the knee with a modular titanium intramedullary nail. *J Bone Joint Surg Am* 1997;79(1):26-35.

Brodersen MP, Fitzgerald RH, Lowell FA, Peterson MD: Arthrodesis of the knee following failed total knee arthroplasty. *J Bone Joint Surg Am* 1979;61(2):181-185.

Callaghan JJ, Brand RA, Pedersen DR: Hip arthrodesis: A long-term follow-up. *J Bone Joint Surg Am* 1985;67: 1328-1335.

Charnley J, Lowe HG: A study of the end-results of compression arthrodesis of the knee. *J Bone Joint Surg Br* 1958;40:633-635.

Damron TA, McBeath AA: Arthrodesis following failed total knee arthroplasty: Comprehensive review and meta-analysis of recent literature. *Orthopedics* 1995; 18(4):361-368.

Ellingsen DE, Rand JA: Intramedullary arthrodesis of the knee after failed total knee arthroplasty. *J Bone Joint Surg Am* 1994;76(6):870-877.

Hagemann WF, Woods W, Tullos HS: Arthrodesis in failed total knee replacement. *J Bone Joint Surg Am* 1978;60:790-794.

Hak DJ, Lieberman JR, Finerman GA: Single and bi-plane external fixators for knee arthrodesis. *Clin Orthop Relat Res* 1995;316:134-144.

Knutson K, Hovelius L, Lindstrom A, Sidgren L: Arthrodesis after failed knee arthroplasty. *Clin Orthop Relat Res* 1984;191:202-211.

Lai KA, Shen WJ, Yang CY: Arthrodesis with a short Huckstep Nail as a salvage procedure for failed total knee arthroplasty. *J Bone Joint Surg Am* 1998;80(3):380-388.

McClenaghan BA, Krajbich JI, Pirone AM, Koheil R, Longmuir P: Comparative assessment of gait after limb-salvage procedures. *J Bone Joint Surg Am* 1989;71(8): 1178-1182.

Rand JA: Alternatives to reimplantation for salvage of the total knee arthroplasty complicated by infection. *J Bone Joint Surg Am* 1993;75(2):282-289.

Scheid KD, Hanel DP, Strege D: Limb salvage reconstruction in severe knee infections with associated large soft tissue and bony defects. *J Orthop Trauma* 1991;5(1): 60-65.

Segawa H, Tsukayama DT, Kyle RF, Becker DA, Gustilo RB: Infection after total knee arthroplasty. *J Bone Joint Surg Am* 1999;81(10):1434-1445.

Sponseller PD, McBeath AA, Perpich M: Hip arthrodesis in young patients: A long-term follow-up study. *J Bone Joint Surg Am* 1984;66:853-859.

Vahvanen V: Arthrodesis in failed knee replacement in eight rheumatoid patients. *Ann Chir Gynaecol* 1979; 68(2):57-62.

Vlasak R, Grearen PF, Petty W: Knee arthrodesis in the treatment of failed total knee replacement. *Clin Orthop Relat Res* 1995;321:138-144.

Waldman BJ, Mont MA, Payman KR, et al: Infected total knee arthroplasty treated with arthrodesis using a modular nail. *Clin Orthop Relat Res* 1999;367:230-237.

Chapter 28

Computer-Aided Navigation for Total Hip and Total Knee Arthroplasty

Andrew B. Mor, PhD

Branislav Jaramaz, PhD

Anthony M. DiGioia III, MD

Kenneth A. Krackow, MD

Navigation in Total Hip Arthroplasty

Introduction

Computer-aided navigation for total hip arthroplasty (THA) became a reality in the late 1990s, when the use of CT-based systems resulted in an increase in the accuracy of component placement compared with conventional mechanical guides. Since that time, experiences with surgical navigation systems for THA have not only increased the overall accuracy of the procedure, but have greatly reduced the incidence of outliers. Although a variety of methods are used to model the patient's anatomy and to develop a surgical plan, all systems share the same basic concept of showing the surgeon the relative position and orientation between the patient's pelvis and femur and the surgical tools that shape the bones and hold the implant components for insertion. By providing real-time information to the surgeon regarding the position of the implant, computer-assisted orthopaedic surgery systems for THA can help reduce short- and long-term complications caused by improper implant positioning and can enable the development of less invasive surgical techniques.

Conventional Implant Placement

Positioning the acetabular cup and femoral stem in the optimal position is important in reducing the risk of wear, dislocation, and impingement, and in maximizing joint longevity. Since the introduction of the Charnley implant, continual improvement has occurred in the design and construction of the implant components, leading to decreased complications and increased implant longevity. A safe zone, defined as $40° \pm 10°$ of abduction and $15° \pm 10°$ of anteversion, has been commonly adopted as a goal for cup alignment. However, implant alignment remains a challenge as standard mechanical guides have not eliminated component malpositioning. The surgeon's experience as well as variations in the patient's anatomy can greatly affect the apparent position of the implanted components. Conventional mechanical guides assume that the patient's trunk and pelvis are aligned in a known orientation with respect to the operating room table, thereby locating the patient's longitudinal and coronal axes. However, the orientation of the patient's pelvis varies throughout the surgical procedure, and is rarely aligned with the axes of the table. Studies have shown that the patient's pelvis can rotate on the operating room table 20° or more from the time of dislocation to the time of cup placement. Navigation systems were developed to address these variations in orientation that conventional guides were unable to accommodate.

Systems

Navigation systems for THA were initially developed after recognizing the intraoperative difficulties inherent in active robotic systems. Using bulky robots in the operating room presented certain logistical issues and adversely impacted the standard surgical flow. Passive navigation systems were envisioned as providing similar improvements in the accuracy of implant positioning, while minimizing the impact on surgical routine and allowing surgeon involvement in all aspects of the procedure. By tracking the location of the patient and the surgical tools, these systems report the relative position of the implant to the surgeon, allowing fine control of implant positioning. The preoperative planning components of some CT-based systems allow simulation of postoperative biomechanical results, allowing the surgeon to optimize the position of the implant to maximize the patient's range of motion. Navigation systems also can help the surgeon visualize the patient's anatomy that cannot be directly viewed through the incision, thus facilitating surgery through smaller incisions with less soft-tissue trauma.

Navigation in Total Knee Arthroplasty

Accuracy of performance also is of paramount importance in total knee arthroplasty (TKA). Components must be placed as precisely as possible. Each component must be correctly positioned in all six degrees of freedom. The soft-tissue connections, capsule, and ligaments need to be considered when placing components in or-

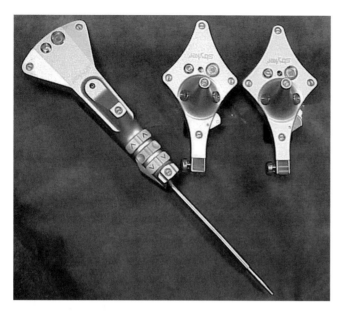

Figure 1 A navigation pointer (*left*) and separate tibial and femoral infrared markers (*right*) are shown (Stryker, Kalamazoo, MI).

der to achieve stability and to ensure that range of motion will be as full as possible. The capabilities of infrared, ultrasound, and electromagnetic position-detection instruments, and the speed, memory capacity, and computational capabilities of modern digital computers make these devices appropriate for use in TKA.

The personal experience of orthopaedic surgeons and literature that describes 90% to 95% good and excellent clinical results for knee replacement surgery over a 10- to 15-year period may lead some surgeons to believe that mechanical instruments are adequate for use in TKA. However, errors of component rotation, postoperative instability, and patients who are dissatisfied with limitations of motion are still commonly reported. Also, it cannot be concluded that axial alignment is optimal because postoperative long-standing weight-bearing radiographs are not typically obtained and measured.

A completely navigated, computer-assisted TKA was first described in August 1997. A navigation system for TKA, like a system for THA, involves the use of computer-based equipment in combination with highly technical devices with sensing and locating capabilities, which are used to navigate to the component position and result desired. Several different computer-assisted navigation systems for TKA are currently available from a variety of manufacturers.

Navigation Systems for THA and TKA

Current navigation systems can be divided into three different categories based on the type of information source used to model the patient's anatomy and to establish anatomic references: three-dimensional imaging,

fluoroscopic imaging, and image-free systems. Three-dimensional imaging typically consists of CT images acquired preoperatively, and fluoroscopic imaging consists of two or more intraoperative fluoroscopic images. Image-free systems use intraoperatively located landmarks and kinematic information and function without the use of radiographs, CT scans, or fluoroscopy. The surgeon indicates bony landmarks, which allow determination of position, alignment, and rotation. For THA, the main outcome of each information system is the orientation of the pelvic and femoral reference systems. With this information, the navigation systems can display the position of bone-shaping or implant-placing tools relative to the patient. These navigation systems also provide other relevant information such as the distance of the reamer to the medial wall of the acetabulum, orientation of the acetabular cup, femoral stem anteversion, limb length, and femoral offset.

Similarly, navigation systems for TKA provide real time observation of the position of each bone and instrument in the field. Any one point or multiple points at some aspect of the knee can be related to the overall position of both the tibia and the femur at that time. The system accurately reflects the position of each bone to within several millimeters and 1° to 2°.

Intraoperative Tracking of the Patient and Tools

All navigation systems rely on methods of locating the patient's anatomy and tracking the relevant surgical tools during the procedure. These systems typically incorporate an optical position sensor to determine the position of the moving objects. Dynamic rigid bodies, or trackers, are attached to the patient's bones and either attached or incorporated into the surgical tools (Figure 1). The position sensor can then "see" these trackers as they move in space, and report their position to the underlying computer software program. If the navigation system knows where the anatomy or implant is located with respect to its tracker, then the tracker position in space will convey the location and orientation of the anatomy or implant.

A typical surgical setup for a navigation system will incorporate a position sensor, a computer monitor, tools with tracking bodies integrated with them, and additional tracking bodies mounted to the patient's bony anatomy (Figure 2). The position sensor usually consists of a pair of very accurate cameras mounted in a rigid housing that views the scene looking for infrared signals. Trackers can be either active or passive, with the first using infrared light-emitting diode markers, and the second using retroreflective markers. The computer system, which holds the software particular to that system, has been programmed to recognize the geometry of such equipment. For example, the system knows the location of the tip of a point probe and usually is pro-

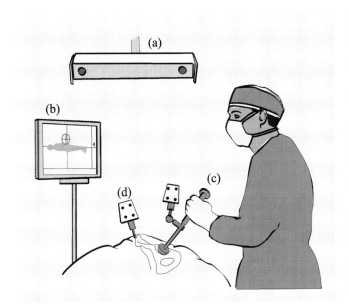

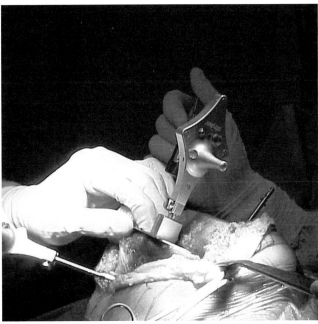

Figure 2 A typical operating room setup for a navigation system will incorporate a position sensor (a), a computer monitor (b), tools with tracking bodies mounted to them (c), and additional tracking bodies mounted to the patient's bony anatomy (d).

Figure 3 A marker/tracker joined with a metal plane is used to assess the plane of resection at the tibia.

grammed with information on the line that is the longitudinal axis of the pointer. The pointer can indicate a bony landmark that is defined by a single point. The pointer also can be used to input an axis such as the "anatomic AP axis" of Whiteside. Markers can be combined to create a plane detector (Figure 3), and markers may be embedded in system instruments (Figure 4). For example, once a navigated reamer has been calibrated, the system will know where the reamer itself is located relative to the tracker mounted to the tool handle. Patient anatomy is tracked in the same manner, although the calculation of the position of the anatomy with respect to the tracker is performed differently based on the information source used for the individual system. In all systems, the tracker must be rigidly attached to the patient's anatomy at the beginning of the surgical procedure. These trackers are fixated with heavy-duty clamps, pairs of Kirschner wires or Steinmann pins, or with bicortical screws with antirotation devices to prevent rotation of the tracker as the anatomy is manipulated. By tracking both the patient and the surgical tools, the systems can report the relative position of tools and implants to the surgeon.

CT-Based Navigation

CT-based systems were the first type of navigation system developed in the mid to late 1990s. These systems are considered the gold standard for surgical navigation. CT-based systems allow the use of highly accurate models of the patient's anatomy because a full three-dimensional model of the relevant anatomy can be built from the volumetric scan obtained preoperatively. With

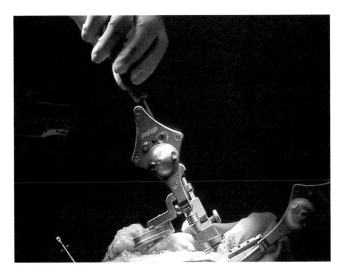

Figure 4 An adjustable femoral jig with a mounted infrared marker is shown. Such adjustable jigs permit setting the cutting slot to the desired depth and angular orientations by navigation.

this full three-dimensional model, an accurate patient-specific preoperative plan can be generated that takes into account the variations in the anatomy of patients, and does not rely on the default orientation specified by the manufacturer of the implant. After a plan is generated, it is used in the operating room for the intraoperative portion of the procedure. The patient's anatomy is located and tracked, and the implant components are then inserted by the surgeon, with feedback from the system on their real-time position. CT-based systems, using the above steps, allow the surgeon to gather as much

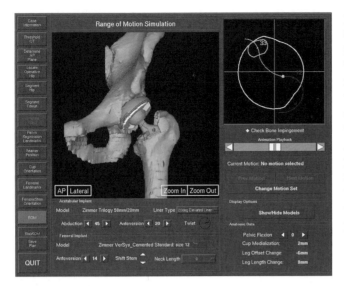

Figure 5 A photograph of a computer screen showing a preoperative planner from a CT-based system that shows the surface models of the patient's pelvis and femur, with an implant model inserted. The range-of-motion simulator shows the location of implant and bony impingement when the femur follows proscribed motion paths that mimic everyday activities.

data about the patient as possible to generate the best possible patient outcome.

The first step in using a CT-based system for THA is to acquire a CT scan of the patient's anatomy, usually consisting of a full pelvic scan, and typically including the distal and proximal portions of the femur. These scans can be obtained in 3 to 4 minutes using current helical CT scanners. The reference frame for the pelvic measurement used by the CT-based system is the anterior pelvic plane, defined by the superior anterior iliac spines and pubic tubercles. All locations and orientations are measured relative to this frame. The landmarks used for the anterior pelvic plane are automatically located in the CT data, with the surgeon verifying the accuracy of their positions. A reference frame for the femur also is defined, although there is less consensus regarding which landmarks to use.

The CT scan is then automatically segmented, to identify the bone of interest, and then triangle-based surface models of the pelvis and femur are built. These surface models are used by the surgeon to help generate the surgical plan, and, in some systems, to perform a range-of-motion simulation with potential implant positions. To generate the initial surgical plan, a model of the implant is located on the CT cross-sectional views. The acetabular cup is located within the outline of the acetabulum, taking into account the press-fit or cement mantle used to affix the cup in the pelvis. The initial plan for the femoral component is performed in a similar manner, with feedback on anteversion, medialization, limb-length change, and offset, as the model of the implant is moved relative to the scan data. After the im-

plant components are initially placed, a range-of-motion simulation may be performed to determine impingement locations between the implant components and the patient's bones. This simulation is performed while moving the leg through either straight flexion or through any selected motion paths (for example, flexion of 90°, followed by internal rotation) that the patient will want to perform during the activities of daily living. An example of the range-of-motion simulation in one preoperative planner is shown in Figure 5. Impingement is viewed as a conservative predictor of implant dislocation, and can be used by the surgeon to adjust implant selection, position, and orientation to maximize the expected range of motion for an individual patient. After the surgeon is satisfied with the surgical plan, the information is saved for use in the intraoperative portion of the system.

For the intraoperative component of a CT-based navigation system for THA, the first step is to verify the accuracy of the tool tracking, such that the tools are correctly calibrated and were not bent or damaged before the procedure. Trackers are then attached to the patient's pelvis on the iliac wing; if the femur is being tracked, another tracker is fixed to the femur typically midshaft or distally, from lateral to medial. Registration of the computer model to the tracked bony anatomy is then performed. Registration simply means that the software calculates the position and orientation of the CT scan and preoperative plan relative to the position of the patient on the operating room table, so that the system can track the position of the anatomy as the patient is manipulated throughout the procedure. For CT-based systems, registration is performed by using a point probe to collect several points on the bone surface. The preoperative three-dimensional model of the anatomy is then translated and rotated to fit the location of that set of points. Navigational feedback provided through a computer monitor can allow the surgeon to verify the accuracy of the registration by seeing the position of the tools relative to the patient's pelvis or femur. Feedback on orientation and position can then be provided to the surgeon during preparation of the patient's bones. When placing the implant, a simple "aim and shoot" interface of lining up two circles is used to orient the acetabular cup in the preoperatively planned position; a similar interface can be used to show alignment of the femoral stem, including version, offset, and changes in limb length. The requirement of a preoperative CT scan is the main drawback of these types of systems, because scheduling and reimbursement for the scan must be arranged.

Using a CT-based system for TKA involves similar procedures, advantages, and disadvantages. The surgeon surveys the CT scan and selects bony landmarks such as the epicondyles and looks at the outline of the tibial plateau to set neutral tibial rotation. It is possible to in-

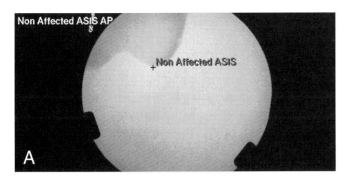

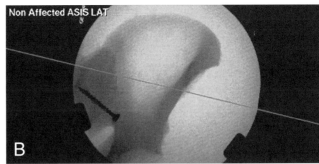

Figure 6 The basic concept of landmark localization from two fluoroscopic views, where the same anatomic point is located in each view, and the location in three-dimensional space is then calculated. **A,** AP fluoroscopic view with the anterior-superior iliac spine point located. **B,** The line along which the anterior-superior iliac spine point is located in this lateral fluoroscopic view based on the location in the AP view. (Courtesy of Medtronic SNT.)

dicate cut lines and levels and visualize different sized components on the cuts. Registration and navigation then proceed in a manner similar to the process used for THA.

Fluoroscopy-Based Navigation

Fluoroscopy-based navigation eliminates the need for preoperative imaging because all of the required images are obtained intraoperatively. Two or more fluoroscopic images, from a C-arm that is itself tracked, are acquired for each landmark point after the trackers are affixed to the patient's anatomy. These images are calibrated to remove any artifacts and image warping and to ensure the geometric accuracy of the surgical guidance. The registration process is intrinsic (as compared with the CT-based system) because the location of the images relative to the patient's anatomy is known when the images are acquired. The anatomic landmarks used for the surgical plan are located on the fluoroscopic images (Figure 6). Each landmark must be identified in a pair of images to properly locate its location in space; the images should be as orthogonal as possible. This technique is used to locate the anterior pelvic plane used for acetabular cup guidance, and the reference frame used for orientation of the femoral component. At this point, the fluoroscopy-based system can report the position of all of the tracked surgical tools relative to the surgical plan, and can project their outlines onto the original fluoroscopic images. This system provides the surgeon with a virtual fluoroscopic image of the patient's anatomy with the tools and implants in use, without the need for additional ionizing radiation. The system can now be used in the same manner as the CT-based system, reporting the position of the tools and implants relative to the patient's anatomy, and can help guide the surgeon in shaping the bones and placing the implants in a safe position.

The main difficulties with fluoroscopy-based systems include the need for intraoperative imaging for a procedure that does not normally require such imaging; a sur-

gical flow impacted by the need to interact directly with the system to locate the landmark points; and potential difficulty in accurately locating the anatomic landmark points in the fluoroscopic views. In addition, the accuracy of the navigation system is very dependent on obtaining accurate images because navigation is based on these two-dimensional images and not on the patient's actual anatomy. No simulation of postoperative results is possible with these systems, although the need for such a simulation may only be required for patients with anatomy that varies greatly from the norm. No preoperative imaging is required because registration is automatic; the system knows the location of the anatomy at all times relative to the fluoroscopic images. The fluoroscopic views can be updated during the procedure to reflect modifications to the anatomy or to verify implant positioning.

Image-Free Navigation

Image-free navigation is similar to fluoroscopy-based navigation in that no preoperative planning is performed and anatomic information is collected during surgery. However, image-free systems do not require imaging either preoperatively or intraoperatively, and may be quicker to set up and run. Information on the anterior pelvic plane is acquired through palpation or visual point selection instead of by locating it on fluoroscopic images or in the CT data. For THA, the procedure is typically performed with the patient supine so that the anterior superior iliac spines and the pubic tubercles are accessible, but may also be collected in the lateral decubitus position. A tracker is attached to the iliac crest, and points on the spine and pubic tubercle are then collected percutaneously. The patient can be rotated if the procedure is being performed from a lateral approach. After the incision is made, femoral landmarks can be located. Resection of the femoral head is performed and points are then collected along the crest of the acetabulum and along the medial wall, to aid in the guidance of the reamer. As with the fluoroscopy-based system, the procedure continues from this point in the same manner as the CT-based system. The limitations of image-free systems are similar to those of fluoroscopy-based systems, with one significant difference. Locating the position of the landmarks through palpation can be difficult, especially in obese patients. The error in locating these landmarks can be significant, which can introduce large inaccuracies into the navigation system. Also, the need to install the tracker and determine the location of the anatomic landmarks before rolling the patient into a lateral position can be a significant drawback. These systems, however, do not require imaging and their cost and intraoperative surgical time may be less compared with the other two types of systems.

One hybrid approach recently has been developed that combines palpation of the superior anterior iliac spines with fluoroscopic localization of the pubic tubercle points. The theory is that the iliac spine points are easily palpable, whereas the pubic tubercle points are not, especially on patients who are more overweight. To locate the pubic tubercle points without a CT scan requires fluoroscopic imaging. This system avoids some of the radiation that the pure fluoroscopic systems use, but still involves the intrusion of the C-arm into the operating room that the image-free systems avoid. It is hoped that these systems will achieve a higher degree of accuracy than the image-free systems, while not requiring preoperative imaging.

Results

Computer-aided navigation in THA and TKA, first used in a research setting, has been in use for less than one decade. Therefore, long-term results are not yet available. Reports of postoperative alignment of the implant components and short- to mid-term results for different systems do exist. The initial study describing the development of the first CT-based system showed all orientations for the first 10 patients to be within 10° of the planned orientation. As the technology has developed, results have improved, with a more recent study showing average abduction of 46° (range, 42° to 48°) and average flexion of 22° (range, 18° to 25°) when the planned orientation was 45° of abduction and 20° of flexion.

A study of a fluoroscopy-based system showed a mean error in abduction of 3.9° with a range of 0° to 9°. These results were similar to those found with a CT-based system that was concurrently tested. A comparison between the systems found a greater increase in surgical time for the fluoroscopy-based technique and better feedback on the location of anatomic landmarks. A hybrid system that uses percutaneous pointer-based digitization for easily accessible landmarks combined with fluoroscopy for less accessible landmarks showed good results. Postoperative inclination was 43° ± 3.0°

(range, 37° to 49°) and anteversion was 19° ± 3.9° (range, 10° to 28°).

One of the first studies on a pure image-free navigation system showed inclination at 42° ± 5° and anteversion of 11° ± 5°. The range of postoperative angles was 34° to 50° of inclination and 3° to 22° of anteversion, which are predominately within the safe zone. This system showed poorer results with anteversion, with approximately twice as many patients outside the safe zone in anteversion when compared with inclination. It should be noted that these results were measured on postoperative radiographs in which the influence of pelvic tilt during the acquisition of the radiograph is not taken into account.

Summary

Results from computer-aided navigation have shown a narrowing and a near elimination of outliers and a marked decrease in the variation of postoperative axial alignment for THA. Computer-aided navigation for the hip has produced distinct improvements in postoperative orientation and positioning of the implant components in THA. The positive outcomes of more accurate placement include the potential for optimal surgical plans for individual implant placement, reduced soft-tissue trauma because of the reduced necessity of large exposures for visualization, and a reduced risk for revision surgery caused by grossly misplaced components. Most surgeons who use navigation systems note that the positioning initially determined by standard mechanical instrument is frequently inaccurate. Small to moderate errors using mechanical positioning can occasionally combine to produce significant inaccuracy (up to 6° to 10°). With the ability to intraoperatively report implant positioning and alignment, computer-aided navigation systems help the surgeon to achieve more accurate and less invasive surgical outcomes for patients undergoing THA or TKA.

Annotated Bibliography

Navigation in Total Knee Arthroplasty

Muir PF, DiGioia A III, Jaramaz B, Picard F: Computer-assisted orthopedic surgery: Tools and technologies in clinical practice. *MD Comput* 2000;17(5):34-43.

The authors report on some of the earliest experiences using computer-assisted orthopaedic surgery.

Saragaglia D, Picard F, Chaussard C, Montbarbon E, Leitner F, Cinquin P: Computer-assisted knee arthroplasty: Comparison with a conventional procedure: Results of 50 cases in a prospective randomized study. *Rev Chir Orthop Reparatrice Appar Mot* 2001;87:18-28.

This is one of the earliest studies on TKA navigation, and the authors report unequivocal alignment improvement using this surgical technique.

Whiteside LA: Soft tissue balancing the knee. *J Arthroplasty* 2002; 17(4, suppl 1)23-27.

The author describes a technique to align the knee during TKA in which distal femoral cuts are aligned in 5° to 7° valgus to the long axis of the femur, and the tibial surface is cut perpendicular to the long axis of the tibia. The author reports that although this technique generally results in a knee that is balanced to varus and valgus stresses in flexion and extension, it often results in AP and rotational instability, which may require a more highly conforming tibial component or posterior-stabilized knee prosthesis.

Results

DiGioia AM III, Plakseychuk AY, Levison TJ, Jaramaz B: Mini-incision technique for total hip arthroplasty with navigation. *J Arthroplasty* 2003;18(2):123-128.

This study compared a mini-incision technique with the standard posterior approach, with navigation of the acetabular component only. Incision length was reduced to an average of 11.7 cm, and all cups were placed within 5° of the desired orientation, with abduction ranging from 42° to 48°, and flexion ranging from 18° to 25°.

Hube R, Birke A, Hein W, Klima S: CT-based and fluoroscopy-based navigation for cup implantation in total hip arthroplasty (THA). *Surg Technol Int* 2003;11: 275-280.

Two different techniques of acquiring patient information for navigation of THA were compared. The CT-based system achieved a mean error in cup orientation of 2.7° (0° to 8°) while the fluoroscopy-based system achieved a mean error of 3.9° (0° to 9°). For patients having routine THA, therefore, the authors recommend the fluoroscopy-based system with the CT-based system used for patients with congenital and post-traumatic deformities.

Kiefer H: OrthoPilot cup navigation: How to optimise cup positioning? *Int Orthop* 2003;27(suppl 1):S37-S42.

An image-free, kinematic based system that uses palpation of the bony landmarks to define the location of the anterior pelvic plane is described. The mean intraoperative error of the acetabular cup was 41° (range, 29° to 48°), whereas the post-operative results based of pelvic radiographs had a mean error of 42° (range, 34° to 50°).

Wentzensen A, Zheng G, Vock B, et al: Image-based hip navigation. *Int Orthop* 2003;27(suppl 1):S43-S46.

A hybrid CT-free image-guided technique was described. The anterior pelvic plane is defined with the anterior superior iliac spines captured with a pointer device, whereas the center of the pubic tubercles is identified on two oblique fluoroscopic views. Acetabular alignment was measured on a postoperative CT, with the mean value for inclination of 43° (range, 37° to 49°) and anteversion 19° (range, 10° to 28°). Correlation between intraoperative measurements and postoperative measurements of cup alignment were within 6°.

Classic Bibliography

Arima J, Whiteside LA, McCarthy DS, White SE: Femoral rotational alignment, based on the anteroposterior axis, in total knee arthroplasty in a valgus knee: A technical note. *J Bone Joint Surg Am* 1995;77:1331-1334.

Delp SL, Stulberg SD, Davies B, Picard F, Leitner F: Computer assisted knee replacement. *Clin Orthop Relat Res* 1998;354:49-56.

DiGioia AM, Jaramaz B, Blackwell M, et al: Image guided navigation system to measure intraoperatively acetabular implant alignment. *Clin Orthop* 1998;355:8-22.

Jaramaz B, DiGioia AM III, Blackwell M, Nikou C: Computer assisted measurement of cup placement in total hip replacement. *Clin Orthop* 1998;354:70-81.

Kennedy JG, Rogers WB, Soffe KE: el al: Effect of acetabular component orientation on recurrent dislocation, pelvic osteolysis, polyethylene wear, and component migration. *J Arthroplasty* 1998;13(5):530-534.

Krackow KA, Bayer-Thering M, Phillips MJ, Mihalko M: A new technique for determining proper mechanical axis alignment during total knee arthroplasty: Progress toward computer assisted TKA. *Orthopedics* 1999;22: 698-702.

Lewinnek GE, Lewis JL, Tarr R, Compere CL, Zimmerman JR: Dislocations after total hip-replacement arthroplasties. *J Bone Joint Surg Am* 1978;60(2):217-220.

McCollum DE, Gray WJ: Dislocation after total hip arthroplasty: Causes and prevention. *Clin Orthop* 1990; 261:159-170.

Murray DW: The definition and measurement of acetabular orientation. *J Bone Joint Surg Br* 1993; 75(2):228-232.

Chapter 29

Rehabilitation After Total Hip and Total Knee Arthroplasty

Anil Bhave, PT

Introduction

The primary goals of rehabilitation after total hip arthroplasty (THA) and total knee arthroplasty (TKA) are to maximize the range of motion, minimize pain, improve muscle strength, promote ambulation, and to encourage independence in performing the activities of daily living. With these goals, the patients' expectations also have grown; an increasing number of patients are demanding enhanced levels of activity and return to participation in recreational sports activities. There is a widening discrepancy between the results of standardized scoring (such as the modified Harris hip score) and self-reported results of patient satisfaction. The current population of patients is not satisfied with relief from pain and the ability to ambulate with a cane, but expects to engage in recreational sports activities and aspires to function at a significantly higher level than was attained preoperatively. This growing aspiration to function at a higher level demands a carefully planned and aggressive rehabilitation regimen.

Rehabilitation protocols are broadly divided into the early phase of postoperative recovery, which takes place during hospitalization, and an outpatient phase, which occurs after the patient returns home. This phase may include outpatient rehabilitation. Patients who have undergone TKA are in significantly more discomfort than those who have THA. After TKA, patients most commonly report increased pain during flexion exercises. Despite pain, early flexion range-of-motion exercise is one of the critical factors needed to achieve good postoperative function. All patients who undergo THA must adhere to certain restrictions on weight bearing and activities for approximately 6 weeks postoperatively. After this 6-week postoperative phase, patients having undergone a THA are usually given more aggressive rehabilitation focused on improving ambulation and hip muscle strength, promoting independence in activities of daily living, and promoting a return to functional activities and participation in low-impact recreational sports. Unlike patients who underwent THA, patients who underwent TKA are not restricted by protocol but by their own abilities, tolerance to pain, and improvement in strength and range of motion.

Rehabilitation After Total Hip Arthroplasty

Acute Phase

The acute phase of rehabilitation after THA lasts for up to 4 days after surgery. Patients will have a better outcome in this phase if they had either a preoperative education class or were assessed for risk factors that increase the length of the hospital stay. Patients with risk factors such as obesity, diabetes, preoperative stiffness, and other comorbidities respond well to a more targeted and intensive therapy regimen, such as physical therapy administered twice daily. Patients who are not in the high-risk group do well with physical therapy once per day. In most institutions, therapy services are offered 6 days a week (Monday through Saturday); this schedule is adequate for most patients after THA. Patients in the high-risk group who have surgery on Thursday or Friday will require therapy on Sunday.

Postoperative rehabilitation starts 1 day after surgery. The first day is focused on getting the patient out of bed and on teaching the method of transfer. Sets of moderate intensity isometric exercises for the gluteal muscles and quadriceps, and ankle pumps also are started at this time. Patients are encouraged to do deep breathing exercises. Pain control is usually achieved through intravenous administration of narcotics controlled by the patient. This method allows pain relief within minutes and provides the patient with more security and less anxiety during activities. Cryotherapy is also a very useful method of pain control and has been shown to reduce the length of hospital stay in patients after THA. Although cryotherapy does not reduce the need for narcotic analgesics in the early postoperative phase, it is a useful adjunct and is best used before and after therapy sessions. Day 2 through the day of discharge (day 4) from the acute care setting involves education and rehabilitation to teach hip precautions, ambulation with an assistive device with appropriate weight bearing, progression to moderately active exercise within the constraints of the hip precautions, and instructions on the use of adaptive equipment such as a tool to reach distance objects. Planning for discharge to home or an inpatient rehabilitation institution also occurs.

For up to 6 to 8 weeks postoperatively, patients should use an abduction pillow and supine lying position, adhere to hip flexion restrictions of 90° maximum, and should avoid the use of low chairs. Patients are encouraged to sit on high chairs and are provided raised toilet seats. To avoid excessive forward bending to reach an object, patients are provided with a reaching or grabbing tool. An aid is used to put on socks and a long-handle shoehorn is used to avoid excessive flexion at the hip joint when donning shoes. Regardless of the surgical approach used for THA, resisted hip abduction is not permitted in most patients until 6 weeks after surgery. Ambulation training begins with the use of appropriate assistive devices. Most patients do well using rolling walkers initially and later can transition to bilateral crutches. Weight-bearing restriction in the early postoperative phase are imposed to protect soft tissue and muscles and to avoid out of plane forces on the implant that can cause significant torsional stress. Patients should use bilateral support to avoid torsional stress on the prosthesis. Stair climbing also causes increased torsional stress if the surgical side of the body is used to step up. The patient should step up using the leg on the contralateral side of the body and should ascend one step at a time, always using the leg on the nonsurgical side to step up. Most noncemented implants allow the patient to use partial weight bearing; cemented implants allow weight bearing as tolerated. The use of a weighing scale to provide biofeedback is a useful method to teach a patient how much weight is safe. Patients stand in front of a weighing scale and exert pressure with their foot on the scale to the allowed weight limit. Patients who participate in this exercise have a better understanding of the amount of weight that can be tolerated and better proprioception and control during walking. Many patients are confused by the concept of the amount of weight on the lower extremity compared with joint contact force. For example, the use of a cane reduces the contralateral hip joint contact force by 60% (normal force is three to four times body weight), but the contralateral limb still experiences 85% of the body weight during ambulation. The use of unilateral aids after THA are not recommended because they cannot control weight bearing and may result in out-of-plane forces that cause torsional stress on the prosthesis. After the weight-bearing restrictions are removed, patients should be allowed to gradually reduce bilateral support and replace it with unilateral support. This patient-controlled gradual joint loading limits torsional stress on the prosthesis and allows a relatively pain-free return to activities.

Resisted hip exercise, especially straight-leg raises, also should be avoided for the first 4 to 5 weeks after surgery. This activity leads to increased torsional stress on the implant resulting from out-of-plane loading. Active resistive exercises for knee extension are encouraged

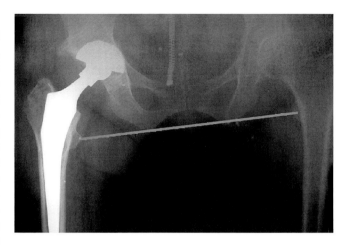

Figure 1 An AP standing radiograph showing an apparent limb-length discrepancy caused by an abduction contracture. Note that the line drawn from the ischial tuberosity passes close to the lesser trochanter on both sides, indicating that there is no true difference in limb length caused by the implant.

early in the rehabilitation process. Patients with atrophy of the quadriceps should use electrical neuromuscular stimulation to augment strength. Patients who have undergone THA have been shown to have quadriceps weakness for up to 1 year after surgery if not treated by a focused rehabilitation regimen. Most THA patients do not need passive range-of-motion exercise except for gentle stretching of the hip flexor and adductor muscles. If not addressed during the early postoperative phase, tightness of these muscles has been shown to cause significant gait deviation after ambulation is undertaken without an assistive device. In the acute phase of rehabilitation, some patients feel that their body is too long on the side that received surgery; this feeling is most often caused by posture and tightness of the hip abductor muscle (Figure 1). With time and better posture, this feeling is eliminated in most patients.

The decision to send a patient home with a program of home therapy followed by outpatient therapy or to discharge the patient to an inpatient rehabilitation unit is based on many physical and social factors. This decision should be made by a team that includes the surgeon, physical therapist, nursing staff, and the social worker. The patient's social background or physical barriers at home (such as too many steps leading to the entry) may require admission to inpatient rehabilitation. Most primary THA patients with no comorbidities are discharged to home therapy followed by an outpatient therapy regimen. Inpatient rehabilitation should be planned for patients with comorbidities, those with postoperative complications, bilateral THAs, those with a high body mass index, and patients with diabetes.

Subacute and Outpatient Phase
The subacute and outpatient phase of rehabilitation begins approximately 6 weeks after surgery. Patients have

Table 1 | Functional Impairments That Require Special Attention for Rehabilitation

Impairment	Symptoms Reported by the Patient	Physical Findings
Knee flexion contracture	Anterior knee pain (retropatellar or patellar tendon) Quadriceps fatigue pain Back pain Limping gait Difficultly in walking long distances Unable to participate in light sports or recreational activities*	Gastrocnemius-soleus complex contracture Hamstrings contracture Posterior capsule and cruciate ligament contracture Hip flexion contracture compensated by knee flexion contracture Foot flat gait with quadriceps avoidance Inflammation of patellar tendon Peroneal nerve entrapment or sciatica Limb-length difference true or apparent
Knee flexion deficit < 90°	Difficulty sitting in a chair Difficulty rising from a chair Difficulty in descending and ascending stairs Difficulty in bicycling Difficulty in participating in sexual activities Unable to participate in light sports or recreational activities*	Rectus femoris contracture Quadriceps or patellar tendon adhesions Retropatellar scarring or adhesions Joint effusion Reflex sympathetic dystrophy Abnormal pain response
Quadriceps weakness	Quadriceps fatigue pain Bucking or giving way especially on uneven ground Difficulty climbing steps Difficulty walking long distances Unable to participate in light sports or recreational activities*	Active extension lag Quadriceps atrophy Anterior trunk lean in stance phase Lack of knee flexion or quadriceps avoidance gait in early stance phase

Peroneal nerve entrapment syndrome	Numbness with weakness in the dorsum of the foot
	Radiating pain in the dorsum of the foot
	Difficulty walking resulting in tripping or stumbling
		Positive Tinel's sign
		Extensor hallucis longus, extensor digitorum longus, and
		  tibial anterior weakness
		Paresthesias of the foot
		Knee extension increases radiating pain
		Fixed flexion posture of the knee to avoid peroneal nerve
		  symptoms

Hip flexion contracture	Deep anterior hip pain Abnormal gait Difficulty in sexual activities Low back pain	Iliopsoas contracture Rectus femoris contracture Sartorius, tensor fascia lata contracture Decreased step length and increases pelvic rotation during gait
Hip abduction contracture	Lateral hip pain Limb-length difference Abnormal gait Back pain Unable to participate in light sports or recreational activities*	Tensor fascia lata tightness Apparent limb-length difference Lateral trunk lean gait Trochanteric bursitis
Hip abductor weakness	Lateral hip pain Abnormal gait Need to use cane Back pain Hip muscles fatigue pain Difficulty walking long distances Unable to participate in light sports or recreational activities*	Weakness of gluteus medius and minimus Positive Trendelenburg's sign and gait Trochanteric bursitis Poor balance Lateral trunk lean during gait

*Light sports or recreational activities = golf, doubles tennis, light dancing, gardening, etc

usually progressed to participation in an outpatient program with goals that include improved muscle strength, normalization of range of motion, return to functional activities, and the initial phase of retraining for low-impact recreational sports activities and return to work. Several functional impairments that need special attention during rehabilitation are listed in Table 1.

Muscle Contractures

Hip flexion contractures are seen in the iliopsoas, rectus femoris, sartorius, and sometimes the tensor fascia lata. Abnormal posture is the most common cause of muscle contractures. In the preoperative phase, patients assume a fixed flexion posture to minimize joint pain; this posture leads to adaptive muscle shortening. Manual therapy

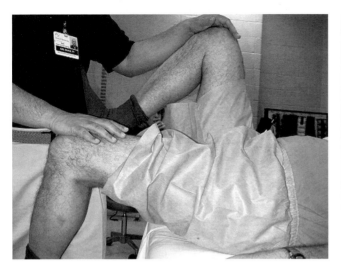

Figure 2 Iliopsoas stretching with the patient stabilizing the lumbar spine and pelvis by maintaining a "back flat" posture. This exercise is best done at the end of the table.

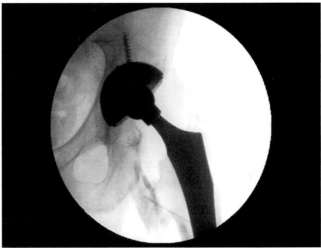

Figure 3 An image-intensified guided injection to the iliopsoas tendon just above the lesser trochanter is shown. Intra-articular and extra-articular hip injections are used to provide pain relief and to decrease inflammation to help the patient tolerate hip flexion contracture stretching and improve range of motion.

may be used to treat hip flexion contractures (Figure 2). This therapy includes aggressive stretching of the involved muscles with a customized protocol of at least five to seven stretches for each muscle per physical therapy session at a frequency of three times per week. All patients also are provided with a home exercise regimen to be performed individually or with the assistance of family members. Injection of the iliopsoas tendon with image-guided assistance is useful in patients with recalcitrant hip flexion contracture with tendinitis (Figure 3). This condition is diagnosed when resisted hip flexion is painful when performed with the patient in a seated position. The normal protocol is to inject 2 mL of triamcinolone along with 3 mL of 1% lidocaine. The contracture of the tensor fascia lata results in an apparent limb-length difference. Patients report the limb-length difference with the tight side being longer by 1 to 2.5 cm. Patients with this condition respond well to a regimen of stretching for the tensor fascia lata, which involves stabilizing the hip either in the prone (Figure 4) or side-lying positions, after which the therapist performs extension and adduction mobilization of the hip joint. In addition to stretching, patients with tensor fascia lata tightness respond well to manual massage and soft-tissue mobilization techniques using deep massage. In patients with tensor fascia lata tightness that results in a limb-length discrepancy, shoe lifts should not be used initially; the patient should be instructed to ambulate to stretch the tensor muscle. The author believes that using a shoe lift prevents effective stretching of the tensor fascia lata during ambulation.

Muscle Weakness

Hip abductor weakness is a major complication for many THA patients. If the muscle weakness is less than grade 3, a therapeutic treatment regimen should begin

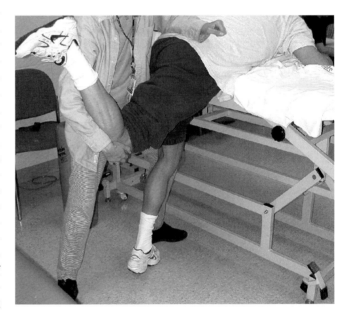

Figure 4 Stretching of the tensor fascia lata with the patient positioned in 90° of opposite limb hip flexion. The table stabilizes the pelvis and the affected limb is stretched into extension and adduction.

with aqua-therapy. Aqua-therapy improves muscle performance by using buoyancy to reduce gravitational forces. The warm temperature of the water also increases blood flow to the affected muscles. Hydrotherapy allows hip muscles to be strengthened and reduces joint contact forces compared with land-based exercise. After muscle strength is increased to more than grade 3 (on a grade 1 through 5 scale), a land-based strengthening regimen can begin. Electrical stimulation should be used to augment the strengthening program for the gluteus minimus and medius muscles (Figure 5). The program should focus on

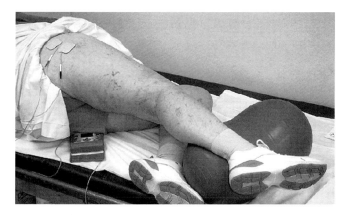

Figure 5 Neuromuscular electrical stimulation is used to strengthen the gluteus medius. The electrodes are placed posterior and posterior/superior to the greater trochanter and the patient is instructed to abduct, extend, and externally rotate the hip while the stimulator is active.

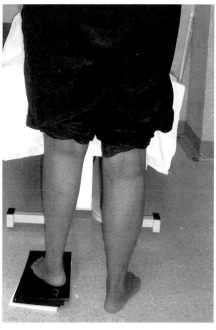

Figure 6 The block method is used to assess limb-length difference. The examiner evaluates the level of the posterior superior iliac spine and spinal curvature.

muscle pattern techniques that strengthen hip abduction using correct positioning to enhance muscle performance rather than using resistance to complete standard hip abduction exercises. For example, the gluteus medius is best strengthened in the side-lying position with the hip in approximately 10° of extension and external rotation while completing the abduction motion. This positioning specifically addresses the role of the gluteus medius in abduction. The gluteus minimus is strengthened in pure abduction in the side-lying position, while the tensor fascia lata is strengthened in the supine position with the hip held in internal rotation with abduction completed in a 45° arc. As the muscle performance improves, weights are applied first at the knee and then at the ankle to increase the lever arm of the resistance. The maximum weight used with this specific regimen should not exceed 10 lb. When an acceptable level of improvement is achieved with these treatment techniques, functional techniques such as a single leg stance in front of a mirror for biofeedback, and devices such as the Biomechanical Ankle Platform System (Spectrum Therapy Products, Jackson, MI) are used to increase total limb function and pelvic stability using a single leg stance. Closed chain position training on the Biomechanical Ankle Platform System emphasizes the role of the gluteus medius and minimus muscles in stabilizing the pelvis. When exercise is performed in the open chain for hip abduction strengthening, the gluteus medius and minimus muscles along with the sartorius, obturator internus, and upper portion of the gluteus maximus are all exercised. When using closed chain exercise, only the gluteus medius and minimus muscles are active. In most patients who have revision THA and in some primary THA patients, the average length of the exercise program (with or without a supervised physical therapy regimen) is 3 to 6 months to achieve return to full function.

In addition to abductor muscle strengthening, attention should be focused on strengthening the quadriceps and hip extension muscles. Weakness in these muscles has been found up to 1 year after THA surgery. This weakness has been correlated with reduced walking speed and abnormal gait with compensation from the knee and ankle joints. Poorer results in outcome self-assessment also have been reported in these patients. Hip and knee extension exercises should begin as closed chain exercise (such as the leg press) and later can progress to open chain exercise.

Limb-length differences caused by hip abductor tightness should be treated with aggressive stretching and manual physical therapy techniques to improve tensor fascia lata length. Patients who have a true limb-length difference with the surgical side longer than the contralateral side report trochanteric pain and pain around the THA incision. These symptoms are caused by pelvic tilt compensation, which places the long leg in adduction and the short leg in abduction. This condition is resolved with appropriate shoe lifts on the contralateral side. When the contralateral side is longer than the surgical side, shoe lifts from 0.5 to 1 cm less than the true limb-length difference are used to aid in foot clearance during walking. It is best to assess the limb-length difference using the block method with the patient standing (Figure 6). The examiner evaluates the level of the posterior superior iliac spine and also examines spinal curvature. The patient should be asked for feedback on the comfort of shoe lifts of varying sizes and should try different lifts before shoes are modified with appropriate lifts.

Return to Activities

Most patients can return to driving a motor vehicle after 6 to 8 weeks if THA has been performed on the left hip.

Patients with THA on the right hip may require additional rehabilitation before returning to driving. The decision to return to driving should be based on improvement in reaction time, ability to sit for prolonged periods, and strength of the surgical side. Gradual return to the activities of daily living followed by graduated joint loading in ambulation leads to good results. Patients are often eager to return to some form of recreational sports activities. Patients should be encouraged to engage in light recreational activities such as swimming, golf, bowling, bicycling, and doubles tennis. Patients who participate in high-impact sports such as singles tennis, jogging, racquetball, and backpacking have twice the risk of early aseptic loosening compared with those who participate in low-impact activities. Patients can resume sexual activity approximately 6 to 8 weeks after surgery. Patients should be informed about safe positions for sexual activities even if specific questions are not asked during clinical visits.

Rehabilitation After Total Knee Arthroplasty
Acute Phase
The acute phase of rehabilitation after TKA lasts for up to 4 to 5 days after surgery. Patients will have a better outcome in this phase if they have had either a preoperative education class or have been assessed for risk factors that increase the length of the hospital stay. Patients with risk factors such as obesity, diabetes, preoperative stiffness, and other comorbidities respond well to a more targeted and intensive rehabilitative regimen in this phase. Therapy should be provided at least once per day; however, twice daily therapy is useful in most patients after TKA. It is best to provide therapy coverage through the weekend days for all patients after TKA. Postoperative rehabilitation begins 1 day after surgery and is focused on getting the patient out of bed and on teaching the method of transfer. Sets of moderate intensity isometric exercises for the gluteal muscles and quadriceps, and ankle pumps are also started. Patients are encouraged to do deep breathing exercises. A gentle regimen of active assistive flexion and passive extension exercise is followed by the slide and flex, tighten, extend (SAFTE) protocol. Active exercise of the hamstring muscles relaxes the quadriceps mechanism by reciprocal inhibition and reduces the pain of flexion exercise. Aggressive passive flexion exercise should be avoided in the early postoperative phase; however, passive knee extension of moderate intensity is recommended to avoid the risk of developing flexion contracture. Patients are positioned with a towel roll under the heel for several hours per day to promote gravity-assisted extension. Patient-controlled administration of intravenous narcotics is usually used to achieve pain control. This method provides the patient with pain relief within minutes and makes them feel more secure and less anxious during

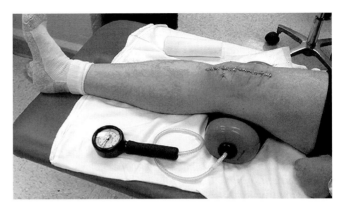

Figure 7 A simple cuff method to promote knee extension exercise using the biofeedback principle is shown.

activities. Cryotherapy is also a useful method of pain control and has been shown to reduce the length of the hospital stay and to improve walking velocity. Although cryotherapy does not reduce the need for narcotic analgesics in the early postoperative phase, it a useful adjunct and is best used before and after therapy sessions.

The routine use of continuous passive motion (CPM) in all patients after TKA is unwarranted. Several studies in the literature have shown no additional benefit from routine use of CPM in patients after TKA compared with the use of a standardized physical therapy regimen. CPM should be reserved for patients with preoperative stiffness, poor tolerance to pain, and inadequate participation in therapy. These patients also benefit from continuous epidural analgesia. Patients with preoperative stiffness with reduced flexion range of motion may benefit from an early flexion protocol with CPM (70° to 110° flexion followed by increased extension as tolerated daily). Patients with preoperative flexion contractures are better treated with periods of extension bracing followed by CPM that ranges from full extension to flexion, or the surgical side should dangle at several sessions per day. Care should be taken to avoid the development of flexion contracture because most CPM machines allow the knee to stay flexed. The use of additional padding under the heel avoids the flexion position while using CPM. Electrical neuromuscular stimulation of the quadriceps is a very useful modality to promote knee extension and improve the strength of the quadriceps. In the early postoperative phase, the intensity of the stimulator can be sufficient to produce submaximal contractions for a longer duration. In the outpatient setting, the stimulator can produce maximal contractions for short duration. Simple biofeedback measures such as inflated cuffs to promote knee extension with sets of isometric exercises for the quadriceps are also useful (Figure 7).

Most patients use bilateral support for ambulation. Patients are typically allowed to bear weight as tolerated after TKA. Early use of a unilateral assistive device such as a cane can cause out-of-plane stress on the joint and increased torsional stress and pain. Patients (especially those with quadriceps weakness) should use a knee immobilizer early in the ambulation process to ensure axial weight bearing and to reduce the risk of out-of-plane forces on the prosthesis. Similar to the recommendations for THA patients, TKA patients should use the leg on the nonsurgical side as the leading leg for stair ascent and should ascend steps one at a time in the early postoperative phase. The decision to send a patient to inpatient rehabilitation should be made in a team setting after evaluating the physical, social, and psychological needs of the patient. There is an increasing trend in many hospitals to refer patients to an inpatient rehabilitation unit to reduce the length of stay in the acute treatment setting. This trend may lead to inadequate therapy for the TKA patient, which could result in the premature onset of stiffness. The reduced length of stay in the acute setting has been correlated with the increased incidence of manipulations under anesthesia for treatment of postoperative loss of flexion range of motion. Unlike THA patients, TKA patients have few restrictions except for a gradual increase in loading of the joint. They are allowed unlimited ambulation on a level surface and are encouraged to participate in at least 1 hour of daily exercise focused on attaining range of motion, strength of the lower extremity, and improved balance and gait.

Subacute and Outpatient Phase

In the subacute and outpatient phase of rehabilitation, quadriceps weakness, flexion contracture, knee flexion deficit, peroneal nerve symptoms, and limb-length difference require special attention (Table 1). Quadriceps weakness is defined as active extension lag exceeding 15° in the early postoperative phase, or less than 50% strength compared with the contralateral limb when tested using a dynamometer in the later stages of recovery. Knee flexion contracture is defined as a lack of extension of 10° or more. A knee flexion deficit is defined as knee flexion of less than 90°. Peroneal nerve entrapment produces burning pain down to the dorsum of the foot, paresthesias of the foot, increased foot pain, mild extensor hallucis longus weakness, and a positive Tinel's sign. In addition to these peroneal nerve symptoms, patients with a previous history of sciatica can develop increased peroneal nerve tension and symptoms postoperatively. After TKA, patients can have a limb-length discrepancy with the TKA side being longer than the contralateral side; this condition results in a flexed knee posture and a resultant flexion contracture. These flexion contractures may develop to compensate for the limb-length difference. At the author's institution, it has been observed that patients with bilateral genu varum deformity after a unilateral TKA develop limb-length differences. This deformity may occur because the surgical side gains length

from the correction of the varus deformity.

The causes of the knee flexion contracture include preoperative loss of motion with muscle shortening, previous surgery with exuberant scar formation, knee effusion resulting in pain and quadriceps inhibition causing hamstring overactivity, unrecognized gastrocnemius tightness, a limb-length difference with a longer TKA side resulting in a knee-flexed posture, periarticular remodeling, joint subluxation, and peroneal nerve entrapment. All patients who develop knee flexion contractures should have aggressive therapy four to five times weekly for the first few weeks. In addition, they should be fitted with a splint to wear at home. Two types of off-the-shelf devices are available. One device uses the low load, prolonged stretch principle and needs to be used for up to 8 hours per day. Another device uses the stress relaxation technique in which the patient applies a greater degree of force across the joint. This device is used for 30 minutes, three times per day. Both methods require preapproval from the patient's health insurance provider and are expensive. A low cost alternative device that can be fitted the same day has been developed. This device, called the customized knee device, allows for knee extension positioning using a resistance band attached in a figure-of-8 fashion to produce an extension moment at the knee (Figure 8). Patients use the customized knee device at a maximally tolerated tension for 30 to 45 minutes, three times per day.

In addition to splinting, recommended aggressive adjunctive therapy consists of moist heat and soft-tissue mobilization to the posterior knee with maximal knee extension. End-range knee extension is promoted by the use of anterior/posterior joint mobilization of grade II to III to the femur with the patient supine and with the proximal tibia supported by a bolster. Gastrocnemius stretching with the patient supine with the heel propped and the knee in maximum extension also is used. Neuromuscular electrical stimulation involves applying electrodes to the quadriceps over the vastus medialis oblique fibers and over the proximal vastus lateralis. This treatment is recommended for 20 to 30 minutes with 5 seconds of stimulation alternating with 15 seconds of no stimulation, and a waveform at 70 to 90 pulses per second with a 400-microsecond pulse duration. Intensity of the stimulation should be at the maximum level the patient can tolerate. After the patient tolerates neuromuscular stimulation at a submaximal intensity, a short duration protocol of the burst superimposition technique with maximal isometric contraction is used to achieve rapid gains in strength. Weight-bearing exercises using leg presses for closed chain end-range knee extension also are used. An aggressive treatment regimen for flexion contracture is successful for most patients. This regimen focuses on joint positioning, careful assessment of joint subluxation, and the use of an anterior drawer maneuver to mobilize the knee into extension. The cus-

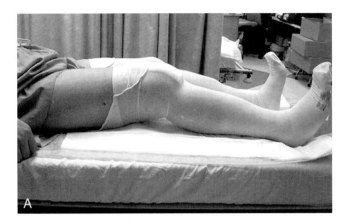
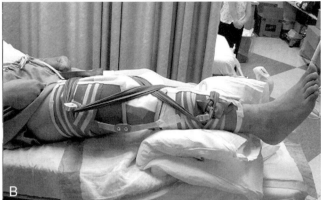

Figure 8 A customized knee device is used to increase knee extension range of motion and to eliminate knee flexion contracture. **A,** The patient lies supine with the knee extended. **B,** The brace is donned with tension produced by a resistance band in a figure-of-8 fashion to create a knee extension moment and a sustained end-range stretch to the posterior knee structures. Patients use the device before physical therapy and three times per day for 30 minutes per session.

tomized knee device or splints are used for prolonged knee extension positioning at home and sometimes at night. Aggressive mobilization of the joint and electrical stimulation of the quadriceps is used to supplement the passive range of motion achieved with active extension. After flexion contracture has resolved, gait training is used to improve active heel strike at initial contact. Any limb-length discrepancy is managed with an appropriate shoe lift. Special attention is given to terminal knee extension strength. Patients who have weakness in this range will flex the knee during walking to put the quadriceps under tension for stance phase stability. This adaptive compensation can result in the reoccurrence of knee flexion contracture.

Knee flexion deficits (less than 90° of flexion) result in functional deficits in stair ascent and descent, rising from a chair, sitting in a chair, prolonged sitting, and participation in sexual activities. These complications are mainly related to joint effusion, quadriceps tightness, rectus femoris tightness, and patellar tendon tightness or inflammation. In a subset of patients in whom physical therapy alone fails to achieve adequate knee flexion, additional mechanical therapy is recommended. A simple adaptation of the overhead pulley system can be used for self-stretching exercises (Figure 9). The customized knee device is used for knee flexion as well as for improving extension (Figure 10). The patients are instructed to use the device for 30 to 45 minutes three times per day to improve knee flexion. In addition to splinting, careful knee joint mobilization with posterior glides of the tibia (Figure 11), inferior patellar mobilization (Figure 12), and mobilization of the quadriceps tendon and patellar tendons all are techniques applied to increase knee flexion. Physical therapy and customized bracing alone are successful treatments for most patients. If these methods fail, manipulation under anesthesia can be used to improve flexion range of motion. Manipulation produces the best result when used 6 to

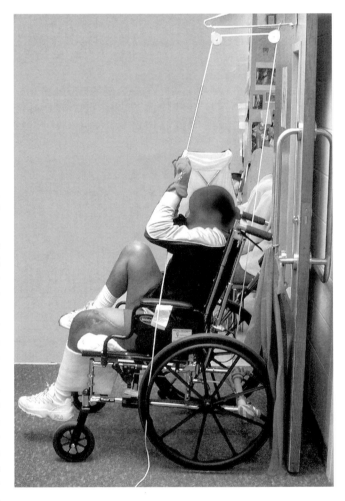

Figure 9 An overhead pulley system is used to improve knee flexion. Adjunctive mechanical therapies are useful in patients after TKA.

12 weeks postoperatively. After 12 weeks, most patients will need either arthroscopic lysis or arthrotomy to treat stiffness of the joint. In most patients who undergo TKA, outpatient therapy for up to 3 months after sur-

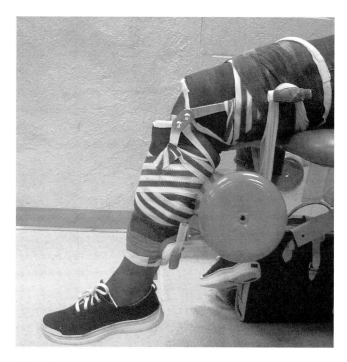

Figure 10 A custom knee device is used to improve knee flexion. The patient sits at maximal knee flexion with a posterior force from the elastic tubing maintaining maximal knee flexion for 30 minutes, two to three times per day. Note the use of a cylindrical tube to achieve a perpendicular flexion force on the tibia.

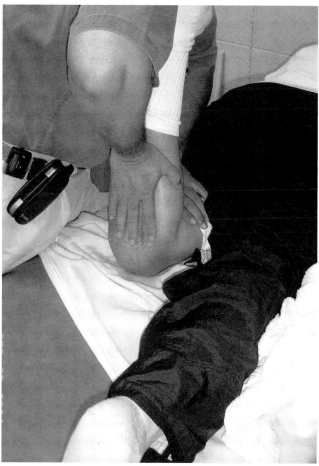

Figure 11 The joint mobilization technique is used to improve knee flexion. Posterior glide of the tibia on the femur mobilizes the knee with the patient prone. This mobilization directly addresses tight structures and increases knee flexion range of motion.

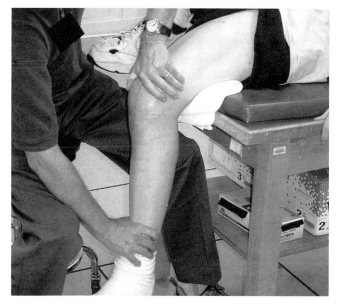

Figure 12 Rectus femoris stretch with inferior patellar mobilization. This technique promotes true elongation of the quadriceps without increasing joint contact forces of the patellofemoral joint. Pain during flexion mobilization is reduced.

gery is required because there is a significant risk of developing stiffness between 3 to 7 weeks postoperatively. Careful monitoring and modification of therapy protocol is warranted to avoid stiffness.

Significant weakness of the quadriceps requires the use of a protocol for muscle stimulation to augment the muscle contraction during strengthening. This regimen is more effective than voluntary contractions alone because of the neural overflow produced by the electrical stimulation. There is a high incidence of weakness in the quadriceps in patients after TKA and this condition will remain unresolved at 2-year follow-up if not specifically treated. Patients should be advised that regular daily activities and walking do not improve quadriceps strength; only a targeted strengthening exercise regimen will improve strength. Closed chain exercises (Figure 13) initially followed by open chain exercises and isokinetic exercises are recommended. In addition to this targeted regimen, functional activities that promote quadriceps strengthening are very beneficial. These activities include step-ups and minisquats. Quadriceps weakness is always noticeable in terminal knee extension because of selective vastus medialis inhibition and the need for greater motor recruitment in terminal extension. Electrical neuromuscular stimulation applied with the knee in the terminal extension position against resistance is beneficial to improve the strength of the quadriceps (Figure 14).

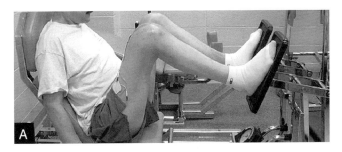 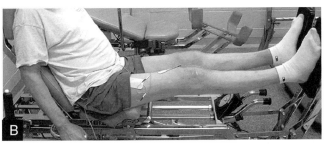

Figure 13 Closed chain exercise for improving concentric and eccentric quadriceps strength. This exercise promotes full knee extension to achieve proper gait, assists in gaining knee flexion range of motion, and provides proprioceptive input. **A,** Shows a patient maximizing the knee flexion range of motion with assistance from a leg press. **B,** Shows a patient performing knee extension exercise with electrical stimulation of quadriceps muscle against resistance from a leg press.

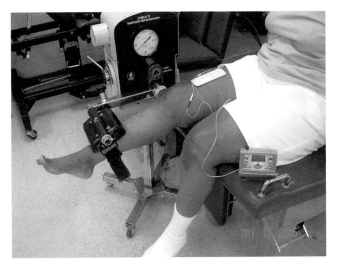

Figure 14 The terminal knee extension exercise is augmented with neuromuscular electrical stimulation.

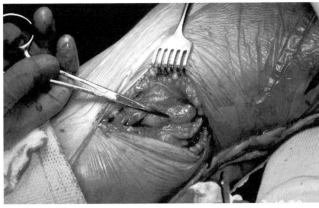

Figure 15 A peroneal nerve release is performed to decrease peroneal nerve symptoms to aid the patient in achieving functional knee extension.

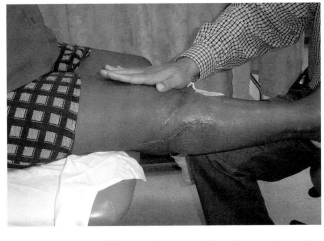

Figure 16 After release of the peroneal nerve, resolution of nerve symptoms allows for therapy to be quickly resumed. Patients can achieve knee extension quickly after the surgical release.

Peroneal nerve entrapment can result in a lack of knee extension. Patients with this complication show no frank motor involvement except for mild weakness of the extensor hallucis longus. Knee extension results in foot pain and knee flexion improves the pain. Peroneal nerve symptoms make rehabilitation difficult and produce poor results. Surgical release of the peroneal nerve (Figure 15) results in quick resolution of symptoms; aggressive rehabilitation can immediately begin (Figure 16).

Return to Activities

Most patients can return to driving a motor vehicle 6 weeks after TKA. As with THA patients, the decision to return to driving should be based on improvement in reaction time, ability to sit for a prolonged period of time, and strength on the surgical side. Gradual return to the activities of daily living followed by graduated joint loading in ambulation produces favorable outcomes. Patients who have undergone TKA should be encouraged to engage in light recreational activities and can resume sexual activity approximately 4 weeks after surgery. TKA patients should be given information about safe positions for sexual activity.

Annotated Bibliography
General
Sicard-Rosenbaum L, Light KE, Behrman AL: Gait, lower extremity strength, and self-assessed mobility after hip arthroplasty. *J Gerontol A Biol Sci Med Sci* 2002; 57(1):M47-M51.

Although most patients are satisfied with pain relief after THA, many express dissatisfaction with their ability to perform domestic and social activities. Reduced walking ability and long-term lower extremity muscle weakness may contribute to decreased mobility. This study compared muscle strength, gait, and functional mobility in 15 adults at 9-month to 6-year follow-up after THA. Results were compared with a group of 15 age- and gender-matched controls. The THA group walked significantly slower than the control group. THA patients had less muscle strength in the lower extremity on the operated side than on the nonsurgical side; the hip abductors were the most affected muscle group. The authors recommend an intervention beyond the initial postsurgical rehabilitation to address long-term residual impairments and disabilities found after THA.

Youm T, Maurer SG, Stuchin SA: Postoperative management after total hip and knee arthroplasty. *J Arthroplasty* 2005;20(3):322-324.

A comprehensive review of protocols for the management of THA and TKA patients is presented. This study is a review of the results of a survey mailed to active members of American Association of Hip and Knee Surgeons. The survey included questions on postoperative rehabilitation and activity restrictions. The information derived from this survey provides a compilation and consensus of responses that can serve as the foundation for a standardized postoperative protocol for THA and TKA surgery.

Rehabilitation After Total Hip Arthroplasty
Bertocci GE, Munin MC, Frost KL, Burdett R, Wassinger CA, Fitzgerald SG: Isokinetic performance after total hip replacement. *Am J Phys Med Rehabil* 2004;83(1):1-9.

The authors of this study evaluated muscle strength differences in isokinetic hip flexion, extension, and abduction muscles of operated versus nonoperated hips in 20 THA patients and in 22 healthy older adults. Results showed that hips of THA patients generated significantly less peak torque per body weight across all exercises compared with the group of healthy older adults. The operated and nonoperated hips of the THA patients showed similar biomechanical performance. THA patients are not restored to the same level of strength as found in the population of healthy older adults.

Erler K, Anders C, Fehlberg G, Neumann U, Brucker L, Scholle HC: Objective assessment of results of special hydrotherapy in inpatient rehabilitation following knee prosthesis implantation. *Z Orthop Ihre Grenzgeb* 2001; 139(4):352-358.

This study evaluated the use of hydrotherapy in the early phase of recovery in TKA patients. Twenty-five patients received hydrotherapy for 3 weeks during inpatient rehabilitation. Electromyogram mapping, ultrasound, and isokinetic muscle strength testing were used to compare this group with 38 patients who received the standard rehabilitation protocol. All of the objective testing was performed at 4, 7, and 26 weeks postoperatively. The results were also compared with those of age-matched healthy individuals. The authors found that patients in the hydrotherapy group showed greater improvements in coordination and strength than patients treated with the standard rehabilitation program. An early hydrotherapy regimen is recommended for patients after TKA.

Gotze C, Sippel C, Rosenbaum D, Hackenberg L, Steinbeck J: Objective measures of gait following revision hip arthroplasty: First medium-term results 2.6 years after surgery. *Z Orthop Ihre Grenzgeb* 2003;141(2):201-208.

After THA, patients have persistent muscle weakness and abnormal gait as measured by three-dimensional gait analysis techniques. Standard measures of THA outcome do not correlate with gait deviations measured with objective techniques. This study evaluated gait and function of 33 patients after revision THA (mean follow-up of 2.6 years). All of the revisions involved acetabular components. Gait analysis showed a decreased range of hip extension movement and reduced hip abductor moment (force generation). This deficit was compensated for by increased muscle activity to stabilize the operated hip. Neither the Harris Hip score (77.8 points) nor the d'Aubigne score (14.9 points) were associated with the gait abnormalities observed in three-dimensional gait studies ($P > 0.05$).

Mahomed NN, Koo Seen Lin MJ, Levesque J, Lan S, Bogoch ER: Determinants and outcomes of inpatient versus home based rehabilitation following elective hip and knee replacement. *J Rheumatol* 2000;27(7):1753-1758.

Patients are often referred to inpatient rehabilitation after joint arthroplasty. This study presents a retrospective evaluation of 146 patients after primary TKA and THA. Ninety-six patients completed a mailed survey consisting of the Western Ontario and McMaster University Osteoarthritis Index, the Medical Outcomes Survey Short Form-36, and a satisfaction questionnaire. At a mean follow-up of 8 months postoperatively, there were no significant differences between the inpatient and home-based rehabilitation groups with respect to the surveys and the satisfaction scores.

Miyoshi T, Shirota T, Yamamoto S, Nakazawa K, Akai M: Lower limb joint moment during walking in water. *Disabil Rehabil* 2003;25(21):1219-1223.

Walking in water is a widely used form of rehabilitation that is based on the belief that the reduction of body weight in water reduces joint reactive forces thus reducing secondary injuries to the lower limb joints. The authors used a three-dimensional kinematic system to measure joint moments at the hip, knee, and ankle joint while volunteers walked in water. Results of the study show that joint moments of the hip, knee, and ankle were reduced during walking in water, and that interjoint coordination was changed. This reduction in moments and change in the inter-joint relationship reduces joint contact forces. Water offers a pain-free medium to exercise joints after joint replacements without the risk of secondary injuries.

Oldmeadow LB, McBurney H, Robertson VJ, Kimmel L, Elliott B: Targeted postoperative care improves discharge outcome after hip or knee arthroplasty. *Arch Phys Med Rehabil* 2004;85(9):1424-1427.

Preoperative risk assessment followed by targeted postoperative care reduces the length of the hospital stay and reduces the number of inpatient rehabilitation admissions. The risk of discharge to extended inpatient rehabilitation was preoperatively assessed for 50 patients with a newly developed Risk Assessment and Prediction Tool. Postoperative treatment was targeted on the basis of the identified level of risk. Results were compared with those of a similar group of 50 patients. The percentage of patients discharged directly home increased significantly, from 34% during 2000, to 64% in 2001 (P =0.002). In addition, the mean acute hospital length of stay decreased by 1.1 days to 7.5 days in 2001 (P = 0.02). The authors recommend preoperative screening followed by targeted intervention during the acute phase after joint arthroplasty to increase the rate of discharge to home and reduced the length of the hospital stay.

Perron M, Malouin F, Moffet H, McFadyen BJ: Three-dimensional gait analysis in women with a total hip arthroplasty. *Clin Biomech (Bristol, Avon)* 2000;15(7):504-515.

This cross-sectional study compared the gait patterns of women with a THA to those of women with healthy hips. A significant decrease (20%) in the hip extensor moment was correlated with a significant decrease of 14% in gait speed. Moreover, a significant decrease of 59% in the range of hip extension was observed together with secondary impairments such as the increase in anterior pelvic rotation, knee flexion, and ankle dorsiflexion. A significant increase in ipsilateral bending of the trunk during single limb support on the operated limb and a significant decrease in the hip abductor moment of force was observed. The authors proposed using these objective measures as guidelines to establish rehabilitation programs designed to restore optimal locomotor function after THA.

Reardon K, Galea M, Dennett X, Choong P, Byrne E: Quadriceps muscle wasting persists 5 months after total hip arthroplasty for osteoarthritis of the hip: A pilot study. *Intern Med J* 2001;31(1):7-14.

This study evaluated vastus lateralis atrophy before and up to 5 months after THA in 19 patients. Evaluation techniques included ultrasound, dynamometry, pain scores, and the use of the Timed Up and Go test. Results showed an improvement in pain and Timed Up and Go test scores. At 5-month follow-up, significant atrophy (measured by ultrasound) and weakness (measured by dynamometry) persisted. Prolonged exercise and other therapeutic strategies to reverse significant atrophy and weakness were recommended.

Rehabilitation After Total Knee Arthroplasty

Avramidis K, Strike PW, Taylor PN, Swain ID: Effectiveness of electric stimulation of the vastus medialis muscle in the rehabilitation of patients after total knee arthroplasty. *Arch Phys Med Rehabil* 2003;84(12):1850-1853.

This prospective randomized trial evaluated the effects of neuromuscular electrical stimulation of the vastus medialis muscle on walking speed in 30 patients after TKA. Patients were randomly assigned to one of two groups. Both groups received standard physical therapy. The treatment group also received neuromuscular electrical stimulation of the vastus medialis during the first 6 weeks after surgery. The patients in the treatment group who received neuromuscular stimulation in addition to standard physical therapy achieved significantly improved walking speeds. A carryover effect was also noted after the discontinuation of treatment.

Branch TP, Karsch RE, Mills TJ, Palmer MT: Mechanical therapy for loss of knee flexion. *Am J Orthop* 2003; 32(4):195-200.

The authors describe a simple technique of adjunctive mechanical therapy to induce prolonged stretch in patients after TKA to improve knee flexion range of motion. Thirty-four patients who had a primary TKA and who did not achieve flexion after therapy alone were fitted with a mechanical device to improve knee flexion range of motion. Improved knee flexion to 115° in 7 weeks occurred in 31 of 33 patients (91%). Only two patients required surgical manipulation. Results of the study show the need for additional therapeutic options to augment knee flexion range of motion in patients who do not improve from physical therapy alone.

Hopkins J, Ingersoll CD, Edwards J, Klootwyk TE: Cryotherapy and transcutaneous electric neuromuscular stimulation decrease arthrogenic muscle inhibition of the vastus medialis after knee joint effusion. *J Athl Train* 2002;37(1):25-31.

This article discusses the role of arthrogenic muscle inhibition of the vastus medialis in the presence of knee joint effusion and also investigates the usefulness of cryotherapy and electrical neuromuscular stimulation to disinhibit arthrogenic muscle inhibition. Thirty neurologically sound volunteers participated in this study. Knee joint effusion was artificially produced by injection of saline solution. Artificial knee joint effusion resulted in significant muscle inhibition. Cryotherapy and transcutaneous electric nerve stimulation both disinhibit the quadriceps after surgery on the knee joint.

Kolisek FR, Gilmore KJ, Peterson EK: Slide and flex, tighten, extend (SAFTE): A safe, convenient, effective, and no-cost approach to rehabilitation after total knee arthroplasty. *J Arthroplasty* 2000;15(8):1013-1016.

This study describes a simple and effective technique to improve functional range of motion after TKA. In a single-radius, posterior-stabilized knee prosthesis, the SAFTE protocol resulted in 70% of patients achieving full extension and at least 90° of flexion. Authors conclude that SAFTE is a safe, effective, and no-cost approach to achieve functional range of motion in the early postoperative phase after TKA.

Lamb SE, Frost H: Recovery of mobility after knee arthroplasty: Expected rates and influencing factors. *J Arthroplasty* 2003;18(5):575-582.

This study evaluated the effect of knee extensor strength, knee flexion range of motion, and pain on mobility (walking speed and stair climbing speed) after TKA in 79 patients at 6 months postoperatively. A marked loss of flexion in the postoperative period was not a significant determinant of mobility speed. At 6-month follow-up, body mass index was the most significant determinant of stair climbing speed, and leg extensor power was the most significant determinant of walking speed.

Lyons CL, Robb JB, Irrgang JJ, Fitzgerald GK: Differences in quadriceps femoris muscle torque when using a clinical electrical stimulator versus a portable electrical stimulator. *Phys Ther* 2005;85(1):44-51.

The efficacy and adequacy of the portable battery-operated muscle stimulator compared with a plug-in stimulator are evaluated as used in the therapy clinics. Peak isometric torque of the quadriceps femoris was measured in 40 patients using two methods of electrical stimulation. The portable stimulator produced comparable levels of average peak torque to those produced by the plug-in stimulator. Based on these data, the authors concluded that plug-in units have the potential to produce adequate levels of torque production for neuromuscular electrical stimulation for quadriceps femoris muscle performance training.

MacDonald SJ, Bourne RB, Rorabeck CH, McCalden RW, Kramer J, Vaz M: Prospective randomized clinical trial of continuous passive motion after total knee arthroplasty. *Clin Orthop Relat Res* 2000;380:30-35.

This prospective randomized clinical trial evaluated the usefulness of CPM in early postoperative rehabilitation after TKA. One hundred twenty patients were randomly assigned to treatment groups that included group I, no CPM; group II, CPM from 0° to 50° and increased as tolerated; and group III, CPM from 70° to 110°. CPM was initiated in the recovery room. All patients began a standardized physical therapy regimen 24 hours after surgery. Patients were assessed preoperatively, during their hospital stay, and at 6, 12, 26, and 52 weeks postoperatively. There were no statistical differences between any of the treatment groups regarding cumulative analgesic requirements, range of motion at any measured interval, length of hospital stay, or Knee Society scores. Routine use of CPM is not warranted in primary TKA. A carefully structured physical therapy program is adequate in most patients after TKA.

Morsi E: Continuous-flow cold therapy after total knee arthroplasty. *J Arthroplasty* 2002;17(6):718-722.

The results of 60 TKAs done on 30 patients are presented. A single surgeon using the same technique did all the surgeries 6 weeks apart. One side received a continuous-flow cooling device immediately applied over the surgical dressing postoperatively. The other TKA in the same patient was done 6 weeks later without a cooling device. The study compared the range of motion, the volume of Hemovac output and blood loss, the visual analog pain score, analgesic consumption, and wound healing. This study showed that continuous-flow cold therapy is advantageous after TKA because it provides better results in all areas of comparison.

Ranawat CS, Ranawat AS, Mehta A: Total knee arthroplasty rehabilitation protocol: What makes the difference? *J Arthroplasty* 2003;18(suppl 1)27-30.

The rehabilitation protocol for 2,000 patients after TKA is reviewed. The goals of any rehabilitation protocol should be to control pain, improve ambulation, maximize range of motion, develop muscle strength, and provide emotional support. Most patients (85%) will recover knee function after TKA regardless of the rehabilitation protocol used. The remaining 15% will have difficulty because of significant pain, limited preoperative motion, or the development of arthrofibrosis. This subset of patients will require a special, individualized rehabilitation program that may involve prolonged oral analgesia, continued physical therapy, additional diagnostic studies, and occasional manipulation.

Silva M, Shepherd EF, Jackson WO, Pratt JA, McClung CD, Schmalzried TP: Knee strength after total knee arthroplasty. *J Arthroplasty* 2003;18(5):605-611.

This study evaluated muscle strength 2 years after TKA in 32 patients and compared it with 52 knees in a control group of healthy individuals. The mean peak torque values for the quadriceps and hamstring were reduced by 30% in the TKA patients. Knee Society functional scores were positively correlated to the average isometric extension peak torque and negatively correlated to the average isometric hamstring-to-quadriceps ratio. Greater quadriceps strength was associated with a better functional score. Older TKA patients (> 70 years of age) had lower isometric extension peak torque values in terminal extension than younger TKA patients. A higher body mass index was associated with relative quadriceps weakness (r = 0.44, $P = 0.007$). The authors concluded that more rehabilitation after TKA to address extensor strength and controlling weight gain would improve functional outcomes.

Stevens JE, Mizner RL, Snyder-Mackler L: Quadriceps strength and volitional activation before and after total knee arthroplasty for osteoarthritis. *J Orthop Res* 2003; 21(5):775-779.

This prospective study evaluated the magnitude of quadriceps weakness (caused by arthrogenous muscle inhibition) at 26 days after TKA. The study differentiated between quadriceps muscle weakness caused by pain versus neurogenic inhibition. Results of this study in 28 patients with unilateral TKAs showed that most quadriceps weakness (65%) is caused by neurogenic inhibition leading to reduced voluntary activation when compared with inhibition that results from pain. The authors recommend a strong muscle contraction regimen and facilitation of the quadriceps mechanism using neuromuscular electrical stimulation and biofeedback to reverse quadriceps atrophy in the early rehabilitation phase after TKA.

Trudelle-Jackson E, Emerson R, Smith S: Outcomes of total hip arthroplasty: A study of patients one year post-surgery. *J Orthop Sports Phys Ther* 2002;32(6):260-267.

Most TKA patients receive instructions on self-help and a self-directed exercise regimen after early postoperative physical therapy. Outcomes of THA 1 year after surgery indicate that current physical therapy programs used during the acute phase of recovery do not effectively restore physical and functional performance. In this study, 15 patients were reviewed 1 year after unilateral THA. Range of motion, muscle strength, and postural stability between the involved hip and uninvolved hip were reviewed. These objective measures were compared with self assessments of function. Measures of postural stability were significantly lower ($P <$ or $= 0.01$) on the side of the replaced hip. Correlations between scores of self-assessed function and hip abductor and knee extensor strength were statistically significant (r $= 0.56$, $P <$ or $= 0.03$). The brief postoperative rehabilitation program for THA patients may not be adequate. A second phase of rehabilitation, implemented 4 or more months after surgery, that emphasizes weight bearing and postural stability, may be advisable.

Classic Bibliography

Mauerhan DR, Mokris JG, Ly A, Kiebzak GM: Relationship between length of stay and manipulation rate after total knee arthroplasty. *J Arthroplasty* 1998;13(8):896-900.

Scarcella JB, Cohn BT: The effect of cold therapy on the postoperative course of total hip and knee arthroplasty patients. *Am J Orthop* 1995;24(11):847-852.

Section 3

The Hip

Section Editors:
Joseph C. McCarthy, MD
Harry E. Rubash, MD

Chapter 30

Surgical Approaches

William A. McGann, MD

Introduction

Virtually all of the surgical approaches used for total hip arthroplasty require accurate and secure positioning of the patient to provide accurate orientation for component insertion and leg length measurements. The lateral or semilateral decubitus position is used for all exposures except the anterior, ilioinguinal, and medial approaches. Positioning, draping, the choice of approach, and the size and location of the skin incision should be chosen to maximize the exposure, and in revision procedures, options should be made available for extending the exposure to treat potential problems.

The position of the acetabulum for total hip arthroplasty depends on initial patient position, which may change during surgery. Variations of pelvic anteversion have been recently reported (lying and standing positions). The error in version may be as high as 20°. As a result of the variation in pelvic reference during surgery and the inaccuracy of freehand positioning of insertion guides, acetabular position has been demonstrated to vary greatly. Computer-assisted component positioning has been recently shown to improve the accuracy of acetabular component insertion and is predicted to become more valuable during hip reconstruction in the future.

In a recent computer navigation study of the abduction angle of the acetabular component, three groups of 50 total hip arthroplasties were assessed. In the first group, a freehand method was used to position the cup component. In the second group, CT-based computer navigation was used. The third group consisted of 50 historical comparison total hip arthroplasties in which a freehand method was used to position the cup. The use of computer navigation helped the surgeon to place the cup component with less variability of the abduction angle; more importantly, no cups were placed in the more extreme positions.

There are several options for the surgical approach to the hip in reconstructive surgery. Several advantages and disadvantages exist for each approach. Most hip surgeons will choose an approach from among several of these approaches to address needs for a patient or functional issue. A more anterior or direct lateral approach may lower the risk for dislocation in the confused patient. A posterior approach may maximize the chance for return of abductor function. A trochanteric osteotomy may be indicated for a large patient for better access, a hip with poor anatomy requiring advancement to tension the abductors, or fragile femoral bone that may not withstand torsion during rotation for posterior approach. It is important, therefore, for orthopaedic surgeons to be familiar with the commonly used surgical approaches for hip reconstruction. Some advantages and disadvantages differentiate each approach and help provide a template for their use.

Anterior Approach

The anterior approach, also known as the iliofemoral or Smith-Petersen approach, dissects the interval between the sartorius and rectus femoris muscles (femoral nerve innervated) and the tensor fascia and gluteus minimus and medius muscles (superior gluteal innervated) and thus is a true internervous approach. At risk during the approach are the lateral femoral cutaneous nerve and the ascending branch of the lateral femoral circumflex artery. The approach allows the hip to be dislocated anteriorly without risk to the femoral head blood supply. This approach is most useful when extensive exposure of the anterior column is necessary, such as in patients undergoing pelvic osteotomy or pelvic fracture repair. The extended exposure provides excellent access to the inner and outer tables of the ilium, anterior femoral head and neck, and acetabulum, but it severely limits posterior acetabular visualization. After release of the inguinal ligament from the anterior-superior iliac spine, the subperiosteal elevation of a portion of the iliopsoas can be extended into the true pelvis to the level of the greater sciatic notch. Extensive release of the abductors results in a high incidence of residual weakness of the abductors and formation of heterotopic bone. These two complications are the main limitations of this approach.

A new abductor-sparing surgical approach has been recently described as the direct anterior exposure. The approach was developed in an effort to eliminate the postoperative abductor morbidity associated with the classic Smith-Petersen approach. It combines the medial portion of the classic Smith-Petersen iliofemoral exposure with or without the second window of the ilioinguinal exposure. An osteotomy of the anterior-superior spine is done routinely to relax the attached sartorius and inguinal ligament origins. In a study of 195 patients, nearly all had demonstrated a return of their abductor function by 3 months after surgery, in distinct contrast to the authors' previous experience with the Smith-Petersen approach. The authors consider the direct anterior exposure to be the surgical approach of choice for periacetabular osteotomy, with the more limited version proving satisfactory in all patients, except the largest and most muscular patients.

The mid- to long-term results in a recent study of the Chiari pelvic osteotomy performed with the iliofemoral approach were found to be inferior to those using the transtrochanteric approach. The study included 135 hips in 129 patients at a mean follow-up of 16.2 years. The anterior iliofemoral approach without a trochanteric osteotomy was used in the initial 31 hips. Thereafter, the transtrochanteric approach was used to ensure that the osteotomy was at the most appropriate level and to advance the high-riding greater trochanter distally. The clinical result was excellent or good in 103 hips (77%). The outcome in 104 hips in which a transtrochanteric approach was used was superior, the osteotomy level was more appropriate, and a Trendelenburg gait was less common than in 31 hips for which an anterior approach was used.

A modification of the anterior approach described by Hueter provides limited access to the anterior hip for procedures such as biopsy, synovectomy, labral excision, or arthrotomy. This approach is essentially a limited Smith-Petersen approach and uses only the distal portion of the classic approach. This approach interval is currently popularized as the anterior portion of the two-incision minimally invasive approach for total hip replacement. The angle of the skin incision is usually rotated to align with the axis of the femoral neck in the minimally invasive surgical technique.

Two-Incision Anterior Approach

Originally conceptualized by Mears, the two-incision approach for total hip replacement has been under development since 2001. One anterior incision is used for the insertion of the acetabular component, and a lateral incision is used for the femoral component.

Two-Incision Approach With Fluoroscopy

This technique is done with the patient positioned supine on a standard radiolucent operating table. A small bolster is placed under the ipsilateral ischium, which el-

evates the acetabulum to aid in acetabular preparation and posterior draping. A fluoroscope is used to locate the anterior incision over the femoral neck (two to three finger breadths distal to the anterior-superior iliac spine). A pin is placed on the skin overlying the axis of the femoral neck, and the incision is marked at the mid-axis beginning at the head-neck junction and extends 1.5 inches distally. With the fluoroscope removed, the incision is made down to fascia. The fascial incision is then made just medial to the tensor fascia lata along the axis of the femur and parallel to the sartorius muscle and tensor fascia lata. Because the lateral femoral cutaneous nerve runs over the sartorius muscle, an incision lateral to the sartorius that is close to the tensor fascia lata avoids injury to the nerve.

Retractors are placed to retract sartorius medially and tensor fascia lata laterally. The medial retractor is repositioned to retract the rectus femoris muscle medially. The capsule is then exposed after coagulation of the lateral circumflex vessels. Two lighted Hohmann retractors are placed medially and laterally to the capsule. The capsule is incised longitudinally just lateral to the middle of the femoral neck from the acetabular rim to the intertrochanteric line. The capsule can be elevated 1 cm medially and laterally along the intertrochanteric line to enhance exposure. The two Hohmann retractors are shifted to the intracapsular position to expose the femoral neck for the osteotomy. The osteotomy is made at the equator of the head perpendicular to the axis of the femoral neck. A second osteotomy cut is made 1 cm distal to the first cut, which allows a wafer of femoral neck to be removed using a Steinmann pin and gentle leg traction. A threaded device is then placed in the femoral head, which is removed with the help of a curved Cobb elevator. If the femoral head cannot be extracted, additional cuts may be made to remove it in pieces. The fluoroscope is used to confirm proper femoral neck resection length and angle. The resection level can also be assessed by direct measurement after exposing the femoral neck and lesser trochanter with a figure-4 maneuver.

Attention is next directed to the acetabulum. Three curved, lighted Hohmann retractors are placed and located superiorly, anteriorly at the anterior margin of the transverse acetabular ligament, and posteriorly around the acetabulum. These specialized instruments have been developed to maximize efficiency and safety of retraction. To visualize the entire acetabulum, the retractors can be shifted slightly anterior or posterior to improve visibility. Specially designed reamers are used to allow easier insertion. A specialized dog-leg acetabular inserter is used to clear soft-tissue restraints and more easily position the acetabular shell. The shell is manipulated into position using both the fluoroscope and direct vision. The femur is prepared with the patient's leg adducted and in neutral rotation. The piriformis fossa is palpated from the anterior incision to determine location of the second incision in the buttocks. A small stab wound is then made and extended in line with the femoral neck approximately 1.25 inches. A Charnley awl is guided posteriorly to the abductors and anteriorly to the piriformis fossa. Because the initial insertion point is usually medial, special lateralizing reamers are used under fluoroscopy. Standard insertion can then be performed with position checks for rotation and length through the anterior incision. Closure of the capsule is performed.

The updated results of a radiographic follow-up study have been recently reported for the first 30 patients who underwent this technique. At an average 17-month follow-up (range, 12 to 25 months), all stems were determined to be between neutral and 3° of valgus. Acetabular component position was a mean of 45°, (range, 36° to 54°). All 30 femoral and acetabular components were reported to be ingrown and without migration.

Two-Incision Anterior Approach Without Fluoroscopy

A two-incision approach has been described without the need for fluoroscopy. This approach evolved from a single small-incision anterior approach, with the goals of sparing the abductors and fascia lata complex, eliminating fluoroscopy, and developing a technique that would be applicable to all patients and all implants. The two incisions mimic the distal one third of the Smith-Peterson approach for the socket and the proximal or medial one third of the Moore posterior approach for the femur. The interval is between tensor fascia lata and sartorius, and the vastus lateralis and rectus femoris more deeply. The posterior incision separates fibers of the gluteus maximus and avoids disturbance of the fascia lata.

For this approach, the patient is placed in the lateral position. The anterior 2-inch incision is made along the medial border of the tensor fascia lata and centered at the lower margin of the greater trochanter and the vastus ridge. The interval between tensor fascia lata and sartorius is developed and cobra retractors are placed. The reflected head of the rectus is released superomedially. In most patients, the anterior capsule is excised. The posterior incision is made with the leg flexed 30° and slightly internally rotated and adducted. A vertical line is drawn two finger breadths posterior to the greater trochanteric line and a transverse line two finger breadths inferior to the line at the tip of the trochanter. The intersection is bisected obliquely. The maximus fibers are split while taking care to avoid any extension into the fascia lata. The piriformis, gemelli, and a variable portion of the quadratus are released. The capsule is released circumferentially around the femoral neck in line with the tendons. The hip is dislocated posteriorly, and the preparation and insertion of components are

carried out as in a standard posterior approach. One advantage of this approach is that it allows both cemented and cementless femoral stem choice of any design (straight or curved) in patients of any size.

Anterolateral Approach

The anterolateral approach, popularized by Watson-Jones, provides limited exposure to the anterior hip. It is an excellent approach for anterior hip arthrotomy, biopsy, and fracture reduction because of its limited dissection of the major muscle groups. Its application for total hip replacement is limited because of poor exposure to the proximal femur for prosthetic insertion. The anterolateral approach dissects between the gluteus medius muscle and tensor fascia muscle, both of which are innervated by the superior gluteal nerve. It is therefore not a true internervous approach. This approach is less invasive to the abductors when compared with the iliofemoral approach.

The Harris lateral approach is similar to the traditional anterolateral approach. It can be performed with or without a trochanteric osteotomy. The exposure is more extensive than the technique of Watson-Jones, and it is useful for pelvic osteotomies and hip reconstruction. To improve medial exposure, the rectus tendon can be released and later reattached. To improve the distal wound exposure of the femoral neck and shaft, a portion of the vastus lateralis muscle origin can either be split or released from the vastus lateralis ridge and intertrochanteric line. Exposure of more superior capsule of the hip can also be accomplished by a partial release of the fibers of the gluteus medius from the distal trochanter as described by Muller.

Most studies demonstrate a lower incidence of postoperative dislocations with the anterolateral approach in total hip arthroplasty when compared historically with the posterolateral and transtrochanteric approaches. This advantage over the posterior and posterolateral approaches should disappear with the use of the newer capsular repairs. In a recent study, patients who had either an anterolateral or posterolateral approach in total hip replacement surgery were compared clinically for limp, dislocation, hospital stay, and discharge disposition. The only statistical difference was that the posterior approach had a statistically higher dislocation rate.

A recent study of a large consecutive series of primary total hip arthroplasties (N = 1,518) for which an anterolateral abductor split approach was used detected an overall dislocation rate of less than 1% (12 of 1,518; 0.79%). By diagnosis, trauma patients and those with congenital dislocation of the hip were found to have the highest risk for postoperative dislocation.

A recent prospective study of 499 primary total hip arthroplasties for which an anterolateral approach was used examined the concept of releasing patients from postoperative restrictions. There were three early dislocations within 6 weeks of surgery. All were reduced closed, and every patient subsequently had a stable hip without further intervention. The results suggest that a low early dislocation rate can be achieved using an anterolateral approach without the need to restrict postoperative mobilization.

The 6-month performance outcomes of the anterolateral and posterior approaches were compared in a recent gait study. The anterolateral approach group had the largest trunk inclination ($3.0° \pm 2.4°$) and the smallest hip range of motion ($34.0° \pm 7.4°$). The gait of 85% of the patients who underwent total hip arthroplasty had not returned to normal at 6 months.

A small incision anterolateral approach has been advocated as an alternative to the larger incision technique to facilitate a faster recovery. The incision is centered 2.0 to 2.5 cm distal to the tip of the trochanter and is canted posterior (proximal incision) 20° for a 3.5- to 4-inch incision and 30° for an incision smaller than 3.5 inches. The anterior portion of gluteus medius is released. This technique can be used in most but not all patients undergoing total hip replacement. Patients with varus femoral neck angles are considered better candidates than those with long valgus femoral necks because of the exposure challenges. Further study is required to determine whether this approach will offer any advantages over more conventional incisions.

To study the advantages of a small incision anterolateral approach, a clinical series was compared with a conventional group of patients; 212 cementless total hip arthroplasties were divided into three groups according to the length of the incision. At the end of surgery, incisions of 10 cm or smaller were defined as mini (N = 115) and incisions of 10 to 15 cm were defined as short (N = 70); these two groups were defined as shorter skin incision groups. Incisions longer than 15 cm in patients undergoing the standard procedure were defined as conventional and served as the controls (N = 27). Statistically significant differences were found with regard to surgical duration and intraoperative blood loss: the shorter the length of the incision, the shorter the surgical duration and the smaller the intraoperative blood loss. There was no significant difference in postoperative bleeding or in the incidence of complications among the three groups.

Direct Lateral Approach

The direct lateral approach, popularized by Hardinge, provides access to the hip joint through the anterior hip capsule. It differs from the anterolateral approach in that the incision releases the anterior portion of the abductor from the greater trochanter. It can provide a similar exposure to the anterolateral approach. With modifications of the approach by distal extension, the direct

lateral method can be quite versatile, especially in patients who require extensive exposure such as those undergoing total joint revision. A low incidence of dislocation, but a higher incidence of limp and heterotopic ossification, has been reported with this approach.

The lateral approach minimizes the incidence of postoperative dislocation in the mobile independent elderly patient. One study assessed the outcomes of displaced subcapital neck of femur fractures in independent elderly patients (age > 70 years) who underwent total hip arthroplasty through a modified Hardinge approach. In 36 consecutive patients, no dislocations were reported, and 80% of patients had a good clinical outcome.

A recent clinical series assessed complications of the lateral approach. Of 1,515 primary total hip arthroplasties (1,333 patients) that were performed using the direct lateral approach, 11.6% of patients had a moderate or severe limp, and 2.5% had severe heterotopic ossification.

A recent prospective comparison study of hip abductor strength after total hip arthroplasty reported favorable results with the lateral approach. In 100 total hip arthroplasties for which a lateral or posterior approach was used, the strength of the hip abductor and the results of the Trendelenburg test improved postoperatively in both groups. No difference was found between the groups in either hip abductor strength or Trendelenburg test results at 3 and 12 months postoperatively.

Perioperative outcomes of the direct lateral approach and mini-incision approach have been compared. Patients who underwent total hip arthroplasty via a mini-incision approach had significantly earlier ambulation, less transfer assistance, and more favorable discharge dispositions than those who underwent total hip arthroplasty via a direct lateral approach. Patients who had a mini-incision approach also had decreased transfusion requirements and better functional recovery with early physical therapy.

Posterolateral/Posterior/Mini-Posterior Approaches

The differences between the various posterior and posterolateral approaches are subtle. The classic posterior (Moore approach) has been termed the Southern exposure (because Moore considered the best exposure for a room to be a Southern exposure). The posterior approach was originally described as extending from the posterior-superior iliac spine to the posterior border of the trochanter and then 10 to 13 cm distally along the axis of the femoral shaft. This approach is excellent for exposure of the posterior capsule, posterior acetabular wall, ischium and posterior trochanter, and upper femur, and allows limited exposure of the acetabulum after excision of the femoral head. The posterolateral approach improves the exposure, especially of the acetabulum, and provides excellent access for total hip arthroplasty.

The posterolateral approach was developed from a combination of the posterior approach described by Langenbeck and a distal limb approach described by Kocher. The Langenbeck incision extends from the posterior-superior iliac spine to the trochanter tip, with the hip held at 45°. Kocher modified the approach by shifting the incision to the anterior aspect of the trochanter and added a distal extension in line with the femur. The Kocher-Langenbeck procedures were combined, and the approach was popularized for pelvic fracture exposure. The distal end was subsequently modified by extending it posterior to improve the exposure. Then the proximal incision to the upper border of the gluteus maximus was modified to preserve the muscle. All of these modifications preserve the abductors, which contribute to excellent functional outcomes with the posterior and posterolateral approaches.

A recent observational study compared the outcomes of 271 total hip arthroplasties for hip osteoarthritis performed by different surgeons. Although the posterior surgical approach was associated with a nonstatistically significant higher rate of dislocation, overall, improved function and reduced pain were associated with this approach in the first 12 months postoperatively when compared with patients who underwent total hip arthroplasty using lateral or anterolateral surgical approaches.

The posterolateral approach has a low rate of reported complications. Results from a recent comparison study of 100 total hip arthroplasties using a transtrochanteric approach and 100 total hip arthroplasties with a posterolateral approach showed that patients undergoing primary total hip arthroplasty by the posterolateral approach were 18.4 times more likely to be free of complications than patients in whom the transtrochanteric approach was used.

In an attempt to improve clinical outcomes, a small-incision approach has been advocated for the posterior approach. There does not appear to be a clear consensus of what size constitutes a mini-incision, nor is there adequate information to confirm the improvement in outcome. One author has advocated a mini-incision posterior approach ranging from 6 to 8.5 cm long. The incision is described as being centered over the greater trochanter or slightly posterior to the center, with 6 cm of the 7-cm incision placed distal to the tip of the greater trochanter.

A recent prospective study compared a mini-incision technique with a traditional posterior approach for total hip arthroplasty. Thirty-three patients who had undergone total hip arthroplasty using a mini-incision approach were matched by diagnosis, gender, average age, and preoperative Harris Hip Score to 33 patients who had undergone total hip arthroplasty using the tradi-

tional posterior approach. The average length of the incision for the mini-incision group was 11.7 cm (range, 7.3 to 13.0 cm); for the traditional posterior approach, it was 20.2 cm (range, 14.8 to 26.0 cm). At 3-month follow-up, patients in the mini-incision group had significant improvement in limp and ability to climb stairs compared with the traditional posterior approach group. At 6-month follow-up, the mini-incision group was significantly better in terms of limp, distance walked, and stair climbing ability. No significant difference was reported between the two groups for pain, function, or range of motion at 1-year follow-up.

Transtrochanteric/Trochanteric Slide Approach

The transtrochanteric approach implies that an osteotomy of the greater trochanter is performed. This procedure can be done through a variety of approaches to the hip, including use of the direct lateral, anterolateral, and posterolateral approach techniques. The level of the osteotomy can be varied to include a small wafer (trochanteric slide), a standard size (at or near to the trochanteric ridge), extended trochanteric (3 to 10 cm distal to the trochanteric ridge), and extended proximal femoral (8 to 16 cm distal to the ridge) osteotomy. The approach is most useful for additional exposure of the acetabulum and pelvis (acetabular revision and allografting), the proximal femur (removal of ingrowth prostheses), and the distal medullary canal (cement removal). Advantages over other approaches include improved exposure, the ability to preserve the blood supply of the femoral head, and the ability to increase tension and offset of the abductors. It also allows exposure of the hip without torque applied to the femur, which could be at risk for fracture in weakened bone in patients with osteoporosis or cortical defects. Disadvantages include increased blood loss, slower rehabilitation resulting from weight-bearing protection, bursitis, hardware breakage, and nonunion.

A transtrochanteric approach can improve the results of a technically demanding surgical procedure such as periacetabular osteotomy. A recent retrospective review reported the results of a modified periacetabular osteotomy in 38 consecutive patients (46 hips) at an average follow-up of 4.2 years. No patient had a neurovascular complication. The early experience with the modified periacetabular osteotomy showed encouraging results in terms of the technical ease of the technique and patient outcome.

The type of fixation of the osteotomy may affect the healing rate. A recent review of the extended trochanteric osteotomy through the modified direct lateral approach in revision total hip arthroplasty found a lower dislocation rate but a higher incidence of trochanteric fracture and migration than described previously. The study included 44 patients (45 procedures) at a minimum of 2-year follow-up. The mean length of the osteotomy was 133.9 mm. The mean migration of the osteotomized fragment was 2.1 mm (range, 0 to 20 mm), with significantly more proximal migration seen with the use of cerclage wires than with the use of cables.

Excellent outcomes were recently reporting using a new bolt-and-plate fixation technique for trochanteric reattachment in revision surgery. Eighteen patients had traditional wiring fixation and a 72% union rate; 111 patients had a bolt-and-plate fixation device and a 94% union rate. Two bolts of a first-generation design broke, and one required removal. Two bolt-and-plate devices disassembled, and one needed removal.

The results of a first-time outcome study of repeat trochanteric osteotomy have been reported. A repeat osteotomy was not associated with any significant morbidity and did not affect the clinical outcome. Remarkably, the overall pseudarthrosis rate decreased from 20 patients (29%) to 10 patients (14%) after the revision surgery.

A recent report of the trochanteric slide approach in 94 revision procedures noted several advantages over standard trochanteric osteotomy. This technique proved to be adequate for removing the components, with few complications. It was found to be versatile because it was extended by a femoral flap (in four patients) or a distal femoral window. The lateral femoral cortex was left intact so that a stem longer than 200 mm was used in only 25% of patients. The trochanteric slide is an approach similar in size to the standard trochanteric osteotomy, but it has a nonunion rate of 4% versus 15%.

Another recent study of the trochanteric slide technique in 127 total hip arthroplasties reported no major complications. A small anterior fragment of greater trochanter was released and the soft-tissue insertions of the gluteus minimus and vastus lateralis muscles were maintained. The entire insertion of the gluteus medius was preserved intact, providing good prosthetic stability and rapid recovery of abductor power and gait. Three months after surgery, 74% of patients had recovered good abductor strength.

A recent electromyographic study of 12 patients who underwent total hip arthroplasty using the trochanteric slide approach on the superior gluteal nerve identified the factors that may lead to injury to the nerve. Irritation of the nerve occurred first during splitting of the gluteus medius muscle, then with increased gluteus medius retraction for exposure of the acetabulum, and finally during positioning of the leg for preparation of the femur. The evidence of alterations on electromyograms was important because it was found in a single patient with persistent abductor muscle weakness after 1 year.

The transfemoral approach accesses the femoral shaft with a longitudinal window to remove hardware and cement during total hip arthroplasty revision surgery. The use of an ultrasonically driven cement removal instrument has been described and has been reported to result in a shorter length of the transfemoral osteotomy, and thus shorten the required length of the prosthesis by 60%.

A transabdominal (transperitoneal) approach has been reported to safely remove an intrapelvic acetabular component in a single patient who underwent revision hip arthroplasty. It was performed in combination with a transtrochanteric approach.

Dislocation While Preserving Femoral Head and Trochanteric Blood Supply

The preservation of vascularity to the femoral head with the type of surgical approach has been recently studied. The traditional anterior and anterolateral approaches are considered appropriate to expose and dislocate the hip safely. The posterior blood anastomoses (crucial or cruciate anastomoses) are critical to this exposure. The femoral head blood supply can be maintained with a trochanteric osteotomy that preserves the medial circumflex vessels. Thorough understanding of the extracapsular anatomy of the medial femoral circumflex artery and its surrounding structures will help to avoid iatrogenic osteonecrosis of the head of the femur in reconstructive surgery of the hip and fixation of acetabular fractures through the posterior approach. Recent anatomic studies further clarify the important vascular anatomy.

A recent cadaveric study described the anatomy of the medial femoral circumflex artery and its branches based on dissections of 24 hips. The authors demonstrated that the obturator externus protects the deep branch of the medial femoral circumflex artery from being disrupted or stretched during dislocation of the hip in any direction after serial release of all other soft-tissue attachments of the proximal femur, including a complete circumferential capsulotomy.

A recent clinical study confirmed the success of preserving the femoral head blood supply while performing a precise trochanteric osteotomy. The technique combines an anterior dislocation through a posterior approach with a trochanteric flip osteotomy. The external rotator muscles are not divided, and the medial femoral circumflex artery is protected by the intact obturator externus. The authors of this study reported using this approach in 213 hips over a period of 7 years, including 19 patients who underwent simultaneous intertrochanteric osteotomy. The perfusion of the femoral head was verified intraoperatively and no patients have subsequently developed osteonecrosis.

The effect of the posterior approach on the greater trochanter blood supply has been studied in patients who underwent cemented or uncemented total hip arthroplasty, with possible implications to bone ingrowth to the proximal femoral prosthesis. Complete detachment of the quadratus femoris was associated with a significant decrease in trochanteric blood flow in both the cementless and cemented total hip arthroplasty groups. The lowest perfusion levels during the procedures were seen transiently with posterior dislocation of the femoral head, after which trochanteric perfusion was decreased by 66% in the cementless total hip arthroplasty group, and by 61% in the cemented total hip arthroplasty group compared with baseline values. Blood flow remained approximately half that of baseline values after insertion of the femoral prosthesis in the cementless and cemented total hip arthroplasty groups.

Pitfalls in Surgical Approaches
Vascular Injuries

Vascular injuries are less common than nerve injuries, but they are more immediately life threatening. The mechanisms of vascular injury include occlusion associated with preexisting peripheral vascular disease and direct vascular injury. Injury can occur during removal of cement and during screw fixation of acetabular components, cages, or structural grafts. Preoperative patient assessment should include vascular evaluation of patients with absent pulses, previous vascular bypass surgery, or dysvascular limbs. In one recent study, CT was recommended in patients with cement or components extending medially into the pelvis.

Another recent study outlined the experience in the diagnosis and management of acute arterial hemorrhagic and limb-threatening ischemic complications associated with total hip arthroplasty and total knee arthroplasty. Between 1989 and 2002, 23,199 total knee arthroplasty procedures (13,618 total; 11,953 primary and 1,665 revision) and total hip replacement procedures (9,581 total; 7,812 primary and 1,769 revision) were performed. Arterial injuries were grouped according to type (ischemia, bleeding, pseudoaneurysm, ischemia plus bleeding) and time of recognition of injury. Acute arterial complications developed in 32 patients (0.13%); 24 of these acute arterial complications were associated with total knee arthroplasty procedures (0.17%) and 8 were associated with total hip arthroplasty procedures (0.08%). Arterial injury was detected on the day of surgery in 18 patients (56%), but it was not recognized until the first to fifth postoperative day in 14 patients (44%). There were no deaths, and limb salvage was achieved in all patients. Use of preoperative arteriography and aggressive revascularization are critical to achieving limb salvage.

Neural/Nerve Injuries

Total joint arthroplasty surgery carries a risk for both central and peripheral neural injury. Central nervous system changes after total hip arthroplasty may be attributed to the fat embolism syndrome. When there is an associated right to left cardiac shunt, paradoxic embolization can occur, which may account for previously unexplained instances of confusion and mental status changes after surgery. Certain maneuvers during surgery are associated with mobilization of marrow fat into the venous system. These maneuvers include impaction of the acetabular component, reaming of the femoral canal, and cement pressurization.

Peripheral nerve injury can include any of the upper extremity nerves that are potentially stretched or compressed during lengthy anesthetic sessions. A recent report has described three patients who developed meralgia paraesthetica (neurapraxia of the lateral femoral cutaneous nerve) after the use of a well-padded and carefully placed patient positioning device during total hip replacement. In vitro and animal experiments have shown that increased tensile strain on peripheral nerves, when applied for a prolonged period impairs nerve function. Hip surgery can affect any of the pelvic and lower extremity nerves, although the sciatic nerve (especially the peroneal portion) is the most common injured nerve after total hip arthroplasty. Fortunately, sciatic nerve palsy is an uncommon complication. Femoral nerve injury is much less common and is most commonly associated with the anterior approach or anterior acetabular retraction. Diagnosis is often delayed, but the prognosis for femoral nerve injury is generally better than that for sciatic nerve palsy.

Attempts to monitor patients for sciatic nerve injury during surgery have been unsuccessful or impractical because of inconsistent results. Motor-evoked potentials and electromyography have been used to study the effects of limb position and retraction on sciatic and peroneal nerve function. Recently, motor-evoked potentials and electromyography have been used in combination with monitoring during revision total hip arthroplasty in 27 consecutive patients to identify intraoperative events that cause conduction abnormalities. Significant electric events occurred, most commonly during acetabular reconstruction. The authors of this study identified specific issues related to potential nerve injury. They reported that hip flexion should be avoided during posterior acetabular retraction when using the posterior approach with posterior dislocation. In addition, the position of the sciatic nerve should be clearly identified when acetabular augmentation with structural allograft is performed.

A recent study of sciatic stretch during surgery suggests that excessive flexion of the hip and extension of the knee should be avoided during total hip replacement. Video extensometry was used to measure strain on the human sciatic nerve during total hip replacement. Ten consecutive patients with a mean age of 72 years who were undergoing primary total hip re-

Table 1 | Dislocation Rates: Effect of Approach and Soft Tissue

No. of Patients	Approach	Soft-Tissue Repair	Dislocation Rate (%)
13,203 (meta-analysis)	Transtrochanteric	NA	1.27
	Posterior	(-)	3.95
	Posterior	(+)	2.03
	Anterolateral	NA	2.18
	Direct lateral	NA	0.55
1,333	Direct lateral	NA	0.4
315	Posterior	(-)	4
395	Posterior	(+)	0
500 (control)	Posterior	(-)	2.8
500	Posterior	(+)	0.6
1,078 (control)	Posterior	(-)	4.8
437	Posterior	(+)	0.7
884	Posterior	(+)	1.36
945	Posterior	(+)	0.85

+ = yes, - = no, NA = not applicable

placement using the posterior approach were recruited, and strains in the sciatic nerve were measured in different combinations of flexion and extension of the hip and knee. Significant increases in strain in the sciatic nerve were observed in flexion of the hip and extension of the knee. The mean increase was 26% (19% to 30%). In animal studies, increases of this magnitude have been shown to impair electrophysiologic function in peripheral nerves.

Dislocations

Dislocation is a leading early complication of total hip arthroplasty (Table 1). To minimize the potential for instability, preoperative planning must not only include radiographic templating, but also identification of patient and surgical variables that could increase the likelihood of dislocation. Rigorous intraoperative tests of hip stability and good repair of soft tissues during closure all help prevent dislocation. The surgical approach has also been considered as a major factor in dislocation risk.

The results of a comprehensive literature review have been reported that correlate the type of surgical approach with the incidence of dislocation in primary total hip arthroplasty. Fourteen studies involving 13,203 primary total hip replacements showed a combined dislocation rate of 1.27% for the transtrochanteric approach, 3.23% for the posterior approach (3.95% without posterior repair and 2.03% with posterior repair), 2.18% for the anterolateral approach, and 0.55% for the direct lateral approach. The authors of this study ad-

vised that larger controlled prospective studies are needed to investigate the potential benefits of the posterior approach because of the high rate of dislocation associated with this approach when compared with the direct lateral approach.

Additional support for the direct lateral approach was provided in a study of 1,515 primary total hip arthroplasties that were done via a direct lateral approach in 1,333 patients. Only six hips (0.4%) had a dislocation or an episode of instability.

An understanding of patient factors and component position is important to minimize the risk of dislocation. In a recent study of 2,023 total hip arthroplasties, 21 patients who had at least one dislocation were compared with a control group of 21 patients without dislocation. The dislocation risk was 6.9 times higher if total anteversion (rotation angle of the limb with socket and stem equatorially matched) was not between 40° and 60°. The rate was 10 times higher in the patients with a high American Society of Anesthesiologists score, which was considered to be an important part of the preoperative assessment for dislocation risk.

Posterior Surgical Approaches and Soft-Tissue Repair

An important recent advance in primary total hip arthroplasty outcome has been the dramatic reduction in the dislocation rate resulting from soft-tissue repair with the posterior surgical approaches. The early dislocation rate (during the first 3 months after surgery) for posterior dislocations is highest in patients who undergo a posterior surgical approach. A recent study of 315 patients undergoing primary total hip arthroplasty with a complete capsulectomy reported a prevalence of 14 acute dislocations (4%). The technical success of soft-tissue repair has been most significant in the posterior and posterolateral approaches. The reduction in the incidence of dislocations in patients who undergo a posterior surgical approach enhances the overall outcome of total hip arthroplasty because posterior approaches generally have the best functional outcomes. Both the early and late dislocation rates have improved with soft-tissue repair.

Several studies have reported that the incidence of dislocation in primary cases has been reduced to less than 1% with the use of soft-tissue repair. A recent study reported lowering the dislocation rate from 4% to 0 in a series of 395 consecutive patients. Several methods of posterior repair have been described, all of which appear to be successful. Generally, the capsule is either sewn together or reattached to bone at the insertion into the greater trochanter. The short rotators are reattached either with the capsule or separately (Figures 1 through 4).

A study of 1,000 patients, 500 of whom were treated with capsulotomy and capsulorrhaphy and 500 of whom

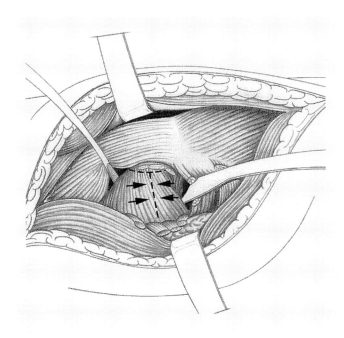

Figure 1 Illustration of the T-capsulorrhaphy technique (posterior view, right hip). The dotted line indicates the incision of the posterior hip capsule. Arrows depict the location of sutures for closure. This technique is most useful for hemiarthroplasty approaches for which visualization of the acetabulum is less important.

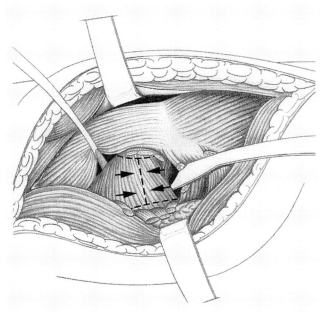

Figure 2 Illustration of the H-capsulorrhaphy technique (posterior view, right hip). The dotted line indicates the incision of the capsule. The "sling" that is created at closure can be tightened by overlap of the capsule edges. Arrows depict the location of sutures to approximate capsule flaps. This technique allows excellent acetabular exposure for total hip arthroplasty.

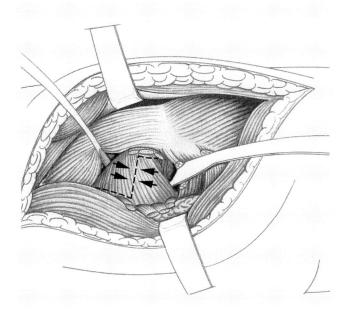

Figure 3 Illustration of the Z-capsulorrhaphy technique (posterior view, right hip). The dotted line indicates the incision of the capsule. The tension of the repair can be adjusted at the midincision by varying the overlap. This technique allows excellent acetabular exposure because the flaps are retractable and can be approximated with high femoral offset prostheses and femoral lengthening, unlike direct repair.

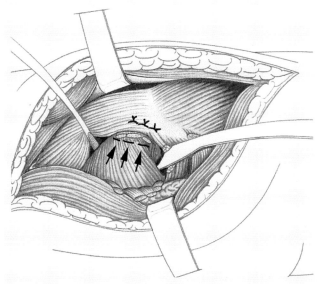

Figure 4 Illustration of the direct capsule repair technique. The capsule and short rotator tendons are reapproximated to the posterior edge of the greater trochanter through drill holes. Arrows indicate three mattress sutures sewn through the capsule (and typically the short rotators) and into the posterior portion of the greater trochanter.

were treated with a simple change to posterior repair (from capsulectomy and capsulotomy with closure of the external rotator muscles, demonstrated a dramatic reduction in the prevalence of dislocation after total hip arthroplasty through a posterolateral approach. The dislocation rate was 2.8% for the capsulectomy and capsulotomy group and 0.6% for the new posterolateral technique ($P < 0.005$).

A recent study compared the incidence of early posterior dislocation (within the first 6 months after surgery) using a complete posterior capsulectomy versus a formal posterior capsular and short external rotator tendon repair. In patients with a complete posterior capsulectomy, 52 of 1,078 primary total hip replacements (4.8%) had an early posterior dislocation. In patients with posterior capsular repair, three of 437 primary total hip replacements (0.7%) had an early posterior dislocation ($P < 0.001$).

The success of the posterior repair in primary total hip replacement appears to be independent of the experience of the surgeon. A study of dislocators in patients who had undergone a previous repair of the soft tissue concludes that less surgeon experience was not associated with a higher dislocation rate. The group included 884 consecutive primary total hip arthroplasties approached via a posterior incision, with repair of the posterior soft tissues. After a mean follow-up of 30 months, the overall dislocation rate was 1.36%. All dislocations were posterior and occurred within 6 months after surgery; 91% dislocated within 6 weeks.

Direct capsular and short external rotator repair to the greater trochanter with nonabsorbable suture has been studied at intermediate- and long-term. Among 945 primary total hip arthroplasties performed with this technique at a mean 6.4-year follow-up (range, 2.0 to 9.3 years), dislocation occurred in 8 patients (0.85%). Of these, dislocation occurred within the first postoperative year in three patients who were subsequently treated without surgery, three patients required revision surgery and placement of a constrained liner, and dislocation after trauma occurred in two patients who were subsequently treated without surgery. With the correct orientation of components and enhanced soft-tissue repair, the posterior surgical approach can result in an extremely low dislocation rate.

Soft-tissue management is not only important in primary total hip arthroplasty, but also provides a solution to recurrent posterior dislocation in the patients who undergo revision. A recent clinical series of recurrent dislocators reported that the most common cause for dislocation was posterior soft-tissue deficiency (N = 17). Thirty-two patients were analyzed at 9-month to 7-year follow-up (average, 3.6 years) after undergoing revision surgery to treat instability. Dislocations were posterior in 26 patients, anterior in 4 patients, and multidirectional in 2 patients. Management of the instability by repair of the soft tissue and modification of the modular components was successful in 25 patients and unsuccessful in 1 patient. Three unstable hips with complete posterior soft-tissue deficiency were treated successfully with a posterior soft-tissue augmentation using an Achilles tendon-bone allograft.

The significant improvement in the incidence of dislocation among patients who undergo total hip arthro-

plasty via a posterior or posterolateral approach has been extrapolated to the hemiarthroplasty procedure. A prospective study was undertaken on 183 patients with a femoral neck fracture. A modified posterior approach was used that preserves the piriformis, the labrum, and the capsule. The dislocation rate for the posterior approach was 7.4% (7 patients) and 1.1% (1 patient) for the modified posterior approach ($P < 0.05$). The authors of this study concluded that the modified posterior approach significantly increased the stability of a hemiarthroplasty when compared with a classic posterior approach.

The results of a cadaveric study of the functional anatomy of two types of posterior repair and its effect on stability after total hip replacement have been reported. Three different repair techniques (no repair, soft-tissue repair, and transosseous fixation) were then consecutively tested on each hip. The transosseous repair was superior with regard to torsion strength (four times stronger than no repair and more than twice as strong as soft-tissue repair). The magnitude of the angle of rotation observed before dislocation increased by 83% compared with that of no repair, and it increased 46% compared with that of soft-tissue repair.

Complications from posterior capsular repair are uncommon; when they do occur, it typically results in low morbidity. In the technique of reattachment of the capsule with the short rotators using drill holes in the greater trochanter, studies have reported external rotation contractures, failure of the repair, and avulsion of a portion of the trochanter. The incidence of avulsion fracture of the greater trochanter is recently reported in 4 of 437 total hip replacements (0.9%). There was no significant morbidity from the complication.

Summary

The risk of dislocation after total hip replacement depends on numerous factors. The recent literature emphasizes the importance of preserving (or repairing if disrupted) the posterior soft tissue of the hip. The favorable effect of repair of the posterior capsule and the short rotators with the posterior approaches is well established. Other direct approaches that do not disrupt the posterior soft tissues, such as the anterolateral and direct lateral approaches, also favorably influence the prevalence of acute postoperative dislocation.

Annotated Bibliography

Anterior Approach

Kennon RE, Keggi JM, Wetmore RS, Zatorski LE, Huo MH, Keggi KJ: Total hip arthroplasty through a minimally invasive anterior surgical approach. *J Bone Joint Surg Am* 2003;85-A(suppl 4):39-48.

The authors describe a surgical technique using a single small incision and an anterior approach.

Two-Incision Anterior Approach

Berger RA: Total hip arthroplasty using the minimally invasive two-incision approach. *Clin Orthop Relat Res* 2003;417:232-241.

This article reports the results of the first 100 patients to undergo total hip arthroplasty using a new minimally invasive two-incision approach.

Posterolateral/Posterior/Mini-Posterior Approaches

Masonis JL, Bourne RB: Surgical approach, abductor function, and total hip arthroplasty dislocation. *Clin Orthop Relat Res* 2002;405:46-53.

From a review of several studies, the authors combine data on dislocation rates and limp for total hip arthroplasty done via the lateral and posterior hip approaches. Concern is raised regarding the rate of dislocation in posterior approaches, even with apparent posterior soft-tissue repair.

White RE Jr, Forness TJ, Allman JK, Junick DW: Effect of posterior capsular repair on early dislocation in primary total hip replacement. *Clin Orthop Relat Res* 2001; 393:163-167.

The authors report a significant reduction in the dislocation rate and an associated low risk of complications and morbidity using posterior capsular repair on early dislocation in primary total hip arthroplasty.

Transtrochanteric/Trochanteric Slide Approach

Ganz R, Gill TJ, Gautier E, Ganz K, Krugel N, Berlemann U: Surgical dislocation of the adult hip a technique with full access to the femoral head and acetabulum without the risk of avascular necrosis. *J Bone Joint Surg Br* 2001;83:1119-1124.

The authors of this study surgically dislocated adult hips using a posterior approach with a trochanteric osteotomy while protecting the medial femoral circumflex artery with the intact obturator externus muscle.

Langlais F, Lambotte JC, Collin P, Langlois F, Fontaine JW, Thomazeau H: Trochanteric slide osteotomy in revision total hip arthroplasty for loosening. *J Bone Joint Surg Br* 2003;85:510-516.

The authors discuss the versatility of this approach in revision surgery and conclude that it provides advantages over extended osteotomies in preserving bone and results in a low rate of trochanteric nonunion.

Dislocation While Preserving Femoral Head and Trochanteric Blood Supply

Gautier E, Ganz K, Krugel N, Gill T, Ganz R: Anatomy of the medial femoral circumflex artery and its surgical implications. *J Bone Joint Surg Br* 2000;82:679-683.

The authors discuss the important anatomic details of the major vascular supply leading to the femoral head. The importance of the obturator externus and proximal border of the quadratus femoris to the medial femoral circumflex artery is also discussed.

Pitfalls in Surgical Approaches

Fleming P, Lenehan B, O'Rourke S, McHugh P, Kaar K, McCabe JP: Strain on the human sciatic nerve in vivo during movement of the hip and knee. *J Bone Joint Surg Br* 2003;85(3):363-365.

In this study, video extensometry was used to measure abnormal strain (mean increase, 26%) to the sciatic nerve during a combination of hip flexion and knee extension at the time of total hip arthroplasty. The authors concluded that excessive positions should be avoided during this procedure.

Classic Bibliography

Crenshaw AH: Surgical approaches, in *Campbell's Operative Orthopaedics*, ed 8. St Louis, MO, Mosby Year Book, 1992, pp 23-116.

Hardinge K: The direct lateral approach to the hip. *J Bone Joint Surg Br* 1982;64:17-19.

Harris WH: A new lateral approach to the hip joint. *J Bone Joint Surg Am* 1967;49:891-898.

Light TR, Keggi KJ: Anterior approach to hip arthroplasty. *Clin Orthop Relat Res* 1980;152:255-260.

Marcy GH, Fletcher RS: Modification of the posterolateral approach to the hip for insertion of femoral head prosthesis. *J Bone Joint Surg Am* 1954;36:142.

McGann WA: Surgical approaches, in Callaghan, JJ, Rosenberg, AG, Rubash HE (eds): *The Adult Hip.* Philadelphia, PA, Lippincott-Raven, 1998.

Pellicci PM, Poss R: Posterior approach to THA using enhanced posterior soft tissue repair. *Clin Orthop* 1998; 355:224-228.

Smith-Peterson MN: Approach to and exposure of the hip joint for mold arthroplasty. *J Bone Joint Surg Am* 1949;31:40.

Watson-Jones R: Fractures of the neck of the femur. *Br J Surg* 1935;23:787.

Chapter 31

Biomechanics of the Hip

Thomas D. Brown, PhD

Introduction

An appreciation of the salient aspects of hip joint biomechanics constitutes an important background for diagnosis and treatment of a wide range of disorders. Among the major synovial joints, the hip is probably the most heavily investigated from a biomechanical standpoint, with much of this research driven to support advances in total hip arthroplasty. Topics of long-standing interest in hip biomechanics include the range of motion and the kinematics of activities of daily living, the loading experienced both statically and during activities of daily living, the transmission of mechanical stress within the articulating members and across their contact interface, and the mechanical interplay of the various tissues and structures comprising the joint.

Functional Loading of the Hip

The subject of functional loading of the hip, as assessed by contemporary gait analysis techniques, was comprehensively reviewed several years ago. Important recent developments in this area have included substantial improvements in the accuracy and reliability of these loading estimates. Earlier work with instrumented prostheses reported peak joint contact forces in the first few months after implantation, spanning the range from 1.8 to 4.3 times body weight for level walking, with most ranging from 2.5 to 3 times body weight. A somewhat higher force range (2.6 to 5.5 times body weight) has been recorded for stair ascent/descent. However, joint contact forces from inverse newtonian analytic models have tended to be substantially higher, in the range of 3.5 to 5 times body weight for level walking, and 6 to 7 times body weight for stairs. This historical tendency for analytic values to be higher is apparently attributable to the assumptions typically built into muscle force estimations; higher values have been derived analytically, even in direct comparisons of the same patient.

The key to improving this situation has been improved techniques for assessing the muscle forces about the hip. Patterns of muscle activity necessarily interact with body-limb segment inertial effects, gravity, and external loadings (foot-floor reaction force) to determine the contact force across the articular surface. Suitable techniques are needed for direct measurement of muscle forces in living human subjects undergoing functional activities. (Indwelling sensors such as tendon buckle transducers and implantable force sensors used selectively in animal experiments are impractical and/or unethical for use in human subjects; muscle force assessments from MRI-assessed tendon strains are not feasible for ambulatory activities.) This information has therefore necessarily been assessed indirectly, relying upon mathematical modeling.

Recent work with a muscle set constructed from the US National Library of Medicine's Visible Human Database that included 95 individual lines of action, had fully anatomic wrap-around effects, and constrained the upper limit of calculated muscle forces to not exceed 85% of theoretic physical maximum has succeeded in reconciling much of this discrepancy. Peak force differences (versus instrumented prosthesis recordings) of only 7% for level walking and 10% for stair climbing were achieved. An extensive database of information regarding this model has been made freely available on compact disk and is widely used within the biomechanics research community. A more tractable version of this rather complex model has recently been developed, based on pooling of some of the logically correlated individual muscle force vectors, without causing undue sacrifice of overall force prediction accuracy. Other noteworthy new studies regarding ease/tractability of hip joint force assessment have documented the relatively modest accuracy compromise to be expected for two-dimensional as opposed to fully three-dimensional inverse dynamics analysis, a tradeoff that may be acceptable in various applications. Also, credible data are now available regarding the higher levels of hip joint loading for normal patients as opposed to those who have undergone total hip arthroplasty, an important distinction because the latter group has been the focus of most research in this area.

Reference Framework Standardization

Another important new development in this area involves standardization. Historically, lack of consistency among investigators regarding reference frameworks for reporting hip joint motions has hindered comparisons among studies; moreover, many of the definitions used have had limited clinical relevance. To improve this situation, the International Society of Biomechanics has recently established a standard definition for a joint coordinate system for the hip joint to facilitate gait analysis, radiographic analysis, in vivo studies, and finite element modeling. This standard, which has widespread acceptance among workers in the field (Figure 1), has anatomic landmarks to define the pelvic coordinate system: the anterior-superior iliac spine, the posterior-superior iliac spine, and the (preferably functionally determined) acetabular center. This standard also has anatomic landmarks to define the femoral coordinate system: the femoral epicondyles and the (preferably functionally defined) femoral head center. Both of these bony reference systems, when positioned with their origins coincident at the hip rotation center, formally define the joint coordinate system.

New Biomechanical Measurement Techniques

Contact stress and/or pressure determinations in the natural hip remain of great interest in the context of cartilage degeneration propensity—for example, with regard to reconstructive osteotomies, reduction of displaced intra-articular fractures, or repair of osteochondral defects. This is an area in which measurement techniques are continuing to evolve, with ideal capabilities again unfortunately still lacking. Precedent techniques have included selective cartilage removal experiments, conventional fluid transducers mounted retrograde up through the subchondral bone, arrays of individual piezoresistive minitransducers embedded in the cartilage, and Fuji pressure-sensitive film (Fuji Photo Film, Tokyo, Japan). Sheet-array sensors (such as those produced by Tekscan, South Boston, MA) that are otherwise attractive for combining high spatial resolution with transient recording capability have not proved adaptable to the hip joint because they crinkle when forced to conform to a spherical surface. Peak local pressures reported for physiologic contact force levels have typically been in the range of 3 to 10 MPa (1 MPa = 145 psi.)

Discrete Element Analysis

Another recently introduced approach that is useful for determining hip joint contact stress is discrete element analysis. This is a computational modeling technique whereby the articulation is represented as an array of a large number (typically many thousands) of linear compression springs, the stiffnesses of which are assigned to mimic that of articular cartilage; the femoral and ace-

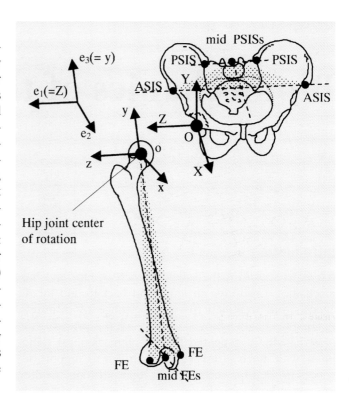

Figure 1 Schematic diagram of the International Society of Biomechanics femoral coordinate system (x,y,z), the pelvic coordinate system (X,Y,Z), and the joint coordinate system for a right hip joint. ASIS = anterior-superior iliac spine, PSIS = posterior-superior iliac spine, FE = femoral epicondyle.

tabular bony members are treated as rigid bodies. With this approach, for a given resultant force applied across the joint, the two bony members assume the unique relative position corresponding to minimum energy storage within the spring array, with local pressures varying in accordance with the amount of local spring compression. (Any springs coming into tension are automatically deleted from the model.) Discrete element analysis solutions execute very expeditiously from a computational standpoint, and thus lend themselves to use in studies in which a large number of parametric influences need to be considered or when an appreciable number of individual patients need to be studied. The primary disadvantage of this approach is that the mechanical characterization of cartilage is simplified because it does not include time- or deformation-dependent stiffness and does not account for stresses in transverse directions within the cartilage layer.

Another expeditious recent mathematical approach—but one that also has its own (different) set of simplifying assumptions—is the iterative computational solution of integral equations, which uses routinely available normative tables that are based on simple parameters (such as body weight and femoral head diameter).

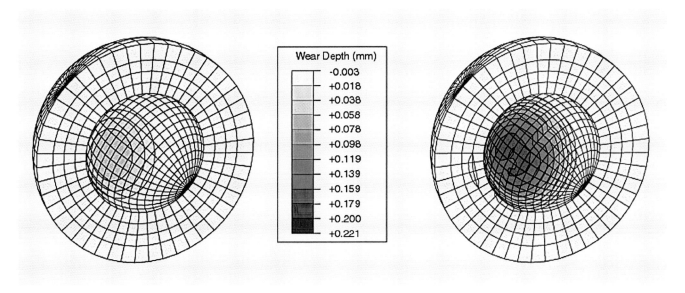

Figure 2 Computed distribution of polyethylene wear depths on the acetabular bearing surfaces after one million cycles of loading. Compared with a nonroughened femoral head (*left*), simulating localized head scratching from third-body debris (*right*) has greatly increased the volumetric wear and appreciable altered the otherwise smooth pattern of polyethylene removal.

Finite Element Analysis

Finite element analyses have continued to rapidly evolve in terms of engineering sophistication and clinical realism, and they now constitute a central pillar of the information base on hip joint biomechanics. The technical basis for this methodology is beyond the scope of this chapter; a recent conceptual overview oriented toward orthopaedic clinicians and nonengineering musculoskeletal research scientists is available elsewhere. Historically, most finite element analysis studies involving the hip addressed issues of stress distribution within prostheses and at their fixation interfaces. Over the past several years, however, the breadth of finite element analysis applications has widened appreciably to include subjects such as estimating wear of prosthesis bearing surfaces (Figure 2), quantifying the influence of implant design and surgical positioning parameters on dislocation propensity (Figure 3), and documenting the contribution to stability provided by the capsule (Figure 4). Recently, in an attempt to compute clinically tractable patient-specific contact stress in the natural hip, a finite element technique was introduced involving voxel-based structural (element) discretizations extracted directly from CT scans. No contact stress measurements in vivo for fully natural hip joints have yet to be reported; the closest to that ideal has been the use of an instrumented femoral endoprosthesis, with which peak pressures of approximately 18 MPa were detected. Another important area in which definitive information is still lacking is the long-term pressure tolerance of hip joint cartilage. Although limited stress analysis data are available for patients with hip dysplasia who were treated nonsurgically, both the stress analysis techniques and

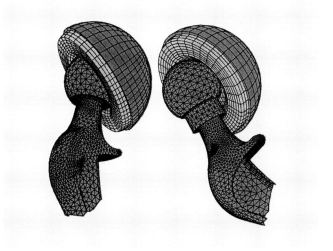

Figure 3 Three-dimensional finite element meshes showing a nonskirted femoral component during stable articulation (*left*) and an impinged, subluxating, skirted modular femoral component just before the instant of dislocation (*right*).

the clinical/radiographic assessments of joint degeneration used were highly simplified.

Poroelastic Finite Element Modeling

The functional significance of the labrum is arguably underappreciated. A plausible explanation for the clinical association between labral pathology and cartilage degeneration has recently been elucidated on biomechanical grounds based on the loss of a sealing effect to contain a fluid layer that otherwise would more smoothly distribute intra-articular contact stress. Using a poroelastic finite element model (accounting for load

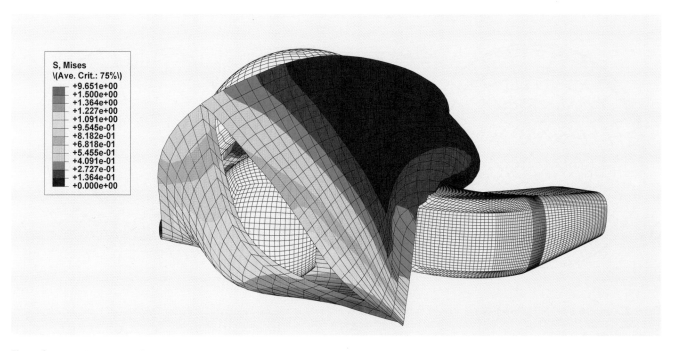

Figure 4 Lateral direction view of computed capsule stresses and implant component position for a three-dimensional finite element simulation of posterior dislocation of a total hip arthroplasty femoral head component during a leg-crossing maneuver. In this instance, the presence of capsule compromise because of a posteriorly located longitudinal slit allows ready egress of the femoral head component.

carriage by both the fluid and solid constituents of cartilage matrix), loss of labral sealing was found to cause approximately a fivefold increase in peak computed cartilage strains for a quasiphysiologic resultant joint contact force of 1,200 N.

In Vivo Wear Measurements

There have been several significant developments in the area of in vivo wear measurements in patients who have undergone total hip arthroplasty. To improve the subjectivity and limited accuracy of measuring radiographically apparent wear by manual templating techniques, digital edge detection techniques (Figure 5) have been introduced to objectively delineate the images of component margins, leading to order of magnitude improvements in measurement precision and reliability. One such algorithm is now commercially available and is in widespread use. The additional accuracy afforded by digital edge detection techniques has made it possible to discriminate the relatively small amounts of radiographically apparent penetration occurring early in the life of the implant. Coupled with regression analysis, this increased accuracy has enabled researchers to discriminate bedding-in from true wear, and it has enabled researchers to predict relatively long-term (10-year) wear rates based on short-term (2-year) performance. Another noteworthy development, offering even greater precision, has been the use of radiostereometry in conjunction with digital radiographs. This latter approach, however, involves a rather complex and expensive

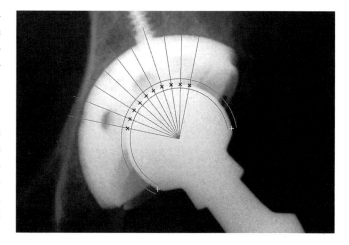

Figure 5 Computer-workstation screen rendition of a typical digitized radiograph from a patient who has undergone total hip arthroplasty, illustrating the procedure for digital edge detection of the articular surface of the femoral head component. Along each search ray (for clarity, only 10 are shown here, whereas several hundred are used in actual practice), the edge detection algorithm identifies the site at which image intensity changes most markedly, as ascertained mathematically by the gradient of a gray scale value of the image pixels. To expedite computation, the algorithm samples only at the radii in the vicinity of the provisional edge of the femoral head component (black Xs).

equipment installation, and requires permission for beadlet augmentation of the implants, thus largely restricting its use to specialty centers. Another important imaging advance that is pertinent to hip joint biomechanics is the application of pose fluoroscopy to track in vivo kinematics. This modality has indicated that head-cup separation is commonplace during abduction events that do not require weight bearing, such as the swing phase of gait. Presumably, adverse implications include edge wear of the components themselves, in-drawing of potentially third-body laden joint fluid during the separation event, and impaction loading when the components subsequently reseat.

Fragility and Fracture Risk Assessment

An additional area of recent advance in hip joint biomechanics has involved fragility and fracture risk. Although traditional screening measures such as dual-energy x-ray absorptiometry provide reliable estimates of bone mass, failure by fracture is fundamentally a mechanical rather than a material phenomenon, and thus depends on bony structural competence rather than simply on the amount of material present. The two primary clinical entities stimulating work in this area have been aging fragility fractures caused by osteopenia and pathologic fractures caused by neoplasms. Over the past several years, advances in clinical imaging, mechanical characterization of bone, computational techniques, and processing power have made it feasible to estimate the structural competence of individual bones on a patient-specific basis. The proximal femur has been the focus for much of this work because of the high (and increasing) societal importance of hip fractures. Key enabling technology in this area includes the advent of CT voxel-based finite element meshing, with which highly automated structural analyses can be directly performed with minimal intervention needed to preprocess the finite element model. Although early applications of this approach involved relatively coarse, low-resolution structural models with just a few thousand individual elements, progressively more advanced and refined models have emerged. Recently, the more advanced models include millions of individual elements and have reached the stage of representing every individual trabeculum within entire proximal femora of normal versus osteoporotic proximal femurs. Concurrently, mechanical characterization of trabecular and cortical bone tissue has allowed researchers to formally account for the role of local tissue architecture on multidirectional stress development and material failure. Bench experiments have documented reasonably accurate predictions of global failure load and site of fracture. Complementary experimental work has documented the external loadings from fracture-prone fall events, data that have proved to be useful in identifying relative failure risk for different impact challenges. For patients with metastatic bone defects, this structurally based approach, even when somewhat simplified, provides substantially more reliable assessments of failure risk than those traditionally made from the morphologic appearance of the lesion.

Annotated Bibliography

Functional Loading of the Hip

Alkjaer T, Simonsen EB, Dyhre-Poulsen P: Comparison of inverse dynamics calculated by two- and three-dimensional models during walking. *Gait Posture* 2001; 13:73-77.

In this study, gait analysis was performed for 15 healthy male subjects; sagittal plane joint moments were computed at the hip, knee, and ankle for otherwise similarly conceived two-dimensional versus three-dimensional inverse Newtonian dynamic analyses. The data showed that the differences between the two-dimensional and three-dimensional models were relatively modest when compared with other sources of variation, thus justifying two-dimensional modeling for many practical applications.

Bergmann G (ed): *HIP98 – Loading of the Hip Joint.* Compact Disc. Berlin, Germany, Free University of Berlin, 2001.

This freeware compact disc was made widely available to members of the orthopaedics and biomechanics research communities. It contains in-depth biomechanical data on a wide range of parameters for various activities of daily living. These datasets have come into wide use among biomechanics researchers, serving as de facto standard input data for many research studies (for example, loading inputs for implant stress analyses).

Heller MO, Bergmann G, Dueretzbacher G, et al: Musculoskeletal loading conditions at the hip during walking and stair climbing. *J Biomech* 2001;34:883-893.

Four patients with instrumented total hip implants were studied experimentally and modeled computationally based on CT and radiographic data and a muscle force optimization algorithm. The authors found that agreement of experimentation and computation was within 12% for level walking and 14% for stair climbing.

Heller MO, Bergmann G, Kassi JP, Claes L, Haas NP, Duda GN: Determination of muscle loading at the hip joint for use in pre-clinical testing. *J Biomech* 2005; 38(5):1155-1163.

Because explicit representation of all of the individual muscles exerting forces about the hip is often unwieldy or impractical for routine preclinical testing or modeling of implants, the authors developed a formulation in which functionally similar muscles were segregated into four distinct groups. This was done in a manner that induced less than a 10% margin of error versus average values of peak loading for four patients with instrumented total hips.

Stansfield BW, Nicol AC: Hip joint forces in normal subjects and subjects with total hip prostheses: Walking and stair and ramp negotiation. *Clin Biomech (Bristol, Avon)* 2002;17:130-139.

Because a void has existed in the gait analysis literature for forces about the hip (most work has focused on total hip arthroscopy subjects), the authors captured data for five male and six female subjects in the 40- to 60-year age range for level walking and stair and ramp negotiation. These healthy subjects had substantially higher joint contact forces, cadence, speed, and stride length than age-matched total hip arthroplasty patients.

Reference Framework Standardization

Wu G, Siegler S, Allard P, et al: ISB recommendation on definitions of joint coordinate system of various joints for the reporting of human motion: Part I. Ankle, hip, and spine. *J Biomech* 2002;35(4):543-548.

This article describes the formal mathematical anatomic and functional definition for a coordinate reference system for measuring and reporting motions and loadings at the hip joint as set forth by the International Society of Biomechanics. This standard has gained wide acceptance within the biomechanics research community.

New Biomechanical Measurement Techniques

Bayraktar HH, Morgan EF, Niebur GL, Morris GE, Wong EK, Keaveny TM: Comparison of the elastic and yield properties of human femoral trabecular and cortical bone tissue. *J Biomech* 2004;37(1):27-35.

The authors of this article report that high-resolution voxel-based finite element modeling at the individual trabecular level makes it possible to relate the intrinsic mechanical properties of bone tissue and the local trabecular architecture to multiaxial deformation of the local trabecular lattice.

Bragdon CR, Estok DM, Malchau H, et al: Comparison of two digital radiostereometric analysis methods in the determination of femoral head penetration in a total hip replacement phantom. *J Orthop Res* 2004;22(3):659-664.

The increased usage of radiostereometric analysis for measuring in vivo wear in modern total hip arthroplasty constructs has stimulated the development of various algorithms for postprocessing the marker data. Moreover, the advent of digital radiography has changed the performance characteristics of radiostereometric analysis compared with its performance with conventional radiographic source images. The influence of these factors was systematically compared in this study using a physical surrogate as the gold standard.

Brown TD: Finite element modeling in musculoskeletal biomechanics. *J Appl Biomech* 2004;20:336-366.

The author outlines the conceptual basis for the finite element analysis of load transmission through musculoskeletal tissues and orthopaedic constructs. Various examples are presented. The author provides perspective on the capabilities and limitations of this type of analysis for clinicians and for researchers who have not directly worked in this area.

Daniel M, Antolic V, Iglic A, Kralj-Iglic V: Determination of hip stress from nomograms based on mathematical model. *Med Eng Phys* 2001;23(5):347-357.

Because techniques for mathematically estimating hip joint contact stresses span a range of complexities and simplicity of calculation is an important consideration for feasibility of usage in the clinical arena, the authors developed a technique in which contact stresses can be quickly estimated directly from look-up tables, using geometric parameters directly measurable from standard AP radiographs.

Dennis DA, Komistek RD, Northcut EJ, Ochoa JA, Ritchie A: In vivo determination of hip joint separation and the forces generated due to impact loading conditions. *J Biomech* 2001;34(5):623-629.

Fluoroscopy-based image analysis work has demonstrated that femoral head separation occurs in total hip arthroplasty during certain activities that do not require weight bearing. The authors of this article describe an abrupt impaction pulse that occurs when the femoral head reseats within the acetabular cup.

Ferguson SJ, Bryant JT, Ganz R, Ito K: The acetabular labrum seal: A poroelastic finite element model. *Clin Biomech (Bristol, Avon)* 2000;15:463-468.

Because the biomechanical information base is relatively sparse in regard to the function of the labrum, the authors developed a finite element model to address the ability of the labrum to seal a pressurized layer of synovial fluid within the joint. Data from the model showed that the labral sealing function is indeed quite important; when compromised sealing integrity was simulated, cartilage strains rose more than fivefold.

Fleming BC, Beynnon BD: In vivo measurement of ligament/tendon strains and forces: A review. *Ann Biomed Eng* 2004;32(3):318-328.

The authors of this article review the wide range of specialized instrumentation modalities that have been recently developed for measuring soft-tissue distensions in articular and periarticular structures. The theoretical basis, usage, performance characteristics, and limitations of the various types of instruments are critically assessed.

Genda E, Iwasaki N, Li G, MacWilliams BA, Barrance PJ, Chao EYS: Normal hip joint contact pressure distribution in single-leg standing: Effect of gender and anatomic parameters. *J Biomech* 2001;34(7):895-905.

The authors discuss the expedited computational approximations of intra-articular contact stress distributions that have been enabled by a technique known as discrete element analysis, which involves mathematically representing the articular cartilage as an array of equivalently stiff compression springs. Such computations execute hundreds of times more rapidly than traditional finite element models.

Grosland NM, Brown TD: A voxel-based formulation for contact finite element analysis. *Comput Methods Biomech Biomed Engin* 2002;5(1):21-32.

In response to the inability to perform patient-specific computations of contact stress in the natural joint, the authors developed a computational formulation in which source data from CT or MRI can be automatically transformed into finite element meshes in a way that eliminates the "stairstep" jaggedness at the contact surface that otherwise occurs with voxel-based image sources.

Hong J, Cabe GD, Tedrow JR, Hipp JA, Snyder BD: Failure of trabecular bone with simulated lytic defects can be predicted non-invasively by structural analysis. *J Orthop Res* 2004;22(3):479-486.

To predict pathologic fractures resulting from lytic defects, the authors developed models in which structural compromise could be estimated in the neighborhood of the defect based on readily clinically ascertainable geometric measures. The authors report that this technique proved capable of reasonably accurate prediction of the failure loads and failure sites for corresponding benchtop cadaver preparations.

Keyak JH, Rossi A, Jones KA, Les CM, Skinner HB: Prediction of fracture location in the proximal femur using finite element models. *Med Eng Phys* 2001;23(9):657-664.

Advances in automatically generating structural finite element models from CT scans have made it possible to predict osseous material failure under various loading challenges. The authors found application of this approach to predicting fragility fractures of the hip to be encouraging and reported achieving a 72% accuracy rate (versus corresponding cadaver experiments) in predicting bony failure for stance phase loading, and a 67% accuracy rate for trochanteric loading from fall events.

Keyak JH, Skinner HB, Fleming JA: Effect of force direction on femoral fracture load for two types of loading conditions. *J Orthop Res* 2001;19(4):539-544.

Automatically generated finite element models facilitate the systematic study of technologies to reduce fracture risk. In this study, specific direction of the loading to the proximal femur was systematically varied in such a model, allowing determination of the highest-risk loading directions. The authors found that falls in which the impact force was directed onto the posterolateral aspect of the greater trochanter had the greatest fracture risk.

Komistek RD, Dennis DA, Ochoa JA, Haas BD, Hammill C: In vivo comparison of hip separation after metal-on-metal or metal-on-polyethylene total hip arthroplasty. *J Bone Joint Surg Am* 2002;84-A(10):1836-1841.

Video fluoroscopy was used in this study to assess relative motion between the femoral and acetabular components in total hip arthroplasty for a total of 20 patients. The authors report that 10 patients with a metal-on-polyethelene construct consistently showed femoral head sliding/subluxation (averaging 2 mm) during certain activities that did not require weight bearing. By contrast, there was no apparent femoral head sliding/subluxation in the 10 patients with metal-on-metal bearing surfaces.

Lundberg HJ, Pedersen DR, Muste MV, Baer TE, Brown TD: Quantifying fluid ingress to the joint space during THA subluxation, in *Transactions of the 51st Meeting of the Orthopaedic Research Society*. Rosemont, IL, Orthopaedic Research Society, 2004, p 833.

The authors postulated a mechanism to explain how third-body particulate debris suspended in the fluid of the joint space can gain access to the bearing surface of the total hip arthroplasty implant and studied the debris ingress phenomenon quantitatively, using an experimentally validated computational fluid dynamics technique.

Malkani AL, Voor MJ, Rennirt G, Helfet D, Pedersen DR, Brown TD: Increased peak contact stress after incongruent reduction of transverse acetabular fractures: A cadaveric model. *J Trauma* 2001;51(4):704-709.

The relationship between residual fragment displacement and elevations of cartilage contact stress in acetabular fractures was studied in a cadaveric preparation. The authors used Fuji contact film to measure cartilage pressure. They report that digital image analysis enabled high-resolution pressure mapping in the near vicinity of local incongruities.

Nadzadi ME, Pedersen DR, Yack HJ, Callaghan JJ, Brown TD: Kinematics, kinetics, and finite element analysis of commonplace maneuvers at risk for total hip dislocation. *J Biomech* 2003;36:577-591.

The authors of this study used finite element analysis (experimentally validated) to assess how total hip arthroplasty dislocation resistance is influenced by individual factors of mechanical design or surgical component placement for various hip maneuvers and postures that are commonly associated with dislocation.

Sparks DR, Beason DP, Etheridge BS, Alonso JE, Eberhardt AW: Contact pressures in the flexed hip joint during lateral trochanteric loading. *J Orthop Res* 2005;23(2):359-366.

Encouraging success with computational models of fracture risk from falls and from impacts has informed and motivated supporting physical testing work; experimental validation of computer models is one key experimental endeavor. The authors of this study report that pressure-sensitive film inserted into the joint space can identify regions of the acetabulum that are most critically challenged by sideways impact to the greater trochanter.

Stewart KJ, Pedersen DR, Callaghan JJ, Brown TD: Implementing capsule representation in a total hip dislocation finite element model. *Iowa Orthop J* 2004;24:1-8.

The authors of this study assessed capsular contribution to total hip arthroplasty stability using finite element analysis, based on capsule mechanical properties measured cadaverically. They report that this computational technique also provided detailed local information concerning stresses within the capsule itself.

van Rietbergen B, Huiskes R, Eckstein F, Ruegsegger P: Trabecular bone tissue strains in the healthy and osteoporotic human femur. *J Bone Miner Res* 2003;18(10): 1781-1788.

In this study, microfinite element models of a healthy versus osteoporotic human proximal femur were developed automatically from CT data sets. The results showed that tissue-level strains in the osteoporotic femoral head averaged 70% higher than normal and were much less evenly distributed.

Williams S, Butterfield M, Stewart T, Ingham E, Stone M, Fisher J: Wear and deformation of ceramic-on-polyethylene total hip replacements with joint laxity and swing phase microseparation. *Proc Inst Mech Eng [H]* 2003;217(2):147-53.

The authors of this study assessed the microseparation of the femoral head from the acetabular cup during swing phase in a hip simulator study of ceramic-on-polyethylene bearings. They reported that this caused substantial rim deformation of the cups, but involved lower volumetric wear of the polyethylene than that observed for otherwise identical duty cycles lacking microseparation.

Classic Bibliography

Baker KJ, Brown TD, Brand RA: A finite element analysis of the effects of intertrochanteric osteotomy on stresses in femoral head osteonecrosis. *Clin Orthop Relat Res* 1989;249:183-198.

Bergmann G, Graichen F, Rohlmann A: Hip joint loading during walking and running measured in two patients. *J Biomech* 1993;26(8):969-990.

Bergmann G, Graichen F, Rohlmann A: Is staircase walking a risk for fixation of hip implants? *J Biomech* 1995;28(5):535-553.

Brand RA, Pedersen DR, Davy DT, Kotzar GM, Heiple KG, Goldberg VM: Comparison of hip force calculations and measurements in the same patient. *J Arthroplasty* 1994;9(1):45-51.

Brown TD, Pope DF, Hale JE, Buckwalter JA, Brand RA: Effects of osteochondral defect size on cartilage contact stress. *J Orthop Res* 1991;9:559-567.

Brown TD, Shaw DT: In vitro contact stress distributions in the natural human hip. *J Biomech* 1983;16(6): 373-384.

Caldwell NJ, Hale JE, Rudert MJ, Brown TD: An algorithm for approximate crinkle artifact compensation in pressure-sensitive film recordings. *J Biomech* 1993;26(8): 1001-1009.

Crowninshield RD, Johnston RC, Andrews JG, Brand RA: A biomechanical investigation of the human hip. *J Biomech* 1978;11:75-85.

Day WH, Swanson SAV, Freeman MA: Contact pressures in the loaded human cadaver hip. *J Bone Joint Surg Br* 1975;57:302-313.

English TA, Kilvington M: In vivo records of hip loads using a femoral implant with telemetric output: A preliminary report. *J Biomed Eng* 1979;1(2):111-115.

Ford CM, Keaveny TM, Hayes WC: The effect of impact direction on the structural capacity of the proximal femur during falls. *J Bone Miner Res* 1996;11(3):377-383.

Hadley NA, Brown TD, Weinstein SL: The effects of contact pressure elevations and aseptic necrosis on the long-term outcome of congenital hip dislocation. *J Orthop Res* 1990;8(4):504-513.

Hodge WA, Carlson KL, Fijan SM, et al: Contact pressures from an instrumented hip endoprosthesis. *J Bone Joint Surg Am* 1989;71(9):1378-1385.

Huiskes R, Chao EY: A survey of finite element analysis in orthopedic biomechanics: The first decade. *J Biomech* 1983;16(6):385-409.

Huiskes R, Hollister SJ: From structure to process, from organ to cell: Recent developments of FE-analysis in orthopaedic biomechanics. *J Biomech Eng* 1993;115(4B): 520-527.

Hurwitz DE, Andriacchi TP: Biomechanics of the hip, in Callaghan JJ, Rosenberg AG, Rubash HE (eds): *The Adult Hip*. Philadelphia, PA, Lippincott-Raven Publishers, 1998.

Keyak JH, Meagjer JM, Skinner HB, Mote CD Jr: Automated three-dimensional finite element modeling of bone: A new method. *J Biomed Eng* 1990;12(5):389-397.

Kotzar GM, Davy DT, Goldberg VM, et al: Telemeterized in vivo hip joint force data: A report on two patients after total hip surgery. *J Orthop Res* 1991;9:621-633.

Lewis JL, Lew WD, Schmidt J: A note on the application and evaluation of the buckle transducer for the knee ligament force measurement. *J Biomech Eng* 1982; 104(2):125-128.

Livermore J, Ilstrup D, Morrey B: Effect of femoral head size on wear of the polyethylene acetabular component. *J Bone Joint Surg Am* 1990;72:518-528.

Maxian TA, Brown TD, Pedersen DR, McKellop HA, Liu B, Callaghan JJ: Finite element analysis of acetabular wear: Validation, and backing and fixation effects. *Clin Orthop Relat Res* 1977;344:111-117.

Maxian TA, Brown TD, Weinstein SL: Chronic stress tolerance levels for human articular cartilage: Two non-uniform contact models applied to long-term follow-up of CDH. *J Biomech* 1995;28(2):159-166.

Martell JM, Berdia S: Determination of polyethylene wear in total hip replacements with use of digital radiographs. *J Bone Joint Surg Am* 1997;79:1635-1641.

Mizrahi J, Solomon L, Kaufman B: A method for direct measurement of the local pressures in the human cadaver hip joint. *Phys Med Biol* 1980;25:1181.

Olson SA, Bay BK, Hamel A: Biomechanics of the hip joint and the effects of fracture of the acetabulum. *Clin Orthop Relat Res* 1997;339:92-104.

Paul JP: Approaches to design: Force actions transmitted by joints in the human body. *Proc Res Soc London* 1976;192:163-172.

Pedersen DR, Brown TD, Hillis SL, Callaghan JJ: Prediction of long-term polyethylene wear in total hip arthroplasty, based on early wear measurements made using digital image analysis. *J Orthop Res* 1998;16(5):557-563.

Rydell NW: Forces acting on the femoral head prosthesis: A study on strain gage supplied prostheses in living persons. *Acta Orthop Scand Suppl* 1966;88:37.

Seireg A, Arvikar RJ: The prediction of muscular load sharing and joint forces in the lower extremities during walking. *J Biomech* 1975;8:89-102.

Shaver SM, Brown TD, Hillis SL, Callaghan JJ: Digital edge-detection measurement of polyethylene wear after total hip arthroplasty. *J Bone Joint Surg Am* 1997;79:690-700.

Sychterz CJ, Engh CA Jr, Yang A, Engh CA: Analysis of temporal wear patterns of porous-coated acetabular components: Distinguishing between true wear and so-called bedding-in. *J Bone Joint Surg Am* 1999;81(6):821-830.

Chapter 32

Bearing Surfaces

Michael T. Manley, FRSA, PhD

John Dumbleton, PhD, DSc

Introduction

The articulating joint of hip prostheses generates wear debris. The accumulation of wear particles in the local tissues can result in osteolysis, necessitating replacement of the prosthesis. Osteolytic defects may compromise fixation and complicate the revision procedure. The goal of new hip bearing materials is to extend implant life by substantially decreasing the amount of wear debris generated, thus greatly reducing or even eliminating the incidence of osteolysis.

Bearing combinations include polymeric, ceramic, and metallic materials. Materials are categorized as hard or soft, with polymeric materials classified as soft and ceramic and metallic materials classified as hard. Both hard/soft and hard/hard combinations have been used for total hip prostheses. The hard/soft (cobalt-chromium alloy/ultra-high-molecular-weight polyethylene [UHMWPE]) combination prevailed after initial experience with metal/metal bearings in the 1970s and remained dominant until recently. With increasing demand on hip prostheses imposed by younger patients and greater patient activity, hard/hard (alumina/alumina and cobalt-chromium alloy/cobalt-chromium alloy) combinations that have material and design improvements over earlier implants have been reintroduced. Advances in the existing class of hard/soft bearings have also been made. Although all bearing combinations have strengths and potential weaknesses, the new bearing combinations exhibit reduced wear compared with that of earlier hip bearings.

Hard/Soft Bearings

Wear Mechanisms

Clinical studies of total hip replacements indicate a relationship between the level of bearing wear and the occurrence of periprosthetic osteolysis. Wear greater than a threshold value of 0.1 mm/yr appears to increase the incidence of osteolysis, whereas wear substantially below this threshold value makes osteolysis uncommon. However, the threshold may be modified by intracapsular pressure, bone interface access, and patient reaction to debris. Different wear mechanisms contribute to the generation of debris. Adhesion occurs during contact of the opposing bearing surfaces. Sliding breaks these contacts. However, if the strength of the adhesion exceeds the strength of the material, particles (wear debris) are pulled from the material. This is adhesive wear debris, and it is typically generated from the polyethylene acetabular component because polyethylene is the weaker of the two bearing materials. Two-body abrasive wear occurs when a hard projection on one surface cuts into the opposing surface. Again, abrasive wear is generally observed with polyethylene components. Hard particles such as bone or polymethylmethacrylate cement can also cause abrasive damage if trapped between the bearing surfaces. This is referred to as third-body wear. Scratching of metallic femoral heads is commonly observed during revision surgery and is usually thought to be caused by third-body wear. Wear can also be caused also by bearing material fatigue failure (fatigue wear), which may result from the repetitive loading of the bearings during articulation.

Not all wear debris is generated at the articulating surface. Wear debris can be produced at any modular junction where there is relative motion between the components (for example, backside wear between the inside of a metal acetabular shell and the outside of a polyethylene liner). Unintentional contact, such as impingement at the femoral neck on the acetabular bearing, can also generate debris. These wear mechanisms apply not only to hard/soft bearings, but also to hard/hard bearings. However, the relative contribution to joint wear from the femoral head and cup, the level of total wear, and the wear particle size may be different for different bearing types.

Femoral Head Materials

The metallic alloys that have been used with UHMWPE bearings are stainless steel, cobalt-chromium alloy, and titanium alloy. Laboratory and clinical studies have shown the wear rates of UHMWPE and either stainless steel or cobalt-chromium to be comparable. In the

United States, cobalt-chromium alloy was chosen over the 316 L stainless steel in use at the time because the cobalt-chromium alloy was more resistant to corrosion. Stainless steel continues to be used outside the United States, and newer, more corrosion-resistant stainless steel alloys introduced in the early 1980s remain in use. Titanium alloys are more vulnerable to abrasion than cobalt-based alloys; therefore, they are no longer used as bearings. It was proposed that hardening of the surface of the titanium alloy using techniques such as gas nitriding, solution nitriding, or ion implantation may improve performance, but wear can still occur if the hardened layer is penetrated.

Cast or forged cobalt-chromium alloy predominates as the choice of femoral head material for articulation against UHMWPE. Cobalt alloy components can be produced by either investment casting or by forging. Forged components have a smaller grain size and greater hardness than cast components. Components manufactured using both methods have been used widely as bearing surfaces. The wear of the cobalt-chromium alloy against UHMWPE bearing combination is the standard against which the wear of all other bearing combinations is measured.

Alumina and zirconia ceramics have also been used as femoral head materials with polyethylene cups. The hardness of ceramic femoral heads reduces the incidence of scratching and surface damage to the head and is therefore believed to reduce polyethylene wear. Alumina is used widely. Zirconia is not used as widely because of reports of phase transformation of the material in vivo, protruding ceramic grains, surface roughening, and increased polyethylene wear rates. Laboratory and clinical studies provide conflicting reports on whether the wear of polyethylene is indeed reduced with ceramic ball heads. Recently, oxidized zirconium femoral heads have been introduced. Laboratory studies indicate lower polyethylene wear and higher resistance of the femoral head surface to abrasion with oxidized zirconium, but clinical experience is too short to indicate whether this material is superior to those ceramics already in use.

Conventional UHMWPE

Most UHMWPE components are machined from powder that is converted into solid form. The solid form is produced either by ram extrusion or by compression molding. Rods are produced by ram extrusion, and blocks are produced from compression molding. Sometimes components are machined from near net shape molding of powder or by directly performing compression molding of the powder to the shape of the final component.

The final step in the manufacturing process is sterilization. Although ethylene oxide was used initially and gas-plasma was used more recently, most polyethylene

components implanted between 1975 and 1995 were sterilized using gamma radiation (2.5 to 4 mrad) in air. Sterilization of UHMWPE by gamma radiation introduces cross-linking of the polyethylene molecules from the interaction of the free radicals formed during irradiation. Laboratory and clinical studies have shown improved wear resistance of gamma sterilized UHMWPE compared with UHMWPE sterilized using nonionizing means (ethylene oxide or gas plasma) because the latter methods do not produce cross-linking. Gamma air sterilized UHMWPE components have demonstrated excellent clinical outcomes in a variety of settings. However, by the early 1990s, research on the structure and properties of UHMWPE identified the potential for oxidation of polyethylene gamma sterilized in air because of the existence of free radicals that are not cross-linked. Oxidation reduced the mechanical properties of these components. Consequently, some manufacturers changed the sterilization process to gamma irradiation in an inert atmosphere, such as nitrogen, argon, or vacuum. The lack of oxygen prevented the oxidation process from commencing. Other manufacturers either switched to nonionizing sterilization methods or continued with them, despite the potential disadvantage of lower wear resistance.

Research on the link between polyethylene structure and wear continues. Additional exploration of the role of cross-linking in reducing wear led to the development of highly cross-linked polyethylenes that were introduced in the late 1990s.

Highly Cross-Linked UHMWPE

The cross-linking found in traditional polyethylene was a fortuitous byproduct of the sterilization process using ionizing radiation. Because cross-linking reduced wear, it was theorized that increased cross-linking would result in an even more wear-resistant UHMWPE. In these new processes, cross-linking is produced using higher doses of radiation followed by or combined with heat to enhance the cross-linking process and the removal of free radicals. There are many variables that can be manipulated in the production of a highly cross-linked UHMWPE. However, the key variables are radiation dose and the temperature of heating applied to the material. Heating above the polyethylene melting range is known as remelting, and heating below the melting range is known as annealing. Manufacturers have introduced different highly cross-linked polyethylenes by making different choices in variables, such as radiation dose and selection of remelting or annealing. From hip simulator tests, the greatest reduction in UHMWPE wear has been shown to occur as the radiation dose increases from 0 to 5 mrad. An additional smaller decrease occurs between 5 and 10 mrad, and there is little reduction thereafter. Because UHMWPE is a semicrys-

Table 1 | Comparison of Commercially Available Cross-Linked Polyethylenes

Brand Name	Manufacturer	Radiation Type (Temperature)	Radiation Dose	Cross-linking Temperature	Sterilization
Crossfire	Stryker Orthopaedics	Gamma (ambient)	7.5 mrad with subsequent dose of 3 mrad	Below melt temperature at 120°C to 135°C for a minimum of 8 hours	Gamma at 2.5 to 3.5 mrad (in nitrogen)
Durasul	Zimmer	Electron beam (125°C)	9.5 mrad	Remelted at ~150°C for approximately 2 hours	Ethylene oxide
Longevity	Zimmer	Electron beam (ambient)	10 mrad	Remelted at ~150°C for approximately 2 hours	Gas plasma
Marathon	DePuy	Gamma (ambient)	5 mrad	Remelted at 155°C for 24 hours	Gas plasma
Reflection XLPE	Smith & Nephew	Gamma (ambient)	10 mrad	Remelted at ~150°C for approximately 2 hours	Ethylene oxide

talline polymer, its mechanical behavior is affected by its crystalline morphology. Heating UHMWPE above its melting temperature eliminates free radicals, but changes material morphology. Heating UHMWPE below its melting temperature preserves its morphology and thermal processing history, but can leave some free radicals behind. In general terms, highly cross-linked UHMWPE that is annealed maintains its mechanical and fatigue properties but contains free radicals, whereas remelted materials have lower mechanical and fatigue properties but do not contain detectable free radicals. General details and characteristics of each type of polyethylene are included in Table 1.

Marathon (DePuy, Warsaw, IN), Reflection XLPE (Smith & Nephew, Memphis, TN), Longevity and Durasul (Zimmer, Warsaw, IN), UHMWPEs are remelted and do not contain detectable free radicals. The manufacturers of these materials believe that free radicals are more of a concern than altered mechanical and fatigue proper- ties. Crossfire (Stryker Orthopaedics, Mahwah, NJ) UHMWPE is annealed and contains free radicals. Its manufacturer is more concerned with preserving the crystalline morphology and mechanical and fatigue properties than in eliminating all free radicals. Crossfire UHMPWE is terminally sterilized in nitrogen and vacuum packed to avoid oxidation.

Laboratory studies demonstrate that highly cross-linked polyethylenes have significantly lower wear rates than conventional polyethylene. Although highly cross-linked polyethylenes have been in clinical use for about 5 years, early clinical measurements indicate that in vivo wear rates are greatly reduced with these new materials.

When making a choice between the different highly cross-linked polyethylenes, the compromises inherent in their properties must be considered. The mechanical and fatigue properties of remelted highly cross-linked polyethylenes are reduced in comparison with the properties of annealed material. Reports from the US Food

and Drug Administration (FDA) Medical Device Reporting database detail some rim failures of remelted polyethylene acetabular liners when the cup was placed in a vertical position. Retrieval analysis of annealed highly cross-linked hip bearing liners shows oxidation and reduction in mechanical properties in regions of the liner rim exposed to body fluids. However, the finding of no evidence of in vivo degradation in the contact regions of these retrieved bearings suggests that the femoral head partially protects the bearing surface from oxidative changes, at least for the period (0.02 to 4.8 years) in which these devices were implanted.

Metal-on-Metal Bearings

Concerns regarding osteolysis caused by polyethylene wear debris created a renewed interest in metal-on-metal bearings for total hip replacement. Metal-on-metal designs were introduced 40 years ago, but their clinical performance overall was compromised by poor implant and bearing design. However, some of these original metal-on-metal hip implants were found to be functioning well after 20 to 30 years in vivo, which suggests that metal-on-metal hip implants may be a viable treatment option if design and bearing deficiencies are addressed. Consequently, manufacturers made improvements to the design of the so-called first-generation metal-on-metal hip implants, and early clinical data are now available on the performance of these second-generation metal-on-metal hip implant designs, which were cleared in 1999 for clinical use by the FDA.

Laboratory studies conducted on these second-generation metal-on-metal components showed decreased wear when compared with first-generation metal-on-metal components. Measurements of second-generation components retrieved after clinical use indicated levels of wear comparable to first-generation long-term survivors. The volume of wear debris released by metal-on-metal bearings is about 100 to 200 times lower than that of traditional polyethylene gamma sterilized in air. The actual metal-on-metal wear rate apparently depends on the type of cobalt-chromium alloy used, its surface finish, and the bearing clearance and sphericity. Cobalt-chromium alloys may be wrought or cast, and some have higher carbon content than others. Although implant manufacturers use different bearing alloys, it appears that the bearing design parameters rather than the alloy itself play the most important part in determining the level of wear. This is because the bearing size, clearance, sphericity, and surface finish determine the degree of fluid film lubrication attained. Alloy characteristics may be of consequence only if contact between the articulating surfaces occurs. Laboratory studies indicate that larger femoral head diameters provide a greater assurance of fluid film lubrication. However, a clinical study showed that patients had lower metal ion levels in blood serum with small femoral heads than large femoral heads, possibly as a result of nonoptimal clearance with large heads.

One of the main concerns surrounding metal-on-metal bearings is the long-term biologic effect of metal ions released from the metal-on-metal articulation. The literature indicates that patients with second-generation metal-on-metal hips have higher levels of cobalt and chromium in their blood and urine than patients with metal/polyethylene bearings or patients without implants. The metallic constituents of orthopaedic alloys are biologically active. The cobalt and chromium in metal-on-metal bearings have been noted to be sensitizers with mutagenic and, in some ionization states, carcinogenic effects, and cobalt-chromium wear debris is toxic to cells. Several studies have reported on the level of metal ions in body fluids for patients with metal-on-metal total hip prostheses. Red blood cells are a reservoir for cobalt and chromium, and excretion of cobalt and chromium in the urine is important to control metal ion levels. The loss of efficacy of ion clearance with increasing age may result in further elevation of metal ion levels, and it is possible that continued stress on the kidneys from the metal load could result in earlier compromised kidney function. In one study, researchers stated that they no longer used metal-on-metal articulations in patients with chronic renal disease because of these concerns.

Overall, second-generation metal-on-metal bearings exhibit substantially better wear properties than traditional metal-on-polyethylene bearings. However, the number of published clinical studies with second-generation metal-on-metal bearings is relatively small, the follow-up period is medium term, and the populations studied are not large. Additionally, the effects of metal ion release over time remain a concern, and longer-term studies with larger populations are needed.

Ceramic-on-Ceramic Bearings

Solid ceramic materials such as alumina are attractive for use as hip bearing components because of their hardness, high wear resistance, and chemical inertness. A potential shortcoming of these bearings is the low tensile strength of the ceramic materials. Early designs of alumina-on-alumina hip implants that were introduced more than 30 years ago had unacceptable performance because of wear and fracture. These shortcomings were the result of designs that allowed stem impingement on the ceramic and the relatively poor mechanical properties of early alumina (first-generation) materials.

Second-generation alumina ceramics were introduced after 1977. The average grain size was reduced and porosity was lowered, resulting in improvements in strength. In 1980, the FDA allowed alumina-ceramic bearing components (Autophor/Xenophor, Osteo, Selzach, Switzerland) to be marketed in the United States based on European data. Despite improved alumina properties, this design was unsuccessful because of pain, neck-socket impingement, ceramic fracture, and loosening. Data have indicated that the improved bearing properties cannot compensate for the design shortcomings of a hip implant.

Over the past two decades, there has been a substantial improvement in prosthesis design, implantation technique, and the quality of the alumina components. Third-generation alumina materials were introduced in 1994 (for example, Biolox Forte, CeramTec, Plochingen, Germany). Biolox Forte has a small grain size (< 1.8 μm) and increased density because of hot isostatic pressing during manufacture. Identification marks are placed via laser etching to avoid stress concentrations. All components are proof tested to ensure that they meet the manufacturer's specifications for strength. With these improvements, the manufacturer estimates that the incidence of fracture will be 1 in 25,000 (0.00004%) for alumina bearings. Recent analysis of clinical data suggests the actual fracture rate is about 0.012% for balls and liners. However, to meet these low levels of fracture, several precautions must be taken: impingement should not occur, the femoral head should be carefully placed on a clean taper, and the taper should not be reused for a ceramic head during revision.

Several hip simulator studies conducted in the late 1990s identified the steady-state wear rate for alumina-alumina bearings to be between 1 and 2 μm/million cycles, which is equal to or lower than that of metal-on-metal bearings. Wear measurements on retrievals of first- and second-generation alumina components demonstrated a strong direct relationship between wear and grain size. The wear pattern on the retrievals was described as a wear stripe with a visible dull area of contact. Stripe wear can only be reproduced on a hip joint simulator if the components are allowed to separate during the swing phase of gait. Clinically, stripe wear has been demonstrated to occur with third-generation alumina ceramics and is probably caused by edge loading during rising from a chair. Wear within the strips is estimated to be about 0.3 mm/yr.

The wear debris from alumina-alumina bearings is comparable in size to metallic wear debris from metal-on-metal bearings. However, in contrast to metallic debris, there is no ion release, and the debris appears to be well tolerated by the body. Alumina-alumina total hip prostheses were introduced to the United States via clinical trials in the mid 1990s and were approved by the FDA in 2003. Short- to mid-term results for these implants have been good. In one study of more than 300 patients at 4-year follow-up, no wear-related fractures or complications were reported. Although the follow-up time is short- to medium-term in the United States, 20-year clinical data from France on earlier generation alumina materials and designs have been reported.

Comparison of Bearing Options

Hard/hard bearings, whether of metallic or ceramic material, have different characteristics than hard/soft bearings. In particular, hard/hard bearings are less forgiving under impingement conditions. Impingement can lead to ceramic fracture or notching of the femoral neck by the hard acetabular component. Impingement may also lead to the fracture of bearing components as has been reported with some isolated ceramic designs and more recently with isolated highly cross-linked remelted polyethylene inserts.

Ceramic-ceramic, metal-on-metal, and metal/highly cross-linked polyethylene hip prostheses are available with large diameters femoral heads. One advantage of a large diameter femoral head is a reduction in the incidence of impingement and dislocation. Hip simulator studies have demonstrated that large diameter femoral heads may be used with highly cross-linked polyethylenes without increasing wear. However, the clinical probability of failure of thin polyethylene liners associated with these large femoral heads is not known.

Second-generation metal-on-metal hip implants have been in widespread use for more than 10 years; however, few definitive clinical data are available regarding their performance. Investigational device exemption studies for FDA approval of ceramic-ceramic hip implants with third-generation alumina are now at 7-year follow-up. One study in which patients were randomized to receive ceramic-on-ceramic or metal-on-conventional polyethylene implants reported data at 5-year follow-up. Both bearing combinations currently demonstrate clinical equivalency for implant survival and performance, but there are fewer secondary signs of wear debris release with the ceramic bearings (such as localized proximal osteolysis) and no ceramic failures.

Because scant clinical information is available regarding these hip implants, reliance must be placed on conclusions from the characteristics of each class of materials, laboratory studies, and clinical reports from earlier generations of a device (Table 2). Laboratory studies show that the degree of wear of metal-metal, ceramic-ceramic, and metal/highly cross-linked polyethylene is low, and that all three combinations meet the threshold criterion for wear (< 0.1 mm/yr) to substantially reduce osteolysis. With metal-on-metal bearings, runaway wear has been demonstrated in the laboratory; however, the clinical incidence is not known. Squeaking and clicking have been reported for both metal-on-metal and ceramic-ceramic prostheses. The incidence of squeaking and clicking is low (approximately 1 in 700 patients with implants). The cause of the noise is not known. Impingement is suggested as the cause of clicking, whereas squeaking is most likely caused by breakdown of the fluid film within the bearing during certain activities. The wear debris particle size is much smaller with metal-metal and ceramic-ceramic bearings than it is for implants with a metal-polyethylene articulation. Ceramic-ceramic bearings may have a bimodal particle size distribution if microseparation of the joint occurs. Adverse, long-term biologic effects from metal ion release with metal-on-metal hip prostheses remain a concern, but clinical consequences have not been demonstrated, even with first-generation hip implants that were in place for many years. The effects may be subtle in nature and may only be apparent following careful study.

Ceramic-ceramic, metal-on-metal, and metal/highly cross-linked polyethylene are three choices of materials for total hip replacements because all have low wear rates and a lower incidence of osteolysis than articulations with a conventional UHMWPE bearing. Each combination has strengths and potential shortcomings. Long-term follow-up with a large number of patients is required to demonstrate whether any of these bearing combinations is superior to the others. Table 3 provides a comparison of the different bearing options along with the associated volumetric wear rate.

Future Directions With Bearing Materials

The current generation of highly cross-linked polyethylenes falls into one of two classes depending on whether the heating to further cross-link the material and quench (eliminate) free radicals takes place above (remelting) or below (annealing) the melting temperature of the polymer. Both remelted and annealed highly cross-linked polyethylenes demonstrate low wear rates clinically. However, remelting changes the microstructure of the polymer. Remelted highly cross-linked polyethylenes have undetectable levels of residual free radicals but have reduced fatigue properties. Cracking and

Table 2 | Comparison of Hip Implant Materials

Material Properties	Ceramic-on-Ceramic	Metal-on-Metal	Metal-on-Highly Cross-Linked UHMWPE
Hardness (MPa)	2300	350	Low
Fracture of components	Reported	No	Reported for remelted material
Tribology			
Running-in wear	1 μm	25 μm	100 μm creep
Steady-state wear (linear/year)	0 to 3 μm	5 μm	10 to 20 μm
Runaway wear	Not reported	Reported	Not reported
Particle size (mean)	< 0.02 and > 0.2 μm	0.05 μm	0.4 μm
Three-body wear	Not reported	Reported	Reported
Metal ion level in body fluids in well-fixed prosthesis	Not increased	Increased in blood and urine	Not increased
Biologic Effects			
Cell toxicity	No	Yes	No
Local tissue reaction	Low	Low	Low
Chromosomal changes	Not reported	Reported	Not reported
Hypersensitivity	Not reported	Reported	Not reported
Carcinogenicity	Not reported	Consideration	Not reported
Other Considerations			
Squeaking	Reported	Reported	Not reported
Clicking	Reported	Reported	Not reported
Seizing	Not reported	Reported	Not reported
US clinical introduction	1996 IDE/2003 approval	1996 IDE/2002 approval	1998 approval

IDE = Investigational device exemption

Table 3 | Hip Simulator Wear of Various Bearing Combinations*

Bearing Combination	Wear Rate (mm³/million cycles)
Cobalt-chromium/polyethylene gamma sterilized in nitrogen	46.0
Cobalt-chromium/UHMWPE sequentially irradiated and annealed	1.3
Cobalt-chromium/cobalt-chromium	2.0
Alumina/alumina	0.1

All wear measurements were made on hip joint simulator with crossing path motion. A physiologic loading pattern (Paul curve) with a maximum load of 2,450 N and minimum load of 150 N was applied. The arrangement of components was anatomic with the cup placed superior to the articulating femoral component. Frequency was 1 Hz. Alpha fraction bovine calf serum was used as the joint fluid. Weight loss measurements were made for the polyethylene components and dimensional changes determined for the hard-on-hard bearings.

fatigue failure have been reported. The microstructure of the material is maintained with annealed highly cross-linked polyethylenes, providing fatigue properties that are superior to those of remelted materials. However, annealed highly cross-linked polyethylenes have residual free radicals and retrieved components have demonstrated oxidation.

In the past several years, research efforts have been directed toward the development of the next generation of highly cross-linked polyethylenes. The goal has been to combine the advantages of the two existing classes of materials without the disadvantages of reduced fatigue strength or residual free radicals. The limitation of remelting has been acknowledged and annealing has been used in the new processes for producing highly cross-linked polyethylenes.

One approach for cross-linking polyethylene has been the use of sequential irradiation and annealing. In this method, UHMWPE is gamma irradiated to 30 kGy followed by annealing. The cycle is repeated twice more to give a cumulative radiation dose of 90 kGy. This sequentially irradiated and annealed material (X3, Stryker Orthopaedics, Mahwah, NJ) was approved for acetabular component use in February 2005.

A second approach has been the combination of irradiation and solid-state deformation by extrusion below the melting temperature. In one development, a gamma radiation dose of 50 kGy is used. This material (ArCom XL, Biomet, Warsaw, IN) was approved in March 2005 for use in the hip.

Avoidance of remelting has been suggested using vitamin E (α-tocopherol) as an antioxidant. The diffusion of α-tocopherol into polyethylene may be combined with cross-linking to give a material with good wear and fatigue properties. The FDA has recently approved such a product containing vitamin E.

For metal/metal bearings the early femoral heads were of smaller diameter, typically 28 mm in size. Thus, longer-term clinical results reflect this experience. An increase in femoral head size produces a great sliding velocity and may increase the probability of fluid film lubrication with a concomitant decrease in wear. Furthermore, large diameter heads reduce the risk of impingement and dislocation. This led to a general increase in the size of the femoral head (32 mm and larger). Whether these efforts will result in lower levels of wear and improved clinical results is not yet known. The use of ceramic-on-metal bearings has been proposed. One simulator study demonstrated that an alumina head articulating against a cobalt-chromium alloy cup produced a 100-fold reduction in wear compared with that of the metal-on-metal construct. Clinical studies are underway.

With ceramic materials, research has been directed toward increasing the toughness of alumina. Zirconia is tougher than alumina, but it is softer and has lower structural stability (potential for phase transformation). Efforts have been directed at combining zirconia and alumina to see whether the best of both materials can be retained in the composite. The result of this research is Biolox Delta (CeramTec, Plochingen, Germany), which is a transformation-toughened and platelet-reinforced alumina containing 75% alumina, 24% zirconia, and 1% chromium oxide and strontium oxide. Although slightly softer than Biolox Forte, this material has much greater bending strength and may have a lower wear rate at the expense of added manufacturing complexity and higher cost. Whether this added increase in strength and wear resistance is necessary for clinical performance will only be known after considerable follow-up with the current ceramic-ceramic hip prostheses.

An alternative approach for hard-on-hard bearings uses the surface transformation of metallic alloys or surface coatings. The goal is to combine the best features of metal-on-metal and ceramic-on-ceramic bearings to result in bearings without fracture risk and without risk of long-term metal ion release. As with all hard-on-hard bearings, it is not yet known whether some or all of these new bearings will produce noise during patient activity. Noise, a previously rare patient complaint with traditional metal/polyethylene bearings, may eventually revitalize the research into hard/soft and soft/soft bearing combinations.

Summary

When deciding which bearing to use in a given patient, all of the modern bearings produce far less wear than the conventional gamma/air irradiated metal/polyethylene couple. For young and/or active patients, hard/hard bearings will produce less wear debris than metal/highly cross-linked polyethylene, but bearing noise remains a possible complication. For hard-on-hard bearings, cup placement is important to reduce the risk of impingement, excessive wear, and fracture (particularly with ceramic bearings). Metal-on-metal bearings release metal ions and corrosion products and probably should not be used for patients with impaired kidney function or women of childbearing age. Perhaps the most recent generation of annealed highly cross-linked polyethylene bearings will prove to be the conservative option. Currently, all modern bearings appear to meet the clinical goal of reducing debris load on surrounding tissues and reducing the incidence of periprosthetic osteolysis. Therefore, the choice of bearing may be a compromise between individual patient need and the costs of the different bearing options.

Acknowledgment

The authors want to thank Kate Sutton, MA, ELS, and Aigui Wang, PhD, for their assistance in the preparation of this manuscript.

Annotated Bibliography

Hard/Soft Bearings

Clarke IC, Manaka M, Green DD, et al: Current status of Zirconia used in total hip implants. *J Bone Joint Surg Am* 2003;85-A(suppl 4):73-84.

This is an extensive review of the structure and properties of zirconia and a clinical history of its use as a femoral head articulating against UHMWPE. The ongoing controversy over the potential for phase transformation leading to high wear or to ball fracture is comprehensively discussed.

Collier JP, Currier BH, Kennedy FE, et al: Comparison of cross-linked polyethylene materials for orthopaedic applications. *Clin Orthop Relat Res* 2003;414:289-304.

This article compares the characteristics and properties of highly cross-linked polyethylenes from different manufacturers. The compromises made for each material are discussed, and each manufacturer contributed a comment on its material. The comparison is limited to structural and mechanical properties and to free radical content; wear is not discussed.

Dorr LD, Wan Z, Longjohn DB, Dubois B, Murken R: Total hip arthroplasty with the use of the Metasul metal-on-metal articulation: Four to seven-year results. *J Bone Joint Surg Am* 2000;82(6):789-798.

Between 1991 and 1994, 70 patients (70 hips) were implanted with a metal-on-metal articulation prosthesis and a Weber cup; 56 of the patients (56 hips) were available for follow-up at an average of 5.2 years. The average Harris Hip Score was 89.6 points. Clinical results were found to be similar to those of patients with metal-on-polyethylene articulation prostheses.

Dumbleton JH, Manley MT, Edidin AA: A literature review of the association between wear rate and osteolysis in total hip arthroplasty. *J Arthroplasty* 2002;17(5):649-661.

This is an extensive review of clinical series published in the literature for which survivorship, osteolysis incidence, and bearing wear are reported. Despite the difficulty of comparing studies that use different methodologies, the authors concluded that the threshold wear level for polyethylene above which osteolysis is highly likely to occur is 0.1 mm/yr.

Harris WH: Cross-linked polyethylene: Why the enthusiasm? *Instr Course Lect* 2001;50:181-184.

The author discusses the relationship between polyethylene debris and osteolysis, arguing that highly cross-linked polyethylenes provide greatly reduced wear with the potential to substantially reduce the incidence of osteolysis.

Hopper RH, Young AM , Orishimo KF, Engh CA: Effect of terminal sterilization with gas plasma or gamma radiation on wear of polyethylene liners. *J Bone Joint Surg Am* 2003;85 (3):464-468.

In this comparison of the wear rate of 61 polyethylene hip inserts that were sterilized by gamma radiation and 63 hip inserts sterilized by gas plasma, the authors reported that at clinical follow-up between 1 and 5.5 years, significantly less bearing wear occurred with the gamma-sterilized hip inserts ($P < 0.001$). Additionally, no correlations were identified between wear and the shelf life of the polyethylene hip insert or wear and hip insert age.

Kurtz SM, Hozack W, Turner J, et al: Mechanical properties of retrieved highly cross-linked Crossfire liners after short-term implantation. *J Arthroplasty* 2005;20(7):840-849.

This study reports mechanical and oxidation measures of Crossfire liners (Stryker Orthopaedics) that were retrieved for reasons other than wear at less than 5 years after implantation. Minimal wear and no association between the time of implantation and either mechanical properties or oxidation near the worn bearing surface were found. Lower mechanical properties and higher oxidation were found in unworn locations exposed to body fluids.

Kurtz SM, Manley M, Wang A, Taylor S, Dumbleton J: Comparison of the properties of annealed crosslinked (Crossfire) and conventional polyethylene as hip bearing materials. *Bull Hosp Jt Dis* 2003;61(1-2):17-26.

The authors discuss the development of cross-linked polyethylenes, focusing on Crossfire polyethylene. The merits of annealing versus remelting polyethylene to maintain the physical properties of the bearing material are also discussed, as are the radiation and sterilization processes. A discussion on

the role of free radicals is included, and the results from testing in a commercial laboratory are presented.

Manley MT, Capello WN, D'Antonio JA, Edidin AA: Highly cross-linked polyethylene acetabular liners for reduction in wear in total hip replacement, in *Proceedings of the 67th Annual Meeting*. Rosemont, IL, American Academy of Orthopaedic Surgeons, 2000, p 605.

This scientific presentation focused on the reduction of abrasive wear in the hip. The structure and mechanical properties of cross-linked polyethylenes and the role of free radicals in oxidative degradation are discussed. The authors also present test results on sterilizing cross-linked polyethylene in an oxygen-free environment.

Manley MT, D'Antonio JA, Capello WN, Edidin AA: Osteolysis: A disease of access to fixation interfaces. *Clin Orthop* 2002;405:129-137.

This article discusses the role of particle access to the bone interface in the development of osteolysis. Osteolysis depends not only on the rate of particle generation but also on design factors that may limit access.

McKellop HA: Bearing surfaces in total hip replacements: State of the art and future developments. *Instr Course Lect* 2001;50:165-179.

Wear mechanisms such as adhesion, abrasion, and fatigue are defined and discussed. Information is provided on wear studies of metal-on-metal bearings, ceramic-on-ceramic bearings, metal-on-polyethylene bearings, and ceramic-on-polyethylene bearings. Special attention is given to cross-linked polyethylene.

McKellop H, Shen FW, Lu B, Campbell P, Salovey R: Effect of sterilization method and other modifications on the wear resistance of acetabular cups made of ultra-high molecular weight polyethylene: A hip simulator study. *J Bone Joint Surg Am* 2000;82(12):1708-1725.

A hip joint simulator was used to assess whether it is preferable to sterilize UHMWPE with gamma radiation with the cups packaged in a low-oxygen environment to avoid oxidation or without gamma radiation to avoid radiation-induced oxidation. Sterilizing UHMWPE without radiation was found to avoid immediate- and long-term oxidative degradation, but wear resistance was not improved. Sterilizing UHMPWE with radiation in a low-oxygen environment increased cross-links and improved wear resistance, but concerns were expressed that long-term oxidation resulting from the presence of free radicals may result in significantly reduced wear properties.

Muratoglu OK, Bragdon CR, O'Connor D, et al: Larger diameter femoral heads used in conjunction with a highly cross-linked ultra-high molecular weight polyethylene. *J Arthroplasty* 2001;16(8):24-30.

This article describes the wear performance in a hip simulator of an electron-beam highly cross-linked polyethylene with a femoral head diameter ranging from 22 to 46 mm. Bearing wear was reduced compared with conventional polyethylene. For the highly cross-linked material, wear was found to be independent of femoral head size.

Wannomae KK, Christensen SD, Freiberg AA, Bhattacharyya S, Harris WH, Muratoglu OK: The effect of real-time aging on the oxidation and wear of higly cross-linked UHMWPE acetabular liners. *Biomaterials* 2005; November 3 [Epub ahead of print]. Available at: http://www.sciencedirect.com/science?_ob=ArticleURL&_udi=B6TWB-4HGM7BW-2&_coverDate=11%2F04%2F2005&_alid=337800445&_rdoc=1&_fmt=&urlVersion=0&_userid=10&md5=a9815e3c81b228508954d5d5809895b2. Accessed November 21, 2005.

The results of aging in real time in an aqueous environment to simulate the in vivo environment are described. After 95 weeks, annealed samples demonstrated oxidation, whereas remelted samples did not.

Metal-on-Metal Bearings

Lhotka C, Szekeres T, Steffan I, Zhuber K, Zweymüller K: Four-year study of cobalt and chromium blood levels in patients managed with two different metal-on-metal total hip replacements. *J Orthop Res* 2003;21:189-195.

This article addresses the effect of metallic wear debris on whole-blood metal levels and the potential adverse effects. The study included 259 patients (age- and gender-matched to healthy, unimplanted control subjects) who were implanted with metal-on-metal bearings. Compared with control subjects, all study patients had significantly higher cobalt and chromium levels.

MacDonald SJ, McCalden RW, Chess DG, et al: Metal-on-metal versus polyethylene in hip arthroplasty: A randomized clinical trial. *Clin Orthop* 2003;406:282-296.

In this blinded clinical trial, 41 patients undergoing hip arthroplasty were randomized to receive either a metal-on-metal (N = 23) or a polyethylene (N = 18) bearing. Femoral and acetabular components were the same for all hip implants. The authors reported no significant differences in radiographic outcomes or outcome measurements in the two groups. All patients who received a metal-on-metal bearing had significantly elevated erythrocyte and urine metal ion levels compared with the polyethylene bearing group.

Savarino L, Granchi D, Ciapetti G, et al: Ion release in patients with metal-on-metal hip bearings in total joint replacement: A comparison with metal-on-polyethylene bearings. *J Biomed Mater Res* 2002;63:467-474.

The authors of this study compared the metal ion levels of four groups of patients: those who underwent total joint replacement with metal-on-metal implants, those who underwent total joint replacement with metal-on-polyethylene implants, a third group of patients who had the preoperative status of representative patients from the first two groups, and a fourth group of control subjects. Follow-up was between 14

and 38 months. The authors found that the patients with metal-on-metal bearings had a significantly higher systemic release of cobalt and chromium when compared with patients in all of the other groups.

Yew A, Jagatia M, Ensaff H, Jin ZM: Analysis of contact mechanics in McKee-Farrar metal-on-metal hip implants. *Proc Inst Mech Eng [H]* 2003;217(5):333-340.

The authors of this study used the finite element method to predict the contact area and the contact pressure distribution at the bearing surfaces of metal-on-metal hip implants. The effects of cement and underlying bone, radial clearance between the acetabular cup and femoral head, cup thickness, and design issues were assessed. The authors found that design optimization of the geometric parameters in terms of the cup thickness and the radial clearance was found to be important for minimizing contact stress at the bearing surfaces and avoiding equatorial and edge contact.

Ceramic-on-Ceramic Bearings

D'Antonio J, Capello W, Manley M: Alumina ceramic bearings for total hip arthroplasty. *Orthopedics* 2003; 26(1):39-46.

This article presents the results of a prospective, randomized study comparing alumina-on-alumina ceramic bearings to chromium-cobalt/polyethylene bearings at a minimum 3-year follow-up. Concerns about fracture of alumina components were addressed by using improved alumina ceramic material (Biolox Forte) and an acetabular component design that protects the ceramic insert in case of impingement. Excellent results with the alumina ceramic components were reported.

D'Antonio J, Capello W, Manley M, Bierbaum B: New experience with alumina-on-alumina ceramic bearings for total hip arthroplasty. *J Arthroplasty* 2002;17(4):390-397.

The authors conducted an investigation device exemption study of ceramic-on-ceramic bearings that included 514 hips in 458 patients from 16 sites. Patients were randomized to participate in one of three arms of the study: the first and second arms used alumina-on-alumina bearings, and the third arm used a cobalt-chromium-on-polyethylene bearing. A fourth arm of the study in which a ceramic-on-ceramic bearing with a titanium sleeve on the ceramic cup was used was added subsequently. The authors reported that four insertional chips occurred with the alumina cup, but no alumina ceramic fractures and no alumina bearing surface–related failures occurred.

Garino JP, Marks R, Dinh V, Leyen S: Modern ceramic component fracture: Trends and recommendations based on improved reporting methods, in *Proceedings of the 72nd Annual Meeting*. Rosemont, IL, American Academy of Orthopaedic Surgeons, 2005, p 352.

The database of the largest supplier of medical grade ceramics was analyzed from 2000 through 2003. After reviewing data on more than 1 million components produced during that period, the overall fracture rate of the ceramic balls and liners was found to be 0.012%.

Good V, Ries M, Barrack RL, Widding K, Hunter G, Heuer D: Reduced wear with oxidized zirconium femoral heads. *J Bone Joint Surg Am* 2003;85-A(suppl):105-110.

Wear results of oxidized zirconium and chromium-cobalt heads articulating against conventional and highly cross-linked polyethylene were compared under smooth conditions and after a roughening protocol. Testing was conducted using a physiological hip simulator. The zirconium heads produced fewer polyethylene particles than the chromium-cobalt heads when sliding against either highly cross-linked or conventional polyethylene because of the greater hardness of the oxidized zirconium material and its higher resistance to surface damage during roughening.

Prudhommeaux F, Hamadouche M, Nevelos J, Doyle C, Meunier A, Sedel L: Wear of alumina-on-alumina total hip arthroplasties at a mean 11-year follow-up. *Clin Orthop* 2000;379:113-122.

The authors investigated the surface topography of 11 alumina-on-alumina bearing couples retrieved for aseptic loosening at a mean 11-year follow-up. Microscopic wear and the microstructure of the alumina were evaluated. Alumina quality assessed by grain size measurements and porosity percentages showed progressive improvement from 1977 to 1988. On a macroscopic scale, load increase or impairment in load distribution over components surfaces increased the penetration rates.

Tipper JL, Hatton A, Nevelos JE, et al: Alumina-alumina artificial hip joints: Part II. Characterization of the wear debris from in vitro hip joint simulations. *Biomaterials* 2002;23(16):3441-3448.

The authors discuss clinically relevant wear rates and wear patterns from in vitro wear simulations. When comparing alumina ceramic wear particles generated from standard simulator testing and microseparation simulator testing with wear particles generated in vivo, the authors found that stripe wear that was occasionally observed on the in vivo on femoral heads was reproducible in vitro when microseparation was introduced into the wear simulation.

Walter WL, Insley GM, Walter WK, Tuke MA: Edge loading in third generation alumina ceramic-on-ceramic bearings: Stripe wear. *J Arthroplasty* 2004;19(4):402-413.

In this report on 16 retrieved alumina ceramic bearings exhibiting a stripe pattern of wear, none of the bearings was retrieved for failure. Mapping of the wear stripes on the femoral heads indicated that the stripes were caused most likely by rising from a chair or climbing steps and not during normal walking.

Comparison of Bearing Options

Berry DJ: Periprosthetic fractures associated with osteolysis: A problem on the rise. *J Arthroplasty* 2003; 18(3):107-111.

The author discusses periprosthetic fractures associated with osteolysis that occur in the pelvis, peritrochanteric area, or femoral diaphysis. To prevent fractures, the author suggests exchanging loose implants when appropriate and grafting osteolytic lesions. More frequent radiographic monitoring is encouraged for younger, active patients. Treatment options for fractures are addressed.

Future Directions With Bearing Materials

Bradford L, Baker DA, Graham J, Chawan A, Ries MD, Pruitt LA: Wear and surface cracking in early retrieved highly cross-linked polyethylene acetabular liners. *J Bone Joint Surg Am* 2004;86:1271-1282.

This study assessed in vivo wear mechanisms to determine whether they can be predicted accurately by hip simulators. Twenty-four liners were examined: 21 explanted liners, 1 unimplanted highly cross-linked liner, and 2 explanted ethylene oxide–sterilized non–cross-linked liners. The explanted liners were retrieved an average of 10 months after implantation and showed signs of surface damage that was not predicted by the wear simulators. The authors theorized that the difference might be the result of the variability in cyclic loading and in vivo lubrication.

Digas G, Karrholm J, Thanner J, Malchau H, Herberts P: Highly crosslinked polyethylene in total hip arthroplasty: Randomized evaluation of penetration rate in cemented and uncemented sockets using radiostereometric analysis. *Clin Orthop Relat Res* 2004;429:6-16.

Highly cross-linked polyethylene was evaluated in two prospective, randomized clinical studies. In one study, highly cross-linked polyethylene liners were compared with a control group of conventional polyethylene. The other study consisted of conventional cemented all-polyethylene and highly cross-linked polyethylene cups. At 6-month follow-up, the penetration rate for the study and control groups was virtually the same. However, at 2-year follow-up, the highly cross-linked polyethylene liners and cemented cups showed substantially lower penetration than conventional polyethylene.

Dorr LD, Wan Z, Shahrdar C, Sirianni L, Boutary M, Yun A: Clinical performance of a Durasul highly-crosslinked polyethylene acetabular liner for total hip arthroplasty at five years. *J Bone Joint Surg Am* 2005;87: 1816-1821.

The authors theorized that a Durasul highly cross-linked polyethylene liner would exhibit less wear at 5-year follow-up than a conventional polyethylene line used in the same acetabular implant. Clinical results comparing the Durasul and conventional polyethylene groups did not differ, but the annual linear wear rate for the Durasul liner was reported to be 55% less than that of conventional polyethylene.

Firkins PJ, Tipper JL, Ingham E, Stone MH, Farrar R, Fisher J: A novel low wearing differential hardness, ceramic-on-metal hip joint prosthesis. *J Biomech* 2001; 34:1291-1298.

In a physiologic anatomic hip joint simulator, ceramic-on-metal articulations were compared with metal-on-metal articulations. The ceramic-on-metal articulations had a wear rate that was approximately 100 times lower than that of the metal-on-metal articulations. The ceramic-on-metal articulations also produced smaller volumetric particle loads than the metal-on-metal articulations.

Halley D, Glassman A, Crowninshield RD: Recurrent dislocation after revision total hip replacement with a large prosthetic femoral head. *J Bone Joint Surg Am* 2004;86:827-830.

This case report details the experience of the authors in treating the left hip of a 65-year old woman. The hip, implanted with a large femoral head, had dislocated several times within 6 months after surgery and had been treated with closed reduction. Prior to revision, the hip was tested for stability and was found to be unstable anteriorly. During revision surgery, the liner was observed to be cracked anteriorly and was replaced. The revised liner also cracked anteriorly within the subsequent 10 months. At the re-revision surgery, the cup, liner, and head were all replaced. A smaller head (28 mm) was used with a thicker polyethylene liner. The hip was re-evaluated 6 months after re-revision surgery and was stable.

Heisel C, Silva M, dela Rosa MA, Schmalzried TP: Short-term in vivo wear of cross-linked polyethylene. *J Bone Joint Surg Am* 2004;86:748-751.

In this article, the authors report on the use of moderately cross-linked polyethylene. Of two groups of patients, one received conventional polyethylene liners, and the other received cross-linked polyethylene liners. At a minimum follow-up of 2 years, wear in the cross-linked polyethylene group was reported to be 81% lower than that in the conventional polyethylene group.

Kurtz SM, Mazzucco D, Rimnac CM, Schroeder D: Anisotropy and oxidative resistance of highly cross-linked UHMWPE after deformation processing by solid-state ram extrusion. *Biomaterials* 2006;27(1):24-34.

The authors reported on a solid-state deformation process as a possible new technique for modifying the physical and mechanical properties of highly cross-linked UHMWPE. The anisotropy and oxidative resistance of the material were evaluated. Testing indicated that the processed material had significantly enhanced strength along the long axis of the rod. Free radicals were detected in the processed material, but at a concentration that was 90% less that that found in gamma-inert–sterilized UHMWPE, which was used as the control. The authors concluded that the oxidative stability observed in the processed material suggests it might be suitable for air-permeable packaging and gas sterilization.

Oral E, Wannomae KK, Hawkins N, Harris WH, Muratoglu OK: Alpha-tocopherol-doped irradiated UHMWPE for high fatigue resistance and low wear. *Biomaterials* 2004;25:5515-5522.

The authors theorized that a lipophilic antioxidant (α-tocopherol) might protect UHMWPE against oxidation and improve fatigue strength thereby eliminating the need for post-irradiation melting of cross-linked polyethylene. The UHMWPE used underwent 5 weeks of accelerated aging. Testing showed doping with alpha-T eliminated the need for post-irradiation melting of UHMWPE to protect it from long-term oxidation. The fatigue strength of the α-tocopherol–doped, 100-kGy irradiated UHMWPE improved by 58% compared with irradiated and melted UHMWPE. This improvement was attributed to the positive effects caused by the lipophilic nature of α-tocopherol, which increased the plasticity of the UHMWPE.

Stewart TD, Tipper JL, Insley G, Streicher RM, Ingham E, Fisher J: Long-term wear of ceramic matrix composite materials for hip prostheses under severe swing phase microseparation. *J Biomed Mater Res B Appl Biomater* 2003;66:567-573.

In this study, the long-term wear performance of alumina matrix composite heads and inserts was tested in a hip joint simulator incorporating severe swing phase joint microseparation. Alumina matrix composite on alumina was used as the control. The alumina matrix composite bearing couple had a lower wear rate at the end of 5 million cycles than the alumina matrix composite on alumina bearing couple. The wear mechanisms and debris generated by both bearing couples were similar to those found with retrieved alumina-on-alumina bearings exhibiting stripe wear.

Wang A, Manley M, Serekian P: Wear and structural fatigue simulation of cross-linked ultra-high molecular weight polyethylene for hip and knee bearing applications, in Kurtz SM, Gsell R, Martell J (eds): *Crosslinked and Thermally Treated UHMWPE for Joint Replacements.* West Conshohocken, PA, ASTM International, 2003.

The authors examined the theoretic correlation between the deterioration of mechanical properties of remelted highly cross-linked polyethylene and clinical performance during a worst case scenario. Both remelted highly cross-linked polyethylene and annealed highly cross-linked polyethylene were tested. Two clinically relevant worst case scenario tests were conducted on highly cross-linked polyethylene. The first test used a cemented all-polyethylene patellar component that was tested under simulated stair climbing conditions. The second test used metal-backed thin acetabular liners rim loaded in a hip simulator. The post-irradiation remelted hip and knee components both experienced catastrophic fractures. The liners fractured at the rim, and the patellar components fractured at the pegs. The annealed highly cross-linked polyethylene components did not fracture when subjected to the same testing conditions as the remelted highly cross-linked polyethylene. Ultimate tensile strength was found to correlate with the structural fatigue performance of the highly cross-linked polyethylene, but tensile elongation within the 250% to 400% range had no impact on structural integrity. The authors concluded that long-term clinical follow-up is needed to make a clinically valid assessment of the performance of highly cross-linked polyethylene in vivo.

Williams S, Isaac G, Hatto P, Stone MH, Ingham E, Fisher J: Comparative wear under different conditions of surface-engineered metal-on-metal bearings for total hip arthroplasty. *J Arthroplasty* 2004;19(8, suppl 3)112-117.

The authors hypothesized that modifying the surface of metal bearings by applying a thick layer of chromium nitride could further reduce wear and ion release. Although the chromium nitride on chromium nitride bearings produced particles that were similar in size to those produced by metal-on-metal bearings, the chromium nitride wear particles were less cytotoxic when co-cultured with macrophage and fibroblast cells. Additionally, the chromium nitride on chromium nitride bearings had lower wear rates compared with the metal-on-metal bearings.

Yau SS, Wang A, Essner A, Manley MT, Dumbleton JH: Sequential irradiation and annealing of highly cross-linked polyethylenes resist oxidation without sacrificing physical/mechanical properties, in *Proceedings of the 51st Annual Meeting of the Orthopaedic Research Society*. Rosemont, IL, Orthopaedic Research Society, 2005, p 1670.

The authors discuss the benefits of a sequential irradiation and annealing process for highly cross-linked polyethylene. They reported that after irradiation-induced cross-linking, annealed UHMPWE retains its original mechanical properties, but still contains a measurable amount of free radicals. Moreover, remelted UHMWPE has reduced mechanical and fatigue properties, but the remelting process essentially removes the free radicals. They concluded that the sequential irradiation and annealing process reduces the free radical content of UHMWPE substantially, providing a material that resists oxidation, yet retains its original mechanical and fatigue properties.

Classic Bibliography

Bono JV, Sanford L, Toussaint JT: Severe polyethylene wear in total hip arthroplasty: Observations from retrieved AML PLUS hip implants with an ACS polyethylene liner. *J Arthroplasty* 1994;9(2):119-125.

Boutin P, Christel P, Dorlot JM, et al: The use of dense alumina-alumina ceramic combination in total hip replacement. *J Biomed Mater Res* 1988;22(12):1203-1232.

Clarke IC: Role of ceramic implants: Design and clinical success with total hip prosthetic ceramic-to-ceramic bearings. *Clin Orthop Relat Res* 1992;282:19-30.

Meyeroff WJ: Metal-on-metal hip implants. *Orthop Tech Rev* 1999;1(4):27.

Willmann G: Ceramics for total hip replacement: What a surgeon should know. *Orthopedics* 1998;21(2):173-177.

Chapter 33

Hip Designs

Carlton G. Savory, MD

William G. Hamilton, MD

Charles A. Engh, Sr, MD

Craig J. Della Valle, MD

Aaron G. Rosenberg, MD

Jorge O. Galante, MD, DMSc

Cemented Femoral Components

During the past four decades, since its introduction, cement has been the most widely used form of primary femoral fixation in total hip arthroplasty. Throughout the world, it continues to be the standard by which all other methods of stem fixation are judged. The Swedish National Hip Arthroplasty Registry is the world's most complete data repository for total hip arthroplasty, and in a 2002 report, the revision burden (the fraction of revisions and the total number of primary and revision total hip arthroplasties) for cemented prostheses that were implanted from 1979 through 2000 was reported to be 7.4% compared with 27.3% for cementless implants (implanted from 1992 through 2000). Cemented total hip arthroplasty continues to provide the best long-term results available. Although cemented fixation of the acetabulum has been questioned, cement fixation of the stem has traditionally been considered the criterion standard.

Design Considerations

Successful long-term results of total hip arthroplasty depend on many factors. However, the consensus is that the durability of the cemented femoral stem is highly dependent on the quality of the cement technique and the design of the implant. Cemented technology has been and continues to be both evolutionary and controversial. Some of the evolution with regard to stem design and materials could be considered trial and error, that is, changes have been made in response to early failures or complications. Over the years, there has been a proliferation of stem designs—both cemented and cementless—that have not stood the test of time. Changes in philosophy and design to address one problem often created others. Many of these failed innovations came at a high cost to the patient, the health care systems, and the surgeon.

After more than 40 years of total hip arthroplasty experience, much has been learned about the complex interactions among biomechanics, surface finish, and geometry with regard to cemented stem fixation. From this experience, two separate design philosophies have emerged: the taper slip and the composite beam models for femoral design, both of which have produced good long-term results.

With the taper slip design, slight stem subsidence is thought to take advantage of the viscoelastic behavior of cement (creep). Cement continues to deform under constant load; therefore, subsidence results in tighter wedging of the loaded taper, which, in turn, results in compressive stresses within the cement and reduced shear at the bone-cement interface.

In the composite beam model, features are designed to strengthen the mechanical bond between the stem-cement interface that is thought to be the weak link in femoral fixation. These features include roughened stem surfaces or precoating the stem with polymethylmethacrylate (PMMA). Collars were believed to strengthen the stem-cement bond by pressurizing the cement, reducing subsidence, and transferring load to the proximal femur.

Materials and cross-sectional geometry of cemented stems have an effect on cement stresses. Stiff materials, such as cobalt-chromium alloys and stainless steel, decrease cement stresses. They are also harder and more resistant to abrasion. Sharp corners in a material are undesirable. Broad medial borders reduce proximal cement strain, and broad lateral borders increase component strength.

Cement Technique

Contemporary techniques for cementing femoral stems are also the products of an evolutionary process (Table 1). Although the techniques for the use of bone cement have been refined, the basic chemical composition of cement has remained the same. So-called first-generation cement techniques did not include bone lavage or drying before cement insertion. The cement was delivered in an antegrade fashion with attempts at pressurization limited to finger packing without distal restriction. These techniques tend to allow for cement lamination, creation of voids within the cement, inadequate or in-

Table 1 | Femoral Stem Cementing Techniques

Technique	First-generation	Second-generation	Third-generation
Filling	Antegrade	Retrograde	Retrograde
Cement gun	No	Yes	Yes
Distal femoral restriction	No	Yes	Yes
Proximal femoral restriction	No	No	Yes
Hand mixing cement	Yes	Yes	No
Vacuum mixing/ centrifugation of cement	No	No	Yes
Canal brushing	No	Yes	Yes
Pulsed lavage	No	No	Yes
Distal centralization	No	Yes	Yes
Proximal centralization	No	No	Yes/No

Table 2 | Postoperative Radiographic Grading System

Grade	Radiographic Appearance
A	Complete filling of the medullary cavity by cement; whiteout at bone-cement interface
B	Slight radiolucency of the cement-bone interface
C	Radiolucency involving 50% to 99% of the cement-bone interface or a defective or incomplete cement mantle
D	Radiolucency at the cement-bone interface of 100% in any projection or a failure to fill the canal with cement such that the tip of the stem was not covered

complete cement mantles, and poor penetration of the cement into the cancellous bone. In spite of what is now considered poor cement technique, many authors have reported good long-term survivorship. Other reports, particularly in North America, revealed unacceptable rates of early femoral loosening with these techniques. At 5-year follow-up, reported radiographic loosening rates ranged from 20% to 24%. At 10-year follow-up, these rates increased to 30% to 40%.

Because bone cement has no adhesive characteristics, it functions as a grout, not a glue. Pressurization increases its penetration into the interstices of cancellous bone. It is this intrusion of cement into the bone that is responsible for the shear strength of the interface. Pressurized cement was shown to have better tensile and shear strengths at the bone-cement interface than finger-packed cement.

Bone preparation (removing fat, blood, and debris) has been shown to promote better cement preparation by improving mechanical interlock and interface and shear strength. Based on these findings, cementing techniques evolved throughout the 1980s, and the second-generation techniques predominated. Bone was cleaned and dried before cement insertion, an intramedullary plug was used, and cement was introduced in a retrograde fashion, thus reducing lamination and voids. Second-generation cementing techniques resulted in marked reduction in the incidence of femoral loosening.

One study described a radiographic grading of cement technique to be used when assessing follow-up of procedures using cemented femoral stems. This widely accepted grading system for initial cementing techniques (Table 2) provides a baseline for comparison with other studies regarding outcomes.

Contemporary or third-generation techniques introduced the concept of maintaining pressurization of the cement before and during stem insertion by adding

proximal restriction to distal femoral occlusion. Retrograde filling, proximal restrictions, and use of the cement gun allow increased pressurization of the cement into the interstices of the cancellous bone. In addition, centrifugation and vacuum mixing of bone cement have been recommended to decrease porosity and remove the noxious fumes of the monomer. The amount of reduction of porosity of the cement remains somewhat controversial. Although voids can act as crack initiators, they can also be crack terminators. Nonporous cement can exhibit excessive contraction after polymerization, and this contraction can compromise fixation by diminishing microinterlock.

The Cement Mantle
The long-term success of cemented femoral stems is highly dependent on creating, maintaining, and protecting the integrity of the cement mantle and its interfaces. Minimizing mantle stresses can be achieved by creation of an optimally thick, symmetric, complete, and homogenous cement mantle.

Early development of stem-cement interface separation and subsequent fracture are believed to be the beginning of aseptic loosening. This debonding as an initiating event has been shown to be the result of stresses at the cement mantle that exceed the fatigue strength of both the stem-cement interface and the actual cement material. Although the stresses of weight bearing experienced by the normal intact femur are quite uniform, these stresses are permanently altered after cemented total hip arthroplasty.

Multiple investigations have shown that stresses experienced in the cement mantle are highest at the stem tip and secondarily at the proximal medial cement mantle. Stem malposition produces nonuniform cement mantle thickness in critical areas. Defects in the mantle also reduce cement thickness and can have a significant effect on cement stresses, as can variations in stem geometry. Optimizing these variables is important to obtain a quality cement mantle, thereby avoiding the potential negative consequences attributed to elevated cement mantle stresses.

Debonding at the stem-cement interface has been directly associated with and attributed to areas of deficient or thin cement mantles. This debonding occurs early after cemented total hip arthroplasty, is seen on most all retrieved specimens, and commonly occurs in the areas that experience the highest cement mantle stresses (the distal tip and proximal medial femur). At some point, early debonding probably accelerates further debonding. These increased stresses and subsequent debonding are directly associated with development of cement mantle fractures. The development of these fractures has been associated with sections of thin cement thickness (< 1 mm). Cement mantle fractures, rarely seen on radiographs, are found in most retrieval specimens.

Aseptic femoral loosening is a late event following the earlier mechanical changes just described and associated with thin or deficient cement mantles. Late symptomatic stem loosening occurring at the bone-cement interface is probably initiated by osteolytic reaction resulting from debris generated at an area of compromise at the stem-cement interface.

Although studies have determined that cement thickness is an important factor in optimizing cement mantle stresses, specific recommendations for optimal cement thickness vary. Proximal medial cement mantle thickness of greater than 10 mm has been associated with an increase in cement fracture, radiolucencies, and progressive component loosening when compared with cement mantles that are 2 mm to 5 mm in thickness. Preserving less than 2 mm of proximal medial cancellous bone for a distance of 30 mm distal to the neck cut decreased proximal medial cement stresses and reduced the incidence of cement fractures and progressive implant loosening compared with patients in whom more than 2 to 5 mm of bone was retained.

It has been suggested that a stem occupying 80% to 90% of the proximal canal optimizes cement stresses. Femoral anatomy and stem geometry dictate to some degree the space available for the cement mantle. Proper preparation of the canal along with choice and placement of the stem should ensure a proximal medial cement mantle of 2 to 5 mm. This can be accomplished, in part, by using stems with smaller mediolateral dimensions, avoiding varus stem positioning, and lateralization of the proximal stem.

Cement stresses increase proximally to distally. Defects or deficiencies (< 2 mm thick) near the stem tip increase the risk of stem failure. Numerous studies (clinical, laboratory, and finite element analyses) have determined that distally it is important to have a uniform cement mantle of more than 2 to 5 mm.

Malpositioning of the stem within the canal produces asymmetric cement mantles that can be marked enough to prejudice the overall results. When compared with neutral or slight valgus stem alignment, stems placed in greater than 5° of varus have been associated with increased risk of cement fracture, radiographic lucencies, and loosening. The use of proximal and distal cement centralizers has improved stem alignment and centralization, as well as maintenance of cement mantles of greater than 2 mm when compared with systems without centralizers. Voids in the cement mantle affect the thickness and homogeneity of the cement and the cement stresses at these defects. Peripheral defects are considered detrimental, but the affected voids in the mid-cement mantle remain controversial. Large voids up to 5 mm in diameter are often detrimental, whereas smaller voids are considered less significant. The location of these voids has been shown to be important because small voids in areas of high stress can result in early failure. Stem introduction with or without centralizers can create voids at the tip of the prosthesis. Heat generated during cement polymerization can expand trapped air, thereby enlarging voids. Coating the distal stem tip and centralizer with cement before insertion into the cement column can reduce the incidence of these distal voids.

Surface Finish

Surface finish for cemented stems is a topic that continues to generate controversy with regard to contemporary implants. Although rougher surfaces can improve mechanical interlock with cement, they can also cause abrasive damage to the cement mantle. In the presence of stem loosening, a rough surface can generate more particulate debris. Movement of a debonded rough-surface stem also provides a potential channel for debris particles to the distal portion of the stem.

One study reported on stem wear in 172 retrieval specimens, 74 of which had been stable in vivo. Wear at the surface was found in 93% of stems, with the surface finish determining the mechanism of wear. Matte surfaces showed abrasive wear patterns associated with cement damage and the release of debris from the cement and metal surfaces. Polished stems showed a typical fretting appearance with retention of wear debris on the stem surface without significant damage to the cement. The distribution of wear was the same in both matte and polished stems and was unaffected by the stem alloy. The wear affects the anterolateral and posterolateral aspects of the stem in regions where contact forces are highest, and it results from torsional force applied through the femoral head.

Another study suggested that any stem with a surface roughness of 0.4 μm or greater wears by an abrasive mechanism. The clinical significance of stem wear and surface finish as a factor in septic failure has yet to be completely defined. Others believe that in the instance of a debonded stem the long-term survival of the implant may depend on its ability to minimize cement wear during micromotion.

Table 3 | Cemented Femoral Component Revision Results

Author	No. of Hips	Mean Follow-up (Years)	Cement Technique (Generation)	Re-revision Rate (%)	Radiographic Loosening Rate (%)
Amstutz et al (1976)	66	2.1	First	9.0	29.0
Pellicci et al (1985)	110	3.4	First	5.4	13.6
Pellicci et al (1985)	99	8.1	First	19.0	29.0
Kavanagh and Fitzgerald (1987)	166	4.5	First	6.0	44.0
Kavanagh and Fitzgerald (1987)	210	10.0	First	30	–
Rubash and Harris (1988)	43	6.2	Second	4.0	11.0
Estok and Harris (1994)	38	11.7	Second	10.5	10.5
Katz et al (1997)	79	11.9	Second	5.4	16.6
Izquierdo et al (1994)	148	6.5	Second	3.3	8.8
Collis (1993)	110	4.6	Second	3.6	5.0
Raut et al (1996)	399	6.0	Second	6.1	8.5

It has been also shown that surface finish has a profound effect on clinical outcome. In patients with stems of similar or identical geometry that have different surface finishes, a poorer clinical outcome is exhibited in patients with the implants with the rougher surface finish. The Swedish Registry states that the controversy over surface finish and the presence or absence of collars in cemented total hip arthroplasties cannot be resolved using Swedish Registry data. In a recent report, investigators examined the importance of roughness with respect to fixation of cemented femoral stems. Three cohorts of patients (age range, 60 to 80 years) were examined. In the first cohort, 130 patients underwent total hip arthroplasty with a Charnley prosthesis (Johnson and Johnson, Raynham, MA) and first-generation techniques, including a distal plug. In the other two cohorts, 275 patients underwent total hip arthroplasty with the Omnifit system (Osteonics, Allendale, NJ) and 180 patients underwent total hip arthroplasty with the Ranawat-Burstein Interlok prosthesis (Biomet, Warsaw, IN) and modified third-generation techniques. Kaplan-Meier survivorship of the femoral component, using failure for all causes as the end point, was 90% ± 5.1% at 20 years for the Charnley prosthesis, 95.1% ± 3.4% at 15 years for the Omnifit system, and 99.5% ± 0.5% at 9 years for the Ranawat-Burstein Interlok prosthesis. Comparisons showed statistically significant differences when the patients with the Charnley prostheses were compared with those with the Omnifit system and Ranawat-Burstein Interlok prostheses, but there was no significant difference between the latter two groups.

Long-Term Results

Early total hip arthroplasty was performed with hand packing of cement, and most long-term (> 20 years)

follow-up results reflect the use of this technique (Table 3). One recent study examined 93 Charnley total hip arthroplasties; 69 of the patients were younger than 50 years at the time of surgery. The duration of follow-up for this cohort was a minimum of 25 years after surgery or until death. At the last follow-up evaluations, the combined prevalence of radiographic failure or revision for aseptic loosening was 13% for the patients with femoral components and 34% for those with acetabular components. Another series of 68 Charnley total hip arthroplasties in young patients who were followed for a minimum of 20 years or until death revealed similar results. With radiographic loosening or revision as an end point for these patients, 30.9% of those with acetabular components and 12.7% of those with femoral components experienced implant failure. In a study of the Exeter polished, tapered, collarless stem, a 92.13% survival rate at 33 years was reported for primary stems, using revision for aseptic loosening as an end point. When stem fracture, aseptic loosening, and patients lost to follow-up were combined as an end point, the survival rate of this stem was 82.72% at 33 years. In this study, the authors noted an interesting trend: less aseptic loosening occurred in stems that were implanted with cement mixed at 5 to 6 Hz (extremely porous cement) than in those implanted with cement mixed at 2 Hz. Although there is probably no statistically significant difference between the survival rates of these two subgroups, the findings suggest that cement porosity is not a drawback with this particular stem and may be an advantage.

In general, second-generation femoral cement techniques used since the late 1970s include distal occlusion with an intramedullary plug, pulsatile lavage of the medullary canal, the use of a canal brush, drying the canal, retrograde filling using a cement gun, and pressurization

Table 4 | Cemented Femoral Stem Results

Author (Year)	Prosthesis	No. of Hips	Length of Follow-up (Years)	Femoral Component Survivorship (%)
Nercessian et al (2005)	Charnley	98	18.9 mean	98.6[‡]
Howell et al (2004)	Exeter	433	33 minimum	92.1[*]
				82.7[†]
Callaghan et al (2000)	Charnley	330	30 minimum	82.0[‡]
Halley and Glassman (2003)	Charnley	68	22.0 mean	85.2[*]
Issack et al (2003)	Spectron	120	16.0 mean	93.9[§]
				90.3[‖]
Berry et al (2002)	Charnley	2,000	25.0 mean	89.8[*]
Keener et al (2003)	Charnley	93[‖]	25 minimum	87.0[‡]
Garcia-Cimbrelo et al (2000)	Charnley	67[¶]	21.7 mean	87.0[#]
Sochart and Porter (1997)	Charnley	226[¶]	19.7 mean	81.0

Aseptic loosening as end point
[†]*Stem fracture, aseptic loosening, and lost to follow-up as failures and end point*
[‡]*Revision or radiographic loosening as end point*
[§]*Revision for aseptic loosening as end point*
[‖]*All patients younger than 50 years*
[¶]*All patients younger than 40 years*
[#]*Revision for aseptic loosening or radiographic evidence of loosening as end point*

of the cement. Stems implanted with these techniques showed improved results over first-generation techniques at 10- to 15-year follow-up. The Swedish Registry reports a 94.8% 10-year survivorship with revision for aseptic loosening as an end point in primary total hip arthroplasty performed for osteoarthrosis. Revisions for other causes reduce the survivorship by 1% to 2%. One study reported on 325 hips with a 12-year survivorship of 91.7% with revision for any cause as an end point. With femoral revision for aseptic loosening as the end point, survivorship was 100%.

In an attempt to continue to improve femoral stem fixation, third-generation cementing techniques and femoral design changes were introduced. The cement techniques include proximal and distal stem centralization and methods to reduce cement porosity. Design changes in the femoral stems were directed toward improving the bond between the stem and cement. The design rationale for this was based on laboratory evidence that debonding of the cement from the stem was the initiating cause of failure for many cemented stems. The result of this finding was the increase in stem surface roughness, the addition of a thin layer of polymethylmethacrylate (precoating), or both. There have been few evidence-based clinical series that show the superiority of third-generation cementing techniques over second-generation techniques. Several studies have demonstrated similar midterm results in the 5- to 10-year follow-up period. Studies involving precoated stems have shown conflicting midterm results—some reporting stem failure rates of 2% to 3%, and others reporting increased loosening and osteolysis.

Long-term studies of cemented femoral components are limited to a few successful stem designs using early cementing techniques (Table 4). Studies with more than 20 years of follow-up demonstrate the durability of these implants and have helped to identify certain product-related factors that affect this durability. One of the most important factors is the age of the patient at the time of the index surgery. In general, the younger the patient, the lower the 25-year survivorship of the femoral implant. Men have higher rates of loosening than do women—nearly a twofold increase as reported in a recent study. Diagnosis affects femoral component loosening rates as well. In patients undergoing total hip replacement, one study found a 25-year survival rate of 89% when the diagnosis was hip dysplasia, 85% when the diagnosis was rheumatoid arthritis, and 74% when the diagnosis was osteoarthritis. Analysis of such studies can help surgeons who perform total joint arthroplasty make decisions regarding patient selection and alternative technologies.

Cement in Femoral Revision

The use of cement in femoral revision surgery has been limited because of discouraging revision rates and radiographic loosening. These poor results used first-generation techniques, with approximately 20% revision and 30% primary failure rates in patients with follow-up of less than 10 years. Results improved with the intro-

Table 5	Femoral Bone Loss Classification
Mallory (1988)	
Type I	Medullary contents and cortical bone intact
Type II	Medullary contents deficient and cortical bone intact
Type IIIA	Medullary contents deficient, cortical bone deficient to greater trochanter
Type IIIB	Medullary contents deficient, cortical bone deficient to level between lesser trochanter and isthmus
Type IIIC	Medullary contents deficient, most of proximal part of femur deficient
Paprosky et al (1999)	
Type I	Defects are minimal
Type II	Defects have mostly metaphyseal damage with minimal diaphyseal damage
Type III	Defects have metaphyseal and diaphyseal damage
Type IV	Extensive metaphyseal and diaphyseal damage, thin cortices, and widened canal

Table 6	Prosthesis Loosening Classification
Definite loosening	Stem migration (medial collar to calcar; if not collar, then tip of prosthesis to calcar), stem/cement mantle fracture
Probable loosening	Continuous radiolucent line surrounding entire cement mantle on any view
Possible loosening	Radiolucent zone involving 50% to 99% of cement-bone interface on any view and radiolucency not present immediately postoperatively
Stable	None of the above criteria met

duction of second-generation techniques. At 7- to 12-year follow-up, failure rates because of aseptic loosening ranged from 0 to 11% and radiographic loosening rates ranged from 6% to 21%.

Comparing results of revision hip arthroplasty is considerably more difficult than comparing those of primary procedures. Bone quality, bone defects, and adjunctive surgical technique (for example, grafting) make for difficult outcome comparisons. The use of descriptive classifications can help in making such comparisons. There are two widely used classifications. Femoral bone loss can be classified according to the system described by Mallory or Paprosky and associates, which is based on the extent and location of bone loss (Table 5). Most studies incorporate evaluation of radiographic loosening as part of the analysis and use the Harris classification to assess loosening (Table 6).

In a recent study, 129 revision total hip arthroplasties were reviewed. The 10-year survival rate was 91% with re-revision of the femoral component because of aseptic loosening as the end point and 71% with mechanical failure as the end point. Patients older than 60 years had greater long-term component survival and better clinical results than younger patients. A good quality cement mantle correlated with better long-term radiographic signs of fixation. Poor femoral bone quality was associated with an increased rate of re-revision for aseptic loosening. The total hip arthroplasties in this study were performed with first-generation, second-generation, and third-generation techniques, which allowed for some comparison. The 10-year survival rate for hips implanted with third-generation cementing techniques was significantly better than that for hips implanted with second-generation techniques when re-revision for aseptic loos-

ening was used as an end point (94% [95% confidence interval, 89% to 99%] compared with 85% [95% confidence interval, 79% to 91%]; $P = 0.049$). Compared with second-generation techniques, first-generation techniques were associated with a significantly higher rate of re-revision for aseptic loosening and re-revision for any reason ($P < 0.01$).

In another study, investigators revising failed cementless femoral components with cemented revision stems found that although this technique provided pain relief and improved function, the rate of loosening at intermediate follow-up (a minimum of 5 years) was higher than commonly reported after revision with the use of cementless extensively porous-coated implants. The 6-year survival rate for the femoral component was 72% with revision for aseptic loosening as the end point and 67% with mechanical failure as the end point.

The consensus of these more recent studies is that cemented femoral revisions are probably best suited for elderly patients with short life expectancy and with only minor bone loss. The positive correlation between quality of cementation and advanced age at the time of revision and long-term survival of revision has been demonstrated, and deterioration of bone stock influences survival of the cemented revision femoral component.

Other types of cemented revisions include the tap-in/tap-out technique used in a situation in which a well-fixed stem and an intact cement mantle exist and stem removal is required to gain acetabular exposure or adjust neck length. In this instance, the stem is removed, leaving an intact cement mantle; then it is recemented into the mantle. Limited follow-up results are encouraging.

Femoral Impaction Grafting
Femoral impaction grafting with cement has proved to be another successful technique in revision total hip arthroplasty. Intermediate and long-term results have been encouraging. The use of this technique in patients who have significant bone loss (Paprosky type III and IV femora) or in patients in whom distal fixation is not practical provides the revision surgeon with an addi-

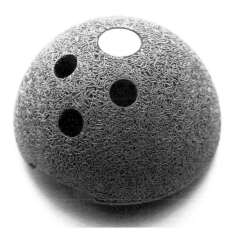

Figure 1 Photograph of a cementless pure titanium acetabulum component with fiber metal coating and dome screws for adjunctive fixation (Trilogy Acetabular Shell, Zimmer).

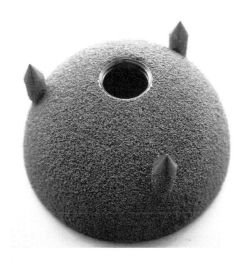

Figure 2 Photograph of a beaded cobalt-chromium cementless acetabular component with three spikes for fixation (Duraloc 300 Acetabular Shell, DePuy).

tional treatment option in this patient population. One study described the technique and advocates use of the taper-slip principle as it applies to femoral impaction grafting with cement. Using a polished double-taper stem for revision of the femoral component in 487 patients (540 hips), survivorship at 15-year follow-up was 90.6%. Others studies have reported success with implants that use the composite-beam principle. Reports of significant subsidence and complications exist and appear to be technique-related. Proper technique is demanding, but the results of the procedure and avoidance of complications are technique-dependent.

Cementless Acetabular Components

Cementless acetabular components were introduced in the early 1980s in an attempt to improve the results of using cemented implants in total hip arthroplasty. Although cemented acetabular components provided reliable early results, long-term studies noted increased rates of radiographic and clinical loosening. In addition, the surgical technique for the implantation of a cemented all-polyethylene cup was demanding, with difficulties noted in routinely obtaining a bloodless field and providing for optimal cement pressurization, even among experienced surgeons. Consequently, a variety of novel designs were implemented, including threaded components and hemispherical designs. A variety of strategies for gaining initial implant stability were used, including dome screws, peripheral screws, peripheral threads, dome spikes, peripheral fins, and insertion with a press-fit technique in which the component is oversized compared with the diameter of the prepared acetabulum. These cementless components were used in North America and rapidly became the most popular type of acetabular implant because the surgical technique was easier (when compared with that of acetabular fixation

with cement) and the theoretic advantages of biologic fixation and modularity were viewed as attractive.

Unfortunately, new problems arose with increased polyethylene wear and osteolysis being the most commonly reported complications of cementless acetabular reconstruction. Furthermore, modularity of the polyethylene liner introduced problems with backside wear of the liner, and early locking mechanisms were prone to catastrophic failure. Over the past two decades, significant knowledge has been gained, and the attributes of the more successful designs have been incorporated into most current cementless acetabular components (Figures 1 through 4). In addition, more wear-resistant bearing surfaces have been developed and refined, including highly cross-linked ultra-high molecular weight polyethylene, ceramic-on-ceramic components, and metal-on-metal components. These bearing surfaces may have a major impact on the long-term results of cementless acetabular reconstruction.

Factors Critical to Initial and Long-Term Success

The most critical factors for obtaining bone ingrowth or ongrowth of a cementless acetabular component include initial implant stability, the presence of an appropriate apposition surface that is receptive to bone ingrowth or ongrowth, and intimate contact of that surface with the host bone. Stability of the implant relative to host bone allows for bony ingrowth into porous surfaces. Micromotion of less than 28 to 50 µm is consistent with reliable bony ingrowth, whereas larger amounts of motion tend to lead to ingrowth of fibrous tissue and occasionally early catastrophic failure. Similarly, the implant must be in intimate contact with the concave acetabular bony bed with which it is intended to osseointegrate, with gaps as small as 0.5 to 2 mm impairing osseointegration. In addition to an implant that is stable and

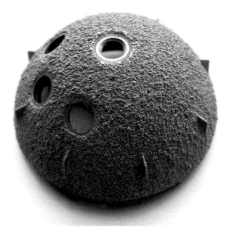

Figure 3 Photograph of a titanium alloy acetabular component with closed pore, plasma spray porous coating and peripheral fins and dome screws for adjunctive fixation (Mallory-Head Radial Acetabular Shell, Biomet).

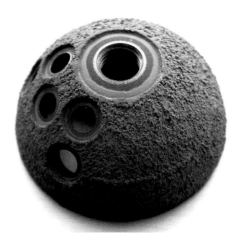

Figure 4 Photograph of an arc-deposited titanium shell with HA coating, an enlarged peripheral rim, and dome screws for adjunctive fixation (Secur-Fit HA PSL Shell, Stryker, Mahwah, NJ).

closely apposed to the host bony bed, the metallic surface itself must be receptive to bony ingrowth or ongrowth, with a pore size of 100 to 400 μm having been shown to lead to optimal osseointegration. Appropriate component positioning (both abduction and anteversion) is critical to not only avoid postoperative instability, but also to maximize contact between the component and the bony acetabular bed.

Clinical Results

Several studies have reported on the results of cementless acetabular reconstruction with a mean follow-up of more than 10 years. A review of these studies reveals several trends. First, cementless implants that have achieved osseointegration, when compared with components inserted with cement, show an improved rate of successful fixation, particularly in younger patients. All cementless components, however, do not behave the same, and components coated with titanium fiber metal mesh have shown to have the lowest rates of revision for loosening over the longest periods when compared with reported results on other components.

These studies also show that with longer follow-up, the prevalence of osteolysis rises substantially, with rates reported to range from 2% to 56% in patient cohorts followed for more than 10 years. Osteolysis occurs when particulate debris (predominantly polyethylene debris) is phagocytized by mononuclear cells and leads to the release of cytokines that stimulate bone resorption. In most studies, the prevalence of osteolysis is associated with both patient- and implant-related factors. Younger patient age and higher activity levels are consistently associated with higher rates of osteolysis secondary to higher rates of wear of the bearing surface. Design-related factors include inadequate polyethylene thickness (components with a liner thinner than 7 mm have

been associated with poorer performance), femoral head size (particularly as it relates to polyethylene thickness), and components with a poor polyethylene liner locking mechanism that allows for motion between the liner and the shell, causing backside wear of the liner. The quality of the polyethylene itself, the method of sterilization used, and the shelf-life of the liner are additional and potentially the most important factors that determine wear rates and osteolysis. Titanium femoral heads have also been associated with higher rates of osteolysis and have generally been abandoned because of their poor wear characteristics. Component positioning, particularly cup abduction, has also been shown to be a critical factor because more vertical components are subject to higher stresses in the polyethylene and accelerated wear. In one long-term study of the cementless Harris-Galante I (Zimmer, Warsaw, IN) acetabular component, excessive acetabular abduction (a more vertical component position) was found to be a significant, independent risk factor for reoperation and failure.

Autopsy Retrieval Studies

Autopsy retrieval studies are critical to obtain a more thorough understanding of the behavior and failure mechanisms of cementless acetabular components. Studies of various component designs have shown that bony ingrowth into clinically successful cementless acetabular components ranges from no bony ingrowth to more than 80%, with an average ingrowth of approximately 15% to 30%. Areas of maximal bony ingrowth tend to be present in the vicinity of fixation screws, spikes, or pegs. In general, these studies have also shown that screws are more effective than spikes in augmenting bony ingrowth, which may be related to both increased stability and greater apposition to host bone because screws tend to draw the metallic surface closer to the bony bed.

Implant Material

Although some early attempts were made to implant cementless acetabular components manufactured from nonmetallic materials, such as all-polyethylene and all-ceramic threaded cups, these experiments were met with unacceptable rates of failure and have been abandoned. The primary implant materials used today include titanium and cobalt-chromium alloys. Autopsy retrieval studies and animal models have both shown that although these materials are biocompatible and support bone ingrowth, titanium implants have been associated with higher amounts of bone ingrowth; however, qualitatively the bone formed around implants made of both implants appears to be the same. Additional benefits of titanium include a lower modulus of elasticity that theoretically may lead to less stress remodeling of the host pelvic bone, a more flexible implant that may lead to greater ease of insertion if a press-fit technique is used, and the potential for a lower risk of insertional fracture. Furthermore, titanium is generally easier to work with than cobalt-chromium from a manufacturing perspective, and it is also less expensive.

A newer implant material that has been implemented in cementless acetabular components is tantalum (trabecular metal). Tantalum is an elemental material that has a highly porous structure (80% porosity), an elastic modulus that is closer to bone than cobalt-chromium or titanium, a high coefficient of friction that aids its ability to gain initial implant stability, and biocompatibility, allowing for high amounts of bony ingrowth as well as soft-tissue attachment. Initial clinical experience with a monoblock acetabular shell made from tantalum has been reported to be favorable; however, increased experience and longer follow-up will be necessary to determine whether a clinical advantage exists to using tantalum on a routine basis in primary total hip replacement.

Implant Geometry

As previously mentioned, cementless acetabular components have been produced in various geometries, including hemispherical, dual geometry (where the radius of the component is larger at the periphery than at the dome), oblong, and threaded. Most threaded acetabular implants do not have a biologic surface for bone ingrowth or ongrowth and rely on a mechanical interlock with the host acetabular bed. Different designs, including all-polyethylene, ceramic, cobalt-chromium, and titanium implants, have been tried, with few designs having shown acceptable survivorship; consequently, most have been abandoned. These components have been shown to have poorer mechanical stability than hemispherical components and a smaller amount of surface area in contact with the native acetabulum. Despite these factors, implants with a biologic surface for bony ingrowth

or ongrowth, such as those using grit-blasted titanium (Zweymuller threaded cup), those using titanium beads with optional screw fixation (S-ROM Super Cup, Joint Medical Products Co, Stamford, CT), and those using hydroxyapatite (HA)-coated titanium (Omnifit Threaded HA cup, Osteonics, Allendale, NJ) have been associated with acceptable clinical results. An additional problem with these components is the relative difficulty of preparation of the acetabular bed and insertion when compared to hemispherical designs. In particular, many components included an awkward insertional handle that predisposes to vertical acetabular cup positioning, particularly in obese patients.

Dual geometry components that have an enlarged radius at the rim of the component were developed in an attempt to maximize the contact of the biologic surface at the rim of the acetabulum with the use of a press-fit technique. These designs were developed in response to concerns over the use of screws for fixation and attempt to maximize initial component stability without the use of adjunctive forms of fixation. Although the intermediate-term results with components that have used this design have been acceptable, there is a concern that this design may decrease total contact between the component and surrounding host bone (particularly in the dome of the implant) and lead to decreased amounts of total bone ingrowth.

Most cementless acetabular implants currently in use have a hemispherical design, and the clinical results thus far are promising. Advantages of this design include ease of acetabular preparation and component insertion.

Surface Coating

The surface of a cementless acetabular component has been shown to be critical to both short- and long-term success. Although initial cementless designs included components without a metallic surface for ingrowth or ongrowth of bone, most modern designs include an ingrowth or ongrowth surface. Pore size has been shown to be a critical factor.

The most commonly used three-dimensional surface coatings are composed of sintered titanium fiber metal mesh and cobalt-chromium beads. These surfaces have been studied at intermediate-term follow-up with acceptable clinical results. Titanium fiber metal mesh was used in one of the earliest implant designs and continues to show excellent long-term success for implant fixation. When compared in animal studies, the histologic appearance of bone ingrowth around cobalt-chromium beaded and titanium fiber metal mesh components are similar; however, bone ingrowth seems to occur more reliably into components with a fiber metal mesh coating.

Several acetabular component designs have incorporated the use of an HA coating to improve bony ingrowth or ongrowth. HA is an osteoconductive material that has been shown in animal models to optimize bony attachment to fixation surfaces. The theory behind these components was that the surrounding bony surface would bond to the HA coating, which in turn was bonded to the acetabular cup. The most popular initial designs that incorporated an HA coating were smooth, hemispherical components that relied on a press fit for obtaining initial implant stability without screws for fixation. Unfortunately, these components have been associated with poor intermediate-term results because the HA resorbed with time, and without a biologic surface available for osseointegration or screws for adjunctive fixation, aseptic loosening ensued. In one comparative study of HA-coated smooth press-fit acetabular components and HA-coated threaded screw-in components, the highest rate of failure (11%) was reported with the HA-coated smooth press-fit cup at a minimum 5-year follow-up. In response to the problems of early failure, HA has since been applied in a thinner layer to grit-blasted implants, with acceptable results being reported at short- and intermediate-term follow-up.

HA has also been used in combination with tricalcium phosphate (TCP) in an attempt to enhance bone ingrowth into metallic surfaces when used as a surface coating that resorbs rapidly. One clinical trial compared a titanium fiber metal mesh component with and without a HA-TCP coating in 23 pairs of patients. Although the clinical results were similar, the components with HA-TCP coating were associated with less migration and fewer radiolucencies when studied with radiostereometry analysis. No clear clinical benefits were identified. Animal studies have suggested that a HA-TCP coating applied to a titanium fiber mesh enhances early bone ingrowth, but there may not be a longer-term benefit in terms of overall implant stability.

Adjunctive Fixation

Initial implant stability is critical for osseointegration to occur. Although various modes of achieving this have been used, a press fit is commonly used to obtain initial implant stability when cementless acetabular components are inserted. The surgical technique typically includes a variable amount of underreaming of the acetabulum compared with the diameter of the component to be inserted. Although good clinical results have been reported, the major concerns with using this technique include insertional fractures of the acetabulum or pelvis and incomplete seating of the component. In a cadaver study, fractures occurred in 14 of 15 specimens when the component was oversized by 4 mm; however, fractures occurred even with underreaming by 2 mm (4 of 15 specimens). Other studies have shown that a similar amount of underreaming in a smaller acetabulum can lead to a higher rate of fracture; thus, in small acetabulums it may be more appropriate to underream by only

1 mm, whereas large acetabulums may require up to 3 mm of underreaming to obtain the same interference fit. Clinical reports have shown that these insertional fractures can be difficult to identify, and that when they occur and are unrecognized intraoperatively, the associated rate of failure is high. These fractures have been seen most commonly in older, female patients and in patients with inflammatory arthritis. Various methods have been used to determine component stability and assess the amount of contact between the host bed and the component intraoperatively (prior to placing the final component), including the use of trial components and reamers in which the back of the reamer can be removed to visualize the amount of contact present.

Threaded screws were used in many of the earliest implant designs to either provide or augment initial stability, and biomechanical studies support this as being the strongest mode of fixation. Screw holes can be placed in the dome of the component or at the periphery; however, because peripheral screws often require a wider exposure to insert, most modern primary total hip arthroplasty devices use dome screws. Concerns with the use of screws include the potential for neurovascular injury during drilling or screw insertion, concerns that screws and screw holes may act as access channels for polyethylene wear debris, and the potential for fretting corrosion and material loss between the screw head and the metal shell. A better understanding of pelvic anatomy as it relates to screw placement has been gained, and the risk of neurovascular injury can be dramatically decreased by placing screws in the posterosuperior quadrant of the acetabulum and by careful measurement of screw length.

Spikes placed in the dome of the component or fins placed at the periphery have been used as alternatives to screws; however, both of these methods of gaining adjunctive fixation can lead to incomplete seating of the component, whereas screws tend to pull the ingrowth surface closer to the host bone when fully tightened. No clear clinical benefit has been shown by avoiding the use of screws because periacetabular osteolysis has been reported to occur in association with components that use these alternative methods of fixation. It is also important to recognize, however, that the longest-term follow-up studies, which have shown excellent results, used line-to-line reaming with the insertion of multiple screws and current techniques may not provide the same results.

Modularity

Advantages of a modular polyethylene liner include the potential for exchange of the bearing surface in the event of wear without the need to disrupt a stable component and the ability to fine tune the construct intraoperatively to optimize factors such as stability, offset, and limb length. Nonetheless, modularity introduced new problems to these components, including backside wear of the polyethylene liner that can lead to osteolysis and, in some designs, frank failure of the locking mechanism that can lead to dislodgement of the liner from the shell. As these phenomena were recognized, several modifications were made, including better locking mechanisms that more securely captured the liner, increased congruity between the liner and the shell itself, and a smooth inner surface of the component to further prevent abrasive wear on the backside of the liner.

Most modern components provide the ability to use elevated rim, oblique, and offset options to optimize stability and when necessary restore femoral offset. As more revisions for polyethylene wear-related problems are encountered, it is important for surgeons performing revision surgery to be familiar with the technique of cementing a new polyethylene liner into a well-fixed, appropriately positioned shell when faced with a component that has a poor locking mechanism or if replacement liners are not available. The basic tenets of this technique include downsizing the liner to allow for an adequate cement mantle and texturing the back of the liner (and in some instances the inner surface of the metal shell) with a burr to provide for a roughened surface that enhances stability of the construct.

Cementless Femoral Components

Cementless femoral components were first introduced in North America in the 1970s in an attempt to improve the long-term survivorship of cemented femoral stems. Cementless technology was initially met with skepticism, but over the past 25 years has grown in popularity because of the accumulation of successful long-term outcome study data. A wide variety of implant designs have been introduced over the past decade, and new implants continue to be developed. Although there have been sporadic reports of poor performance of cementless femoral components, most 10- to 15-year follow-up studies show very low rates of aseptic loosening. Nonetheless, problems with polyethylene wear and osteolysis have emerged as the most common long-term complications, regardless of the design of the component. This has led to an array of modifications intended to decrease the amount of wear and particulate debris at the bearing surface, whereas the component design has remained largely unchanged. Minor design modifications are being made, but newer issues have come to the forefront of cementless fixation technology, such as minimizing complications and cost and minimally invasive surgery.

Design Rationale

The introduction of the concept of bone ingrowth into metallic implants in the early 1900s led to an array of basic science studies confirming the ability of bone to form a bond with porous surfaces. The process of bone ingrowth has been shown to resemble primary fracture healing, with initial hematoma replaced by woven bone, leading to lamellar bone remodeling into the porous surface. The effect of pore size on ingrowth has been widely studied using a canine model. Furthermore, implant stability with micromotion less than 50 to 150 µm was found to be an important factor in obtaining bone ingrowth, and current implants are designed to obtain a tight fit at the time of surgery. The addition of a biologic coating to the surface of the stem such as HA has been used to improve the initial implant stability and bone ingrowth. Currently available implants and surgical techniques use these principles to optimize outcomes.

Avoiding Complications

The complications commonly associated with total hip arthroplasty include infection, dislocation, limb-length inequality, aseptic loosening, and fracture. Since the advent of prophylactic intravenous antibiotics, infection rates in immunocompetent patients have remained acceptably low. To lessen the problems of dislocation and limb-length inequality, most implant manufacturers have made design changes to femoral components to decrease these complications, including increasing the head to neck ratio, offering more neck-shaft angle and offset options, and having components available with variable degrees of anteversion to decrease impingement and improve stability.

Cost

The issue of cost has remained an overwhelming focus for hospitals and surgeons alike over the past decade. As overall costs of total hip arthroplasty have risen modestly, the costs of implants have skyrocketed. The increasing manufacturing cost of cementless implants has contributed to this, and some have questioned the cost-effectiveness of cementless implants when cheaper cemented components have provided reasonable results. Recent reports have suggested that when all associated costs are considered, such as the cost of cement and related equipment as well as the increased operating room time required to cement components, the difference in cost for cemented and cementless components is negligible. Furthermore, the cost of performing revision surgery in patients with implant loosening is overwhelming; therefore, maximizing long-term survivorship is the most important variable in determining the lifelong cost of the implant.

Results

Over the past 10 years, multiple studies have reported mid- to long-term results using cementless femoral components (Table 7). A variety of so-called first-generation designs have been used for many years, some with design flaws that have been abandoned in favor of newer designs, and others with successful long-term results with their original designs. A variety of reports using second- and third-generation designs show good long-term results. Many material and design factors should be considered when evaluating the performance of any particular stem because these factors may influence initial and long-term stability, durability, and ease of use. These factors include stem material, stem shape, type and extent of surface coating, and the use of modularity.

Stem Material

Historically, cementless femoral stems have been fashioned from primarily two alloys: cobalt-chromium and titanium. There are advantages and disadvantages to using each of these materials, and comparable long-term results have been reported using both materials in cementless stems.

Compared with cobalt-chromium, implants made of titanium have a lower modulus of elasticity that more closely approximates that of native cortical bone. The advantages that this theoretically provides include more predictable patterns of bone remodeling, less stress shielding, and better long-term stability. Studies using dual energy x-ray absorptiometry have shown a significant decrease in bone density around cementless femoral stems, with the most pronounced proximal bone loss occurring in stems designed to obtain distal fixation and fashioned from cobalt-chromium. Furthermore, in patients with preexisting osteoporosis or in those in whom large diameter stems (> 18 mm) are used, the amount of subsequent stress shielding appears to be more pronounced. Stems designed to obtain proximal fixation and made from titanium have demonstrated less overall stress shielding with relative maintenance of proximal bone density on dual energy x-ray absorptiometry scans.

Table 7 | Cementless Femoral Stem Results

Stem	Design Features	Study Location (Date)	No. of Hips	Years Follow-Up (Average)
AML	Straight, cobalt-chromium fully porous coated	Alexandria, VA (2001)	211	2 to 18 (13.9)
Anatomic	Anatomic, titanium, proximal fiber metal porous coating circumferential	Chicago, IL (2001)	78	8 to 11 (10)
Mallory-Head	Collarless, dual-tapered, wedge-shaped titanium; proximal third plasma sprayed.	Columbus, OH (2001)	120	Minimum 10 (12.2)
		Chonju, Korea (2003)	76	9 to 13 (10.3)
Omnifit HA	Straight, titanium, proximal HA-coated	Multicenter, (2003)	111	9.6 to 13.8 (11.25)
PCA	Anatomic, cobalt-chromium proximal bead porous coated	Korea (1999)	116	10 to 12 (11.2)
		London, Ontario, (2001)	187	10 to 14
Profile	Anatomic proximal fit, titanium, sintered beads proximal one third	Seoul, Korea (2003)	118	8 to 11 (9.8)
S-ROM	Straight, modular titanium, proximal porous, distal fluted	Montreal (2001)	59	6 to 12.1 (8.4)
Taperloc	Straight, titanium, tapered proximal plasma spray	Neenah, WI (2000)	100	8 to 13 (10.2)
Trilock	Straight, cobalt-chromium wedge-fit, tapered, 60% proximal sintered bead coating	Philadelphia, PA (1999)	71	10 to 14 (11.5)
Zweymuller Alloclassic	Tapered, rectangular, titanium stem (Ti-6Al-7Nb), sand blasted surface roughness 4 to 6 μm; relies on distal, metadiaphyseal fixation	Vienna, Austria (2002)	133	Minimum 10
		Madrid, Spain (2003)	104	Minimum 10 (11.3)

Regardless of the material used or the amount of stress shielding present, the long-term clinical results have not been affected by these changes. Extensively coated stems made from cobalt-chromium (Anatomic medullary locking [AML], DePuy, Warsaw, IN) have been reported to have a 15-year survivorship that equals or exceeds that of tapered, titanium stems. Rates of aseptic loosening have remained consistently low, regardless of adjacent bone remodeling once bone ingrowth is achieved. Furthermore, as long-term follow-up studies become available, no evidence of late failure or other complications related to bone remodeling or stress shielding has been reported in patients with well-fixed cementless femoral stems. Therefore, although different implant materials may provide theoretic advantages, these benefits have yet to be realized in long-term outcome studies.

Implant Shape

The shape of the femoral implant can be either tapered, cylindrical, or anatomic, depending on the method of fixation intended for that particular component. Varying degrees of mediolateral and anteroposterior taper are built into these stems based on the particular design.

Tapered Stems

Tapered stems are designed with a significant proximal to distal taper and are intended to interlock into the metaphyseal region with little or no diaphyseal fixation. Proximal porous coating or plasma spray macrotexturing is used to confer initial stability and allow for bony ingrowth into the proximal region of the stem. These stems are usually manufactured with a collarless design to allow wedging of the prosthesis into the metaphyseal region to obtain optimal fit and bone ingrowth. Because

Table 7 | Cementless Femoral Stem Results (cont)

Revision: Stems Loose	Radiography Results	Comment
2.0% revision for loosening	3.4% overall loosening	27% femoral osteolysis, all proximal
0	0 loosening 5% proximal osteolysis, none distal	9% mild to severe thigh pain associated with large stem
2.5% revision for aseptic loosening	Radiographic loosening not reported 32.4% osteolysis	3.4% thigh pain
1.3% revision for subsidence	93.4% bone ingrown 3.9% stable fibrous	4.4% thigh pain
0.9% revision rate for aseptic loosening, 4.5% overall revision rate	0 of unrevised stems loose 47% proximal osteolysis 0 distal lysis	Osteolysis in Gruen zones 1, 7, 8, and 14 41 hips lost to follow-up since original report
11% revision rate for loosening	11% loosening 59% osteolysis in stem	28% thigh pain Author abandoned use of implant
5.3% stems revised	10% loosening 3% fibrous stable 42% osteolysis 4% distal	36% overal thigh pain Author abandoned use of implant
0 loosening, 1 hip revised for recurrent dislocation	0 loosening 2.5% stable fibrous ingrown	Patients younger than 50 years 4% proximal fractures intraoperatively 3% spiral fractures 10% transitory thigh pain
1.6% (modular fluted stem disengaged from ingrown sleeve)	0 loosening 42% focal proximal osteolysis	11.9% dislocation rate
0 revision for loosening	0 loosening 2% stable fibrous	Young patient population (average age, 37 years) 56% acetabular component revision rate
0 loosening, 9.8% revised at time of socket revision for nonmodularity	5 unstable 3.2% proximal osteolysis, none distal	1.4% thigh pain, none in loose stems High socket revision rate (37.1%)
0 loosening, 1% revised for other causes (infection, malpositioning, multiple acetabular revisions)	0 loosening	3% thigh pain 107 of 208 hips available for 10-yr radiographic follow-up
0 revision for loosening	0 loosening	15 hips lost to follow-up 7 proximal femur fractures 12 hips with mean 8.9-mm nonprogressive subsidence

of the viscoelastic nature of bone and the tapered geometry of the stem, it can subside into a position of tightest fit and subsequently enhance proximal load sharing of the device. Proponents of this design argue that bone ingrowth and stress shielding will be optimized because of these design characteristics. Successful results have been obtained with this design using both titanium (Mallory-Head and Taperloc, Biomet, Warsaw, IN) and cobalt-chromium (Tri-lock, DePuy) stems. Long-term results (> 10 years) have shown a very low (1%) rate of revision, thigh pain, and radiographic loosening (Table 7). Longer-term (15 to 20 years) results are becoming available, which include only sporadic reports of aseptic loosening caused by proximal osteolysis.

Cylindrical Stems
Stems fashioned with a cylindrical design usually have circumferential porous coating over most of the surface area of the stem. Both proximal and distal coating is applied to these stems in an effort to maximize the region of potential bone ingrowth and increase the long-term stability. The primary mechanism for initial stability is dependent on a tight diaphyseal fit. Authors favoring this design argue that machining the tubular diaphysis can be reproducibly performed in all patients, thus maximizing bone-coating contact and providing the best chance of bony ingrowth. Although tapered stems rely on a wedge fit over a relatively small surface area of bone in a variably shaped metaphysis, a tubular diaphysis can easily be machined to accommodate a cylindrical stem. This technique also allows for relative intraoperative flexibility to restore normal hip anatomy, including the ability to raise or lower and rotate the stem without compromising fixation to bone. This stem design has been in use since the late 1970s, and 15-year survivorship with the AML stem has shown excellent results (Table 7).

Anatomic Stems
Stems designed to fit the anatomy of the proximal femur have also been in use since the early 1980s, and multiple studies have reported results. With significant rates of thigh pain and osteolysis, some authors have abandoned the use of anatomic stems (for example, Porous-Coated Anatomic [PCA] first-generation implants, Stryker Howmedica Osteonics, Allendale, NJ) in favor of one of the designs described previously. Crucial to their success is the adequate fill of the metaphyseal region in both the coronal and sagittal planes; high rates of thigh pain have been reported when this is not achieved. Whereas later-generation designs have shown improved results (APR-II, Centerpulse Orthopaedics, Austin, TX; PCA E-Series, Stryker Howmedica Osteonics; Profile, DePuy; Anatomic, Zimmer), the expected benefits of matching the implant shape to the anatomy of the femur have not surpassed other available designs.

Surface Coating
There is a wide variety of different surface coatings available for femoral implants, and different methods are available to distribute this coating over the implant. The main distinction to be made when evaluating stem coating is whether the stem has coating just over the proximal portion of the stem or coating over the length of the implant. Furthermore, it should be determined whether the coating is restricted to patches, whether there is circumferential coverage, and what type of coating the stem has (fiber mesh, sintered beads, plasma spray, or HA coating).

Extent of Surface Coating
The placement of surface coating over the proximal area only or extensive surface of the stem is determined by the region of the native femur that is intended to withstand most of the load in normal gait. Coating confined to the proximal region of the stem is usually paired with stems that are tapered or anatomically shaped to the host femur. Load transfer in these stems is focused on the metaphyseal region, and the distal portion of the stem is left smooth, with little expectation that bone ingrowth will occur.

In theory, because the stress transfer occurs in the more physiologic metaphyseal region, the amount of stress shielding and thigh pain will be significantly less than with stems intended to obtain diaphyseal fixation. Because these stems are entering their third decade of use, longer-term outcome study data are just becoming available. Revision rates, loosening rates, thigh pain, and stress shielding all appear to be consistently low as follow-up periods lengthen. Although reports of stems loosening as a result of proximal osteolysis have been published for implants such as the Omnifit HA, Mallory-Head, and PCA, further follow-up is necessary to establish significant trends.

Stems with extensive porous coating are more commonly cylindrical in shape, and they are intended to obtain a diaphyseal scratch fit for stability. The AML is the most widely used and reported of this design. As the load is transferred more distally, proximal stress shielding has occurred. However, with 15-year follow-up data available, there are no reports of clinical consequences from this stress shielding, and no reports of stem loosening as a result of osteolysis. Critics of this stem design argue that higher rates of thigh pain are reported in distal fit cobalt-chromium stems, but because of the number of reports of proximal and distally coated stems available and the wide range of thigh pain incidence reported, no clear correlation can be made at this time.

Circumferential Versus Noncircumferential Coating
Cementless stems without circumferential coating have essentially been abandoned. Because of the higher rate

of failure of proximal patch-coated stems, circumferential coating has become a critical and uniform design feature in currently available cementless stems. When coating was only applied in patches in the proximal stem, polyethylene debris could traverse along the smooth portion of the stem and cause osteolysis and loosening of the adjacent porous patches. As longer-term follow-up data have become available, the extremely low rate of distal osteolysis in circumferentially coated stems has confirmed that this feature limits the distal access of polyethylene debris and lowers rates of loosening.

Type of Coating

There are several surface coatings available for cementless stems, and many now have 10- to 15-year outcome data showing excellent rates of bone ingrowth and low rates of loosening. The type of coating applied is partly dependent on the metal used, with sintered beads more commonly used in cobalt-chromium stems such as the Trilock (DePuy), PCA, or AML, and mesh, plasma spray, and grit blasting as a substrate for ingrowth more commonly used in titanium stems.

The addition of HA to the surface coating suggests improved bone ingrowth, and excellent results with the Omnifit HA stem (Stryker Howmedica Osteonics) support this contention. Several recent basic science and clinical studies have focused on the use of HA coating in total hip arthroplasty. Animal studies have compared HA-coated stems to both grit-blasted and porous-coated stems and have shown that HA coating improves the extent of bone contact, ingrowth, and pull-out strength of these stems at different times after implantation. In a bilateral study in a sheep model, plasma spray implants coated with HA were found to have superior shear strength when compared with grit-blasted implants. HA coating also appears to enhance osseointegration in the early period after implantation, theoretically lessening the chances of early loosening.

Clinical studies have shown more variable results when comparing HA-coated to noncoated stems. Although excellent clinical results have been obtained using HA-coated stems such as the Omnifit HA, equally successful results have been obtained with noncoated cementless stems. In a study of patients undergoing bilateral hip replacement using the S-ROM modular hip system with a porous-coated sleeve in one hip and an HA-coated sleeve in the other hip, no difference was found with regard to clinical outcomes, thigh pain, or radiographic evidence of bone remodeling. Conversely, two different prospective, randomized clinical studies have shown significant benefits with HA coating. In one study comparing grit-blasted versus HA-coated anatomic stems with the same design, a much higher rate of clinical failure was noted with the grit-blasted stems at 8- to 10-year follow-up. An additional prospective, randomized study compared HA-coated and grit-blasted

stems of the same geometry at 8-year follow-up and found significantly less subsidence in the stems coated with HA. Despite these findings, long-term clinical outcomes of noncoated cementless stems continue to have excellent survivorship, indicating that a multitude of design features are important for obtaining long-term success.

Modularity

Modular femoral heads are available for most implant designs, and they are routinely used in cementless total hip arthroplasty. The intraoperative flexibility that this allows has strengthened the surgical armamentarium in improving intraoperative stability and restoring limb length. With the advent of alternative bearing surfaces such as highly cross-linked polyethylene, metal-on-metal, and ceramic-on-ceramic designs, there is less concern for volumetric polyethylene wear. Consequently, large femoral heads are being used with increasing frequency to improve stability and decrease the overall dislocation rate. Recent evidence has confirmed what has been theorized for many years, that a larger ball size decreases the overall dislocation rate. Furthermore, modularity can be useful in situations in which modular component exchange is necessary, such as patients with recurrent dislocation or polyethylene wear.

Some femoral stem designs incorporate modularity into the design of the stem, such as the S-ROM implant, which uses a metaphyseal sleeve and separate stem-neck segment. This provides certain theoretic advantages, such as more precisely matching the component size to the patient's anatomy and altering the rotational version of the neck independent of the metaphysis to maximize stability. Although 10-year follow-up of patients with this stem has been shown to have low rates of aseptic loosening, no statistically significant difference in aseptic loosening rates over nonmodular stems has been demonstrated. Likewise, dislocation rates have not been significantly lower, with one report on the S-ROM showing dislocations in 7 of 59 patients (11.9%). Although there are certain clinical scenarios in which this stem design offers advantages, such as in patients with hip dysplasia, routine use of modular femoral stems offers no clear advantage over monoblock designs.

The greatest concern for modularity is corrosion at the junction between the modular parts, particularly between dissimilar metals such as a cobalt-chromium head and a titanium trunion. The generation of particulate debris can lead to local tissue hypersensitivity and cause third-body wear at the bearing interface. Recent studies have highlighted the role of mechanical loading in the corrosion process at the head-neck junction, showing that once crevice corrosion is initiated, it can continue even without mechanical loading. Implantation time and flexural rigidity of the neck are predictors of head and neck corrosion and head fretting, with large diameter femoral necks showing less overall corrosion. The benefit of decreased corrosion with large diameter femoral necks needs to be weighed against the loss of motion and instability that occurs with these designs.

There is also concern for particulate debris from the more distal modular interface in modular femoral stems such as the S-ROM, although definitive evidence for consequences from debris generated by these interfaces is lacking. Laboratory studies have shown that metallic debris can be released under cyclic loading conditions from these junctions. Reports of revisions of these stems has not shown evidence of visible fretting or tissue metallosis, but one long-term follow-up report showed evidence of proximal osteolysis in 42% of patients, some of whom had little evidence of polyethylene wear. Whether this higher rate of osteolysis can be attributed directly to the metallic debris or to increased third-body wear from the metallic debris is unknown at this time.

Summary

Cemented total hip arthroplasty continues to be a highly successful and cost-effective treatment of end-stage arthropathies of the hip. If surgeons understand and apply the principles of appropriate stem design, contemporary cement techniques, and optimization of the cement mantle, the long-term results of cemented femoral stems should continue to improve. Combining these principles with improvement in bearing technology and the potential reduction of particulate wear will continue to make cemented femoral fixation the gold standard of total hip arthroplasty well into the future.

Contemporary cementless acetabular components have incorporated lessons learned from the successes and failures observed in earlier designs and provide for a straightforward surgical technique that is applicable to most reconstructions. These components have been associated with high rates of osseointegration and long-term stability, making them the reconstructive modality of choice for most surgeons in North America. The use of more wear-resistant bearing surfaces may further improve the long-term results of cementless acetabular components.

The success of cementless femoral implants continues to increase their usage both in North America and worldwide. Incremental design modifications have improved the survivorship, ease of use, and applicability to a wide variety of clinical scenarios. The exceedingly low rates of aseptic loosening and ever-increasing number of long-term follow-up studies have allowed this technology to become the favored technique with most surgeons in North America. As data continue to accumulate showing consistently low rates of loosening, the focus for improvements in hip arthroplasty has shifted toward other aspects of the surgery and implants.

Annotated Bibliography

Cemented Femoral Components

Ayers D, Mann K: The importance of proximal cement filling of the calcar region: A biomechanical justification. *J Arthroplasty* 2003;18(7 suppl 1)103-109.

The results of this study support the intraoperative removal of proximal medial cancellous bone from the calcar region to increase cement mantle thickness and remove cement mantle stresses to improve long-term fixation of cemented femoral components.

Berry DJ, Harmsen WS, Cabanela ME, Morrey BF: Twenty-five-year survivorship of two thousand consecutive primary Charnley total hip replacements: Factors affecting survivorship of acetabular and femoral components. *J Bone Joint Surg Am* 2002;84:171-177.

The authors analyzed the effects of demographic factors and diagnoses on the long-term survivorship of the acetabular and femoral components used in Charnley total hip arthroplasty. The 25-year rates of survivorship free of revision, free of revision or removal of the implant for any reason, and free of revision or removal for aseptic loosening were 77.5%, 80.9%, and 86.5%, respectively.

Breusch SJ, Lukoschek M, Kreutzer J, Brocai D, Gruen TA: Dependency of cement mantle thickness on femoral stem design and centralizer. *J Arthroplasty* 2001;16:648-657.

In this cadaveric study on 48 left femora with 4 different stem designs (1 anatomic, 3 straight), the authors studied the influence of stem design, centralizer, and femur type on cement mantle thickness. They found that anatomic stems respect the anatomy, allow for more even cement mantles, minimize the risk of thin cement mantles without the use of centralizers, and may be considered for use in a femur with marked proximal bow.

Breusch SJ, Norman TL, Schneider U, Reitzel T, Blaha JD, Lukoschek M: Lavage technique in total hip arthroplasty: Jet lavage produces better cement penetration than syringe lavage in the proximal femur. *J Arthroplasty* 2000;15:921-927.

In this cadaveric study, cancellous bone was irrigated with pulsed lavage and syringe lavage in femora for comparison. Specimens received vacuum-mixed cement applied in a retrograde manner. The use of jet lavage yielded significantly improved ($P < 0.0001$) cement penetration and the ratio of the area of supported to unsupported cancellous bone compared with syringe lavage.

Callaghan JJ, Albright JC, Goetz DD, Olejniczak JP, Johnston RC: Charnley total hip arthroplasty with cement: Minimum twenty-five-year follow-up. *J Bone Joint Surg Am* 2000;82:487-497.

The authors evaluated the results of the senior author's 25-year experience with Charnley total hip arthroplasty with cement in 316 hips. Of the 62 hips in 51 patients who were alive at 25-year follow-up, 14 (23%) had been revised. The prevalence of revision because of aseptic loosening of the femoral component in the living patients was 7%, and in all 316 hips the prevalence was 3%.

Chambers IR, Fender D, McCaskie AW, Reeves PC, Gregg PJ: Radiological features predictive of aseptic loosening in cemented Charnley femoral stems. *J Bone Joint Surg Br* 2001;83:838-842.

Several features were found to be associated with a greater than twofold increase in the risk of implant loosening in patients who had undergone Charnley total hip replacements; inadequate cementation was reported to be the most significant feature.

Collis DK, Mohler CG: Comparison of clinical outcomes in total hip arthroplasty using rough and polished cemented stems with essentially the same geometry. *J Bone Joint Surg Am* 2002;84:586-592.

In the study of 244 total hip arthroplasties, the stems inserted in 122 hips had a grit-blasted surface and the stems in 122 hips had a polished surface. At an average follow up of 5.65 years, there was a significant difference ($P = 0.05$) between the grit-blasted and polished stems with regard to revision. The results favor the use of a polished stem when cement is used for fixation of the femoral component.

Davis CM III, Berry DJ, Harmsen WS: Cemented revision of failed uncemented femoral components of total hip arthroplasty. *J Bone Joint Surg Am* 2003;85:1264-1269.

This article reports the experience of 47 consecutive patients (48 hips) at one institution in which a failed primary cementless femoral component was revised with use of cement. The 6-year rate of survival of the femoral component was 72% with revision for aseptic loosening as the end point and 67% with mechanical failure as the end point. Bone removal at the time of initial surgery and bone loss because of subsequent failure of the cementless implant may explain the high rate of loosening in the first 10 years after revision.

Estok DM II, Harris WH: A stem design change to reduce peak cement strains at the tip of cemented total hip arthroplasty. *J Arthroplasty* 2000;15:584-589.

In studies designed to assess different femoral stem tip designs, a stem with a narrow tip profile that would accept an externally applied polymethylmethacrylate centralizer (shaped similar to a napkin ring) and had a gradual transition zone to join the body of the implant was shown to achieve the objectives of positioning the component in a neutral position centered in a uniform mantle of adequate thickness.

Garcia-Cimbrelo E, Cruz-Pardos A, Cordero J, Sanchez-Sotelo J: Low-friction arthroplasty in patients younger than 40 years old: 20- to 25-year results. *J Arthroplasty* 2000;15:825-832.

A total of 67 low-friction arthroplasties were performed in patients younger than 40 years. The femoral stem proved to be durable, but acetabular cups had poorer results in younger patients than in older patients.

Gramkow J, Jensen TH, Varmarken JE, Retpen JB: Long-term results after cemented revision of the femoral component in total hip arthroplasty. *J Arthroplasty* 2001;16:777-783.

The authors of this study, using re-revision because of aseptic loosening or radiographic loosening as end point, found a 10-year survival of 80.7% in patients undergoing primary arthroplasty. The authors concluded that simple recementation is indicated in elderly patients with only minor bone loss.

Halley DK, Glassman AH: Twenty- to twenty-six-year radiographic review in patients 50 years of age or younger with cemented Charnley low-friction arthroplasty. *J Arthroplasty* 2003;18(7 suppl 1)79-85.

In this radiographic study at 20- to 26-year follow-up of patients who were age 50 years or younger and underwent Charnley low-friction arthroplasty, the mean 22-year survival rate was 78.8% for the stem (all causes). For aseptic loosening, the mean 22-year survival rate was 85.2% for the stem.

Haydon CM, Mehin R, Burnett S, et al: Revision total hip arthroplasty with use of a cemented femoral component: Results at a mean of ten years. *J Bone Joint Surg Am* 2004;86:1179-1185.

To determine component survival, the authors reviewed the results in 129 patients who underwent revision total hip arthroplasties with a cemented femoral stem. The 10-year survival rate was 91% with re-revision of the femoral component because of aseptic loosening as the end point and 71% with mechanical failure as the end point.

Howell JR Jr, Blunt LA, Doyle C, Hooper RM, Lee AJ, Ling RS: In vivo surface wear mechanisms of femoral components of cemented total hip arthroplasties: The influence of wear mechanism on clinical outcome. *J Arthroplasty* 2004;19:88-101.

To assess the appearance and mechanism of femoral stem wear, the authors studied 172 retrieved femoral components. Loss of stem surface in response to wear was found in 93% of stems; matte surfaces showed abrasive processes that damage cement, and polished stems showed a fretting appearance without significant damage to cement.

Issack PS, Botero HG, Hiebert RN, et al: Sixteen-year follow-up of the cemented Spectron femoral stem for hip arthroplasty. *J Arthroplasty* 2003;18:925-930.

This cohort of 105 patients underwent 120 total hip arthroplasties with a straight, cobalt-chromium femoral stem using a second-generation cementing technique. Sixteen-year survivorship of the component was 93.9% when revision for aseptic loosening was used as the end point or 90.3% when either revision for aseptic loosening or radiographic evidence of loosening was used as the end point.

Keener JD, Callaghan JJ, Goetz DD, Pederson DR, Sullivan PM, Johnston RC: Twenty-five-year results after Charnley total hip arthroplasty in patients less than fifty years old: A concise follow-up of a previous report. *J Bone Joint Surg Am* 2003;85:1066-1072.

In this study, the authors assessed the durability of cemented total hip replacements in a young (age < 50 years) population. Sixty-nine percent of the original hip replacements were functioning well at the latest follow-up examination (minimum follow-up, 25 years) or at the time of death. Only 5% required more than one revision arthroplasty.

Malchau H, Herberts P, Eisler T, Garellick G, Soderman P: The Swedish Total Hip Replacement Register. *J Bone Joint Surg Am* 2002;84(suppl 2):2-20.

In this 2002 report from the world's most complete data repository for total hip arthroplasty, the revision burden (the fraction of revisions and the total number of primary and revision total hip arthroplasties) for cemented prostheses implanted from 1979 through 2000 was reported to be 7.4% compared with 27.3% for cementless implants implanted from 1992 through 2000.

Meding JB, Nassif JM, Ritter MA: Long-term survival of the T-28 versus the TR-28 cemented total hip arthroplasties. *J Arthroplasty* 2000;15:928-933.

The authors of this study compared the performance of cemented prostheses of either shot-blast chrome or polished stainless steel used in 550 total hip arthroplasties. They concluded that surface finish may be an important contributor to the survival of cemented femoral stems.

Nercessian OA, Martin G, Joshi RP, Su BW, Eftekhar NS: A 15- to 25- year follow-up study of primary Charnley low-friction arthroplasty: A single surgeon series. *J Arthroplasty* 2005;20:162-167.

In this study, 447 primary Charnley hip arthroplasties were performed. Ninety-eight of the hips (75 patients) were available for an average 18.9-year follow-up. Seventy-two hips (73.5%) survived clinically. Of these 72 hips, 71 stems (98.6%) and 60 sockets (83.3%) survived radiographically. Kaplan-Meier survival analysis on all 447 hips using revision as an end point revealed 66.2% ± 5.7% survival at 20 years. Twenty-six hips were revised. The main reason for revision was failure of the socket.

Ramaniraka NA, Rakotomanana LR, Leyvraz PF: The fixation of the cemented femoral component: Effects of

stem stiffness, cement thickness and roughness of the cement-bone surface. *J Bone Joint Surg Br* 2000;82:297-303.

The authors evaluated titanium and chromium-cobalt stems. Micromovement was minimal with a cement mantle 3- to 4-mm thick. The relative decrease in surface roughness augmented slipping but decreased debonding at the cement-bone interface.

Rasquinha VJ, Ranawat CS: Durability of the cemented femoral stem in patients 60 to 80 years old. *Clin Orthop Relat Res* 2004;419:115-123.

The authors studied surface roughness and durability of fixation of the cemented femoral stem in patients undergoing total hip replacements. Comparisons of survivorship curves for failure from all causes showed significant differences between the Charnley compared with the Omnifit and Ranawat-Burnstein Interlok series respectively, with no significant differences between the Omnifit and the Ranawat-Burnstein Interlok series. The cemented femoral stem, with a good cement mantle and surface roughness ranging from 30 to 150 microinches, did not show any significant differences in mechanical failure.

Rorabeck CH, Bourne RB: The revision hip: Cemented stem revision. Less we forget! *Orthopedics* 2003;26:933-934.

With aseptic loosening as the end point, 91% of cemented femoral revisions in 95 patients had a 10-year survivorship. Significant risk factors for failure were age greater than 60 years, male gender, and use of first-generation cementing techniques.

Settecerri JJ, Kelley SS, Rand JA, Fitzgerald RH Jr: Collar versus collarless cemented HD-II femoral prostheses. *Clin Orthop Relat Res* 2002;398:146-152.

Eighty-four patients received a collared (44 hips) or collarless (40 hips) femoral component at the time of their primary total hip arthroplasty. Kaplan-Meier survivorship analysis predicted an overall survival rate free of revision of 86% at 10 years. The authors found no statistically significant differences in survival rates between the two groups.

Wroblewski BM, Siney PD, Fleming PA: Charnley low-frictional torque arthroplasty in patients under the age of 51 years: Follow-up to 33 years. *J Bone Joint Surg Br* 2002;84(4):540-543.

In this study, 1,092 patients underwent 1,434 primary Charnley arthroplasties. At a mean follow-up of 17 years and 5 months, 220 patients (220 hips) had undergone revision. The indication for revision was aseptic loosening of the cup (11.7%), aseptic loosening of the stem (4.9%), a fractured stem (1.7%), deep infection (1.5%), and dislocation (0.4%). Survivorship was 93.7% with revision for any indication as the end point.

Cementless Acetabular Components

Capello WN, D'Antonio JA, Feinberg JR, Manley MT: Ten-year results with hydroxyapatite-coated total hip femoral components in patients less than fifty years old: A concise follow-up of a previous report. *J Bone Joint Surg Am* 2003;85-A(5):885-889.

Although the focus of this report was the outcomes of the femur, the first-generation, cementless acetabular component that were used (including both porous- and HA-coated components) had a predicted survivorship of 70% at 168-month follow-up.

Della Valle CJ, Berger RA, Shott S, et al: Primary total hip arthroplasty with a porous coated acetabular component: A follow-up note at fifteen to eighteen years. *J Bone Joint Surg Am* 2004;86-A(11):1217-1222.

In a series of 204 consecutive patients followed for 15 to 18 years after undergoing primary total hip arthroplasty with a porous-coated acetabular shell, survivorship of the acetabular component at 15 years was 99%. Ten hips (7%) required a change of the modular polyethylene liner because of excessive wear or osteolysis.

Gaffey JL, Callaghan JJ, Pedersen DR, Goetz DD, Sullivan PM, Johnston RC: Cementless acetabular fixation at fifteen years: A comparison with the same surgeon's results following acetabular fixation with cement. *J Bone Joint Surg Am* 2004;86-A(2):257-261.

When compared with a consecutive series of cemented all-polyethylene cups inserted by the same surgeon and followed-up for a similar amount of time, the rate of revision was significantly lower for cementless acetabular components. No cups were revised because of loosening.

Kawamura H, Dunbar MJ, Murray P, Bourne RB, Rorabeck CH: The porous coated anatomic total hip replacement: A ten to fourteen-year follow-up study of a cementless total hip arthroplasty. *J Bone Joint Surg Am* 2001;83-A(9):1333-1338.

Eighty-three percent of the cobalt-chromium alloy cementless acetabular components that were used showed definite signs of bone ingrowth. Eight acetabular components were revised secondary to loosening. Survivorship of the acetabular component was 92.7% at 14-year follow-up.

Udomkiat P, Dorr LD, Wan Z: Cementless hemispheric porous-coated sockets implanted with press-fit technique without screws: Average ten-year follow-up. *J Bone Joint Surg Am* 2002;84-A(7):1195-1200.

In this study, one hip required revision secondary to loosening and osteolysis was identified in four. The 12-year survivorship was 99.1% with loosening as the end point, but it was 76.9% when any revision for a problem related to the cup was considered as an end point.

Wasielewski RC, Galat DD, Sheridan KC, Rubash HE: Acetabular anatomy and transacetabular screw fixation at the high hip center. *Clin Orthop Relat Res* 2005;438: 171-176.

The authors report that a quadrant system at the high hip center can demarcate safe zones for screw placement and that at the high hip center only the peripheral half of the posterior quadrants are safe for screw placement.

Cementless Femoral Components

Archibeck MJ, Berger RA, Jacobs JJ, et al: Second-generation cementless total hip arthroplasty: Eight to eleven year results. *J Bone Joint Surg Am* 2001;83:1666-1673.

This study followed 92 total hip arthroplasties using the Anatomic stem. This titanium, anatomically designed femoral component features a circumferential proximal porous coating with a titanium fiber metal mesh. The mean follow-up was 10 years, and there were no femoral revisions or femoral components with radiographic evidence of loosening. There was a 9% incidence of thigh pain, although only 2% of these were moderate to severe. The presence of thigh pain was associated with a large femoral stem. A significant percentage of prostheses had radiolucent lines adjacent to the smooth regions of the stem that did not indicate the presence of loosening. Osteolytic lesions were observed adjacent to 5% of the femoral stems, and none of these lesions were located distal to the lesser trochanter, indicating that circumferential coating limited the access of polyethylene particles distally.

Engh CA, Claus AM, Hopper RH, Engh CA Sr: Long-term results using the anatomic medullary locking hip prosthesis. *Clin Orthop Relat Res* 2001;393:137-146.

This report extends the follow-up of a previously reported cohort of patients with AML femoral prostheses to a mean of 13.9 years. The overall loosening rate of the femoral components in this study was 3.4%. Although the focus of this study was to describe the reasons for revision and the effect of osteolysis, no femoral stems in this series became loose or required revision because of progressive osteolysis.

Goldberg JR, Gilbert JL, Jacobs JJ, Bauer TW, Paprosky W, Leurgans S: A multicenter retrieval study of the taper interfaces of modular hip prostheses. *Clin Orthop Relat Res* 2002;401:149-161.

This multicenter retrieval analysis of 231 modular hip implants was conducted to investigate the effects of material combination, metallurgic condition, flexural rigidity, head and neck moment arm, neck length, and implantation time on corrosion and fretting of modular taper surfaces. Moderate to severe corrosion was observed in 28% of the femoral heads of similar alloy couples and 42% of the femoral heads of mixed alloy couples. Corrosion and fretting scores tended to be higher for femoral heads than necks. Implantation time and flexural rigidity of the femoral necks were predictors of femoral head and neck corrosion and femoral head fretting. The results of this study suggest that in vivo corrosion of modular hip taper interfaces is attributable to a mechanically assisted crevice corrosion process.

Grubl A, Chiari C, Gruber M, Kaider A, Gottsauner-Wolf F: Cementless total hip arthroplasty with a tapered, rectangular titanium stem and a threaded cup: A minimum ten-year follow-up. *J Bone Joint Surg Am* 2002;84:425-431.

This report summarizes the Austrian experience with a tapered, rectangular titanium stem and a threaded cup in a cohort of 208 consecutive hips with a minimum 10-year follow-up. The stem is made of titanium and has a sand-blasted surface with an average surface roughness of 4 to 6 μm Ra[5]. Only three femoral stems required revision, and none because of loosening. All stems had radiographic evidence of bone ingrowth, but only 107 of the original 208 hips were available for radiographic review.

Kim YH, Oh SH, Kim JS: Primary total hip arthroplasty with a second-generation cementless total hip prosthesis in patients younger that fifty years of age. *J Bone Joint Surg Am* 2003;85:109-114.

This report on a so-called second-generation femoral component followed-up on 118 hips for a minimum of 9.8 years. The Profile stem is made of titanium, has a sintered bead coating on the proximal one third, and is shaped to maximize stem canal fill in both the coronal and sagittal planes proximally. The rate of survival with loosening as an end point was 100%, and no patient had long-term thigh pain. By using a 22-mm femoral head in all patients, the volumetric wear and subsequently the rate of osteolysis was quite low (12% of patients).

Mallory TH, Lombardi AV, Leith JR, et al: Minimal 10-year results of a tapered cementless femoral component in total hip arthroplasty. *J Arthroplasty* 2001;16(suppl 1): 49-54.

A tapered titanium femoral component coated with titanium plasma spray over its proximal one third was used in 120 consecutive hips. With a mean follow-up of 12.2 years, the survivorship of this stem was 97.5% with revision as an end point. Three femoral components loosened, but two loosened secondary to progressive proximal osteolysis. Osteolysis was noted in 32.4% of patients, and the authors attributed this to the use of 32-mm titanium heads and inferior quality polyethylene. The incidence of thigh pain was relatively low, with no or mild thigh pain reported in 96.6% of patients.

Sinha RK, Dungy DS, Yeon HB: Primary total hip arthroplasty with a proximally porous-coated femoral stem. *J Bone Joint Surg Am* 2004;86-A(6):1254-1261.

This study reports the results of 123 patients implanted with the multilock femoral stem. This titanium prosthesis incorporates a circumferential fiber-metal porous coating that extends into the metaphyseal-diaphyseal junction and a smooth distal stem with flutes to improve rotational stability and decrease bending stiffness. With a minimum 5-year follow-up, the rate of survivorship using revision as an end point was

99%; the rate of bone ingrowth was 95%, with 3% of stems fibrous stable. Although proximal stress shielding and osteolysis were observed, this was of no clinical significance at this follow-up interval.

Tanzer M, Chan S, Brooks E, Bobyn JD: Primary cementless total hip arthroplasty using a modular femoral component: A minimum 6 year follow-up. *J Arthroplasty* 2001;16(suppl 1):64-70.

In this study, 59 patients who underwent primary cementless total hip arthroplasty using a modular femoral component were followed for an average of 8 years and 5 months. All patients showed evidence of bone ingrowth, and no instances of femoral loosening were noted. Stress shielding in Gruen zone 7 was noted in most of the patients studied. One femoral revision was performed in a recurrent dislocator, and at the time of surgery, the femoral stem was disengaged from the metaphyseal sleeve. There was no obvious tissue metallosis, but fretting at the stem-sleeve junction was apparent. Of interest in this study was the relatively high incidence of proximal osteolysis (42% of patient). The authors hypothesized that their longer follow-up and use of large diameter heads could explain this incidence. However, the effect of metallic debris from corrosion between the modular components could not be ruled out as a contributing factor. Five patients were noted to have osteolysis without significant polyethylene wear, indicating that some factor other than polyethylene wear may have contributed to these lesions.

Classic Bibliography

Ahmed AM, Raab S, Miller JE: Metal/cement interface strength in cemented stem fixation. *J Orthop Res* 1984;2: 105-118.

Amstutz HC, Markolf KL, McNeice GM, Gruen TA: Loosening of total components: Cause and prevention, in *Proceedings of the 4th Meeting of The Hip Society*. St Louis, MO, CV Mosby Co, 1976, p 6.

Askew MJ, Steege JW, Lewis JL, Ranieri JR, Wixson RL: Effect of cement pressure and bone strength on polymethylmethacrylate fixation. *J Orthop Res* 1984; 1(4):412-420.

Ballard WT, Callaghan JJ, Johnston RC: Revision of total hip arthroplasty in octogenarians. *J Bone Joint Surg Am* 1995;77:585-589.

Barrack RL, Castro F, Guinn S: Cost of implanting a cemented versus cementless femoral stem. *J Arthroplasty* 1996;11:373-376.

Barrack RL, Mulroy RD, Harris WH: Improved cementing techniques and femoral component loosening in young patients with hip arthroplasty. *J Bone Joint Surg Br* 1992;74:385-389.

Beckenbaugh RD, Ilstrup DM: Total hip arthroplasty. *J Bone Joint Surg Am* 1978;60:306-313.

Berger RA, Seel MJ, Wood K, Evans R, D'Antonio J, Rubash HE: Effect of a centralizing device on cement mantle deficiencies and initial prosthetic alignment in total hip arthroplasty. *J Arthroplasty* 1997;12:434-443.

Bobyn JD, Pilliar RM, Cameron HU, Weatherly GC: The optimum pore size for the fixation of porous-surfaced metal implants by the ingrowth of bone. *Clin Orthop Relat Res* 1980;150:263-270.

Callaghan JJ, Heekin RD, Savory CG, Dysart SH, Hopkinson WJ: Evaluation of the learning curve associated with uncemented primary porous-coated anatomic total hip arthroplasty. *Clin Orthop Relat Res* 1992;282:132-144.

Callaghan JJ, Salvati EA, Huo MH, et al: Advances in total hip reconstruction. *Instr Course Lect* 1991;40:115-197.

Collis DK: Revision total hip replacement with cement. *Semin Arthroplasty* 1993;4:38-49.

Collis DK, Mohler CG: Loosening rates and bone lysis with rough finished and polished stems. *Clin Orthop Relat Res* 1998;355:113-122.

Crawford RW, Evans M, Ling RS, Murray DW: Fluid flow around model femoral components of differing surface finishes: in vitro investigations. *Acta Orthop Scand* 1999;70:589-595.

Crawford RW, Gie GA, Ling RSM: An 8-10 year clinical review comparing matt and polished Exeter stems. *Orthop Trans* 1998;22:40.

Crowninshield RD, Jennings JD, Laurent ML, Maloney WJ: Cemented femoral component surface finish mechanics. *Clin Orthop Relat Res* 1998;355:90-102.

Dall DM, Learmonth ID, Solomon MI, Miles AW, Davenport JM: Fracture and loosening of Charnley femoral stems. Comparison between first-generation and subsequent designs. *J Bone Joint Surg Br* 1993;75:259-265.

Dohmae Y, Bechtold JE, Sherman RE, Puno RM, Gustilo RB: Reduction in cement-bone interface shear strength between primary and revision arthroplasty. *Clin Orthop Relat Res* 1988;236:214-220.

Ebramzadeh E, Sarmiento A, McKellop HA, Llinas A, Grogan W: The cement mantle in total hip arthroplasty. Analysis of long-term radiographic results. *J Bone Joint Surg Am* 1994;76:77-87.

Elting JJ, Mikhail WE, Zicat BA, Hubbell JC, Lane LE, House B: Preliminary report of impaction grafting for exchange femoral arthroplasty. *Clin Orthop Relat Res* 1995;319:159-167.

Engh CA, Bobyn JD: The influence of stem size and extent of porous coating on femoral bone resorption after primary cementless hip arthroplasty. *Clin Orthop Relat Res* 1988;231:7-28.

Engh CA, Massin P, Suthers KE: Roentgenographic assessment of the biologic fixation of porous-surfaced femoral components. *Clin Orthop Relat Res* 1990;257:107-128.

Engh CA, McGovern TF, Bobyn JD, Harris WH: A quantitative evaluation of periprosthetic bone-remodeling after cementless total hip arthroplasty. *J Bone Joint Surg Am* 1992;74:1009-1020.

Estok DM II, Harris WH: Long-term results of cemented femoral revision surgery using second-generation techniques. An average 11.7-year follow-up evaluation. *Clin Orthop Relat Res* 1994;299:190-202.

Estok DM, Orr TE, Harris WH: Factors affecting cement strains near the tip of a cemented femoral component. *J Arthroplasty* 1997;12:40-48.

Fisher DA, Tsang AC, Paydar N, Milionis S, Turner CH: Cement-mantle thickness affects cement strains in total hip replacement. *J Biomech* 1997;30:1173-1177.

Garellick G, Malchau H:, Regnér H, Herberts P: The Charnley versus the Spectron hip prosthesis. *J Arthroplasty* 1999;14:414-425.

Gie GA, Linder L, Ling RS, Simon JP, Slooff TJ, Timperley AJ: Contained morselized allograft in revision total hip arthroplasty: Surgical technique. *Orthop Clin North Am* 1993;24:717-725.

Gie GA, Linder L, Ling RS, Simon JP, Slooff TJ, Timperley AJ: Impacted cancellous allografts and cement for revision total hip arthroplasty. *J Bone Joint Surg Br* 1993;75:14-21.

Gie GA, Ling RS: Femoral bone grafting: intramedullary impaction grafting, in Steinberg ME, Garino JP (eds): *Revision Total Hip Arthroplasty.* Philadelphia, PA, Lippincott Williams and Wilkins, 1999, pp 281-297.

Goldberg BA, al-Habbal G, Noble PC, Pavavic M, Liebs TR, Tullos HS: Proximal and distal femoral centralizers in modern cemented hip arthroplasty. *Clin Orthop Relat Res* 1998;349:163-173.

Halawa M, Lee AJ, Ling RS, Vangala SS: The shear strength of trabecular bone from the femur, and some factors affecting the shear strength of the cement-bone interface. *Arch Orthop Trauma Surg* 1978;92:19-30.

Hanson PB, Walker RH: Total hip arthroplasty cemented femoral component distal stem centralizer. Effect on stem centralization and cement mantle. *J Arthroplasty* 1995;10:683-688.

Harrigan TP, Kareh JA, O'Connor DO, Burke DW, Harris WH: A finite element study of the initiation of failure of fixation in cemented femoral total hip components. *J Orthop Res* 1992;10:134-144.

Harris WH: Is it advantageous to strengthen the cement-metal interface and use a collar for cemented femoral components of total hip replacements? *Clin Orthop Relat Res* 1992;285: 67-72.

Harris WH, McCarthy JC Jr, O'Neill DA: Femoral component loosening using contemporary techniques of femoral cement fixation. *J Bone Joint Surg Am* 1982;64: 1063-1067.

Hernigou P, LeMouel S: Do voids in a femoral cement mantle affect the outcome? *J Arthroplasty* 1999;14:1005-1010.

Howie DW, Middleton RG, Costi K: Loosening of matt and polished cemented femoral stems. *J Bone Joint Surg Br* 1998;80:573-576.

Izquierdo RJ, Northmore-Ball MD: Long-term results of revision hip arthroplasty: Survival analysis with special reference to the femoral component. *J Bone Joint Surg Br* 1994;76:34-39.

James SP, Schmalzreid TP, McGarry FJ, Harris WH: Extensive porosity at the cement-femoral prosthesis interface: A preliminary study. *J Biomed Mater Res* 1993;27: 71-78.

Jasty M, Maloney WJ, Bragdon CR, O'Connor DO, Haire T, Harris WH: The initiation of failure in cemented femoral components of hip arthroplasties. *J Bone Joint Surg Br* 1991;73:551-558.

Jasty M, Rubash HE, Paiement GD, Bragdon CR, Parr J, Harris WH: Porous-coated uncemented components in experimental total hip arthroplasty in dogs: Effect of plasma-sprayed calcium phosphate coatings on bone ingrowth. *Clin Orthop Relat Res* 1992;280:300-309.

Katz RP, Callaghan JJ, Sullivan PM, Johnston RC: Long-term results of revision total hip arthroplasty with improved cementing technique. *J Bone Joint Surg Br* 1997; 79:322-326.

Kavanagh BF, Fitzgerald RH Jr: Multiple revisions for failed total hip arthroplasty not associated with infection. *J Bone Joint Surg Am* 1987;69:1144-1149.

Kawate K, Maloney WJ, Bragdon CR, Biggs SA, Jasty M, Harris WH: Importance of a thin cement mantle. Au-

topsy studies of eight hips. *Clin Orthop Relat Res* 1998; 355:70-76.

Kawate K, Ohmura T, Hiyoshi N, Natsume Y, Teranishi T, Tamai S: Thin cement mantle and osteolysis with a precoated stem. *Clin Orthop Relat Res* 1999;365:124-129.

Kendrick JB II, Noble PC, Tullos HS: Distal stem design and the torsional stability of cementless femoral stems. *J Arthroplasty* 1995;10:463-469.

Kerboull M: L'athroplastie totale de hanche. *Maîtrise Orthopédique* 1999;83:6.

Kerboull L, Lefevre N, Hamadouche M, et al: Influence de l'etat de surface des implants femoroux cimentés: Etude statistique comparative á 9 ans de deux séries homogènes de arthroplasties totales de hanche. *Rev Chir Orthop Reparatrice Appar Moteur* 1999;85(suppl 3):117.

Kim YH, Kim JS, Cho SH: Primary total hip arthroplasty with a cementless porous-coated anatomic total hip prosthesis: 10- to 12-year results of prospective and consecutive series. *J Arthroplasty* 1999;5:538-548.

Krause WR, Krug W, Miller J: Strength of the cement-bone interface. *Clin Orthop Relat Res* 1982;163:290-299.

Kwak BM, Lim OK, Kim YY, et al: An investigation of the effect of cement thickness on an implant by finite element stress analysis. *Int Orthop* 1979;2:315-319.

Lee IY, Skinner HB, Keyak JH: Effects of variation of prosthesis size on cement stress at the tip of a femoral implant. *J Biomed Mater Res* 1994;28:1055-1060.

Lieberman JR, Moeckel BH, Evans BG, Salvati EA, Ranawat CS: Cement-within-cement revision hip arthroplasty. *J Bone Joint Surg Br* 1993;75:869-871.

Majkowski RS, Miles AW, Bannister GC, Perkins J, Taylor GJ: Bone surface preparation in cemented joint replacement. *J Bone Joint Surg Br* 1993;75:459-463.

Mallory TH: Preparation of the proximal femur in cementless total hip revision. *Clin Orthop Relat Res* 1988; 235:47-60.

Maloney WJ, Jasty M, Burke DW, et al: Biomechanical and histologic investigation of cemented total hip arthroplasties: A study of autopsy-retrieved femurs after in vivo cycling. *Clin Orthop Relat Res* 1989;249:129-140.

Maloney WJ, Jasty M, Rosenberg A, Harris WH: Bone lysis in well-fixed cemented femoral components. *J Bone Joint Surg Br* 1990;72:966-970.

Maloney WJ, Sychterz C, Bragdon C, et al: Skeletal response to well fixed femoral components inserted with and without cement. *Clin Orthop Relat Res* 1996;333:15-26.

Marti RK, Schuller HM, Besselaar PP, Vanfrank Haasnoot EL: Results of revision of hip arthroplasty with cement: A five- to fourteen-year follow-up study. *J Bone Joint Surg Am* 1990;72:346-354.

Mulroy RD Jr, Harris WH: The effect of improved cementing techniques on component loosening in total hip replacement: An 11-year radiographic review. *J Bone Joint Surg Br* 1990;72:757-760.

Mulroy WF, Estok DM, Harris WH: Total hip arthroplasty with use of so-called second-generation cementing techniques: A fifteen-year-average follow-up study. *J Bone Joint Surg Am* 1995;77:1845-1852.

Murray DW, Rushton N: Mediators of bone resorption around implants. *Clin Orthop Relat Res* 1992;281:295-304.

Noble PC: Contributions of basic and applied sciences to hip replacement in the older patient. *Instr Course Lect* 1994;43:381-392.

Noble PC, Collier MB, Maltry JA, Kamaric E, Tullos HS: Pressurization and centralization enhance the quality and reproducibility of cement mantles. *Clin Orthop Relat Res* 1998;355:77-89.

Otani T, Whiteside LA, White SE: The effect of axial and torsional loading on strain distribution in the proximal femur as related to cementless total hip arthroplasty. *Clin Orthop Relat Res* 1993;292:376-383.

Paprosky WG, Greidanus NV, Antoniou G: Minimum 10-year-results of extensively porous-coated stems in revision hip arthroplasty. *Clin Orthop Relat Res* 1999;369:230-242.

Pellicci PM, Wilson PD Jr, Sledge CB, et al: Long-term results of revision total hip replacement. A follow-up report. *J Bone Joint Surg Am* 1985;67:513-516.

Pierson JL, Harris WH: Effect of improved cementing techniques on the longevity of fixation in revision cemented femoral arthroplasties: Average 8.8-year follow-up period. *J Arthroplasty* 1995;10:581-591.

Pilliar RM, Lee JM, Maniatopoulos C: Observations on the effect of movement on bone ingrowth into porous-surfaced implants. *Clin Orthop Relat Res* 1986;208:108-113.

Powers CM, Lee IY, Skinner HB, Keyak JH: Effects of distal cement voids on cement stress in total hip arthroplasty. *J Arthroplasty* 1998;13:793-798.

Raut VV, Siney PD, Wroblewski BM: Outcome of revision for mechanical stem failure using the cemented Charnley's stem: A study of 399 cases. *J Arthroplasty* 1996;11:405-410.

Retpen JB, Jensen JS: Risk factors for recurrent aseptic loosening of the femoral component after cemented revision. *J Arthroplasty* 1993;8:471-478.

Rubash HE, Harris WH: Revision of nonseptic, loose, cemented femoral components using modern cementing techniques. *J Arthroplasty* 1988;3:241-248.

Sakalkale DP, Eng K, Hozack WJ, Rothman RH: Minimum 10-year results of a tapered cementless hip replacement. *Clin Orthop Relat Res* 1999;362:138-144.

Snorrason F, Karrholm J: Early loosening of revision hip arthroplasty: A roentgen stereophotogrammetric analysis. *J Arthroplasty* 1990;5:217-229.

Sochart DH, Porter ML: The long-term results of Charnley low-friction arthroplasty in young patients who have congenital dislocation, degenerative osteoarthrosis, or rheumatoid arthritis. *J Bone Joint Surg Am* 1997;79:1599-1617.

Sporer SM, Callaghan JJ, Olejniczak JP, Goetz DD, Johnston RC: The effects of surface roughness and polymethylmethacrylate precoating on the radiographic and clinical results of the Iowa hip prosthesis: A study of patients less than fifty years old. *J Bone Joint Surg Am* 1999;81:481-492.

Star MJ, Colwell CW Jr, Kelman GJ, Ballock RT, Walker RH: Suboptimal (thin) distal cement mantle thickness as a contributory factor in total hip arthroplasty femoral component failure: A retrospective radiographic analysis favoring distal stem centralization. *J Arthroplasty* 1994;9:143-149.

Stauffer RN: Ten-year follow-up study of total hip replacement. *J Bone Joint Surg Am* 1982;64:983-990.

Stromberg CN, Herberts P: A multicenter 10-year study of cemented revision total hip arthroplasty in patients younger than 55 years old: A follow-up report. *J Arthroplasty* 1994;9:595-601.

Stromberg CN, Herberts P: Cemented revision total hip arthroplasties in patients younger than 55 years old: A multicenter evaluation of second-generation cementing technique. *J Arthroplasty* 1996;11:489-499.

Stromberg CN, Herberts P, Palmertz B: Cemented revision hip arthroplasty: A multicenter 5-9-year study of 204 first revisions for loosening. *Acta Orthop Scand* 1992;63:111-119.

Sutherland CJ, Wilde AH, Borden LS, Marks KE: A ten-year follow-up of one hundred consecutive Müller curved-stem total hip replacement arthroplasties. *J Bone Joint Surg Am* 1982;64:970-982.

Turner TM, Sumner DR, Urban RM, Rivero DP, Galante JO: A comparative study of porous coatings in a weight-bearing total hip-arthroplasty model. *J Bone Joint Surg Am* 1986;68:1396-1409.

Verdonschot N, Huiskies R: Cement debonding process of total hip arthroplasty stems. *Clin Orthop Relat Res* 1997;336:297-307.

Xenos JS, Hopkinson WJ, Callaghan JJ, Heekin RD, Savory CG: Osteolysis around an uncemented cobalt chrome total hip arthroplasty. *Clin Orthop Relat Res* 1995;317:29-36.

Chapter 34

The Difficult Primary Total Hip Arthroplasty

Joseph C. McCarthy, MD

Thomas R. Hackett, MD

Jo-ann Lee, MS

Introduction

Total hip arthroplasty for patients with primary osteoarthritis and normal femoral and acetabular geometry has a proven track record for improving the patient's quality of life by providing a dramatic improvement in pain, range of motion, and function. The goal of total hip arthroplasty is to restore hip biomechanics and secure rigid implant fixation. Conditions that present a particular challenge in primary total hip arthroplasty include developmental dysplasia, metabolic disease, inflammatory processes, primary or metastatic tumors, structural deformities, and cognitive dysfunction. Each of these disorders increases the likelihood of intraoperative or perioperative complications. Careful preoperative planning and templating along with classifying bone defects and their biomechanical significance is crucial to obtaining proper positioning and fit of the implants during surgery.

Prosthetic fixation becomes considerably more challenging when, in addition to cartilage damage, there is distortion of the bony anatomy or deficient bone stock of the femur, the acetabulum, or both. Structural joint abnormalities are often associated with congenital dislocation or dysplasia, inflammatory collagen diseases, posttraumatic or postosteotomy conditions, or metabolic bone diseases. These entities can produce not only anatomic bony changes, but also limb-length discrepancy, synovial abnormalities, osteopenia, muscular changes, and on occasion, neurovascular distortion. Perioperative risks associated with these conditions include an increased dislocation rate, infection rate, fracture of the femur, prolonged muscle weakness, neurovascular injury, or heterotopic bone formation. Awareness of the increased difficulty involved as well as different surgical options available will help surgeons minimize these risks and more consistently achieve successful outcomes.

Developmental Dysplasia

Developmental dysplasia consists of a spectrum of bony and soft-tissue abnormalities. Anatomic distortions that may present with this condition include coxa valga or vara, shortening of the femoral neck, proximal position of the femoral head in Crowe grade IV dislocation (> 100% of subluxation), posterior trochanteric rotation, gracile femoral cortex, narrow femoral canal, and at times dramatic femoral anteversion (Figure 1). In addition, the muscular envelope about the hip is often hypotrophic, and the capsule may be patulous.

Earlier reports on outcomes have been unfavorable. One study reported a 26% revision rate on 29 hips at an average 16-year follow-up. Another study reported an acetabular component loosening rate of 20%. With improved technique, however, recent reports have been more encouraging. One study reported good to excellent results and a 2% revision rate with a hybrid component fixation at an average follow-up of 10.6 years. Another study reported a 94% survival rate at an average 13.3-year follow-up.

Preoperative Planning

A thorough physical examination to assess the presence of contractures and measurement of true and apparent limb lengths is imperative. Radiographs should include an AP view of the pelvis and hips and AP and lateral views of at least the proximal half of the affected femur. Occasionally, Judet views or a CT scan with derived pelvic reconstruction formatting is valuable in assessing Crowe grade III (75% to 100% of subluxation) and IV deficiencies. Digital imaging or radiographs with magnification markers are needed for preoperative templating with several types of implants to determine which equipment and implants will be used for the reconstruction. Acetabular component positioning is determined first. The center of rotation of the acetabular implant, whether in anatomic or high hip center position, will help to determine the axial position and type of femoral prosthesis to restore limb length and offset. Assessment of pelvic tilt and the flexibility of the lumbar spine are also important. Preoperative planning for an extensile exposure facilitates safe exposure of the femur and acetabulum.

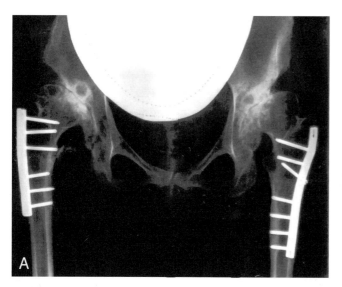

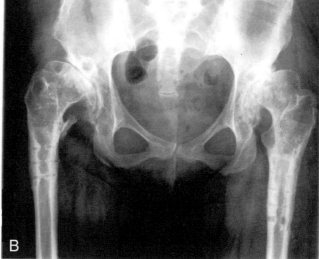

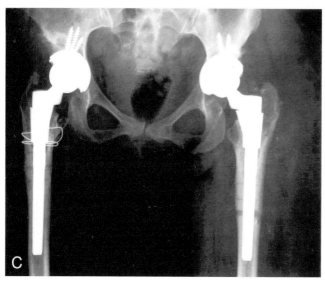

Figure 1 **A,** Preoperative radiograph of a 47-year-old woman with developmental dysplasia of the hip who underwent corrective osteotomies at age 15 years. **B,** Radiograph of the same patient obtained after stage 1 hardware removal. **C,** Radiograph of the same patient obtained after stage 2 total hip arthroplasty was performed with a modular femoral component and hemispherical acetabular component.

Surgical Considerations

Additional surgical time may be required intraoperatively because of the distorted anatomy. Adequate surgical exposure is needed for identification and protection of the abductors and sciatic nerve. Soft-tissue changes can alter the location of both the femoral and sciatic nerves. If the femoral head is proximally located, the femoral nerve may loop proximally, making it susceptible to surgical or traction injury. Contracted and/or shortened hip musculature may create substantial limblength inequality. Severe contractures may require tenotomy.

If the patient is in the lateral decubitus position, the pelvis must be adequately secured to avoid intraoperative pelvic rotation or tilt. The posterolateral approach is often used, but it may be necessary to osteotomize and translate the position of the greater trochanter. A transtrochanteric approach is used when the femoral head is located in a false acetabulum. If there is suffi-

cient posterior bone stock, the acetabulum may be moved a bit proximally without posterior breakout. The true acetabulum should be identified and centrally reamed first while avoiding violation of the anterior or posterior columns. It is important to use the true acetabulum because the ilium is thin, more proximal, and lacks posterior bone stock. Acetabular reamings or the resected femoral head can be used to graft defects if the medial wall is violated. It is important to carefully expand the reamers before anatomic positioning to avoid damage to the lateral rim. A small portion of the cup can be left uncovered superiorly. A conventional osteotomy is advantageous if pelvic bone grafting is needed. This approach avoids tethering of the superior gluteal neurovascular structures. Increased femoral anteversion and trochanteric distortion may cause impingement of the prosthetic neck and greater trochanter during rotation of the limb. To minimize this risk, a modular stem with adjustable anteversion or a cemented congenital

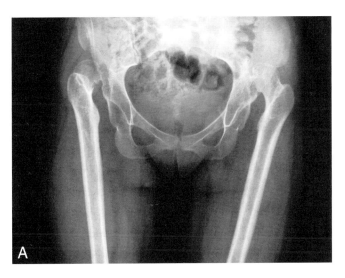
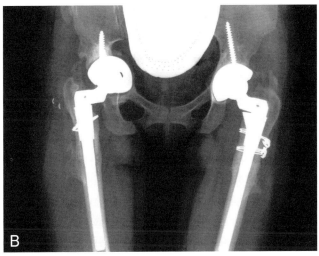

Figure 2 **A,** Preoperative radiograph of a 27-year-old woman with Crowe grade IV developmental dysplasia of the hip. **B,** Postoperative radiograph of the same patient obtained 2 years after total hip arthroplasty was performed shows healed corrective subtrochanteric osteotomies.

dysplasia of the hip stem with offset is advantageous. Coxa valga or coxa magna along with a high hip center and limb-length discrepancies may require an additional procedure at the time of total hip arthroplasty. In patients with severe subluxation, the trochanter may need to be advanced distally. If the femur needs to be lengthened, caution must be taken not to overly stretch the sciatic nerve.

A trochanteric slide osteotomy can be advantageous for limb-length adjustment of up to 3 cm or for anterior transposition of a posteriorly positioned trochanter. This procedure offers more reliable fixation, and the blood supply to the trochanter is less affected. Alternately, a subtrochanteric osteotomy is recommended for patients with high-riding dysplasia when there is insufficient bone to create a high hip center such that considerable femoral shortening and derotation will be necessary. The advantages of the subtrochanteric osteotomy include increased acetabular exposure, better access to the distal femoral canal, and preservation of the superior gluteal nerve and femoral head blood supply. In addition, the greater trochanter can be derotated and the femoral metaphysis preserved. Disadvantages include increases in surgical dissection, blood loss, and surgical time. Potential complications include nonunion and bony migration.

A subtrochanteric derotation osteotomy is also indicated if a monolithic femoral implant would overlengthen the limb or if there is greater than 45° of femoral anteversion. This osteotomy allows distal and medial translation of the socket position while shortening the femur in the diaphysis rather than the metaphysis (Figure 2). Once the femoral head has been resected, the femoral medullary canal should be prepared to the size of the chosen implant. The femoral shaft is then exposed, and rotational marks are scribed with methylene

blue or with an osteotome. The linea aspera is also a reference point. The osteotomy level should be made distal to the coating of a proximally coated implant or within 2 inches of the lower end of the lesser trochanter for extensively coated implants. Once the socket reconstruction has been completed, a trial femoral component is seated within the proximal fragment, the hip is reduced, the leg is placed on traction, and the femoral bony overlap is resected. The real femoral component is then impacted with the trochanter in the true lateral position with the osteotomy ends abutting.

The choice of implants for patients with a dysplastic hip depends on several factors: surgeon preference, size of the medullary canal, thicknesses of the femoral cortices, the amount of anteversion present, whether an osteotomy is necessary, and acetabular bone stock.

Cementless stems used may be proximally or extensively coated, modular, monolithic, or custom-made. Cemented stems should be forged to allow for sufficient strength and offset while minimizing impingement. This is an important consideration because of the higher dislocation potential with reconstruction for this disease. Potential joint instability may also be addressed by a low femoral neck osteotomy or use of a modular cemented or custom-made stem. If a derotation femoral osteotomy is required, a cementless or modular stem will allow compaction of the bony edges on weight bearing. Cemented stem fixation is preferred when the intact diaphyseal canal is stenotic or gracile. Excessive lumbar lordosis, often associated with developmental dysplasia of the hip, increases the risk of posterior dislocation. The components must be placed in more anteversion and range of motion checked with the trial components in place. On the acetabular side, hemispheric porous ingrowth components have been shown to provide reliable fixation with less need of a structural graft.

A prospective study showed no loosening, acetabular migration, or revision surgery at a 6-year follow-up. This technique was also used in acetabular revision surgery to treat failed primary arthroplasty in patients with developmental dysplasia of the hip and yielded overall good results after an intermediate duration of follow-up of 8 years in 53 patients.

Postoperative care must be individualized for each patient. For patients undergoing a femoral osteotomy, protected weight bearing may need to be prolonged and therapy managed as it is with those who undergo a revision procedure.

Inflammatory Arthritis

Inflammatory conditions affecting the hip joint including rheumatoid arthritis, chondrocalcinosis, systemic lupus erythematosus, ankylosing spondylitis, gout, Sjögren's syndrome, and ochronosis are all associated with premature cartilage destruction. Joint destruction in juvenile rheumatoid arthritis can occur during adolescence and be accompanied by multiple contractures.

One study reported overall excellent results of total hip arthroplasties at 66-month follow-up in a series of 43 hips (31 patients with systemic lupus erythematosus). Complications included superficial infections and delayed wound healing that could not be correlated with corticosteroid use.

Results for patients with rheumatoid arthritis have been favorable. One such study compared the 25-year results of a large series of patients with osteoarthritis, rheumatoid arthritis, or developmental dysplasia of the hip. Of the three groups, the patients with rheumatoid arthritis had the lowest rate of implant loosening and the highest rate of implant survival. Although all of the acetabular components were cemented in this series, other reports on the use of cementless acetabular components have also shown favorable results, with no loosening or migration of implants at 9-year follow-up.

Preoperative Planning

Upper extremities are often affected with these diseases and may impact postoperative rehabilitation. The femur can be considerably more osteopenic, thus increasing the risk of fracture, especially during initial dislocation of the hip. Long-term steroid use, which is common in this patient population, increases the extent of osteopenia and the potential for osteonecrosis and infection.

In patients with juvenile rheumatoid arthritis, the metaphysis of the femur is often large, whereas the femoral canal is very small. Increased anteversion and femoral bowing is also common in this patient population, and the joint capsule may be adherent to the underlying bone. The anteroposterior measurement is disproportionate to the mediolateral measurement and may require a custom-made or mini stem. Soft-tissue releases

and tenotomies are often necessary to address contracture deformities. Acetabular protrusio is often present in patients with inflammatory joint disease.

The cervical spine should be assessed for evidence of C1-C2 subluxation before intubation. Collaboration with the patient's rheumatologist is advisable with regard to medications and care planning.

Surgical Considerations

Careful attention should be given to patient positioning. Excessive lordosis of the lumbar spine may potentially predispose patients to malposition of the acetabular component. The component should be placed in proper anteversion, and the range of motion should be checked with trial components in place.

Conventional trochanteric osteotomy should be avoided if possible because of the high incidence of nonunion in this patient population. An in situ femoral neck osteotomy may be necessary to avoid femoral fracture during dislocation. Occasionally, a derotational osteotomy may be necessary to address femoral deformities. When necessary, a trochanteric slide offers more reliable fixation and the blood supply to the trochanter is less affected.

If severe acetabular protrusio is present, a transtrochanteric approach should be considered. If an in situ femoral neck osteotomy is performed, the diaphyseal shaft should be mobilized, and the femoral head can then be readily removed with a corkscrew and curved osteotomes. To restore the acetabular center of rotation to a more normal lateral position, maximal anteroposterior rim contact with the component is needed. Structural or morcellized graft can be used, depending on the extent of the medial defect. The peripheral rim is slightly overreamed to create concentric convergence of the anteroposterior column walls. Medial convergence of the acetabular wall helps attain component stability.

Significant contractures of the rectus or adductors should be released. Rotational force on the femur should be gentle to avoid fracture. If the joint capsule is densely adherent to bone, a complete capsulectomy should be performed.

The choice of femoral component depends on available bone stock, neck anteversion, and surgeon experience. Although cementless fixation may be successful in patients with nondistorted canals, miniature gracile or conversely capacious femurs are preferably fixed with cemented stems. A cemented or modular component is advantageous for those femurs with increased anteversion (Figure 3).

There remains some controversy regarding acetabular component choice in patients with inflammatory arthritis. Again, the amount of bone stock available, the extent of osteoporosis, and the need for bone graft (morcellized or bulk) determines the choices. One study

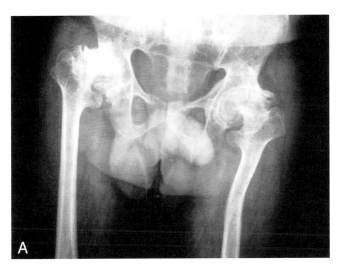
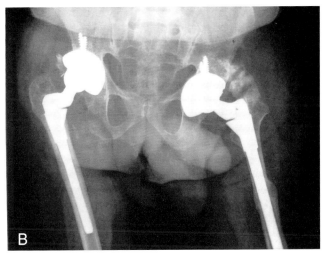

Figure 3 **A,** Preoperative radiograph of a 48-year-old man with rheumatoid arthritis and secondary degenerative arthritis of both hips, posttraumatic deformity of the left femur, and autofusion of the right hip. **B,** Postoperative radiograph of the same patient obtained 2 years after total hip arthroplasty and corrective femoral osteotomy of the left femur were performed.

reported a 60% to 70% survival rate of cemented cups at 15-year follow-up. Another study reported an 86% survival rate of porous-coated implants at mean 4.5-year follow-up.

Spondyloarthropathies

Patients with ankylosing spondylitis often have remarkable joint arthritis and soft-tissue contractures, resulting in severe stiffness and deformity. The lumbar spine can be dramatically deformed where lumbar lordosis is often lost, and nonankylosed segments may function as a fulcrum, thereby increasing the risk of spinal fracture and neurologic sequelae. Arthropathy of the hips usually occurs in the later stages of the disease. The extent of spinal involvement may make it unrealistic to achieve a full range of hip motion, especially in patients with long-standing flexion deformity.

Additionally, the fixed pelvic hyperextension that these patients develop can exaggerate anteversion in the standing position, thus predisposing them to anterior dislocation. Acetabular positioning must be adjusted to account for the pelvic deformity. Some studies have recommended obtaining a weight-bearing lateral radiograph of the pelvis preoperatively to plan patient and acetabular component positioning. Survivorship analysis has revealed that the probability of survival of the femoral component was 91% at 20 years and 83% at 30 years; the probability of survival of the acetabular components was 73% at 20 years and 70% at 30 years. The probability that both components would survive was 91% at 10 years, 73% at 20 years, and 70% at 30 years.

Preoperative Planning

The treating clinician should consider a preoperative CT scan or bone model in patients with severe defor-

mity. Because these patients are at high risk for heterotopic bone formation, preoperative radiation should be used (a single dose of 700 rads is typically administered within 24 hours of surgery). These patients are also at greater risk for pulmonary complications because of fibrotic changes and chest wall constriction. A thorough preoperative evaluation is therefore recommended to screen for cardiopulmonary involvement.

Surgical Considerations

When surgery is performed with the patient in the lateral decubitus position, particular attention should be given to the flexibility of the lumbar spine. If lumbar lordosis has been lost, acetabular component positioning should be adjusted accordingly. A trochanteric osteotomy or slide may be required to gain sufficient acetabular visibility. The final acetabular component positioning should be in 15° to 20° of anteversion. Overflexion of the cup should be avoided to decrease the risk of anterior dislocation. Because of soft-tissue contractures, tenotomy may be necessary and a partial or complete capsulectomy necessary to gain extensile exposure. If soft-tissue adhesions prevent ready femoral head dislocation, an in situ neck osteotomy should be performed to avoid intraoperative fracture. Both cemented and cementless femoral implant fixation have demonstrated satisfactory reults.

The long-term results of patients with ankylosing spondylitis showed acceptable clinical outcomes, with a low rate of complications and revisions. The probability of survival of the femoral component was 91% at 20 years and 83% at 30 years. The probability of survival of the acetabular components was 73% at 20 years and 70% at 30 years.

Metabolic Bone Disease

Patients with osteogenesis imperfecta who survive to adulthood may develop an extensive range of conditions, including premature cartilage degeneration, protrusio acetabuli, femoral bowing, and limb-length discrepancy. Multiple fractures with malunion and shortening of the extremity are also common in patients with osteogenesis imperfecta.

Preoperative Planning

Preoperative templating with many systems will be helpful. A corrective femoral osteotomy may be necessary depending on the extent of the deformity. Multiple joints are often involved, making rehabilitation challenging.

Surgical Considerations

Reconstruction of the femur may require incremental osteotomies to correct angular or torsional deformity. A modular stem can provide adjustable offsets and femoral neck lengths to achieve symmetric leg measurements. Because of bone softening, an extensively coated or cemented stem may be chosen. A well-fixed primary length stem above a bowed femur can work well in a low-activity or elderly patient. Conversely, a corrective osteotomy together with a longer stem is preferred in younger, active patients or those who are at high risk for fracture. Obtaining intraoperative radiographs after correction is recommended. Few published reports have reported the outcomes of arthroplasty in patients with osteogenesis imperfecta. Because of the tenuous quality of medial acetabular bone stock, bipolar hemiarthroplasty is not recommended in this patient population because of significant medial migration. As in other patient populations with deficient and or severely osteopenic acetabular bone, a jumbo cementless component has been shown to achieve satisfactory intermediate results and may be a viable treatment option for this specific group of patients.

Paget's Disease

In patients with Paget's disease, the alteration of subchondral bone results in weakened trabecular bone. The femur is often bowed with an enlarged femoral canal. The brittle bone subjects these patients to a high risk of perioperative fracture.

Preoperative Planning

Collaboration with the patient's rheumatologist will optimize medical therapy to minimize bone hyperactivity. Patients may have bowing of the femur as well as coxa vara deformities. Radiographs of the entire pelvis and femur should be obtained for templating. There is an increased risk of intraoperative hemorrhage in patients with this disease. Preoperative blood donation, erythro-

poietin, and/or blood cell salvage should be used, especially if an osteotomy is planned.

Surgical Considerations

Wide joint exposure during surgery may require a trochanteric slide osteotomy. If a closing wedge diaphyseal osteotomy is required, it should be performed so that the stem, whether cementless or cemented, bypasses the cut surfaces by at least 10 cm. Use of onlay femoral allograft to further buttress the junction should also be considered. As mentioned previously, blood salvage or use of a cell saver device is recommended because of the increased vascularity of bone in patients with Paget's disease.

One recent study reported on 18 patients with Paget's disease (average age, 71 years) who underwent total hip arthroplasty using cementless components. Surgery was reported to be technically demanding because of hard sclerotic bone and excessive bleeding in some patients; estimated blood loss averaged 996 mL. At an average 7-year follow-up, hip scores improved significantly, and there was clinical and radiographic evidence of bone ingrowth in all patients. No revisions for component loosening were required, and no clinical or radiographic evidence of implant loosening was identified.

Previous Trauma or Surgery

Posttraumatic arthritis is often accompanied by a combination of scarring and distorted anatomy. Significant deformity may also be present in the metaphyseal region, and/or patients may have total obliteration of the medullary canal. Posttraumatic or postoperative situations may produce significant femoral malunion, broken hardware, and canal stenosis or occlusion and stress risers at the base of the greater trochanter.

A recent study evaluated patients who underwent total hip replacement after previous fixation of a femoral neck fracture. A 92% survivorship (end point, free of revision) was reported at 10-year follow-up. Major perioperative complications occurred in 45% of patients and included intraoperative femoral fractures and dislocations. Twenty-five percent of the patients with intraoperative femoral fractures experienced femoral component loosening at a later time.

Hip arthroplasty as a salvage procedure after fixation of an intertrochanteric fracture has recently shown more promising results. Preoperative planning is essential in that many of these patients require specialized components. A calcar replacement design, extended femoral neck stem, or long-stem implant was used in 51 of 60 hips in a recent series. Forty-four patients were available for follow-up at an average of 5 years. Thirty-nine of these patients (89%) had no pain or mild pain, and five had moderate or severe pain in the region of the greater trochanter. Forty patients were able to walk,

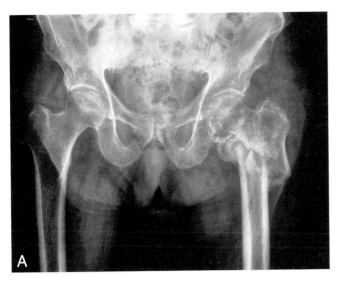
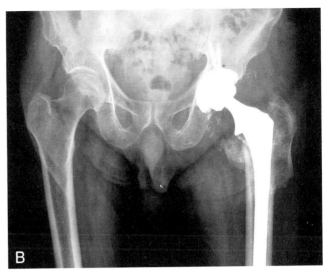

Figure 4 **A,** Preoperative radiograph of an 82-year-old man who was unable to undergo surgery until 4 months after his fracture because of medical comorbidities. **B,** Postoperative radiograph of the same patient after undergoing total hip arthroplasty using an extensively coated stem.

26 with one-arm support or no support. Five patients required revisions that included one rewiring procedure because of trochanteric avulsion, one late removal of trochanteric hardware, and one débridement of fat necrosis. Kaplan-Meier survivorship analysis with revision of the implant for any reason as the end point revealed a survival rate of 100% at 7-year follow-up and 87.5% at 10-year follow-up (95% confidence interval, 67.3% to 100%).

Preoperative Planning
Radiographs of the entire femur and pelvis should be obtained preoperatively to locate residual hardware. Moreland hooks should be available during surgery to remove sclerotic bone and membrane. Broken screws usually can be removed with a crown drill. If the retained hardware is not painful and will not impede implant seating or range of motion, it may be best to leave it in place. Preoperative radiation may be indicated to avoid heterotopic bone. To ensure proper equipment availability and reduce surgical time, it is beneficial to obtain prior surgical notes, especially if there is hardware present.

If hardware removal is required, several studies have shown that when done as a single procedure additional risks are present. One study suggested the use of two-stage implantation to optimize healing and reduce the risk of infection associated with definitive arthroplasty. A trochanteric osteotomy or slide for extensile exposure may be required because of surgical scarring and to prevent inadvertent intraoperative fracture.

The arthroplasty is greatly affected by the type of hardware fixation (such as multiple screws, blade plate, and AO cobra plate), the quality and quantity of the abductor muscles, and the quality of trochanteric fixation.

The clinician should take care to assess the leg lengths and the status of the spine and ipsilateral knee.

Preoperative radiation therapy should be considered to reduce the likelihood of heterotopic bone development. The increased risk of postoperative dislocation can be minimized by use of a hip brace and patient conditioning.

Surgical Considerations
A trochanteric osteotomy is often warranted with a complete capsulectomy. Osteotomy of the femoral neck should be performed with careful preservation of the posterior and superior acetabular bone stock. The anterior-inferior iliac spine, the teardrop, and the ischium are helpful landmarks to accomplish this goal.

The patient's own femoral head can be used as an autograft to address deficiencies from previous hardware. A calcar neck or modular implant can be used for proximal bone deficiencies, and a long-stem prosthesis can be used to bypass other defects in the femoral shaft as well as restore proper anteversion and balance leg lengths. The femoral stem, whether cemented or cementless, should bypass the lowest screw hole by at least two canal diameters. If cemented, cortical polymethylmethacrylate extravasation should be prevented by the occlusion of the screw holes. Alternatively, an extensively coated porous stem can achieve fixation in the distally intact diaphyseal bone (Figure 4).

Hip Arthrodesis
Preoperative Planning
Historically, arthrodesis of the hip has been shown to provide both satisfactory pain relief and provide patients with the ability to maintain ambulatory function

in the posttraumatic or septic hip. However, functional load transfer to adjacent joints (knees, spine, and contralateral hip) may hasten degenerative change in these joints. Arthrodeses typically are performed in younger or high-load occupation individuals. As this population ages and adjacent joints become symptomatic, a takedown of the arthrodesis may be a joint-preserving procedure for adjacent joints as symptoms develop.

Surgical Considerations

If arthrodesis of the hip is performed, the osteotomy should be performed as close to the acetabulum as possible. A trochanteric slide may be necessary for exposure. Following femoral neck osteotomy and shaft mobilization, the acetabular reamers should be centered around the fovea. The depth of reaming is established at the medial extent of residual foveal soft tissue by use of a depth gauge via a drill hole through the medial wall. On the femoral side, a high-speed drill may be necessary to open the intramedullary canal. A long intramedullary guide rod and cannulated reamers can help establish a neutral femoral axis. It is advantageous for the femoral stem to have sufficient offset to restore abductor biomechanics and improve range of motion. It is important to obtain intraoperative radiographs with trial components in place.

The most common complications after conversion to total hip arthroplasty include femoral shaft perforations, trochanteric nonunions, dislocation, wound infection, and peroneal nerve palsy. Preoperative radiation should also be considered. Conversion of a fused hip to a total hip arthroplasty typically has a favorable outcome; however, the technically demanding nature of the procedure should not be underestimated.

In a recently reported series of patients who underwent conversion of a fused hip to total hip arthroplasty, complications included 15 nerve palsies in 24 hips. Twenty-eight hips had heterotopic ossification, but it was not associated with a recurrence of ankylosis or a marked reduction of motion. Revision arthroplasty was performed in 12 hips. The probability of survival of the implant was 96.1% at 10 years, 89.9% at 15 years, and 72.8% at 26 years.

Limb-Length Discrepancies

Limb lengthening or shortening is often indicated for many of the previously mentioned conditions.

Preoperative Planning

Preoperative measurements can be obtained from weight-bearing AP pelvis films. If mechanical devices are used for intraoperative measurement, it is crucial that the leg is repositioned accurately. If limb lengthening is necessary, up to 3 cm can be functionally gained.

Surgical Considerations

Careful attention needs to be given to the sciatic nerve in limb-lengthening procedures, and intraoperative monitoring may be beneficial. Measuring must be meticulous both preoperatively and intraoperatively to avoid overlengthening. In addition to sciatic nerve palsy, low back pain can also result from overlengthening. Overshortening can result in impaired abductor function, with a potential increase in dislocation potential.

One study reported on 85 consecutive patients who had primary total hip arthroplasty in which calipers were used and showed that 43 patients had limb-length discrepancy preoperatively and 14 had limb-length discrepancy after surgery. Eleven limbs had been lengthened from 0.5 to 1 cm compared with the contralateral limb. Of the 42 patients with equal limb lengths preoperatively, 3 had a lengthened limb postoperatively compared with the contralateral limb.

An alternative technique for measuring intraoperative limb lengthening in which a vertical Steinmann pin is used at the infracotyloid groove of the acetabulum was studied in 100 consecutive primary total hip arthroplasties. The predicted intraoperative correction was correlated with postoperative radiographic measurements. Preoperative limb-length discrepancy had a mean of −4.2mm and postoperative limb-length discrepancy had a mean of 1.9 mm. None of the patients had to use shoe lifts for equalization of limb lengths.

More recently, navigation has been used to accurately measure leg length and offsets. Several studies have demonstrated remarkable precision and consistency with this technology. However, current methods and additional surgical time are expensive. The utility of this tool requires additional design, iterations, and clinical outcomes.

Summary

Orthopaedic surgeons must be aware of the potentially increased complication rate for total hip arthroplasty in patients with congenitally abnormal hips or those who have undergone previous hip surgery. Successful management of these challenging patients requires close attention to detail. If surgical hardware is retained, the prior surgical record and appropriate extraction equipment should be available. Additionally, patients who are at risk for heterotopic bone formation should undergo radiation treatment preoperatively. Radiographs of the entire femur and pelvis should be obtained preoperatively and used to template several different systems to determine the best fit. If bone distortion is severe, a CT scan and/or bone model may be necessary. Limb-length discrepancies should be measured preoperatively with weight-bearing radiographs and markers, and the correction should be confirmed intraoperatively. For limb lengthening greater than 3 cm, intraoperative monitoring or navigation should be considered, and overlengthening should always be avoided. When necessary, intraoperative radiographs should be obtained with the trial components in place. Surgeons should also always have a contingency plan. Favorable surgical outcomes are attainable with meticulous preoperative planning and adherence to surgical principles.

Annotated Bibliography

Developmental Dysplasia

Bono JV, McCarthy JC, Turner RH: Complications in total hip arthroplasty, in Pellicci PM, Tria AJ, Garvin KL (eds): *Orthopaedic Knowledge Update : Hip and Knee Reconstruction 2*. Rosemont, IL, American Academy of Orthopaedic Surgeons, 2000, pp 155-166.

This chapter reviews potential complications following total hip arthroplasty, including infection, thromboembolism, heterotopic ossification, trochanteric nonunion, intraoperative fracture, dislocation, stem failure, and nerve and vascular injury. The authors reported that the incidence of nerve palsy increases from 3.7% to 5.2% for patients with congenital dislocation.

Cabanela ME: Total hip arthroplasty for developmental dysplasia of the hip. *Orthopedics* 2001;24(9):865-866.

The author of this article discusses the surgical options available to address bony deformities and soft-tissue abnormalities associated with developmental dysplasia of the hip.

Cameron HU, Lee OB, Chou H: Total hip arthroplasty in patients with deficient bone stock and small femoral canals. *J Arthroplasty* 2003;18(1):35-40.

This study reported outcomes and complications for 34 patients with developmental dysplasia of the hip who had inadequate bone stock. Two acetabular revisions were performed for polyethylene wear, and one femoral component fracture occurred that remained asymptomatic at 7.8-year follow-up.

Dearborn JT, Harris WH: Acetabular revision after failed total hip arthroplasty in patients with congenital hip dislocation and dysplasia: Results after a mean of 8.6 years. *J Bone Joint Surg Am* 2000;82-A(8):1146-1153.

This study reported that the mechanical failure for cementless hemispherical acetabular components was 3% (2 of 61) for the entire series and 4% (2 of 52) for patients with a primary diagnosis of dysplasia at mean follow-up of 8.6 years.

DiFazio F, Shon WY, Salvati EA, Wilson PD Jr: Long-term results of total hip arthroplasty with a cemented custom-designed swan-neck femoral component for congenital dislocation or severe dysplasia: A follow-up note. *J Bone Joint Surg Am* 2002;84-A(2):204-207.

The authors of this study reported on 19 total hip arthroplasties with custom femoral components in patients with congenital dislocation at a mean 13.3-year follow-up. Radiograph evidence of acetabular loosening was identified in 33% of pa-

tients. The total rate of cup failure (radiographic loosening and revision) was 43%.

Ito H, Matsuno T, Minami A, Aoki Y: Intermediate-term results after hybrid total hip arthroplasty for the treatment of dysplastic hips. *J Bone Joint Surg Am* 2003;85-A(9):1725-1732.

In this study, clinical and radiographic evaluation was done on 100 hips at mean 10.6-year follow-up after hybrid total hip arthroplasty in patients with dysplasia. Structural acetabular allograft was used in 15 hips. Early migration of the acetabular component was seen in 6 of the 15 hips with allograft but then stabilized. Two acetabular revisions were done to treat recurrent dislocation.

Masonis JL, Patel JV, Miu A, et al: Subtrochanteric shortening and derotational osteotomy in primary total hip arthroplasty for patients with severe hip dysplasia: A 5-year follow-up. *J Arthroplasty* 2003;18(suppl 1)68-73.

Total hip arthroplasties were performed in the hips of 21 patients with Crowe grade III or IV hip dysplasia using a subtrochanteric shortening osteotomy. The authors reported that 33% of patients required structural acetabular autograft. Ninety-one percent of femoral osteotomies healed without complication. Two osteotomy nonunions required revision. Two acetabular revisions were performed to treat malposition and polyethylene failure. Three patients experienced postoperative dislocation. One cemented femoral component was revised for loosening.

Sanchez-Sotelo J, Trousdale RT, Berry DJ, Cabanela ME: Surgical treatment of developmental dysplasia of the hip in adults: I. Nonarthroplasty options. *J Am Acad Orthop Surg* 2002;10(5):321-333.

The authors describe acetabular reconstruction in dysplasia based on available acetabular bone stock and discuss whether bone grafting is necessary. They recommend that acetabular reconstruction take place at the normal anatomic acetabular location by medializing the component with or without a lateral bone graft. Limb-length discrepancy and the location of the acetabular component determine the femoral component choice. If femoral shortening is necessary, it is performed by metaphyseal resection with a greater trochanteric osteotomy and advancement or by a shortening subtrochanteric osteotomy. The authors report that the results of total hip arthroplasty demonstrate a high rate of pain relief and functional improvement and that the results of cementless implants are promising for early and mid-term intervals.

Inflammatory Arthritis

Katsimihas M, Taylor AH, Lee MB, Sarangi PP, Learmonth ID: Cementless acetabular replacement in patients with rheumatoid arthritis: A 6- to 14-year prospective study. *J Arthroplasty* 2003;18(1):16-22.

This study of 63 patients with rheumatoid arthritis who underwent total hip arthroplasty with a porous coated hemispherical acetabular component at mean 9.1-year follow-up reported six revisions (five to treat polyethylene wear) and concluded that 32-mm femoral heads may have contributed to the high rate of wear.

Spondyloarthropathies

Parvizi J, Schall DM, Lewallen DG, Sim FH: Outcome of uncemented hip arthroplasty components in patients with Paget's disease. *Clin Orthop* 2002;403:127-134.

The authors conducted a clinical and radiographic review of 19 patients who underwent total hip arthroplasty; bone ingrowth was reported in all patients at mean 7-year follow-up. Six of 19 hips had heterotopic bone. One hip was unstable (subluxating) at the latest follow-up. The authors concluded that these patients may be at higher risk for heterotopic bone formation and increased perioperative blood loss because of hypervascularity of the bone.

Tang WM, Chiu KY: Primary total hip arthroplasty in patients with ankylosing spondylitis. *J Arthroplasty* 2000; 15(1):52-58.

In this study, 95 arthroplasties were followed for an average of 135.4 months. Four deep infections required removal of prostheses, and two of three dislocations were anterior dislocations. Nineteen arthroplasties were revised at an average of 162.0 months, and 9 acetabular components were revised because of aseptic loosening. The authors concluded that hyperextension of the hips can lead to surgical error and predispose the prosthesis to anterior dislocation.

Previous Trauma or Surgery

Haidukewych GJ, Berry DJ: Hip arthroplasty for salvage of failed treatment of intertrochanteric hip fractures. *J Bone Joint Surg Am* 2003;85-A(5):899-904.

This study evaluated the results and complications of hip arthroplasty performed as a salvage procedure after the failed treatment of an intertrochanteric hip fracture in 60 patients at mean 5-year follow-up. A total of five reoperations were performed: two patients had a revision, one had a rewiring procedure because of trochanteric avulsion, one had late removal of trochanteric hardware, and one had débridement of fat necrosis. One patient had two dislocations, both of which were treated with closed reduction.

Sierra RJ, Cabanela ME: Conversion of failed hip hemiarthroplasties after femoral neck fractures. *Clin Orthop* 2002;399:129-139.

The authors performed 132 conversions after failed hemiarthroplasty. At mean follow-up of 7.1 years, 9 hips (6.8%) were revised for loosening and four additional hips (3%) were loose at the last follow-up. Major perioperative complications occurred frequently (45%), including 12 intraoperative femoral fractures (9%) and 13 dislocations (9.8%) Three of 12 of the intraoperative femoral fractures (25%) developed later femoral component loosening, and all occurred during conversion of an uncemented Austin-Moore type hemiprosthesis.

Hip Arthrodesis

Joshi AB, Markovic L, Hardinge K, Murphy JC: Conversion of a fused hip to total hip arthroplasty. *J Bone Joint Surg Am* 2002;84-A(8):1335-1341.

This study reviewed long-term clinical and radiographic results after conversion of a fused hip to a total hip arthroplasty of 187 patients (208 hips) with mean follow-up of 9.2 years. The authors reported that 79% to 83% had good-to-excellent results and function. There were 15 nerve palsies and 28 patients developed heterotopic ossification that was not associated marked reduction of motion. Revision arthroplasty was performed in 12 hips.

Classic Bibliography

Anderson MJ, Harris WH: Total hip arthroplasty with insertion of the acetabular component without cement in hips with total congenital dislocation or marked congenital dysplasia. *J Bone Joint Surg Am* 1999;81(3):347-354.

Benke GJ, Baker AS, Dounis E: Total hip replacement after upper femoral osteotomy: A clinical review. *J Bone Joint Surg Br* 1982;64(5):570-571.

Berry DJ: Total hip arthroplasty in patients with proximal femoral deformity. *Clin Orthop* 1999;369:262-272.

Bisla RS, Ranawat CS, Inglis AE: Total hip replacement in patients with ankylosing spondylitis with involvement of the hip. *J Bone Joint Surg Am* 1976;58(2):233-238.

Borden L, Greenky S: The difficult primary total hip replacement: Acetabular problems, in Steinberg M (ed): *The Hip and Its Disorders*. Philadelphia, PA, WB Saunders, 1991, pp 1007-1019.

Callaghan JJ, Brand RA, Pedersen DR: Hip arthrodesis: A long-term follow-up. *J Bone Joint Surg Am* 1985; 67(9):1328-1335.

Cameron HU: Management of femoral deformities during the total hip replacement. *Orthopedics* 1996;19(9): 745-746.

Cameron HU, Eren OT, Solomon M: Nerve injury in the prosthetic management of the dysplastic hip. *Orthopedics* 1998;21(9):980-981.

Chmell MJ, Scott RD, Thomas WH, Sledge CB: Total hip arthroplasty with cement for juvenile rheumatoid arthritis: Results at a minimum of ten years in patients less than thirty years old. *J Bone Joint Surg Am* 1997;79(1): 44-52.

Dorr LD, Tawakkol S, Moorthy M, Long W, Wan Z: Medial protrusio technique for placement of a porous-coated, hemispherical acetabular component without cement in a total hip arthroplasty in patients who have acetabular dysplasia. *J Bone Joint Surg Am* 1999;81(1): 83-92.

Ebraheim NA, Wong FY: Sliding osteotomy of the greater trochanter. *Am J Orthop* 1997;26(3):212-215.

Edwards BN, Tullos HS, Noble PC: Contributory factors and etiology of sciatic nerve palsy in total hip arthroplasty. *Clin Orthop* 1987;218:136-141.

Ferguson GM, Cabanela ME, Ilstrup DM: Total hip arthroplasty after failed intertrochanteric osteotomy. *J Bone Joint Surg Br* 1994;76(2):252-257.

Firestone TP, Hedley AK: Extended proximal femoral osteotomy for severe acetabular protrusion following total hip arthroplasty: A technical note. *J Arthroplasty* 1997;12(3):344-345.

Garvin KL, Bowen MK, Salvati EA, Ranawat CS: Long-term results of total hip arthroplasty in congenital dislocation and dysplasia of the hip: A follow-up note. *J Bone Joint Surg Am* 1991;73(9):1348-1354.

Gross AE: Management of the dysplastic hip. *Orthopedics* 1997;20(9):789-790.

Hanssen AD, Cabanela ME, Michet CJ Jr: Hip arthroplasty in patients with systemic lupus erythematosus. *J Bone Joint Surg Am* 1987;69(6):807-814.

Jasty M, Anderson MJ, Harris WH: Total hip replacement for developmental dysplasia of the hip. *Clin Orthop* 1995;311:40-45.

Jasty M, Webster W, Harris WH: Management of limb length inequality during total hip replacement. *Clin Orthop* 1996;333:165-171.

Kim YY, Kim BJ, Ko HS, Sung YB, Kim SK, Shim JC: Total hip reconstruction in the anatomically distorted hip: Cemented versus hybrid total hip arthroplasty. *Arch Orthop Trauma Surg* 1998;117(1-2):8-14.

Lachiewicz PF: Porous-coated total hip arthroplasty in rheumatoid arthritis. *J Arthroplasty* 1994;9(1):9-15.

Lo TC, Healy WL, Covall DJ, et al: Heterotopic bone formation after hip surgery: Prevention with single-dose postoperative hip irradiation. *Radiology* 1988;168(3): 851-854.

Malizos KN, Soucacos PN, Beris AE, Korobilias AB, Xenakis TA: Osteonecrosis of the femoral head in immunosuppressed patients: Hip salvaging with implantation of a vascularised fibular graft. *Microsurgery* 1994;15(7): 485-491.

McCarthy JC, Bono JV, Turner RH, Kremchek T, Lee J: The outcome of trochanteric reattachment in revision total hip arthroplasty with a Cable Grip System: Mean 6-year follow-up. *J Arthroplasty* 1999;14(7):810-814.

McGrory BJ, Bal BS, Harris WH: Trochanteric osteotomy for total hip arthroplasty: Six variations and indications for their use. *J Am Acad Orthop Surg* 1996;4(5): 258-267.

Poss R: Complex primary total hip arthroplasty: The difficult femur. *Instr Course Lect* 1995;44:281-286.

Ranawat CS: Surgical management of the rheumatoid hip. *Rheum Dis Clin North Am* 1998;24(1):129-141.

Reikeraas O, Lereim P, Gabor I, Gunderson R, Bjerkreim I: Femoral shortening in total arthroplasty for completely dislocated hips: 3-7 year results in 25 cases. *Acta Orthop Scand* 1996;67(1):33-36.

Reikeras O, Bjerkreim I, Gundersson R: Total hip arthroplasty for arthrodesed hips: 5- to 13-year results. *J Arthroplasty* 1995;10(4):529-531.

Ritter MA, Helphinstine J, Keating EM, Faris PM, Meding JB: Total hip arthroplasty in patients with osteonecrosis: The effect of cement techniques. *Clin Orthop* 1997;338:94-99.

Scott RD: Total hip and knee arthroplasty in juvenile rheumatoid arthritis. *Clin Orthop* 1990;259:83-91.

Skinner HB: Subtrochanteric osteotomy in total hip revision: Report of two cases. *J Arthroplasty* 1991;6(1):89-93.

Sochart DH, Paul AS, Kurdy NM: A new osteotome for performing chevron trochanteric osteotomy. *Acta Orthop Scand* 1995;66(5):445-446.

Sochart DH, Porter ML: The long-term results of Charnley low-friction arthroplasty in young patients who have congenital dislocation, degenerative osteoarthrosis, or rheumatoid arthritis. *J Bone Joint Surg Am* 1997;79(11):1599-1617.

Sochart DH, Porter ML: Long-term results of total hip replacement in young patients who had ankylosing spondylitis: Eighteen to thirty-year results with survivorship analysis. *J Bone Joint Surg Am* 1997;79(8):1181-1189.

Sponseller PD, McBeath AA, Perpich M: Hip arthrodesis in young patients: A long-term follow-up study. *J Bone Joint Surg Am* 1984;66(6):853-859.

Suominen S, Antti-Poika I, Santavirta S, Konttinen YT, Honkanen V, Lindholm TS: Total hip replacement after intertrochanteric osteotomy. *Orthopedics* 1991;14(3): 253-257.

Walker LG, Sledge CB: Total hip arthroplasty in ankylosing spondylitis. *Clin Orthop* 1991;262:198-204.

Younger TI, Bradford MS, Magnus RE, Paprosky WG: Extended proximal femoral osteotomy: A new technique for femoral revision arthroplasty. *J Arthroplasty* 1995;10(3):329-338.

Zadeh HG, Hua J, Walker PS, Muirhead-Allwood SK: Uncemented total hip arthroplasty with subtrochanteric derotational osteotomy for severe femoral anteversion. *J Arthroplasty* 1999;14(6):682-688.

Chapter 35

Posttraumatic Management of the Hip

William Macaulay, MD

Julie M. Keller, MD

Introduction

The primary goal of the treatment of hip trauma in elderly patients is to allow mobilization with full weight bearing as soon as possible after injury. This goal is facilitated via stable fixation, regardless of the fracture pattern or mode of surgical treatment because of the pain-relieving nature of a sound mechanical treatment construct. Restoring lower extremity limb length and proper rotational orientation with muscle-preserving treatment is of additional importance. The ultimate goal of treatment is to return patients to their prefracture level of function. This goal is difficult to achieve in elderly patients with hip fractures if treatment is not optimized.

It has been estimated that 6.3 million hip fractures will occur worldwide in the year 2050. In the United States alone, more than 238,000 hip fractures occurred in 1984, at a cost of $7.2 billion. In 1999, the number of hip fractures increased to 338,000. The incidence of hip fractures continues to rise and is expected to increase to more than 500,000 per year by 2040. Hip fractures and lower extremity joint pain are the most common reasons for decreased social and leisure activity in elderly patients. Patients with hip fractures or lower extremity arthroplasty make up the second largest group in rehabilitation facilities. The cost of hip fractures with regard to quality of life and health care resources is enormous.

More than 90% of hip fractures in elderly patients result from a simple fall; hip fractures in younger patients typically occur as the result of high-energy trauma. In people older than 90 years, one third of all women and one sixth of all men will experience a hip fracture. Hip fractures occur more frequently in females than males (a ratio of 3:1). This increased frequency is thought to be because of women's decreased bone mass after menopause, lighter overall body weight, and longer life expectancy. The incidence of hip fracture is greater among Caucasians than among Hispanics and African Americans. Urban dwellers, the physically inactive, people who consume excessive caffeine or alcohol, those with senile dementia, and psychotropic drug users are also at increased risk for hip fracture. Osteoporosis and osteomalacia have not been shown to be independent risk factors.

The overall 1-year mortality rate for patients with hip fractures is between 14% and 36%. Risk for mortality is increased by advanced age, number of medical comorbidities, institutionalized living, dementia, and male sex. Other possible but yet unproven risk factors include fracture type, delay of surgical treatment, and dementia.

Femoral Neck Fractures
Epidemiology and Mechanism
More than 350,000 femoral neck fractures occur each year in the United States, 97% to 98% of which occur in people older than 50 years, with the average age at time of fracture being 74 years for men and 79 years for women. This population is younger, more mobile, more independent, and less likely to require an ambulatory aid than those who experience intertrochanteric fractures, although falls from a standing position account for 90% of all femoral neck fractures. As noted previously, femoral neck fracture in a young person is most often the result of high-energy trauma, including motor vehicle crashes and falls from a height.

Osteoporosis has long been associated with hip fractures, but the patient population with femoral neck fractures does not have significantly greater osteoporosis when compared with age-matched control subjects. The progressive loss of bone strength with age leads to decreased ultimate strength and failure at loads 20% less than those required in young control subjects. Osteoporosis can also lead to altered hip geometry, including changed thickness of the femoral neck and shaft cortex, decreased index of tensile trabeculae, a wider trochanteric region, and increased hip axis length, all of which lead to increased risk of fracture.

Relevant Anatomy
The femoral neck is angled 130° ± 7° relative to the shaft and is 10° ± 6.7° anteverted. Articular cartilage, which covers the femoral head, is 4 mm thick at the

weight-bearing surface and tapers at the periphery. The calcar femorale runs from the posteromedial shaft to the cortex of the posterior neck and influences fracture patterns of the neck. The most important vascular supply to the femoral head is the lateral epiphyseal artery, which is supplied by the profunda femoris and medial femoral circumflex arteries. Because the blood supply to the femoral head surrounds the femoral neck, femoral neck fractures can devastate the femoral head blood supply. The degree of displacement of the fracture is predictive of vascular damage and the severity of the risk to the femoral head. Another threat to the blood supply of the femoral head is occlusion of neck vessels secondary to intracapsular hematoma. The hip capsule usually remains intact unless the fracture is displaced more than half the diameter of the neck, allowing for hematoma and an increase in intracapsular pressure that may occlude venous outflow and/or arteriole inflow and cause head ischemia.

Classification

The most commonly used classification system for femoral neck fractures is the Garden classification, which is based on prognosis and incidence of complications (Figure 1). The prominence of this system has persisted despite significant evidence that it is poorly reliable and has poor interobserver reproducibility. There is good intraobserver reproducibility, and evaluation with both AP and lateral radiographs helps to improve intraobserver agreement and decrease intraobserver variability. The most challenging classification seems to be in the differentiation between type III and IV fractures. Fortunately, differentiating between these two fracture types usually does not change management. The best intraobserver and interobserver reliability was found when evaluators were asked only to differentiate between displaced (types III and IV) and nondisplaced (types I and II) fractures. Therefore, it has been suggested that the Garden classification be modified to a two-category system.

Management

Management is determined by fracture type and is almost always surgical. Untreated stable nondisplaced fractures have a 20% to 30% risk of becoming displaced. Internal fixation reduces this risk and allows for early mobilization, eliminating the morbidity and mortality associated with prolonged bed rest. The treatment of choice is placement of three large cannulated screws in parallel within the femoral head and as widely spaced as possible. The inferior and posterior screws should be adjacent to the cortex of the femoral neck (within 3 mm), but drilling of the lateral femoral cortex should not occur below the lesser trochanter because this can lead to subtrochanteric fracture. Similar treatment in

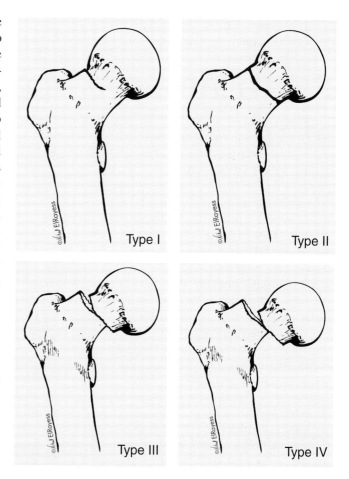

Figure 1 The Garden classification of femoral neck fractures. Type I: incomplete fracture impacted in the valgus position. Type II: nondisplaced, complete fracture. Type III: complete fracture displaced in a varus position. Type IV: completely displaced fracture with the trabeculae of the head realigned with the trabeculae of the acetabulum. *(Copyright © Nihal ElRayess, Medical Illustrator.)*

Scandinavia has been performed with the hook pin osteosynthesis. There is no proven advantage to adding a fourth screw, and all threads should firmly grip the head fragment (not rest traversing the fracture site).

Patients who were completely nonambulatory prior to injury can be treated conservatively, with early mobilization to a chair. The inability to maintain hygiene and discomfort are indications for conversion to hemiarthroplasty or total hip arthroplasty (THA).

For patients with displaced fractures, the primary goal of treatment is return to preinjury level of function. Early mobilization leads to fewer medical complications, improved ultimate function, and decreased length of hospital stay and overall cost. Surgical treatment is therefore indicated for all except the most fragile and bedbound patients. Treatment choices include internal fixation versus arthroplasty (unipolar/bipolar hemiarthroplasty versus total hip replacement) and the debate is ongoing as to which is superior. Internal fixation carries a risk of nonunion and osteonecrosis, in which instance repeat surgery and conversion to a prosthesis may be required, but the native, healed femoral head is usually superior in performance and longevity to prosthetic replacement. One study found that with good reduction and multiple screw fixation, the failure rate of fixation and nonunion was less than 10% and the rate of osteonecrosis was 10% to 30%, with 6.5% of patients having associated segmental collapse. Another study found a 54% relative risk reduction for complications with internal fixation versus arthroplasty, although other studies have reported fewer complications with arthroplasty.

The relative risk reduction for revision to arthroplasty versus repeat internal fixation is 77%. Seventeen percent (10% of low-risk patients and 50% of high-risk patients) of those treated with internal fixation typically require reoperation. Although satisfactory salvage to THA is usually possible, outcomes are worse than with primary replacement. With arthroplasty, there is no risk of osteonecrosis, nonunion, or failure of fixation. There are concerns regarding acetabular erosion with hemiarthroplasty as well as concerns regarding dislocation, infection, loosening, and limb-length inequality with all types of arthroplasty. When choosing among unipolar, bipolar, and THA, the patient's functional demands, life expectancy, and bone quality should be considered. Arthroplasty results in increased blood loss and surgical time compared with internal fixation. Hemiarthroplasty has twice the risk of dislocation compared with THA, and if conversion from hemiarthroplasty to THA is required, the surgery is technically difficult and the outcome is typically poor when compared with primary THA. Bipolar prostheses may decrease the acetabular erosion that occurs with all hemiarthroplasties because they theoretically decrease friction and increase cushioning, but the actual benefits are not clear. A recent prospective randomized trial found no differences in functional outcomes or quality of life at 1-year follow-up for elderly patients with femoral neck fractures. Given these data and the higher cost of bipolar devices, there does not seem to be an advantage to using bipolar instead of unipolar prostheses. Based on existing data, standard recommendations have been established for choosing a treatment modality for patients with displaced femoral neck fractures (Table 1).

Intertrochanteric Fractures
Epidemiology and Mechanism
Intertrochanteric fractures of the femur occur between the extracapsular femoral neck and the area just distal to the lesser trochanter. Approximately half of all hip fractures are intertrochanteric, and the patient population is typically older and has more medical comorbidities and worse ambulatory status than patients with other types of hip fractures. Women are affected two to eight times more often than men. As the longevity of a

Table 1 | Standard Recommendations for the Treatment of Patients With Displaced Femoral Neck Fractures

For young patients with good bone quality and few medical comorbidities, the goal is preservation of the native femoral head. Treatment consists of open reduction and internal fixation with three cannulated screws in parallel. Revision to THA is indicated with failure of fixation and can usually be undertaken with minimal complications.

For community ambulators, the goal is restoration of function. Preinjury functional status, life expectancy, and bone quality should all be considered when planning treatment. For elderly patients with normal anticipated longevity but poor bone density or severe comminution, the rate of osteonecrosis is 36%, and it is unlikely that reduction can be maintained or that internal fixation will be successful. Therefore, hybrid or cementless THA results in the best functional ambulatory outcome and pain control.

For inactive elderly patients with poor bone density, hemiarthroplasty avoids the risk of osteonecrosis and nonunion (which can occur in more than 40% of patients).

For patients with pathologic bone disease, severe chronic illness, rheumatoid arthritis, osteoarthritis, or Paget's disease, THA is the treatment of choice.

For bedbound, nonambulatory patients, a trial of nonsurgical treatment is acceptable. If insufficient routine nursing care is not available or if pain relief is not sufficient, internal fixation, unipolar hemiarthroplasty, or excisional arthroplasty are all treatment options.

For patients with cognitive impairment, arthroplasty has been shown to decrease the rate of mortality and the risk for revision; therefore, it should be strongly considered in treating this patient population. Methods to decrease the risk of dislocation should be undertaken.

population increases, so do the number of unstable, comminuted intertrochanteric fractures. This increase in fracture severity correlates directly with the decrease in bone quality associated with age, independent of sex or menopausal status; osteopenia is an independent risk factor for intertrochanteric fractures.

Most intertrochanteric fractures occur at home after simple falls. The elderly fall more frequently because of decreased visual and hearing acuity, gait disturbances, and the use of psychotropic medications. These falls lead to fracture because of slower ambulatory speed and decreased forward inertia causing a sideways fall. The elderly have impaired protective responses, inadequate soft tissue surrounding the trochanter (to dissipate the energy of the fall), and inadequate bone strength to withstand the residual energy of the fall. An intertrochanteric fracture in a young person is the result of high-energy trauma, and the possibility of additional occult injuries should be excluded by a routine trauma evaluation.

Relevant Anatomy
The intertrochanteric region of the femur is made up of dense trabecular bone that is concentrated at the medial femoral neck and fans out under the dome of the head of

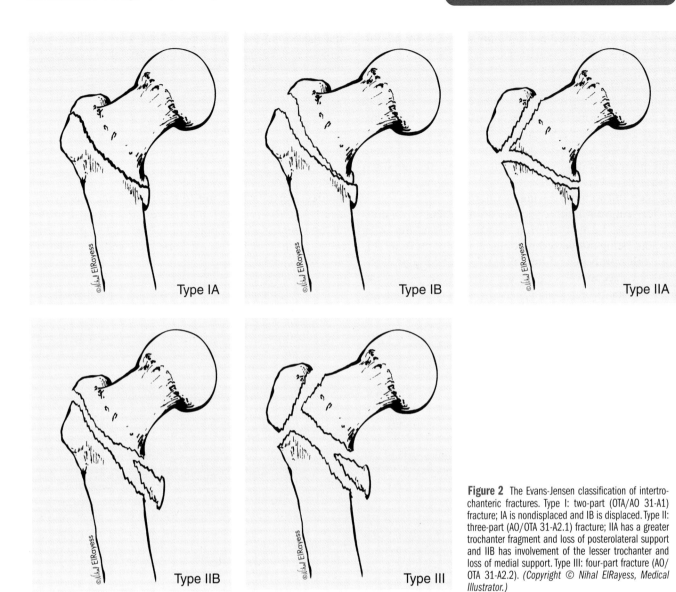

Figure 2 The Evans-Jensen classification of intertrochanteric fractures. Type I: two-part (OTA/AO 31-A1) fracture; IA is nondisplaced and IB is displaced. Type II: three-part (AO/OTA 31-A2.1) fracture; IIA has a greater trochanter fragment and loss of posterolateral support and IIB has involvement of the lesser trochanter and loss of medial support. Type III: four-part fracture (AO/OTA 31-A2.2). *(Copyright © Nihal ElRayess, Medical Illustrator.)*

the femur. The dense cancellous bone transmits body weight to the lower extremities, with the calcar femorale, a vertical wall of bone running from the posteromedial shaft to the posterior femoral neck, providing the strongest stress conduit. The iliopsoas attaches at the lesser trochanter and the hip abductors, and the short internal rotators attach at the greater trochanter, providing strong muscular forces across the region that lead to the characteristic shortening and external rotation with fracture. This bony region has a rich and redundant blood supply. Therefore, osteonecrosis of this area is rare.

Classification

There is no ideal system for the classification of intertrochanteric fractures. The most commonly used system was created by Evans in 1949, which is based on the stability of the fracture pattern and the ability to convert an unstable fracture to a stable reduction (Figure 2).

Evans recognized that fractures with comminution of the posteromedial cortex and calcar femorale are inherently unstable and that medial cortical opposition must be obtained to restore stability. In 1975, Jensen modified this system to include subcategories based on the reducibility of the fracture and the possibility of later loss of reduction. This system is important in that it differentiates stable and unstable fractures and helps to define the characteristics of a stable reduction. Clinical studies have shown poor reproducibility using this system. Therefore, the most valuable characteristic noted using this classification may simply be stable versus unstable.

Management

Relative indications for nonsurgical treatment include nonambulatory status, dementia, adequate pain control, medical instability for surgery, skin breakdown over the surgical site, and chronic asymptomatic fracture. For patients who are definitively nonambulatory, early mobilization out of bed to a chair with adequate pain control should be prescribed to avoid skin breakdown. For patients for whom ambulation is an eventual possibility, traction of 15% of the body weight with a pin through the proximal tibia and balanced suspension with minimal abduction should be used. The goal of this treatment is anatomic union and preservation of function. Traction should be maintained for 8 to 12 weeks; patients should then be advanced to partial weight bearing and then full weight bearing as tolerated.

Surgical treatment is preferred for patients with nondisplaced and displaced intertrochanteric fractures, with the goal being stable reduction and strong internal fixation with a well-placed implant and immediate ambulation. The success of surgical treatment depends on several factors: bone quality, fracture pattern stability, adequacy of reduction, implant design, and aseptic/atraumatic implant placement. Fracture reduction, the first controllable variable, is vital for optimal functioning of the implant and restoration of function. In a stable fracture, reduction can be accomplished with distal traction, abduction, and internal rotation. The intact medial cortex will support the compressive load created by anatomic reduction. If the fracture is unstable, perfect fracture fragment reduction may be more difficult and unnecessary. The goal of reduction (if possible) is to reestablish the anatomic relationship between the proximal fragment containing the head and neck and the shaft of the femur.

An alternative to anatomic reduction is a valgus reduction with high-angled fixation (140° to 150°). This alignment decreases bending forces across the implant, offsets shortening, and increases compressive forces by reorienting the plane of the fracture more perpendicular to the weight-bearing vector. It is also believed that this alignment results in more sliding of the implant, although no clear benefit to this has been determined. A disadvantage is that the implant is in the superolateral portion of the femoral head, which is weaker than the central portion, increasing the risk of cut-out. Overall, there is no indication to use a valgus reduction if anatomic alignment can be achieved.

The original devices used for intertrochanteric fracture repair were rigid nail plate fixation devices, which had a 40% rate of complications. Compression devices were developed to overcome the flaws of the rigid nail plate fixation devices. By allowing for impaction after fixation, the device allowed for immediate stabilization of the fracture and acted as a load-sharing rather than a load-bearing device. Immediate weight bearing was then possible, the complications of prolonged immobility were avoided, and the loss of fixation occurs in only 4% to 12% of patients. Originally, sliding nail and plate devices were used; these were quickly replaced by sliding screw and plate devices. Because of the superior proximal fixation of the screw, these devices are still the most commonly used and are available with angles measuring from 125° to 150°. Theoretic advantages of the 150° plate include shortening offset; the compressive force is closer to the resultant vertically weight-bearing force across the hip, allowing for impaction; and there is a smaller varus moment, which should lead to less implant failure in patients with high-energy injuries (comminuted intertrochanteric fractures). No difference in the amount of impaction or sliding has been reported, and the device is more difficult to insert, with the diaphyseal insertion point resulting in a greater stress riser than the metaphyseal insertion point of a less angled plate. Because of its comparable performance and the relative ease of a central insertion, the use of 135° plate devices is recommended.

Secure placement in the proximal fragment is the most important goal in placement of the device. Central positioning in the head and neck, within 1 cm of subchondral bone is ideal. If this cannot be achieved, posteroinferior placement is preferred over anterosuperior placement to reduce the risk of cut-out. An important measure of placement is the tip-apex distance, which is the sum of the distance of the tip of the lag screw from the apex of the femoral head in both standard AP and lateral radiographs of the hip. It is used to evaluate the position of the lag screw reliably and reproducibly across series of patients. The apex of the femoral head is identified by a line projected from the center of and parallel to the femoral neck. A high tip-apex distance is indicative of deviation from central placement of the screw and is highly predictive of need for reoperation. In patients with fixation failure, the tip-apex distance is significantly higher than in patients without fixation failure. Preoperative impacted reduction is necessary to prevent postoperative collapse that exceeds the sliding capacity of the device, which turns it into the functional equivalent of a fixed device. If excess collapse is anticipated, a short barrel device should be used.

The patient should be placed in the supine position on a fracture table, with both feet in holders and the ipsilateral groin placed against a padded perineal post. The fracture should be reduced with gentle longitudinal traction and internal rotation. The opposite leg should be flexed and abducted to allow for positioning of the image intensifier. Biplanar visualization of the entire proximal femur should be used to assess for varus angulation, posterior sag, and malrotation, all of which should be corrected prior to implant placement. Most fractures can be adequately reduced using a closed technique; if reduction is not possible with few efforts, open reduction rather than excess force should be used.

Plate length should be chosen based on the fracture pattern and the stability of the fixation. Studies have shown that three-hole fixation is adequate, although some surgeons still prefer four-hole fixation. If there is a large posteromedial fragment, reduction using cerclage wires and a lag screw should be used to achieve near-anatomic reduction. Anatomic reduction is not required; instead, the goal should be to position the fragment to act as a buttress against varus displacement. The increase in stability attributable to this repair is proportional to the fragment size. A displaced greater trochanter also requires fixation to restore abductor function. Tension banding with cerclage wires is preferred. Complications with sliding hip screw fixation are not thought to be decreased by delayed or limited weight bearing; therefore, immediate, full weight bearing is recommended.

Intramedullary nailing is an alternative method of fixation. The Ender nail was the most commonly used device, and poor results were common with its initial use. The procedure was technically difficult and resulted in complication rates of 16% to 71% and reoperation rates of 19%. Varus deformity, knee pain caused by distal migration of the nail, and external rotation deformity were problematic, and the nail was only indicated for use in elderly, disabled patients with a stable fracture and low tolerance for surgery. The creation of the Gamma nail, a combination intramedullary nail and compression device, again established a use for intramedullary nails in treatment of intertrochanteric fractures. This device offers the theoretic advantages of limited fracture site exposure, decreased surgical time, decreased blood loss, and a shorter lever arm and bending moment. Clinical trials have not universally demonstrated significant differences when comparing the results of the Gamma nail with those of the sliding hip screw and plate device in regards to blood loss, length of hospital stay, rate of infection, rate of wound complication, or incidence of implant failure. The Gamma nail also has the additional risk of femoral shaft fracture at the tip or the implant or at the site of the distal locking bolts. However, improvements in the device and increased surgeon experience have resulted in improved clinical outcomes with the use of the Gamma nail. In addition, this device is easier to place in the optimal position, as indicated by lower tip-apex distance values compared with those of screw and plate devices, but it has significantly poorer performance than the sliding hip screw device with a high tip-apex distance. Some recent clinical investigations have therefore not recommended regular use of the Gamma nail instead of the sliding hip screw; it is recommended only for specific situations.

The Gamma nail is currently recommended for the treatment of reverse obliquity fractures. The sliding hip screw allows for medial displacement and therefore no impaction in patients with reverse obliquity intertrochanteric fractures, making intramedullary devices a better treatment choice. The Gamma nail is also useful in the treatment of high subtrochanteric and commi-nuted fractures with subtrochanteric extension. As the stability of the fracture decreases, the Gamma nail transmits a decreased load to the calcar femorale so that with a four-part fracture, there is virtually no strain on the bone.

Another option for intramedullary fixation is a device that uses two small-diameter lag screws placed into the femoral head. Theoretically, two proximal screws provide greater rotational control of the femoral head fragment than a single screw. Also, rotational control is inherent in the nail design and not dependent on multiple parts that are likely to increase the risk of mechanical failure. This type of device is technically difficult to insert because it requires the placement of two screws into the femoral neck, which is a challenge in the small, often osteoporotic bones of elderly female patients who most commonly experience this type of fracture. Two such devices, the trochanteric antegrade nail (TAN, Smith & Nephew, Memphis, TN) and the proximal femoral nail (PFN, Synthes, West Chester, PA); each has slightly different characteristics. TAN implants use smaller diameter lag screws and no sleeve (7 mm for the TAN, 9 mm for the Intramedullary Hip Screw [IMHS, Smith & Nephew] [12-mm sleeve]), so the proximal aspects of the intramedullary nail do not need to be as flared (13 mm for the TAN versus 17 mm for the IMHS) to prevent mechanical failure of the nail at the lag screw hole. There are concerns, however, that the smaller diameter screws may be more prone to bending (which would prevent sliding) and migration through the femoral head and thereby increase the incidence of screw cut-out. The PFN has been found to have more secondary varus deformity and a greater incidence of fracture site collapse because of screw migration when compared with the intramedullary nail, but other studies have not supported these results and have found no differences between the devices.

Both nails have a decreased proximal nail diameter that requires little or no reaming of the proximal femur and potentially lowers the incidence of iatrogenic proximal femur fracture. Results from one study found that when compared with the Gamma nail, the PFN resulted in fewer associated diaphyseal and greater trochanteric insertion site fractures, requires equal healing time and achievement of fracture reduction, shorter surgical time, reduced postoperative transfusion, and results in less cut-out. The TAN had a greater ultimate failure load than the intramedullary nail, but otherwise proved equal in all functional parameters. Significant differences in postoperative function have not been found, and the indications for the use of this device versus a sliding hip screw have not been investigated. Indications for the use of these devices and whether these devices are superior to either intramedullary compression devices or sliding hip screws remain unclear.

Primary arthroplasty after an intertrochanteric fracture does not offer advantages over a properly placed sliding hip screw, and because of greater surgical risks, it is not routinely used. In patients with a severely comminuted and unstable fracture, primary arthroplasty may be indicated, but it is otherwise reserved for treating postoperative loss of fixation when internal fixation is not possible or desired. A calcar-replacing prosthesis should be used according to surgical techniques described elsewhere.

The sliding hip screw is the most commonly used device in the repair of intertrochanteric fractures. Common complications associated with this device include varus displacement, malrotation, and nonunion. Varus displacement occurs with an unstable fracture with loss of posteromedial support and cutting out of the screw through the anterosuperior femoral head. This complication is attributable to an unstable initial reduction leading to collapse beyond the sliding capacity of the screw, misplacement of the screw in the weak anterior portion of the head, improper reaming leading to the creation of a second channel, inadequate screw/barrel alignment that disallows sliding, or severe osteoporosis leading to inadequate fixation. Management options include acceptance of the resulting deformity for patients who are nonambulatory or cannot undergo surgery, reattempting internal fixation, or conversion to a hemiarthroplasty or THA.

Malrotation is most often caused by internal rotation of the distal fragment at the time of fixation. An unstable fracture should be reduced to neutral or slight external rotation to avoid this complication. Nonunion occurs in less than 2% of all intertrochanteric fractures. If the bone stock is good, repeat internal fixation with valgus osteotomy and bone graft should be attempted. In most patients, conversion to a calcar-replacing endoprosthesis is required.

Other rare complications include osteonecrosis, screw/barrel disengagement, and screw migration into the acetabulum. Osteonecrosis occurs with extreme comminution and soft-tissue damage; disengagement and migration can be avoided with proper placement of the device.

Polymethylmethacrylate as an adjunct to internal fixation devices can improve screw purchase in osteoporotic bone and replace deficient medial cortex, but the impact of polymethylmethacrylate is not clear. Calcium phosphate cement can be incorporated and remodeled and cured euthermically at a neutral pH. It has been shown by industry-supported research to increase the strength of fixation when injected into a reamed channel, and no clinical complications have been reported in initial studies. Calcium phosphate cement may eventually replace polymethylmethacrylate in the treatment of fractures in patients with osteoporotic bone, but additional investigation is required before it can be recommended for primary repair.

Subtrochanteric Fractures
Epidemiology and Mechanism
Subtrochanteric fractures, which occur between the lesser trochanter and the isthmus of the diaphysis of the femoral shaft, account for 10% to 34% of all hip fractures. They occur in a bimodal distribution, with approximately two thirds occurring in patients 50 years and older and one third in patients 24 to 49 years old. In young patients, subtrochanteric fractures occur as a result of high-energy trauma including motor vehicle collisions, pedestrian-vehicle collisions, falls from significant heights, and penetrating injuries. Ten percent of these fractures are caused by gunshot wounds. Nonpenetrating trauma is most often the result of direct lateral impact or caused by axial loading. These fractures are often severely comminuted, involving large areas of the proximal femur, and the potential for soft-tissue damage and vascular compromise is significant. Ipsilateral patellar and tibial fractures are the most commonly associated injuries, but with all trauma patients a thorough examination is required. In older patients, subtrochanteric fractures typically occur with low-velocity trauma, such as a simple fall. These fractures often involve minimal comminution; transverse, short, oblique, or spiral fractures are common. A significant increase in low-energy subtrochanteric fractures is expected over the next two decades.

Relevant Anatomy
Advances in the understanding of subtrochanteric anatomy and fracture biomechanics and the subsequent development of better implants and new surgical techniques have improved treatment of this notoriously challenging fracture type. The subtrochanteric region displays high interspecimen variation in linear and angular measurements and has an anterior and slightly lateral bow; both factors can affect the choice and efficacy of an implant. The region is circumferentially covered by well-vascularized muscle that ensures good blood supply to the area but may complicate surgical exposure with profuse bleeding. The iliopsoas, gluteus maximus, gluteus medius, gluteus minimus, and hip abductors all insert in the subtrochanteric region, where they contribute powerful forces that act on the individual fragments and can cause shortening and adduction of the distal fragment. The medial and posterior cortex is a site of high compressive forces, and the lateral cortex experiences high tensile stresses. The strong bending, torsional, and axial forces across the region all complicate stabilization of fractures.

Classification
A classification system is useful if it alerts the surgeon to potential complications, recommends specific treatment options, and demonstrates interobserver reproducibility. Systems for subtrochanteric fractures continue to evolve. The Seinsheimer system, developed in 1978, is a concise

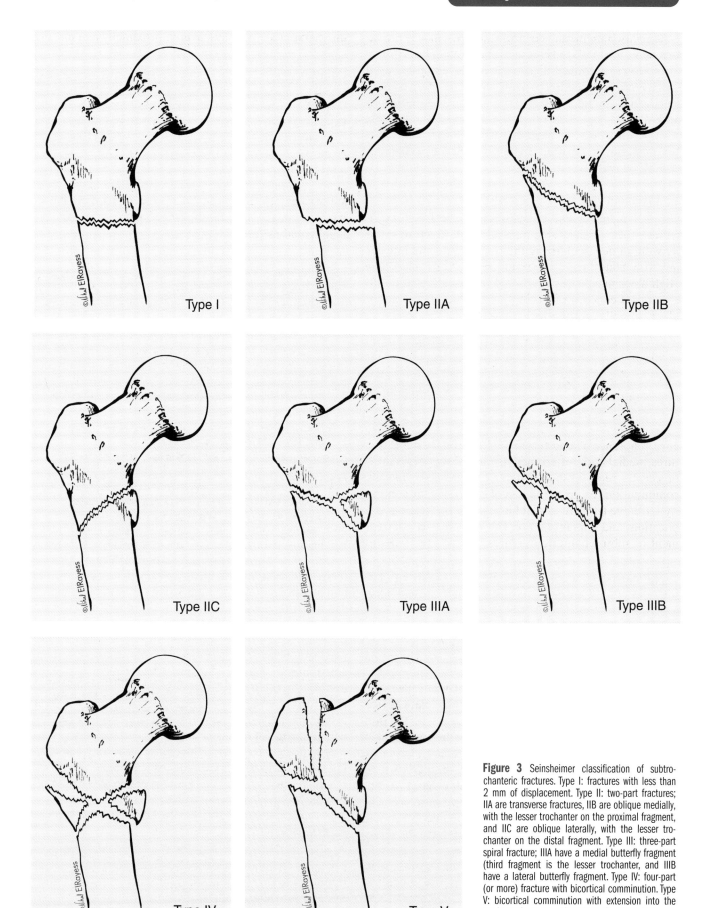

Figure 3 Seinsheimer classification of subtrochanteric fractures. Type I: fractures with less than 2 mm of displacement. Type II: two-part fractures; IIA are transverse fractures, IIB are oblique medially, with the lesser trochanter on the proximal fragment, and IIC are oblique laterally, with the lesser trochanter on the distal fragment. Type III: three-part spiral fracture; IIIA have a medial butterfly fragment (third fragment is the lesser trochanter, and IIIB have a lateral butterfly fragment. Type IV: four-part (or more) fracture with bicortical comminution. Type V: bicortical comminution with extension into the trochanteric mass. (*Copyright © Nihal ElRayess, Medical Illustrator.*)

system based on medial cortical stability, which is predictive of implant failure (Figure 3). The system has poor intraobserver reproducibility, but it is still commonly used. Other systems include the Russell-Taylor system, which is based on guidance toward the type of internal fixation, and the Orthopaedic Trauma Association (OTA)/AO system, which is not specific for subtrochanteric fractures, but can be adapted from OTA/AO pertrochanteric fracture classifications.

Management

Optimal management of subtrochanteric fractures remains controversial. Obtaining adequate fracture stability without devascularizing the fracture site and interfering with bone healing presents a significant challenge. High mechanical stress in the upper one third of the femur raises concern regarding the fatigue life of the implant. Initially, nonsurgical treatment with bracing and traction was advocated to avoid the complications of implant failure and infection, but current surgical treatment is usually successful and has lower complication rates than initial surgical options. Surgical treatment is the first choice unless specific contraindications exist.

The determination of fracture stability is essential in planning treatment. Fracture stability is based on the presence or absence of a posteromedial buttress. In stable fractures, medial and posteromedial cortical support is intact or can be reestablished, whereas in unstable fractures comminution results in the loss of medial cortex continuity. Unstable fractures are at highest risk for healing complications and implant failure. The goals of surgical treatment of subtrochanteric fractures include restoration of normal length and rotation and correction of the femoral head and neck angulations to restore adequate tension to the abductor muscles. To determine which type of fixation is most appropriate, the surgeon must have a thorough understanding of the available devices.

Surgical treatment initially began with Jewett nails. Although good preliminary results were reported, over time concern about implant fatigue increased after failure rates of 20% to 30% were documented, at which time it was recommended that this device not be used. Nail plate devices and blade plates then became popular and, with the popularization of the sliding hip screw for the treatment of femoral neck fractures, this device also gained acceptance. Good results were reported with side plate and sliding hip screw devices, with union rates of greater than 97% and failure rates lower than those of other sliding screw devices. New plate and screw devices for minimally invasive surgery are currently under development and may be the next advance in extramedullary fixation.

Intramedullary nails fall into three categories. Centromedullary nails are contained within the medullary canal and are usually inserted from the piriformis fossa; if the device is interlocking, the screws are inserted into the metaphyseal-diaphyseal area proximally and distally. Condylocephalic nails (such as the Ender nail) are inserted into the femoral condyle and extend into the femoral head and neck. Cephalomedullary nails are derived from Zickel nails and are not represented by interlocking centromedullary nails with screw or nail devices that can be inserted cephalad into the femoral head and neck (for example, Russell-Taylor reconstruction nails, Smith & Nephew; and spiral blade nail, Synthes). Retrograde nailing is rarely indicated for the treatment of subtrochanteric fractures. Each type of fixation device has advantages and disadvantages, some of which are highlighted in Table 2.

Table 2 | Advantages and Disadvantages of Fixation Devices

Dynamic Condylar Screw fixation has a 20% nonunion and delayed union rate and a reintervention rate of 12.5% to 20%.

Sliding screw and nail devices are associated with healing problems in 5% to 9% of patients and a reintervention rate of 9%.

Zickel nails provide inadequate distal rotational control and were reported to have significant mechanical and technical problems in 21% of patients.

Gamma nails have been found to have a complication rate greater than 10% and a reintervention rate of 27%.

Condylar plate fixation has been found to have a reintervention rate of 7%.

A clear advantage of intramedullary locked rods over plate systems in combined bending and compression to failure has been noted.

Although no difference was found in structural stiffness when comparing the Gamma nail and the sliding hip screw for the treatment of stable intertrochanteric and subtrochanteric fractures, the Gamma nail constructs were stiffer when used to treat unstable subtrochanteric fractures.

The strength of the reconstruction nail was found to be significantly greater than that of the short intramedullary hip screw and the long intramedullary hip screw.

Smith & Nephew and Zimmer nails were able to withstand higher loads before failure than Synthes nails.

Second-generation femoral nail constructs were found to be consistently stiffer in compression and torsion than statically locked first-generation femoral nails in a synthetic model of subtrochanteric femur fractures, whereas another study found significant variations in the bending rigidity of the proximal and distal sections of eight different femoral nails.

No difference was found in one study when comparing the Gamma nail and the dynamic hip screw in stress or strain distribution of proximal femur fractures. Other finite element analyses have found that the Gamma nail restricted proximal femur fracture site motion to a greater degree than the 95° condylar plate, particularly in the treatment of more unstable fractures with medial cortex comminution.

The Gamma nail has been reported to carry considerably greater load than a dynamic hip screw. Cyclic testing of the Gamma nail and the dynamic hip screw showed that the Gamma nail had significantly greater fatigue strength and fatigue life.

There is a considerable amount of inconclusive and conflicting evidence regarding which type of device to use in the treatment of subtrochanteric fractures. In simple, well-reduced fractures, the choice of implant is not particularly critical. Interlocking nails are the standard of care because of favorable mechanical characteristics and high rates of union. For fractures with intact trochanters, the most effective management is to use closed insertion of a conventional interlocked centromedullary nail in a static locked mode. As fracture severity increases (comminution, gap, and combined neck fracture), the choice of implant, particularly with reference to proximal nail dimensions and implant materials, is a significant factor in reducing fracture site motion, which is associated with nonunion and delayed union. One study suggested, therefore, that when subtrochanteric fractures are unstable (in patients with comminution or segmental bone loss) and early weight bearing is desirable, the choice of implant is critical and should be restricted to implants that allow minimal fracture site motion, such as the long Gamma nail and Russell-Taylor reconstruction nail.

For fractures with comminution of the greater trochanter, sliding hip screw devices are appropriate, as are cephalomedullary intramedullary nails. The unreamed femoral nail with a spiral blade has been found to have high complication rates in the treatment of fractures with intertrochanteric extension and in reverse obliquity fractures and should not be used in patients with these types of injuries. If a compression screw is used, it should have a locking barrel to limit rotation of the femoral head; if the screw is to function as a dynamically interlocking device, placement through the plate into the proximal fragment must be avoided because this position could maintain distraction. For fractures that extend into the piriformis fossa, cephalomedullary nails are an effective treatment modality, although more technically demanding to place. A locking nail can span the entire length of the femur, making the extent of shaft comminution relatively unimportant, and long nails can help prevent subsequent proximal or distal fractures. The shaft of the intramedullary nail blocks lateral migration of the femoral neck-head fragment and avoids shaft medialization and related shortening. For the treatment of fractures of bone with preexisting deformities or previous implants, plate and screw fixation are indicated.

External fixation is reserved for the treatment of open fractures with severe contamination, for provisional stabilization in the acute injury period, or for intermediate treatment of complications from failed internal fixation. Pathologic fractures are best treated with cephalomedullary devices that allow prophylactic stabilization of the entire femur. Autologous bone grafting is indicated for use during true open reduction of fractures with severe comminution of the medial wall; there are no prospective studies evaluating allograft techniques. Newer closed nailing and indirect reduction techniques have largely obviated the need for bone grafting.

Postoperative care depends on the stability achieved at surgery, which is determined by the strength of the implant and the quality of bone. Patients with reconstruction nails and either a trochanteric portal or piriformis portal are mobilized on the first postoperative day with bed-to-chair transfer and ambulation with a walker or crutches. With comminution, weight bearing is restricted to 10 to 15 kg, but if good bone contact is achieved with surgery, weight bearing as tolerated is acceptable. Range-of-motion exercises should be initiated within the first 2 days after surgery. Removal of implants should not be considered until mature radiographic callus is seen bridging the bone on both AP and lateral radiographs.

If surgical treatment is not possible, balanced (90° to 90°) traction, possibly followed by a hinged-knee hip spica cast brace is an option. Nonsurgical management should be limited to provisional treatment in mass casualty situations, when the patient's medical condition makes the risk of surgery excessive, and in patients in whom bone quality is so poor that there is no hope of secure fixation.

Posttraumatic Pain
Etiology
There can be several possible explanations for pain following surgical fixation of fractures of the proximal femur. These explanations include but are not limited to nonunion, hardware failure, prominent hardware, infection, limb-length inequality, malrotation of the extremity, and alteration of the biomechanics of the limb. The most common cause of hardware failure after surgical treatment of hip fractures is nonunion. Therefore, these two causes of pain often go hand-in-hand: the bone fails to heal prior to fatigue-type failure of the orthopaedic device (such as a blade plate). The fibrous tissue at the fracture site is not strong enough to prevent micromotion on routine weight bearing; thus, the device may fail. A dull pain from nonunion may become a severe sharp pain on hardware fatigue failure. As with any fracture treated openly, infection can be a cause for nonunion and subsequent hardware failure. Prominent hardware, even in the presence of a healed hip fracture, can be a cause of mild to moderate activity-related pain. This can occur in patients with a well-treated hip fracture. For example, the sliding hip screw is designed to allow compression within the metaphyseal portion of the femur after surgery. Severe osteopenia and comminution can cause a well-positioned lag screw to become prominent and palpable under the skin despite a healed hip fracture. Posttraumatic pain (even in the setting of a healed hip fracture) can occur from altered mechanics of the

limb because of (1) a decrease in the abductor moment arm (and resultant early abductor muscle fatigue with simple ambulation) or (2) an overloaded medial or lateral compartment secondary to an altered mechanical axis of the lower extremity.

Nonsurgical Management of Posttraumatic Pain

The most successful treatment of pain is a reversal or direct removal of the cause of pain, which means that such pain after hip fracture repair is often treated surgically. If the patient is too ill to consider surgical intervention or is unwilling to consider surgery, nonsurgical management may be the only available option. Therefore, pain coping and stress reduction techniques such as acupuncture, reflexology, and physical therapy may be helpful in this setting. More traditional pharmacologic treatment with nonsteroidal anti-inflammatory drugs or narcotics may also play a role in pain relief. A pain management specialist may offer some additional insight and relief of pain. Otherwise, surgical treatment to address the direct source of pain is indicated.

Revision Options

Nonunion could be revised with placement of new hardware (such as a blade plate or sliding hip screw) and takedown of the fibrous nonunion with or without bone graft (with or without vascularization) or bone graft substitute. In patients with femoral neck nonunion, it is often prudent to convert to arthroplasty as a definitive method of treatment. THA or hemiarthroplasty (in patients with preserved acetabular cartilage) can often be a more definitive alternative (with a quicker return to full weight bearing and activities of daily living) than an elaborate femoral head salvage procedure. Infection, of course, should be treated in a staged fashion; the first stage consists of débriding all infected or nonviable tissue (possibly including the use of an antibiotic-laden spacer or series of methacrylate beads), and the second stage includes reconstruction in the absence of infected tissue. Prominent hardware pain may be remedied by the removal of the orthopaedic device that is prominent and apparently inducing subcutaneous inflammation.

Osteotomy

Femoral neck nonunion has also been treated with a valgus intertrochanteric osteotomy in conjunction with new hardware and bone grafting; however, this procedure should be reserved for younger, active patients in whom arthroplasty is a less desirable option. Osteotomy can also be useful in patients with an altered mechanical axis of the lower extremity, which raises the possibility that a distal femoral osteotomy or a high tibial osteotomy may be a treatment option. However, if the altered mechanical axis results from altered proximal femoral anatomy alone, it may be unwise to consider osteotomy

elsewhere in the limb because it may become a source of chronic pain itself or alter the alignment of the knee joint with the floor.

Postoperative Considerations

Prophylaxis for Thromboembolic Events

Deep venous thrombosis (DVT) and pulmonary embolism (PE) are the most common causes of morbidity and mortality in orthopaedic patients. Virchow's triad of thrombogenesis (increased coagulability, stasis, and vessel wall damage) are all unfavorably affected by trauma, and the large veins of the thigh are particularly prone to forming clots that can embolize to the lungs. In trauma patients, it is not known when the greatest risk for DVT or PE occurs, and the option to treat patients perioperatively to allow for a given treatment plan is not available. The occurrence of DVT or PE prior to definitive treatment may force alteration of surgical plans when therapeutic anticoagulation is required. One large autopsy study found that DVT occurred in 83% of patients with hip fractures and 86% of those with femur fractures. In addition, PE was found to occur in 46% and 53% of patients with hip and femur fractures, respectively. Other studies have found the incidence of DVT in patients with hip or pelvic fractures to range from 36% to 60% (depending on method of detection) and the incidence of fatal PE to be 0.5% to 12.9%. DVT that forms in the popliteal fossa or at higher levels of the hip results in a high risk for causing PE, although calf thrombi are responsible for 5% to 35% of symptomatic PEs. Two thirds of patients with fatal PE die within 30 minutes of injury. The incidence of fatal PE without prophylaxis during emergency hip surgery ranges from 7.5% to 10%. Other complications of DVT include recurrent thrombosis and postthrombotic syndrome (edema, induration, pain, pigmentation, ulceration, cellulitis, and stasis dermatitis), which is experienced by 20% to 40% of patients with DVT.

DVT is clinically silent in two thirds of the patients in whom thrombi are found on autopsy or by using leg venography; its clinical signs and symptoms are nonspecific. Patients most often have swelling, calf tenderness, positive Homan's sign (pain in the calf with dorsiflexion of the foot), fever, and elevated white blood cell count. Helpful diagnostic signs include changes in color and temperature, venous distention, and edema. With PE, patients who do not die suddenly usually experience slow deterioration and symptoms similar to those of pneumonia, congestive heart failure, or hypotension. Venography is the current standard for diagnosis, with the presence of an intraluminal defect being diagnostic for DVT. However, this test can only be done once, it is painful, and can cause phlebitis, swelling, thrombosis, renal complications, and anaphylactic reactions. Up to 20% of patients cannot undergo venography or have noninterpretable study results. Radioactive fibrinogen is useful for detecting thrombi in the calf, but it is less effective for detecting thrombi in the thigh. Doppler ultrasound is accurate and can be done at the bedside, but it cannot detect nonocclusive thrombi and requires an experienced operator to accurately interpret the results. Compression ultrasound is 97% accurate, 100% sensitive, and 97% specific when performed by an experienced operator, and it can potentially distinguish acute from chronic DVT and visualize the clot. Duplex and color flow duplex ultrasound are also highly effective. In separate studies, MRI was reported to have sensitivities of 90% to 100% and 75% to 100%. MRI is noninvasive, relatively operator-independent, accurately evaluates pelvic and deep femoral veins, simultaneously evaluates both extremities, and images adjacent soft tissue. The main drawback of MRI is cost, which is 2 to 2.5 times that of ultrasound and 1.4 times that of venography.

D-dimer values can be used to screen for the probability of both DVT and PE. If the D-dimer value is low, thromboembolic disease is unlikely, but this test has not been widely accepted as useful. Pulmonary angiography is the gold standard for detection of PE, but ventilation-perfusion scanning with evaluation for DVT is more common. PEs are rare in the absence of DVT, but evidence of DVT and symptoms of PE together justify anticoagulation therapy. Angiography can be used after nondiagnostic ventilation-perfusion scanning and ultrasound with clinical suspicion.

There are three treatment options for DVT: prevent the thrombus, ignore it, or treat it. Prophylaxis for DVT in trauma patients has long been based on guidelines for patients undergoing general surgery or elective orthopaedic surgery, and treatment specific to trauma patients is ongoing. Physical measures can help to limit venous stasis. Careful handling of the extremity during surgery, early active postoperative mobilization, elevation of the extremity, graduated compression stockings, and external intermittent compression devices increase venous velocity and improve the emptying of vascular cusps, which theoretically decreases the chance of thrombus formation. There are data to support the efficacy of these measures during elective surgery and, despite the paucity of data regarding their use in trauma patients, compression stockings and external intermittent compression devices are recommended.

Alterations in coagulability are achieved using prophylactic drugs including dextran, aspirin, warfarin, heparin, low-molecular-weight heparin (LMWH) and thrombin inhibitors. Dextran has been shown to be effective during elective and emergency hip procedures and in the treatment of patients with femur fractures, but there is insufficient information regarding its use for multitrauma patients. It is best started preoperatively and should be limited to less than 500 mL during surgery to avoid increased bleeding. Aspirin has been

shown to decrease the incidence of DVT in patients with hip fractures, but it is insufficient for prophylaxis alone. Warfarin has been shown to effectively minimize DVT in orthopaedic patients when the prothrombin time is increased to an international normalized ratio of 2 to 3 (1.2 to 1.5 times that of control subjects). It must be titrated to this level, however, and it has a narrow therapeutic window and requires intensive monitoring. Subcutaneous heparin at 5,000 U every 8 hours is effective prophylaxis for general surgery patients, but not for orthopaedic patients; it has no role in trauma patients. Adjusted dose heparin, with partial thromboplastin time between 31.5 and 36 seconds is effective at reducing the incidence of DVT, but it can lead to bleeding, allergic reaction, osteoporosis, and thrombocytopenia.

LMWH has a superior risk-to-benefit ratio compared with heparin, aspirin, and warfarin. A study of patients with hip fractures who were immediately given subcutaneous enoxaparin on admission, with therapy continued for a minimum of 5 weeks, reported an incidence of symptomatic DVT and symptomatic PE of 0.6% and 0.2%, respectively. Other studies of patients with hip fractures that used objective evaluation methods found that DVT occurred in 7% to 38% of patients despite prophylaxis. Studies indicate that LMWH (such as enoxaparin) is safe and effective when used preoperatively and can be used in elderly patients with spinal anesthesia and in those treated with aspirin until injury. Its efficacy was significantly improved (incidence of DVT decreased from 17% to 11.7%) when treatment lasted more than 10 days. The risk of bleeding is low with LMWHs (0.9%), and their short half-life, predictable pharmacokinetics, and favorable safety profile make them an excellent choice for prophylaxis in patients with hip fractures.

Thrombin inhibitors (megaltran and hirudin) have been shown to decrease the incidence of DVT in patients undergoing arthroplasty, but they are largely untested in trauma patients. The newest class of antithrombotic compounds, synthetic pentasaccharides, target activated factor X. Fondaparinux is the first agent approved for use as thromboprophylaxis for patients undergoing major orthopaedic surgery. This agent appears to be highly effective; compared with enoxaparin it has been shown to lower the risk of DVT up to day 11 by 55.2%. A meta-analysis of six major trials, all of which used mandatory bilateral venography-detected DVT as the end point, found the overall risk of DVT by day 11 to be 8.3% and a relative risk reduction of 56.4% compared with patients treated with enoxaparin, with no significant difference in the incidence of major bleeding noted. Four weeks of treatment, compared with 1 week of treatment, decreased the risk of venous thromboembolism by 96%, strongly arguing for the continuation of anticoagulation therapy. Fondaparinux is equally effective when administered less than 6 hours before and

Table 3 | Cost of Prophylactic Agents for Thromboembolic Events

Agent	Cost
Pneumatic Compression devices	One-time $18 charge for compression devices $8/day for cycling inflation device
Warfarin	$0.30/pill and $60 per office visit for monitoring
Dalteparin	$13/day
Enoxaparin	$24/day
Fondaparinux	$30/day

6 hours or more after surgery; the incidence of bleeding was significantly lower when treatment was delayed to at least 6 hours postoperatively. Based on these data, it is recommended that fondaparinux therapy be initiated at least 6 hours after skin closure. Overall, at a subcutaneous dose of 2.5 mg daily, fondaparinux has been shown to be more effective than enoxaparin in preventing proximal vein thrombosis and venous thromboembolism. Therapy should start at least 6 hours after surgery, and the optimal duration of treatment is 4 weeks. Fondaparinux has a rapid onset of action, optimal half-life, and highly predictable and reproducible pharmacokinetics, making it an excellent choice for antithrombotic therapy in trauma patients.

In the current health care environment, cost-effectiveness must be considered. Because the treatment and sequelae of DVT and PE can have considerable cost, all prophylaxis for thromboembolic events has proved to be cost-effective. Whether the additional cost of newer, more expensive therapies such as LMWH and fondaparinux is justified requires evaluation of the effectiveness of the drugs, their risk/benefit ratios, and relative costs when compared with other available therapies (Table 3). Several studies have shown that short- and long-term prophylaxis with LMWHs is cost-effective compared with no treatment. Additional studies are required to evaluate the cost-effectiveness of LMWHs compared with other treatment options and to evaluate the cost-effectiveness of synthetic pentasaccharides.

Hardware Removal and Conversion to THA

Following hip trauma, patients may experience one or more complications that merit consideration for treatment with THA. The most common complication is a painful hip or corresponding referred pain. Stiffness, deformity, and limb-length discrepancy are also commonly reported. Pain is sometimes caused by complications of hip fracture fixation, including osteonecrosis, malunion, nonunion, neurogenic pain, or scar tissue. Complicating factors include infection, massive heterotopic bone,

malunion, or neuromuscular weakness, all of which may make reconstruction exceedingly difficult compared with primary THA.

Before initiating treatment, a thorough review of the nature and timing of the initial injury is required, as well as an assessment of late complications and current co-morbidities. Patients with posttraumatic arthrosis are often young men with a history of drug or alcohol abuse, a heavy laboring vocation, and an interest in hobbies such as motorcycling; this type of patient is unlikely to be satisfied following THA and therapeutic options including lifestyle alterations merit consideration. Elderly patients with preexisting degenerative disease and impaired healing are another commonly encountered patient subtype. These patients often have medical comorbidities limiting their surgical tolerance for arduous procedures. In these patients, the goals of treatment must be prioritized to limit the magnitude of the surgical procedure and allow for functional improvement.

Physical examination should assess for the appearance of posttraumatic or surgical scars, muscular atrophy, femoral deformity, limb-length discrepancy, or signs of chronic infection. The strength of the hip abductors and other principal muscles should be assessed, and range of motion should be documented. The pattern of gait and mobility, stability, and neurologic integrity of the contralateral hip, both knees, and the lumbosacral spine should also be assessed. High-quality radiographs should be obtained at known magnification to allow for templating, and sufficient views should be obtained to allow for assessment of deformities.

Contraindications for surgery include medical co-morbidities that jeopardize the life of the patient during or after surgery, neurologic disorders that jeopardize the stability of the hip or render the patient vulnerable to frequent falls, and behavioral problems that compromise the likelihood of prolonged function of the arthroplasty. Younger patients with mild or minimal posttraumatic arthrosis and a nonunion or malunion should undergo attempted salvage of the native femoral head and neck. For elderly patients with osteopenic bone and a large hole around a failed hip screw, salvage is less likely to be successful and THA is often a better option. The same is true for younger patients with limited femoral head or neck bone stock secondary to a failed salvage procedure. Prompt eradication of infection should be undertaken before THA.

Failed fracture fixations requiring conversion to arthroplasty present significant difficulty for the treating surgeon. Internal fixation devices are often very difficult to remove, significant displacement of the upper femur can render preparation of the femoral canal difficult, and there is a risk of fracture of the femur during dislocation in a femur weakened by screw extraction. In general, the hip should be dislocated before removal of plates, screws, and nails because removal can significantly weaken the bone. Removal may be exceedingly difficult or impossible because of osseointegration with screws and filling of bone along the threads. Having the appropriate equipment is vital to successful extraction, and in addition to the proper screwdriver tips and nail extractors, a vice-grip wrench to allow oscillating movements of the screwdriver while torque is applied and a hardened drill to drill a hole into the screw should also be available. If a screw head snaps off, the shaft may be freed by trephining holes to cut the threads free from the surrounding bone; this technique is undesirable, however, because it leaves the femur perforated medially and laterally at several levels. This interferes with cement fixation and can lead to femoral shaft fractures postoperatively. A slight turn in the direction of tightening may loosen the screw before reversing the direction for removal. After removal, the site of the screws and plate must be carefully examined for bacterial infection and osteolysis, and cultures should be taken.

If extraction of fixation from the femoral neck is not possible without extensive damage to the trochanteric area, the femoral head can be removed after dislocation, and then the fixation device can be removed in a retrograde manner. Because of stress shielding, severe osteoporosis, or bone absorption, fracture may occur at the site of a plate and supportive grafting may be required. The application of bone chips under the vastus lateralis has not been found to be effective.

The amount of displacement of the femur can be evaluated using a true lateral radiograph and a routine AP radiograph of the upper third of the femur. The upper femur should be mobilized so that direct access to the top of the femur is possible; the knee should be stabilized and the patella displayed during reaming. Direct palpation and partial detachment of the vastus lateralis can also help in assessing the orientation of the reamer in relation to the medullary canal. If there is marked displacement of the proximal fragment or nonunion of an intertrochanteric fracture, it is possible to excise the entire malunited or nonunited segment down to the level of the lesser trochanter and to use a straight-stemmed prosthesis. The greater trochanter should be osteotomized below the vastus ridge, leaving a large fragment for subsequent fixation. A long neck prosthesis should be used to compensate for loss of length.

Acetabular fractures with poor outcomes secondary to arthritic wear or osteonecrosis may require THA. For patients with gradual onset of arthritis, pain should be the indication for surgery. If the patient shows ongoing wear of the femoral head or acetabulum, surgery should not be delayed because acetabular bone stock and the available femoral head graft are being lost. Although surgical access may be influenced by the approach used in the initial fixation, it usually does not determine the approach for THA.

Bony defects or deformities often complicate THA done after acetabular fracture. The most common bony defect involves the posterior wall. Thorough débridement of nonhealed and necrotic fragments should be carried out to accurately assess the size of the defect. The femoral head and neck are used as a buttress graft against the intact viable bone to substitute for the posterior wall. This block graft should be contoured and fixed with a plate. Nonunions of a transverse fracture or one or both columns must be internally fixed, and it is often best to consider a two-stage procedure, with implantation of the femoral portion of the THA carried out after the bone and graft have healed around the acetabulum. Severe malunions of the innominate bone should be corrected at the time of surgery rather than attempting THA in the presence of such deformity. This can be done as a one- or two-stage procedure. Many patients are at increased risk for dislocation because of partial compromise of soft tissue, in which instance an increased offset neck, large head, and hooded acetabular liner should be considered. Hip arthrodesis should be considered for very young patients with massive associated bone loss and infection.

Postoperative complications associated with conversion to THA include intraoperative and postoperative hemorrhage, sciatic nerve injury, wound infection, thromboembolic events, heterotopic ossification, dislocation, persistent nonunion, premature failure of the THA, and fracture and perforation of the femoral canal. Thorough preoperative planning and careful intraoperative management can reduce the incidence of these potential complications. Postoperative therapy precautions with regard to movement can help limit the incidence of dislocation and premature failure. Anatomic fracture alignment can help prevent nonunion, premature failure and fracture, and perforation of the femoral canal. In addition, postoperative expectations should be discussed with the patient prior to surgery to establish realistic expectations with regard to pain relief and function.

Heterotopic Ossification

Heterotopic ossification, also referred to as ectopic ossification or myositis ossificans, refers to the formation of bone in soft tissue where bone normally does not exist. There are three categories of heterotopic ossification. Myositis ossificans progressive is a rare autosomal dominant metabolic bone disease in children with progressive metamorphosis of skeletal muscle to bone. Myositis ossificans circumscripta, or neurogenic heterotopic ossification, without trauma is localized soft-tissue ossification after neurologic injury or burns. Traumatic heterotopic ossification occurs after musculoskeletal trauma and can occur in any tissue, including abdominal incisions, wounds, kidneys, uterus, corpora cavernosa, and the gastrointestinal tract. Myositis ossificans is a more specific form, in which patients have soft-tissue ossification at sites of trauma adjacent to long bones. Fibrous, cartilaginous, and osseous tissues near bone are affected; the muscle may or may not be involved. Notable but rare occurrences of heterotopic ossification occur in patients with sickle cell anemia, hemophilia, tetanus, poliomyelitis, multiple sclerosis, toxic epidermal necrolysis, and idiopathically. The specific pathophysiology of heterotopic ossification is not known. It is thought to be caused by an interaction between local factors including the pool of available calcium in the adjacent bone, soft-tissue edema, vascular stasis, tissue hypoxia, mesenchymal cells with osteoblastic activity, and unknown systemic factors. The base defect is an appropriate differentiation of fibroblasts to bone-forming cells; early edema and connective tissue proceed to tissue with foci of calcification and then to maturation of calcification and ossification.

Fifty-five percent of patients with hip fractures experience heterotopic ossification, with the incidence increasing to 83% when open reduction and internal fixation is performed. Among patients with hip dislocations and fracture-dislocations, heterotopic ossification occurs in 64%, in up to 62% of patients with acetabular fractures, and in 53% of patients who undergo THA. In patients with severe central nervous system injuries, 10% to 20% experience heterotopic ossification, and the incidence increases with those who undergo open reduction and internal fixation. Clinical evidence of heterotopic ossification may appear as early as 3 weeks or as late as 12 weeks after trauma and is characterized by swelling, pain, and erythema around a stiffening joint. Loss of mobility and the resulting loss of function are the main complications of heterotopic ossification because the joint may become fused and ankylosed. Pressure sores and nerve entrapment may also occur. Eighty percent of instances of heterotopic ossification follow a relatively benign course, without any of these complications, but 10% to 20% of patients with heterotopic ossification experience significant loss of motion and 10% of these patients eventually experience ankylosis.

Diagnosis is difficult because of the nonspecific early symptoms. Alkaline phosphatase can be used as a screening tool, with levels often rising to 3.5 times normal in the acute phase, but it cannot be used indefinitely because the alkaline phosphatase level is sometimes normal and sometimes elevated for years. Measurement of 24-hour prostaglandin E_2 urinary excretion has also been recommended as an early indicator for heterotopic ossification, with an acute increase signaling the need for further investigation. Radiography and three-phase bone scanning provide definitive diagnosis. Heterotopic ossification typically appears as circumferential ossification with a lucent center and is generally visible 4 to 6 weeks after the three-phase bone scan is positive. CT and MRI can both also detect heterotopic ossification.

Prophylaxis for heterotopic ossification is strongly recommended in patients with acetabular fractures, dislocations and fracture-dislocations, and femoral fractures treated with open reduction and internal fixation and approaches to the hip that involve dissection of the gluteus maximus. Diphosphonates and nonsteroidal drugs such as indomethacin are commonly used for prophylaxis. Indomethacin has been shown to significantly reduce the incidence of heterotopic ossification in patients with acetabular and femoral fractures and is regularly recommended for prophylaxis. Radiation therapy also prevents heterotopic ossification when administered 24 hours before surgery or within 72 hours after surgery. No differences in the efficacy of indomethacin versus radiation therapy have been found. No consensus currently exists regarding when prophylaxis should be used and which treatment is most appropriate. One study found that gluteus minimus necrotic muscle débridement diminished heterotopic ossification formation comparably to nonsteroidal drugs and is a safe and adequate prophylaxis for patients with acetabular fractures. Another recent study suggested that indomethacin administration increases the risk of nonunion of long bone fractures in patients with concomitant acetabular and long bone fractures compared with patients who receive neither prophylaxis nor prophylaxis with radiation therapy. It is clear that prophylactic measures are necessary for this patient population, and at this time evidence seems to indicate that treatment with either indomethacin or radiation therapy is appropriate.

If early heterotopic ossification is confirmed, passive range-of-motion exercises are recommended. More aggressive manipulation has also been recommended, but it poses the risk of inciting further heterotopic ossification. Nonsteroidal drugs and radiation therapy are both also used for treatment of heterotopic ossification. To decrease the risk of intraoperative hemorrhage and postoperative recurrence, surgical resection to restore mobility should be delayed for as long as possible—until the process of heterotopic ossification has been completed and there is less metabolic activity.

Rehabilitation

Rehabilitation should begin early for all patients. For trauma patients, joint range-of-motion exercises should begin immediately after stabilization of fractures (passively if the patient is unable to cooperate). Ideally, the patient should participate from the beginning, and the type and duration of exercise should increase as tolerated by the patient. Early bone grafting for injuries at risk of nonunion has been shown to be beneficial, although a soft-tissue envelope is desirable prior to grafting. Deformity correction and bone transport may expedite recovery, but require a significant commitment of time and effort by both the surgeon and the patient, whose active participation is vital. Polytrauma patients are at increased risk of infection, and nonorthopaedic infections should be managed aggressively by a critical care specialist. Orthopaedic wounds should be treated with aggressive excisional débridement of all necrotic bone and soft tissue, and antibiotics that are specific to organisms should be identified at débridement and used to replace broad-spectrum antibiotics initiated at presentation.

Functional Outcomes Assessment

Outcomes have recently become the focus of clinical research, insurance companies, health care delivery systems, and hospitals. This phenomenon seems to have resulted largely from uncertainty regarding the best way to treat patients, and incomplete knowledge of treatment methods and their effectiveness. These uncertainties seem to be a result of the weakness of clinical literature, poor research design, and difficulties in conducting high-quality clinical research in orthopaedic surgery. Clinical outcomes were the focus of clinical research in orthopaedic surgery until the 1990s. Analysis has evolved to include assessment of functional outcomes, including mental health, social function, role function, physical function, activities of daily living, health-related outcomes, and satisfaction with the process of care. Validation scales to assess the efficacy of treatment strategies with regard to outcomes are currently limited. The development of registries of trauma is necessary to provide sufficient data to study the major issues clinicians encounter in optimizing both prevention and treatment.

Several well-validated health instruments are available to assess function following musculoskeletal injury. The four most widely used are the Medical Outcomes Study Short Form 36-Item Health Survey, the Sickness Impact Profile, the Nottingham Health Profile, and the Quality of Well-Being Scale. All assess physical, psychological, social, and role functioning and assess the patient as a whole, rather than by system, disease, or limb. They are internally consistent, reproducible, discriminate between clinical conditions of different severity, and allow for changes in health status over time. None are physician administered, which increases reliability. The American Academy of Orthopaedic Surgeons has also developed a scoring system that is applied to regional or age-specific musculoskeletal populations, and the Musculoskeletal Functional Assessment was developed by the National Institutes of Health and National Institute of Child Health and Human Development to specifically evaluate musculoskeletal injury. All of these systems are broadly accepted and provide the ability to compare the functional impact of various diseases (see chapter 26).

The current gold standard for orthopaedic research is the prospective, randomized, double-blind study.

Some of these study design principles are difficult to apply in surgical interventional studies because double-blinding becomes difficult, and pure randomization can raise ethical questions because of surgeon preference and skills. Because this model has been achieved in some studies and provides the most unbiased and useful data, it remains the standard. Orthopaedic researchers continue to improve their awareness of study design and statistical impact and adequate follow-up of clinical and functional outcomes. Evidence-based medicine is gaining acceptance, and tools such as the Cochrane Collaboration provide systemic reviews to help physicians make informed decisions about health care.

Posttraumatic Arthritis
Clinical and Radiographic Features

Posttraumatic arthritis is a secondary osteoarthritis that can occur after trauma. There is limited research on the pathomechanics of the disease, and several theories exist as to how injury leads to osteoarthritis. The injury may act as the incipient lesion of osteoarthritis by altering the biomechanics across the joint when malalignment, malorientation, and surface incongruities persist after repair. Irreversible cartilage damage may also occur at the time of impact, leading to chondrocyte death and inflammation that ultimately result in osteoarthritis. Trabecular microfracture (bone bruising) followed by bone remodeling and damage to the surrounding musculature may also contribute to posttraumatic arthritis. The injury ultimately leads to biologic and mechanical changes that destabilize the normal coupling of degeneration and synthesis of articular cartilage, chondrocytes, extracellular matrix, and subchondral bone. The interplay of the injury with systemic factors such as age, genetic susceptibility, nutritional factors, and gender; intrinsic factors such as previous damage, bridging muscle weakness, proprioceptive deficiencies, and joint laxity; and external factors such as obesity and injury severity can lead to posttraumatic osteoarthritis.

Studies have established a link between trauma and the development of osteoarthritis. One report found that the adjusted odds ratio (adjusted for age, sex, race, and education) for the development of osteoarthritis after hip trauma compared with the uninjured population is 7.84. The same study also reported a significant association between trauma and hip osteoarthritis for men and in patients with unilateral disease, although the association is not statistically significant for women or in patients with bilateral disease. Another study found that the age-adjusted odds ratio for hip osteoarthritis with a history of injury versus no injury to be 24.2 for men and 4.17 for women. Between 5.6% and 57% of all patients with acetabular fractures, even with anatomic reduction, eventually have posttraumatic osteoarthritis. After anterior dislocation the incidence of posttraumatic osteoarthritis is 17%, whereas the incidence for posterior dislocation is 30% if reduction takes place within 6 hours of dislocation and 76% if reduction takes place more than 6 hours after injury. The disease has significant impact on function and is the most common indicator for elective THA.

Diagnosis of posttraumatic arthritis is symptomatic because radiologic signs correlate poorly with pain and loss of motion. As with all forms of osteoarthritis, the hallmarks are pain relieved by rest, morning stiffness, buckling, instability, and loss of function. Radiographic signs include marginal osteophytes, asymmetrical narrowing of the joint space, subchondral sclerosis, and subchondral cyst formation.

Treatment

Treatment is indicated for pain and is directed toward pain management. Physical and occupational therapy, exercise regimens, nonsteroidal anti-inflammatory drugs, and weight loss can all be helpful. Steroid injections have been used for posttraumatic osteoarthritis of the knee, but are possibly less helpful in posttraumatic osteoarthritis of the hip. Chondroprotective drugs, including inhibitors of degradative metalloproteases, are being developed and may soon offer the opportunity to alter the course of the disease rather than just treat the symptoms. Arthrodesis and arthroplasty are last-resort procedures.

For patients who are young and active, obese, or manual laborers, arthrodesis has been considered as an option for pain relief. As THA techniques and implants continue to improve, and in patients who are unwilling or unable to undergo arthrodesis, THA can also be considered. As a late salvage procedure after hip trauma, THA is commonly used and is currently the best available option for relief of pain and restoration of function, especially in patients who are elderly and sedentary. Excellent short- and intermediate-term results have been reported for THA, although some studies have found high complication rates, including repetitive dislocation, acetabular cement fracture, severe heterotopic ossification, and deep sepsis. Even with these complications, however, one study reported improvements in pain and function.

Summary

Hip fractures are one of the most common causes for a decrease in the quality of life of elderly patients and have a mortality rate of up to 36%. The incidence of hip fractures and the resultant social and health care costs continue to rise. The prevalence and significance of these fractures requires prudent treatment with the goal of functional restoration. Treatment for a hip fracture depends on the type of fracture and the requirements of the individual patient. Knowledge of the epidemiology,

mechanisms of injury, classification, and treatment options for hip fractures are important to achieve treatment goals. The management of posttraumatic pain and postoperative complications including DVT, heterotopic ossification, posttraumatic arthritis, removal of hardware, and revision procedures are all important aspects in the treatment of hip fractures. An understanding of rehabilitation options and the examination of outcome measurements also will improve treatment for patients with hip fractures.

Annotated Bibliography

General

Ottenbacher KJ, Smith PM, Illig SB, et al: Disparity in health service and outcomes for persons with hip fracture and lower extremity joint replacement. *Med Care* 2003;41(2):232-241.

In this study, data from 189 hospitals in 46 states that contributed to the Uniform Data System for Medical Rehabilitation and the National Follow-Up Services were analyzed to determine rehabilitation health services received and outcomes attained by older adults who had a hip fracture or lower extremity joint replacement. The purpose of the study was to examine the disparity in health services and outcomes for adults with these conditions. The authors concluded that disparity in outcomes appeared to be related to family structure and social support.

Urwin SC, Parker MJ, Griffiths R: General versus regional anesthesia for hip fracture surgery: A meta-analysis of randomized trials. *Br J Anaesth* 2000;84:450-455.

This article presents a meta-analysis of 15 randomized trials that compared morbidity associated with the use of general or regional anesthesia for patients with hip fractures. The group receiving regional anesthesia had a 1-month reduction in mortality rate and incidence of DVT compared with the group receiving general anesthesia. Surgery performed using general anesthesia had reduced surgical time. No other outcome measure showed a statistically significant difference. The authors concluded that there are marginal advantages (in terms of mortality and the risk of DVT) in using regional anesthesia for patients with hip fractures.

Femoral Neck Fractures

Bhandari M, Devereaux PJ, Swiontkowski MF, et al: Internal fixation compared with arthroplasty for displaced fractures of the femoral neck: A meta-analysis. *J Bone Joint Surg* 2003;85-A(9):1673-1681.

This study is a meta-analysis of information taken from computerized databases for randomized clinical trials published between 1969 and 2002, and studies identified through hand searches of major orthopaedic journals, bibliographies of major orthopaedic textbooks, and personal files. Of 140 studies that were initially identified, 14 met all eligibility criteria. Results of the analysis comparing internal fixation with arthroplasty for the treatment of a displaced femoral neck fracture showed that arthroplasty significantly reduces the risk of revision surgery. However, arthroplasty increases the risks of infection, blood loss, and surgical time, and possibly increases the rate of early mortality.

Oakes DA, Jackson KR, Davies MR, et al: The impact of the Garden classification on proposed operative treatment. *Clin Orthop* 2003;409:232-240.

Forty radiographs of femoral neck fractures were evaluated independently by five orthopaedic surgeons. Kappa values were calculated for interobserver reliability and intraobserver variability with respect to the readers' ability to assess the fractures using the Garden classification and to determine fracture displacement with and without access to a lateral radiograph. In 69% of the instances in which a reader changed the classification of a fracture, the proposed treatment of the fracture did not change. The Garden classification has poor interobserver reliability but good intraobserver reproducibility. To improve the reliability and usefulness of the Garden classification, the authors suggest that the classification should be modified to have only two stages (Garden A, nondisplaced or valgus impacted, and Garden B, displaced) and to include the use of a lateral radiograph.

Raia FJ, Chapman CB, Herrera MF, Schweppe MW, Michelsen CB, Rosenwasser MP: Unipolar or bipolar hemiarthroplasty for femoral neck fractures in the elderly? *Clin Orthop* 2003;414:259-265.

This prospective randomized trial compared the efficacy of unipolar with bipolar hemiarthroplasty in elderly patients (≥ 65 years) with displaced femoral neck fractures in terms of quality of life and functional outcomes. In this study, 115 patients with a mean age of 82.1 years were randomized to either unipolar or bipolar hemiarthroplasty groups. Results suggest that the bipolar endoprosthesis provides no advantage in the treatment of displaced femoral neck fractures in elderly patients regarding quality of life and functional outcomes.

Shah AK, Eissler J, Radomisli T: Algorithms for the treatment of femoral neck fractures. *Clin Orthop* 2002; 399:28-34.

This article presents a review of femoral neck fracture patterns and the potential risks and benefits of individual treatment modalities for each fracture pattern as well as for pediatric femoral neck fractures.

Intertrochanteric Fractures

Adams CI, Robison M, Court-Brown CM, McQueen MM: Prospective randomized controlled trial of an intramedullary nail versus dynamic screw and plate for intertrochanteric fractures of the femur. *J Orthop Trauma* 2001;15(6):394-400.

This prospective, randomized controlled clinical trial with observer blinding compared the surgical complications and functional outcome of the Gamma nail intramedullary fixation device with the Richards sliding hip screw and plate device for

the treatment of intertrochanteric femoral fractures. All patients admitted from the local population with intertrochanteric fractures of the femur were included in the study. The study included 400 patients; 399 were followed for up to 1 year or until death. Patients were randomly assigned for treatment with either a short-type Gamma nail (203 patients) or a Richards-type sliding hip screw and plate (197 patients). The authors concluded that the use of an intramedullary device for the treatment of intertrochanteric femoral fractures is associated with a higher but nonsignificant risk of postoperative complications. Routine use of the Gamma nail in this type of fracture was not recommended over the current standard treatment using a dynamic hip screw and plate.

Cole PA: What's new in orthopaedic trauma. *J Bone Joint Surg Am* 2003;85-A(11):2260-2269.

This article presents a review of the most important studies in orthopaedic trauma. A study of intertrochanteric fractures that compared treatment using the sliding hip screw with treatment using the intramedullary hip screw did not find any significant differences intraoperatively, radiographically, or clinically between patients treated with each screw type. It was noted that there were no significant differences in the mean number of units of blood given, the number of patients requiring a transfusion for a hematocrit of less than 27, or the incidence of technical problems and postoperative complications.

Herrera A, Domingo LJ, Calvo A, Martinez A, Cuenca J: A comparative study of trochanteric fractures treated with the Gamma nail or the proximal femoral nail. *Int Orthop* 2002;26:365-369.

This prospective study compared the surgical treatment of fractures of the trochanteric region of the femur using the principles of closed intramedullary nailing with the Gamma nail compared with the proximal femoral nail. Both systems enabled early mobilization and ambulation in most patients. There were no significant differences in the use of either nail in terms of the recovery of previous functional capacity or in terms of the time required for fracture healing (average, 12 weeks). Shaft fractures and the cutting-out phenomenon were more common with the use of the Gamma nail, whereas secondary varus occurred more often with the use of the proximal femoral nail.

Kubiak EN, Bong M, Park SS, Kummer F, Egol K, Koval KJ: Intramedullary fixation of unstable intertrochanteric hip fractures: One or two lag screws. *J Orthop Trauma* 2004;18(1):12-17.

This laboratory investigation was undertaken to compare the screw sliding characteristics and biomechanical stability of four-part intertrochanteric hip fractures stabilized with an intramedullary nail using either one large-diameter lag screw (IMHS) or two small-diameter lag screws (TAN). Eight matched pairs of cadaveric human femurs with simulated, unstable intertrochanteric hip fractures were used. One femur of each matched pair was stabilized with an IMHS, and the other was stabilized with a TAN. Femurs were statically, then cyclically loaded on a servohydraulic materials testing machine. All specimens were loaded to failure. The two constructs showed equivalent rigidity and stability in all parameters assessed in elastic and cyclical tests. The TAN had a greater ultimate failure load.

Subtrochanteric Fractures

Broos PL, Reynders P: The use of the unreamed AO femoral intramedullary nail with spiral blade in non-pathogenic fractures of the femur: Experiences with eighty consecutive cases. *J Orthop Trauma* 2002;16(3): 150-154.

This prospective study of 80 consecutive fractures in 80 patients who were followed up at least 10 months after surgery, evaluated the use of the unreamed femoral nail with spiral blade in the treatment of nonpathologic subtrochanteric and segmental femoral fractures. The authors found that there is predictive value of the Seinsheimer classification regarding outcome using this nail. The unreamed femoral nail with spiral blade is an option for the treatment of subtrochanteric or segmental fractures of the femur, especially in patients with a good bone quality. The complications using this device are caused by the characteristics of the implant and the type of fracture for which it is used. The implant should not be used in elderly women with a reversed oblique fracture or a subtrochanteric fracture with an intertrochanteric component.

Browner BD, Jupiter JB, Levine AM, Trafton PG: *Skeletal Trauma: Basic Science, Management, and Reconstruction*, ed 3. Philadelphia, PA, WB Saunders, 2003.

This textbook reviews mechanism of injury, fracture classification, and treatment options. Common complications and outcomes statistics are also presented.

Roberts CS, Nawab A, Wang M, Voor MJ, Seligson D: Second generation intramedullary nailing of subtrochanteric femur fractures: A biomechanical study of fracture site motion. *J Orthop Trauma* 2002;16(4):231-238.

This article presents a review of a laboratory study in which three types of reconstruction nails were inserted in fiberglass composite femurs. Four fracture patterns were studied (transverse subtrochanteric, subtrochanteric with posteromedial wedge comminution, subtrochanteric with a 1-cm gap, and a 1-cm gap with a subcapital neck fracture). Single- and double-leg stance loading was simulated to compare fracture site motion using second-generation intramedullary nails. The authors found the choice of implant was not critical for simple, well-reduced fractures. As the severity of the fracture increased, the choice of implant became a significant factor in reducing fracture site motion. Implants that allow minimal fracture site motion with either the Long Gamma (Howmedica-Osteonics, Rutherford, NJ) or the Russell-Taylor nail had the best performance.

Posttraumatic Pain/Postoperative Considerations

Burd TA, Hughes MS, Anglen JO: Heterotopic ossification prophylaxis with indomethacin increases the risk of long-bone nonunion. *J Bone Joint Surg Br* 2003;85(5): 700-705.

The authors reviewed 282 patients who had open reduction and internal fixation of an acetabular fracture. Patients at risk to develop heterotopic ossification were randomized to receive either radiation therapy or indomethacin. A significant difference in the rate of nonunion was found when comparing patients who received indomethacin with those that did not. Patients with concurrent fractures of the acetabulum and long bones who received indomethacin had a significantly greater risk of nonunion of fractures of the long bones compared with those who had radiation therapy or no prophylaxis.

Burd TA, Lowry KJ, Anglen JO: Indomethacin compared with localized irradiation for the prevention of heterotopic ossification following surgical treatment of acetabular fractures. *J Bone Joint Surg Am* 2001;83-A(12):1783-1788.

The authors of this prospective, randomized study compared the relative effectiveness of local irradiation and the administration of oral indomethacin for prophylaxis to prevent heterotopic ossification following surgical treatment of acetabular fractures. Both local radiation and indomethacin provided effective prophylaxis for heterotopic ossification after surgical treatment of acetabular fractures using the posterior or extensile approach. The authors found no significant difference in efficacy between the two regimens.

Davidson BL, Sullivan SD, Kahn SR, Borris L, Bossuyt P, Raskob G: The economics of venous thromboembolism prophylaxis. *Chest* 2003;124(suppl 6):393S-396S.

This review article lists the important safety and efficacy outcomes of prophylaxis to prevent venous thrombosis after hip and knee replacement and after hip fracture surgery. Estimates of incidences and costs and model comparisons of modalities are presented.

Ennis RS: Postoperative deep vein thrombosis prophylaxis: A retrospective analysis in 1000 consecutive hip fracture patients treated in a community hospital setting. *J South Orthop Assoc* 2003;12(1):10-17.

A retrospective study of 1,000 consecutive hip fractures in patients in a community hospital showed that 95% of patients received a combination of mechanical and pharmacologic prophylaxis for prevention of DVT. Fifty-one patients (18.4%) in the eligible population received no prophylaxis. Aspirin was given to 387 patients (41.2%) as an anticoagulation agent. LMWH (enoxaparin) was given to 429 patients (45.6%). Ten patients (1.1%) were treated with heparin and 17 patients (1.8%) were treated with warfarin. Forty-three patients received a combination of therapies. Concomitant intermittent pneumatic compression and pharmacologic prophylaxis was used to treat 495 patients. Based on outcome results, the authors concluded that enoxaparin is an excellent drug for use in hip fracture patients because of its relatively short half-life and its predictable pharmacokinetics.

Rath EM, Russell GV Jr, Washington WJ, Routt ML Jr: Gluteus minimus necrotic debridement diminished heterotopic ossification after acetabular fracture fixation. *Injury* 2002;33(9):751-756.

This prospective study evaluated the impact of the débridement of the necrotic gluteus minimus muscle on the formation of heterotopic ossification after surgical fixation of posterior wall and associated transverse-posterior wall acetabular fractures using the Kocher-Langenbeck surgical exposure. The authors found that resection of the necrotic gluteus minimus muscle results in a decrease in the formation of heterotopic ossification that is comparable to results found in other studies using nonsteroidal anti-inflammatory drugs. The authors concluded that débridement of the necrotic gluteus minimus muscle was an efficient and safe method of preventing significant heterotropic ossification in the studied patient population.

Schafer SJ, Schafer LO, Anglen JO, Childers M: Heterotopic ossification in rehabilitation patients who have had internal fixation of an acetabular fracture. *J Rehabil Res Dev* 2000;37(4):389-393.

This article describes a study of 94 patients who had posterior surgical fixation of an acetabular fracture. Most patients received irradiation or indomethacin to prevent heterotopic ossification; five patients did not receive prophylaxis. Of the 45 patients who initially received indomethacin, 5 discontinued the use of the medication for various reasons. Of 12 patients who did not receive adequate prophylaxis, 5 developed disabling heterotopic ossification. The authors conclude that adequate prophylaxis is essential to prevent heterotopic ossification.

Shehab D, Elgazzar AH, Collier BD: Heterotopic ossification. *J Nucl Med* 2002;43(3):346-353.

This article discusses symptoms of heterotopic ossification and treatment options including nonsteroidal anti-inflammatory drugs (such as indomethacin), diphosphonate (such as ethane-1-hydroxy-1,1-diphosphate), and local radiation therapy. Surgical resection of heterotopic ossification to preserve joint mobility and possible recurrence caused by resection of the lesion before heterotopic ossification is complete are also discussed.

Thaler HW, Roller RE, Greiner N, Sim E, Korninger C: Thromboprophylaxis with 60 mg enoxaparin is safe in hip trauma surgery. *J Trauma* 2001;51(3):518-521.

This prospective study was undertaken to evaluate clinically apparent DVT, PE, and major hemorrhage in patients receiving thromboprophylaxis with enoxaparin who had hip surgery for a hip fracture. The authors concluded that thromboprophylaxis with 60 mg enoxaparin taken daily in split doses, and started before surgery, is a safe and appropriate in patients with hip fractures. Clinically apparent DVT and PE were rarely observed and bleeding complications were compa-

rable to those occurring with the use of a conventional regimen of thromboprophylaxis.

Turpie AG, Eriksson BI, Bauer KA, Lassen MR: New pentasaccharides for the prophylaxis of venous thromboembolism: Clinical studies. *Chest* 2003;124(suppl 6): 371S-378S.

The benefit-to-risk ratio of preventing venous thrombosis with fondaparinux after major orthopaedic surgery was investigated in four randomized, double-blind international phase III trials of patients undergoing surgery for hip fracture, elective hip replacement, and major knee surgery. Compared with enoxaparin, fondaparinux administered postoperatively at a subcutaneous dose of 2.5 mg daily, reduced the overall incidence of venous thrombosis up to day 11 by 55.2% ($P < 0.001$). The incidence of clinically relevant bleeding was low and did not differ between the two groups. Fondaparinux achieved optimal efficacy and safety when treatment was initiated 6 hours or more after the surgical procedure. In another study, a 4-week course of prophylaxis with fondaparinux after hip surgery reduced the risk of venous thrombosis by 96% compared with 1 week of treatment with prophylaxis.

Turpie AG, Eriksson BI, Lassen MR, Bauer KA: A meta-analysis of fondaparinux versus enoxaparin in the prevention of venous thromboembolism after major orthopaedic surgery. *J South Orthop Assoc* 2002;11(4):182-188.

This worldwide phase III program, consisting of four randomized, double-blind trials, compared the benefit-to-risk ratio of a subcutaneous 2.5-mg once daily regimen of fondaparinux with the use of enoxaparin for patients undergoing surgery for hip fracture, elective hip replacement, or elective major knee surgery. The overall incidence of venous thromboembolism up to day 11 was reduced from 13.7% in the group receiving enoxaparin to 6.8% in the group receiving fondaparinux with a common odds reduction of 55.2% supporting the use of fondaparinux (95% confidence interval: 45.8% to 63.1%, $P = 10(-17)$). Fondaparinux also reduced the incidence of proximal DVT by 57.4%. The overall incidence of clinically relevant bleeding was low and did not differ between the two groups. The benefit of fondaparinux was consistent across all types of surgery and subgroups.

Posttraumatic Arthritis

Felson DT: An update on the pathogenesis and epidemiology of osteoarthritis. *Radiol Clin North Am* 2004; 42(1):1-9.

This review article discusses the causes and risk factors of osteoarthritis. Risk factors include age, obesity, and joint injury. Risk factors for symptoms include bone marrow edema, synovitis, and joint effusion.

Gelber AC, Hochberg MC, Mead LA, Wang N, Wigley FM, Klag MJ: Joint injury in young adults and risk for subsequent knee and hip osteoarthritis. *Ann Intern Med* 2000;133(5):321-328.

This article presents a review of a cohort study to examine the relationship between joint injury and the incidence of knee and hip osteoarthritis. Former medical students (n = 1,321) were evaluated for joint injury during follow-up for incident osteoarthritis. The authors concluded that young adults with knee injuries have an increased risk for osteoarthritis later in life and should be targeted for primary prevention of osteoarthritis.

Classic Bibliography

Creamer P, Hochberg MC: Osteoarthritis. *Lancet* 1997; 350:503-508.

Eftekhar NS: Conversion of failed previous surgery, in Eftekhar NS (ed): *Total Hip Arthroplasty*. St Louis, MO, Mosby, 1993.

Gebhard JS, Amstutz HC: Post-traumatic acute fracture, in: Amstutz HC (ed): *Hip Arthroplasty*. New York, NY, Churchill Livingstone, 1991.

Jimenez ML, Tile M, Schenk RS: Total hip replacement after acetabular fracture. *Orthop Clin North Am* 1997; 28(3):435-446.

Koval KJ, Zuckerman JD: Hip fractures II: Evaluation and treatment of intertrochanteric fractures. *J Am Acad Orthop Surg* 1994;2(3):150-156.

Koval KJ, Zuckerman JD: Trauma: Hip, in Callaghan JJ, Dennis DA, Paprosky WG, Rosenberg OA (eds): *Orthopaedic Knowledge Update: Hip and Knee Reconstruction*. Rosemont, IL, American Academy of Orthopaedic Surgeons, 1995, pp 97-108.

Marchetti ME, Steinberg GG, Coumas JM: Intermediate-term experience of Pipkin fracture-dislocation of the hip. *J Orthop Trauma* 1996;10(7):455-461.

Schonweiss T, Wagner S, Mayr E, Ruter A: Late results after fracture of the femoral head. *Unfallchirurg* 1999; 102(10):776-783.

Seinsheimer F: Subtrochanteric fractures of the femur. *J Bone Joint Surg Am* 1978;60(3):300-306.

Tepper S, Hochberg MC: Factors associated with hip osteoarthritis: Data from the First National Health and Nutrition Examination Survey (NHANES-I). *Am J Epidemiol* 1993;137(10):1081-1088.

Chapter 36

Osteotomy

William M. Mihalko, MD, PhD

Kevin J. Mulhall, MD, MCh, FRCSI (Tr & Orth)

Khaled J. Saleh, MD, MSc (Epid), FRCSC, FACS

Introduction

Osteotomy is a viable option for many pathologic entities of the hip joint. Acetabular and proximal femoral osteotomies are used separately or in conjunction to correct deformity and/or improve the mechanics and the weight-bearing surface of the joint. These pathologic conditions can be identified as those causing mechanical pain without deformity and those that are pain producing in patients with an existing deformity. The goals of osteotomy are essentially to relieve pain and improve function by improving the congruence (sphericity of the joint), coverage (improvement of the center edge angle), and/or containment (the amount of femoral head within the acetabulum) of the joint to obviate or at least substantially delay the need for total hip arthroplasty (THA).

The hip joint withstands millions of gait cycles per year, with a force that is 3 to 10 times body weight depending on the activity being performed. The mechanical axis and weight-bearing profile of the hip must be taken into consideration and optimized when considering a patient for an osteotomy about the hip. When an osteotomy is used to treat hips with congenital or acquired deformity (posttraumatic, nonunion, malunion, slipped capital femoral epiphysis), it should help eliminate impingement, correct the deformity, and create an acceptable range of motion and mechanical profile of the hip.

THA is a viable treatment option for older patients with end-stage osteoarthritis, but for relatively young patients, the option of THA brings about the risk of poorer outcomes. Past studies reporting on the outcomes of younger patients who underwent THA have revealed a lower survival rate at short- and long-term intervals. Therefore, using other native bone procedures that will not significantly compromise the conversion to THA is more appealing. Many osteotomies are performed not as salvage procedures but to prevent or significantly delay the need for prosthetic replacement in the future. These osteotomies are an important tool in the treatment of early osteoarthritis, and they allow reconstruction surgeons to offer an alternative treatment to properly selected patients. In some instances, special-ized training may be required. These procedures can be categorized under two major headings: pelvic osteotomy and femoral osteotomy.

Pelvic Osteotomy

Pelvic osteotomies are commonly used in the treatment of pediatric hip disorders; however, developments in surgical techniques and diagnosis have resulted in the widespread use of pelvic osteotomies in adults as well as joint-preserving surgery in the presence of anatomic and biomechanical hip abnormalities. The basic principle of pelvic osteotomy is to create near-normal hip biomechanics by repositioning normal hyaline articular surfaces so as to increase the surface area's transmitting force and thus reduce articular contact pressures and resultant cartilage damage and ultimately prevent degenerative joint disease.

Residual acetabular dysplasia is the most common cause of degenerative joint disease of the hip (up to 50% of patients), and it is currently the most common indication for pelvic osteotomy. Deficient acetabular coverage of the femoral head and subluxation are a prelude to the development of degenerative joint disease. These abnormalities are in turn associated with abnormally increased joint contact pressures, secondary labral disorders, and ultimately cartilage degeneration progressing from the joint rim. Other common causes of pediatric degenerative joint disease include Legg-Calvé-Perthes disease and slipped capital femoral epiphysis. Many if not most instances of adult idiopathic hip osteoarthritis are actually related to these or other developmental conditions. To best prevent later degenerative joint disease, it is necessary to correct architectural abnormalities as early as possible, often in patients with mild clinical symptoms.

History, Examination, Investigations

Patients with hip dysplasia typically become symptomatic before the development of severe degenerative changes because of abnormal hip biomechanics, mild hip instability, impingement, or associated labral pathol-

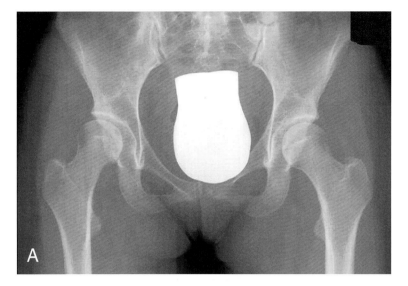

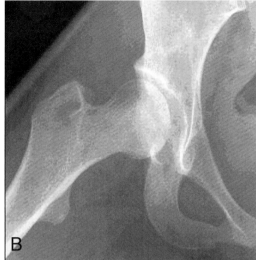

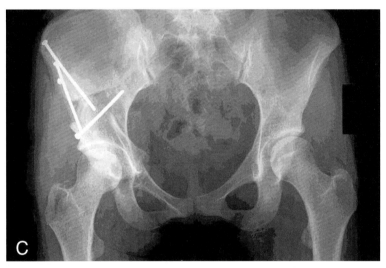

Figure 1 Radiographs of a 27-year-old woman with right groin and lateral hip pain secondary to developmental dysplasia of the hip. **A,** Typical radiographic signs of dysplasia are present, including low center edge angle, inadequate coverage, and increased acetabular inclination. **B,** Abduction view of the right hip demonstrating improved congruency and no anticipated need for femoral osteotomy. **C,** Radiograph obtained after periacetabular (Ganz) osteotomy demonstrating good correction with improved coverage; patient had full resolution of symptoms.

ogy. Pain may be located in the groin or in the area of the greater trochanter, particularly with activity because the abductors experience fatigue and there is trochanteric irritation. Symptoms such as locking or snapping may indicate labral pathology, especially if accompanied by pain on extension from a flexed position, especially with rotation (such as getting out of a car seat or swimming the breaststroke).

Physical examination will determine gait, limb length, range of motion, and abductor dysfunction. Acetabular rim and labral disease may be indicated by a positive impingement test (passive internal rotation while adducting and flexing the hip to 90°). Dysplasia is often accompanied by increased internal rotation; therefore, decrease in this movement with early degenerative changes may be subtle. Symptomatic anterior instability is diagnosed by a positive apprehension test, which is performed with the patient's legs over the end of the examination table. Passive external rotation and extension causes groin discomfort as the antero-

laterally uncovered femoral head subluxates.

Radiographic investigations are crucial and should include a standing orthograde plain film of the pelvis (Figure 1, *A*) and a false profile view of the hip on which joint space, center edge angles, coverage, and subluxation can be assessed. Acetabular retroversion is recognized by the crossover and posterior wall signs.

A functional abduction view (Figure 1, *B*) is obtained to assess potential joint congruency (and whether a femoral osteotomy may be necessary). In some instances, CT may be helpful in surgical planning. MRI and magnetic resonance arthrography can also be helpful to determine labral disorders such as tears and ganglion formation, acetabular rim lesions, and evidence of femoroacetabular impingement, which may all be useful in planning intraoperative maneuvers.

Patient Selection

The most common indication for a reconstructive or reorientation juxta-acetabular osteotomy is symptomatic

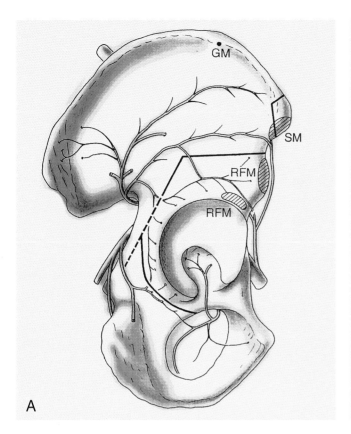

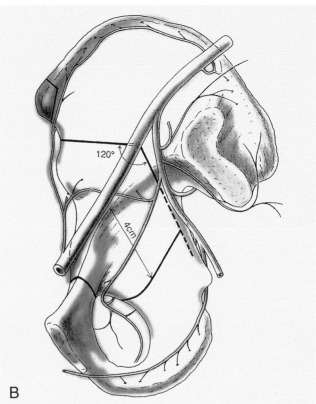

Figure 2 Drawings showing the vascularity to the acetabulum and the sequence of osteotomies at the external **(A)** and internal **(B)** pelvic surface. The abductors are not detached from the external iliac wing. GM = gluteus medius tubercle, RFM = rectus femoris muscle (direct and indirect heads), and SM = sartorius muscle. (Reproduced from Leunig M, Siebenrock KA, Ganz R: Rationale of periacetabular osteotomy and background work. *Instr Course Lect* 2001;50:229-238.)

acetabular dysplasia in a young adult. Because the deformity is typically acetabular in these patients, the acetabulum is the main focus of most interventions. Additionally, proximal femoral osteotomy may be needed and is occasionally indicated as an isolated procedure when most of the deformity is located on the femoral side as with coxa valga subluxans. An open triradiate cartilage is a contraindication to most reconstructive osteotomies, whereas an upper age limit depends on considering each patient's factors, risks, and prognosis for osteotomy and THA. Controversy currently exists regarding the exact radiographic indications. Nonetheless, factors associated with reliably good outcomes generally include relatively young age, good range of motion, early or no degenerative changes, minimal subluxation, and joint congruency or good potential congruency.

Periacetabular (Ganz) Osteotomy

The periacetabular (Ganz) osteotomy has gained great popularity since its introduction approximately 17 years ago because it allows for a large potential correction that is obtainable in all planes through one surgical approach. Additionally, it allows for potential medial translation of the hip center, thus reducing the lever arm of the hip and joint loading. It also does not alter the

shape of the true pelvis or destabilize the pelvis (Figure 1, *C*). There are many detailed descriptions of the surgical technique available in the literature and only recent developments and technical pearls will be considered here.

The procedure essentially involves the following five steps (Figure 2): an incomplete ischial osteotomy, a complete pubic osteotomy, a chevron supra-acetabular osteotomy, a retroacetabular osteotomy, and completion of the whole osteotomy by controlled fracture of the original incompletely osteotomized ischium. Cadaveric study of acetabular landmarks has shown that the posterior margin of the hip is located approximately 2 cm anterior to the sciatic notch. The anatomic guide point for the osteotomy of the ischium has been shown to be on average 14 mm inferior to the distal margin of the hip. Because the posterior column remains mechanically intact, minimal fixation is required. The optimal potential method of fixation has been assessed in cadaver studies that compared three long 4.5-mm cortical screws from the iliac crest to the osteotomized fragment with two such screws supplemented by a transverse screw. Although the latter construct provided greater local stiffness from the acetabular segment to the ilium, neither method allowed immediate weight bearing; therefore, crutch-aided postoperative mobilization is still advised.

Concerns have been expressed regarding the vascularity of the acetabular fragment and the potential for osteonecrosis following periacetabular (Ganz) osteotomy. However, preservation of acetabular fragment blood supply by the supra-acetabular and acetabular branches of the superior gluteal artery, obturator artery, and inferior gluteal artery has been demonstrated in cadaver and injection studies, and also by using MRI and laser Doppler flowmetry.

One of the most challenging aspects of periacetabular osteotomy is performing the actual fragment correction accurately. It has recently been established that, contrary to previous opinion, one in three to six patients with acetabular dysplasia has acetabular retroversion. These patients may also have smaller lateral center edge measurements. Although realignment osteotomy is still appropriate in these patients, the corrective maneuvers must be adjusted to correct for socket retroversion as well as standard anterior and lateral insufficiency.

It is important to perform the intraoperative radiographic assessment of correction by means of an anteroposterior radiograph of the whole pelvis rather than with limited views of the surgical hip or image-intensifier visualization. Anterior capsulotomy, which is almost always indicated, can be performed while waiting for the initial radiograph to be processed. The capsulotomy allows assessment and treatment of labral and articular lesions. Labral tears, typically anterosuperior, may be resected or reattached if suitable or, if small and stable, left untreated. Cartilage flaps should be resected and, if subchondral bone is exposed, drilling or microfracture may be performed. Finally, the range of motion should also be assessed at the time of final correction, with particular attention given to flexion and internal rotation and any anterior impingement. If the latter is present, resection osteoplasty of the femoral head-neck junction to recreate adequate superomedial offset is typically required.

Several authors have demonstrated the significant learning curve associated with performing periacetabular (Ganz) osteotomy, with complication rates decreasing significantly with experience. Complications typically reported include reflex sympathetic dystrophy, motor nerve palsy, heterotopic ossification, delayed or nonunion of the ilium, and rarely incisional abdominal hernias. This has led some to modify the Ganz technique to a more curved periacetabular osteotomy with satisfactory early results. Intraoperative electromyography has also been used in an effort to monitor vulnerable nerves and has shown some promise in its ability to predict postoperative deficits.

In terms of outcomes, significant improvements in both global and disease-specific health outcomes have been demonstrated after this procedure, with high rates of patient satisfaction and improvements in athletic ac-

tivities. Long-term follow-up (minimum 10 years) has also confirmed the maintenance of radiographic correction, such as lateral center edge angle, anterior center edge angle, acetabular index, and lateralization of the femoral head. Good to excellent long-term clinical results have also been reported, with 82% survivorship (hip arthroplasty as end point) of early series of periacetabular (Ganz) osteotomies. Unfavorable outcomes have been associated with patient-dependent factors such as increasing age, moderate to severe osteoarthritis, the presence of labral lesions (supporting the need to address these at the time of surgery), and surgical factors, including less anterior coverage correction and suboptimal postoperative acetabular index.

Traditional indications for periacetabular (Ganz) osteotomies have been limited to younger patients with minimal subluxation, possible congruent reduction, preservation of joint space, and no significant arthrosis. Recent studies have been conducted to determine whether these indications can be extended to include older patients and to those with more severe acetabular dysplasia and subluxation or a secondary acetabulum.

In a study of 16 patients (average age, 17.6 years) with severe acetabular dysplasia (8 with subluxation and 8 with a secondary acetabulum), 11 had good or excellent clinical results postoperatively and were satisfied at more than 4-year follow-up. In another study, it was found that patients with relatively marked degenerative changes have good early results and can thus at least delay the need for THA (provided that there is some evidence of improvement in joint space on preoperative functional radiographs). Good results at 8-year follow-up have also been reported in patients (mean age, 51 years) with early-stage osteoarthritis. Clinical and radiographic improvements of the center-edge angle were achieved in a younger control group. Kaplan-Meier survivorship analysis, with radiographic progression of osteoarthritis as the end point, predicted a 10-year survival rate of 70% in the older group and 93.7% in the younger group, indicating that osteotomy may be appropriate for selected older patients.

A modified periacetabular (Ganz) osteotomy was used to treat dysplasia in a group of patients with Down syndrome (mean age, 16.5 years). During 5 years of follow-up, two patients required secondary varus derotation femoral osteotomies, and one required arthroscopic management of a labral tear. All remained either asymptomatic or symptomatically improved, indicating the potential usefulness of this procedure for these patients.

There has also been increased recognition recently of the importance of acetabular retroversion, identified on AP radiographs and typically caused by deficiency of the posterior wall in association with hip osteoarthritis. This raises the possibility of treating symptomatic anterior femoroacetabular impingement resulting from acetabular retroversion with a periacetabular osteotomy. A recent study of 29 periacetabular (Ganz) osteotomies (22 patients; average patient age, 23 years) that were performed to treat symptomatic acetabular retroversion demonstrated good or excellent clinical and radiographic results in 26 hips at an average 30-month follow-up. There has also been at least one report of the use of periacetabular (Ganz) osteotomy in the treatment of a patient with an unreconstructable posterior wall deficiency and persistent instability after a traumatic hip dislocation.

Other Reconstructive Acetabular Osteotomies

Although the periacetabular (Ganz) osteotomy is probably the most commonly performed, other juxta-acetabular osteotomies may be considered. The most popular alternatives reported in the recent literature include the Steel triple innominate osteotomy and its variations (including the Tonnis osteotomy) and the spherical (and dial) type osteotomies as popularized by Wagner. The indications and patient selection for these procedures are similar to those described above.

Triple osteotomies consist of a Salter osteotomy in combination with superior pubic ramus and ischial cuts. This involves at least two incisions and usually results in a large fragment that may be difficult to position because of the sacropelvic ligaments; a large fragment also tends to lateralize the joint center. Fifteen-year follow-up of this procedure with THA as the end point demonstrated good to excellent clinical results in 64% of patients and a 12% conversion to THA. As with most pelvic osteotomies, poor results occurred in patients with osteoarthritic changes and in those with poor preoperative clinical scores.

Several spherical osteotomies have been described, and the advantages of these over triple osteotomies are similar to the advantages of the periacetabular (Ganz) osteotomy (osteotomy location close to the joint, allowing much better rotation and accurate reconstruction of acetabular coverage, and less fragment displacement for a given correction thus decreasing the risk of nonunion). Spherical osteotomies also allow for joint medialization, produce less secondary pelvic deformity, and are more stable postoperatively. The disadvantages of spherical osteotomies include their relative technical complexity and the increased risk of intra-articular penetration. As a result, the periacetabular (Ganz) osteotomy has generally become the preferred intervention. However, good results are typically achieved with spherical osteotomies when performed by experienced surgeons. Twenty-year Kaplan-Meier survival estimates of 86.4% have been reported with conversion to THA the end point. Joint congruency has been identified as the most important factor for satisfactory long-term outcomes.

Salvage Acetabular Osteotomies

The most comprehensively studied and reported salvage osteotomy is the Chiari osteotomy, with the results of up to 30-year follow-up recently published. It is essentially a modified shelf procedure, of which there are several, involving an iliac osteotomy from the sciatic notch to just proximal to the joint and subsequent medial displacement of the acetabulum. With weight bearing, the capsule undergoes metaplasia to produce weight-bearing coverage, as do the other described shelf procedures, which are less commonly used as definitive procedures in adults. If performed at all, salvage procedures should really only be considered for patients in whom congruous reduction of the hip is not possible because of fixed incongruity or secondary deformity or as a salvage procedure in young patients with advanced degenerative disease related to severe dysplasia. A Chiari procedure may be of benefit in that it can delay the need for THA in these patients, and it may even facilitate later THA by improving acetabular bony coverage.

Technical aspects to consider when performing Chiari osteotomies include use of a transtrochanteric approach that can help ensure that the osteotomy is at an appropriate level and will also facilitate advancement of a high-riding greater trochanter. It is important to avoid intra-articular osteotomy; after the osteotomy, there is typically an osseous defect anteriorly that should be grafted to prevent subsequent anterior instability.

Intra-articular positioning of the labrum can also be problematic after Chiari osteotomy and may be associated with postoperative pain and mechanical symptoms. This is typically secondary to unstable labral tears displacing into the joint in combination with cartilage damage in the acetabulum or femoral head. If a labral tear is present at the time of osteotomy, this should be resected rather than repaired. If symptoms occur postoperatively, treatment with arthroscopic labral resection and chondral flaps with microfracturing of exposed subchondral bone have been shown to be effective.

Recent reports of positive results with these procedures based on long-term follow-up (10 to 30 years) have typically included young patients with minimal dysplasia (and relatively greater center edge angles), those with minimal subluxation, and those with early or no hip arthritis. These patients would now likely be treated with redirectional osteotomies and related procedures. Overall, only satisfactory improvements in mean clinical and pain scores are widely reported. The end point for most studies is conversion to THA, with many studies also demonstrating progression of degenerative joint disease over time. Reported survival rates among heterogeneous populations vary from 72% at 10-year follow-up to 68% to 80% at 18-year follow-up for Chiari osteotomies. Other more limited shelf procedures typically have poorer survival rates free of conversion to THA, with reports of 37% at 20-year follow-up.

Issues for Childbirth

Because most patients undergoing a reconstructive pelvic osteotomy for hip dysplasia are young women of childbearing potential, it is important to have some information with which to effectively counsel these women regarding subsequent childbirth. Whereas the Salter osteotomy seems to have minimal effects on the pelvic dimensions, probably because of the young age at which it is performed and subsequent remodeling, the Steel and Chiari osteotomies tend to decrease pelvic dimensions, particularly the transverse midpelvis diameter, below the threshold required for vaginal delivery, thus increasing the likelihood of cesarean section. An advantage of the Ganz osteotomy is that radiographic studies and MRI pelvimetry have shown that it has little effect on the dimensions of the osseous pelvis.

Proximal Femoral Osteotomy

Patients without significant acetabular deficiency who have either congenital or acquired pathologic anatomy may be candidates for an isolated proximal femoral osteotomy. Proximal femoral osteotomies have been used for many decades and have been described as a salvage procedure for young patients with osteoarthritis, those with posttraumatic arthrosis with or without deformity, and for definitive treatment of symptomatic patients with a slipped capital femoral epiphysis, mild to moderate osteoarthritis, or osteonecrosis.

The etiology of osteoarthrosis is usually associated with an abnormal mechanical profile or abnormal weight-bearing surface of the hip. In patients with a coxa valga deformity, the weight-bearing surface is often shifted laterally and anteriorly on the femoral head. This can cause extrusion of the femoral head and a higher load per unit area on the superoanterior aspect, which is often amenable to a varus derotation type of osteotomy. In patients with a coxa vara deformity, the weight-bearing surface is shifted medially and posteriorly. In this instance, the hip often creates medial and inferior osteophytes on the femoral head and acetabulum, which can often be used to create a weight-bearing surface with a valgus and extension type of osteotomy. When acetabular dysplasia is present and the femoral head is hinging on the lateral aspect of the dysplastic acetabulum, congruency is often improved with a valgus osteotomy. These deformities can cause early arthrosis from the varying mechanical changes about the hip joint, and corrective osteotomy, which improves the weight-bearing surface or congruency of the joint, can delay or possibly halt the progression of the disease.

Osteonecrosis of the femoral head causes pain from abnormal tissue and articular surface geometry as well as from alteration of the mechanical properties of the weight-bearing surface of the femoral head. In some patients, the necrotic area can be rotated out of the main weight-bearing surface of the joint.

Patients with a history of a slipped capital femoral epiphysis are known to progress to early degenerative disease. Extending the proximal femur in these patients (a flexion rotation osteotomy) creates a better weight-bearing surface of the hip and a better mechanical profile of the joint. Thus, regardless of the etiology being treated, the basic principles of proximal intertrochanteric osteotomy can be used to create a better mechanical environment for the hip.

Patient Selection

Changing the weight-bearing surface or orientation of the femoral head with any osteotomy should produce a more congruent joint or a more favorable weight-bearing surface. Regardless of etiology, the ultimate goal of a proximal femoral osteotomy remains the same: to prevent or delay the time until any type of prosthetic replacement in a relatively young patient is required. When trying to determine whether a patient is a candidate for a proximal femoral osteotomy, the surgeon must consider multiple variables to make the proper decision.

A relatively young age is required to outweigh the excellent outcome of THA in patients older than 60 years. The patient must have a range of motion that will not significantly reduce the functional range after an osteotomy. When rotating the proximal femur, patients will have their motion shifted in that direction and overall absolute range of motion will not improve. For example, when performing a valgus proximal femoral osteotomy on a patient with only 10° of hip adduction preoperatively, if a surgeon plans a 10° valgus correction, the patient will have no postoperative adduction. Therefore, functional range of motion is important in determining whether patients are candidates for a proximal femoral osteotomy.

The patient should also have adequate bone stock for fixation, which typically involves a blade type AO plate. A history of inflammatory arthritis is generally considered a contraindication for an osteotomy because the disease process will continue to affect the joint. When considering osteotomy in patients with osteonecrosis, the area of necrosis needs to be taken into consideration. Osteotomy has been found to have a significantly lower rate of success if the angle of the necrotic area on the AP and lateral radiographs of the femoral head exceeds 200°.

Patients must also have improvement of the weight-bearing surface and/or joint congruity. This is determined by preoperative radiographs with the hip in abduction and adduction (Figure 3). Obtaining these ra-

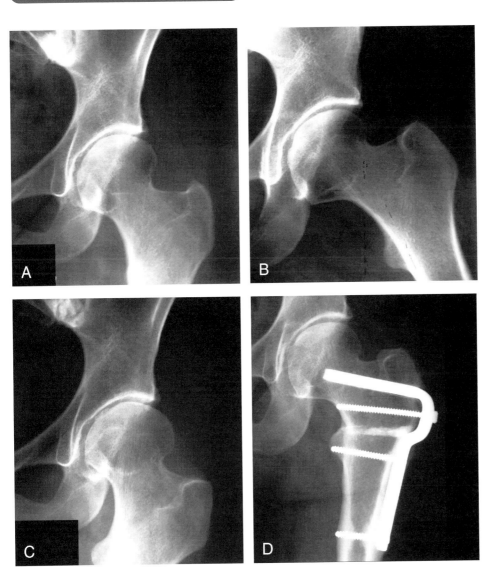

Figure 3 **A,** Preoperative AP radiograph of the hip shows coxa valga and medial osteophytes beginning to form in a young patient with a painful hip. **B,** Abduction radiograph shows improved coverage and congruency. **C,** Adduction radiograph shows less coverage of the femoral head and less congruency of the hip joint. **D,** Postoperative radiograph obtained 4 years after proximal femoral valgus osteotomy shows improvement in coverage of the femoral head. The patient reported significantly less pain.

diographic views is paramount to determine whether patients will have a significant improvement radiographically after the proposed osteotomy. A false profile view will also help the surgeon evaluate any anterior coverage deficiency of the acetabulum on the femoral head.

Other patient factors must also be considered before determining whether a proximal femoral osteotomy is appropriate. Patients must be properly counseled concerning the length of recovery and the long-term outcome of the procedure before proceeding with surgery. Patients must properly understand the consequences of early severe arthrosis or the possible poor outcome of a THA in a young patient population. The patient's occupation, age, and level of activity need to be taken into consideration. When the major symptom is limited functional motion and not pain, there may be an unreasonable level of expectation by the patient. Ideal candidates are typically patients in their third or fourth decade of life without major signs of osteoarthritis in whom the surgery may delay the need for THA until the sixth de-

cade of life. When considering a salvage type of procedure, the risks and benefits must be weighed against those of conversion to THA within a 4- or 5-year time frame.

Preoperative Planning

After the determination has been made that the patient is a candidate for a proximal femoral osteotomy, certain preoperative planning should be done to aid in the successful outcome of the surgery. Abduction and adduction views of the hip are used to determine whether the proposed osteotomy will improve the weight-bearing surface and congruency of the hip joint. If these radiographs do not show improvement of the joint, the patient may be precluded from undergoing a proximal femoral osteotomy or the surgeon may determine that a combined acetabular osteotomy is necessary in a patient with dysplasia. The abduction and adduction radiographs will help identify how much varus or valgus correction is necessary to improve the weight-bearing sur-

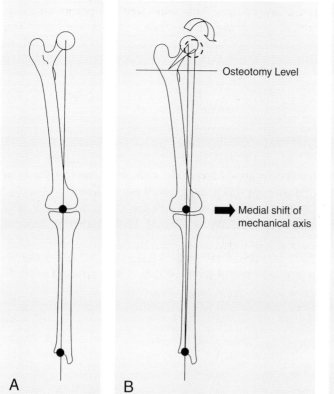

Figure 4 Drawings show that normal coronal mechanical axis alignment **(A)** can be altered with a varus proximal femoral osteotomy **(B)**. In this example, it is evident that the weight-bearing line is shifted into the medial compartment of the knee. Displacement of the lower osteotomy segment medially can correct this alignment.

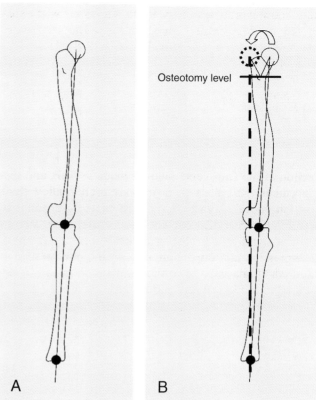

Figure 5 Drawings showing normal sagittal mechanical axis alignment **(A)** and how an osteotomy at the intertrochanteric level **(B)** can adversely effect the normal lower extremity alignment. This example depicts an extension osteotomy and the how it may cause the weight-bearing line of the lower extremity to be located behind the center of the knee.

face characteristics of the hip as well as help determine what effect the procedure will have on the mechanical axis of the lower extremity. Tracing paper is then used to place each segment in the proper location in conjunction with the blade plate. This allows for verification of the preoperative plan.

Surgeons must be aware of mechanical axis changes of the lower extremity from the proposed osteotomy. When considering the mechanical axis effects of the osteotomy, surgeons must consider the correction in all three planes. The remaining placement of the proximal femur may create an abnormal lower extremity mechanical axis and may require displacement at the osteotomy site (Figure 4). In a varus osteotomy, the weight-bearing line will shift medially at the knee, and a valgus proximal femoral osteotomy will shift the weight-bearing line laterally at the knee. These effects need to be taken into account if the patient has a preexisting deformity at the knee and may require long weight-bearing radiographs for proper preoperative planning.

Limb-length changes from different techniques also must be considered as with other lower extremity osteotomies. Surgeons must determine preoperatively whether wedge resection will aid or worsen the limb

length as well as the mechanical axis of the lower extremity. Surgeons must take into consideration that any significant displacement may make the conversion to THA much more difficult in the future.

The sagittal plane alignment may change the mechanical axis when flexion or extension rotations are used to improve the weight-bearing surface. Wedge resection may place the mechanical axis behind (extension) or in front of (flexion osteotomy) the knee. This is yet another reason why wedge resection should be avoided (Figure 5).

Proximal Femoral Osteotomy Technique

Whether performing a varus or valgus osteotomy with or without correction in other planes, the surgical techniques are similar. Once the preoperative planning routine has determined the amount of correction and whether displacement and/or wedge resection are necessary, the standard surgical techniques are used. A fluoroscopic table is used with the patient bumped with a sand bag. The proximal femur is approached via a direct lateral approach, and the vastus lateralis is elevated off its origin. Alternatively, using an anterolateral approach may allow labral pathology to be addressed when suspected or documented preoperatively. The osteotomy site is situated at the proximal portion of the lesser trochanter as identified under fluoroscopy, and a Steinmann pin is placed at this level. A second guide pin is then placed in the position of the blade plate from the preoperative planning template for the coronal plane correction. The blade chisel is then manipulated to allow for the sagittal plane correction, and the four-hole blade plate is inserted. After the osteotomy is made, any correction in the transverse plane is made as well, and displacement and plate type clamps are used to allow shaft fixation to take place. The blade plate insertion site should be 1.5 to 2.0 cm above the osteotomy site to leave a significant bridge of cortical bone for fixation. Compression and impaction at the osteotomy site when the blade plate is fixed to the shaft should also be performed to aid in stability and healing.

The lower extremity alignment can also be checked fluoroscopically with use of a bovie cord to check the colinearity of the center of the femoral head to the center of the knee and ankle. This maneuver can aid in determining whether any displacement of the shaft is necessary to maintain anatomic alignment in the coronal plane.

The changes in the sagittal plane can be minimized by not using a wedge resection, which can shift the weight-bearing line in front of or behind the knee. Instead, the proximal aspect of the osteotomy can be impacted into distal bone to help maintain the mechanical axis. Postoperatively, patients are encouraged to perform heel slides and motion while in bed and initiate crutch walking with toe touch weight bearing. Patients then slowly advance to partial and eventually full weight bearing within 3 to 6 months or once bony union is evident radiographically.

Outcomes

Multiple studies have reported the long-term outcomes of isolated proximal femoral osteotomy. One study reviewed 70 patients with osteoarthritis as a result of acetabular dysplasia who underwent a proximal femoral osteotomy. Inclusion criteria required greater than 60° of flexion and extension, age younger than 60 years, good joint congruity with adduction, and all patients had significant osteoarthritis with a medial osteophyte. All patients underwent a valgus-extension intertrochanteric osteotomy with lateral displacement of the proximal fragment. The mean age of the patients was 44 years, and a mean follow-up of 9.4 years was reported. With revision surgery as an end point, the 10-year survivorship was 82%; in patients younger than 50 years with unilateral disease, the 10-year survivorship was 95%. Another study reviewed 31 hips undergoing a similar osteotomy in 30 patients with a mean follow-up of 12.7

years. Ten of these hips underwent a concomitant acetabular osteotomy for dysplasia and coverage issues. The reported survivorship was 82%, with the pain score as an index for failure. The authors believed a concomitant acetabular osteotomy should be added for patients with poorly developed roof osteophytes. Another study reported on 25 proximal femoral osteotomies in 23 patients who had a mean age of 38 years. Four hips were converted to THA at a mean of 8 years, and the survivorship at 12 years was 67%. The authors believed their results compared favorably with other surgical forms of treatment in this young patient population.

In the treatment of osteonecrosis, a retrospective study reported the results of 17 hips that underwent pure rotational (flexion or extension) osteotomy with the intertrochanteric region left intact to rotate the affected area out of the weight-bearing surface. The study used MRI to define the intact region from a vertical line along the femoral head. Patients with minimal collapse, more than 120° of intact area from the posterior defined line from the center of the femoral head, and age younger than 55 years were considered candidates. At a minimum 42-month follow-up, additional femoral head collapse did not occur, and improvement in pain scores was reported. Another study addressing the amount of involved surface of the femoral head reported on 70 intertrochanteric flexion osteotomies in 64 patients. At a mean 10.4-year follow-up, 27% of patients underwent conversion to THA, and at 5-year follow-up the survivorship was 90% for all stages of disease. Hips with a combined arc of less than 200° of involved pathology on AP and lateral radiographs had a better survivor probability than those with a combined arc of more than 200°. The authors suggested that a combined arc involvement of less than 200° along with Ficat stage 2 or 3 disease were preferable criteria for the procedure.

Conversion to THA

Because many patients who undergo juxta-acetabular osteotomy and proximal femoral osteotomy will eventually undergo THA, it is worthwhile to consider the potential technical difficulties and results of conversion. First, it is clear that THA reliably relieves pain and improves function for patients with progressive disabling osteoarthritis despite earlier osteotomy. Specific technical issues after periacetabular osteotomy include the need for extra vigilance in component positioning. Acetabular retroversion is common in these patients, and adequate exposure and identification of anatomic landmarks (and potentially computer assisted techniques) is required to ensure correct version and joint stability. Given the effects of periacetabular osteotomy, careful reconstruction of the hip center and limb length is important.

If an associated femoral osteotomy has been performed, there may be issues of retained hardware, limb-length inequality, femoral neck resection, and version. In all patients with dysplasia, the proximal femoral anatomy will typically be somewhat abnormal and particularly so if there has been trochanteric overgrowth or an osteotomy in the subtrochanteric region.

Major displacement of the proximal femur at the osteotomy site can produce a misshapen proximal femoral geometry that may preclude stem placement. With intertrochanteric osteotomies this is often not the case. A subtrochanteric osteotomy, however, can create significant difficulty with implant placement. This may necessitate a repeat osteotomy to remove the displacement and correct the canal alignment. A distal fixation type of stem with a modular proximal body is often necessary in this situation. These types of implants (Standard Range of Motion [SROM], DePuy, Warsaw, IN, or a modular revision type of stem) can also be beneficial when transverse plane corrections can make proper anteversion of a primary stem difficult or impossible to achieve. A varus type of proximal femoral osteotomy can also position the trochanter in such a way that access to the canal of the proximal femur can be difficult. In these instances, a trochanteric osteotomy may be necessary to obtain adequate access for stem insertion. For these reasons, careful preoperative planning and templating with specific implants is mandatory.

The intermediate-term clinical and radiographic outcomes of THA after both reconstructive and salvage osteotomies appear to be good and equivalent to reasonably matched populations. Cited advantages at the time of surgery for the osteotomy groups include better cup coverage and less acetabular grafting, relatively shorter surgical times, less intraoperative blood loss, and an equal number of or fewer complications.

Annotated Bibliography

Pelvic Osteotomy

Clohisy JC, Barrett SE, Gordon JE, Delgado ED, Schoenecker PL: Periacetabular osteotomy for the treatment of severe acetabular dysplasia. *J Bone Joint Surg Am* 2005;87:254- 259.

The authors report on 16 patients (average age, 17.6 years) undergoing periacetabular osteotomy for severe acetabular dysplasia (the hips of 8 patients were subluxated and 8 had a secondary acetabulum). Good improvement at 4.2-year follow-up was recorded for all radiographic measures, and despite 1 overcorrection and 1 nonunion, 14 hips had a good or excellent clinical results. These findings suggest that periacetabular osteotomy is an effective technique for severely dysplastic acetabula in adolescents and young adults.

Jingushi S, Sugioka Y, Noguchi Y, Miura H, Iwamoto Y: Transtrochanteric valgus osteotomy for the treatment of osteoarthritis of the hip secondary to acetabular dysplasia. *J Bone Joint Surg Br* 2002; 84(4):535- 539.

The authors of this study present the midterm clinical results of the use of transtrochanteric valgus osteotomy for the treatment of osteoarthritis of the hip secondary to acetabular dysplasia. The surgical procedure included valgus displacement at the level of the lesser trochanter, and lateral displacement of the greater trochanter by inserting a wedge of bone. Of the 70 hips that the authors reviewed (mean patient age, 44 years; range, 14 to 59 years), most (90%) had advanced osteoarthritis. The authors reported that scores for pain and gait improved significantly at a mean follow-up of 9.4 years. The survival rate with additional surgery as the end point was 82% at 10-year follow-up.

Loder RT: The long-term effect of pelvic osteotomy on birth canal size. *Arch Orthop Trauma Surg* 2002;122:29- 34.

This is a retrospective review of the transverse plane birth canal dimensions (inlet, midpelvis, and outlet) as determined using preoperative and postoperative radiographs of 40 patients who underwent pelvic osteotomy (age range, 2.0 to 21.3 years). Although the number of patients in this study was small, the finding that the midpelvis was below the low normal threshold (9.5 cm) in 3 of 21 patients who underwent Salter osteotomies, 2 of 5 patients who underwent Steel osteotomies, and 1 of 2 patients who underwent Chiari osteotomies indicates that counseling regarding the likelihood of needing cesarean section in childbirth may be necessary for patients undergoing these procedures.

Mast J, Brunner R, Zebrack J: Recognizing acetabular version in the radiographic presentation of hip dysplasia. *Clin Orthop Relat Res* 2004;418:48-53.

In a review of the radiographs of 153 patients with developmental hip dysplasia, retroversion of the acetabulum was demonstrated in one third of the patients (and was associated with smaller values of the lateral center edge angle). The importance of this relatively new observation is that it must be taken into account when planning corrective osteotomy of the acetabulum.

Migaud H, Chantelot C, Giraud F, Fontaine C, Duquennoy A: Long-term survivorship of hip shelf arthroplasty and Chiari osteotomy in adults. *Clin Orthop Relat Res* 2004;418:81-86.

In this retrospective study of 145 adult dysplastic hips, the authors reported that survival rates, using hip replacement as the end point, were 37% at 20-year follow-up for shelf arthroplasty and 68% at 18-year follow-up for Chiari osteotomy. The severity of preoperative arthrosis was the main factor impairing survivorship, and the authors concluded that shelf procedures are best for patients with moderate dysplasia without severe arthrosis, whereas Chiari osteotomy is best for those with severe dysplasia and no or slight arthrosis.

Ohashi H, Hirohashi K, Yamano Y: Factors influencing the outcome of Chiari pelvic osteotomy: A long-term follow-up. *J Bone Joint Surg Br* 2000;82:517-525.

The authors report the long-term results of 103 of 126 Chiari osteotomies and conclude that the Chiari osteotomy remains radiologically effective for approximately 25 years. They suggest that the procedure is best suited to patients with subluxated hips with round or flat femoral heads and early or no degenerative change and that intra-articular osteotomy can lead to osteonecrosis and should be avoided. In patients with advanced osteoarthritis, the authors concluded that the Chiari procedure creates an acetabulum that facilitiates later THA and may delay the need for this procedure in younger patients.

Schramm M, Hohmann D, Radespiel-Troger M, Pitto RP: Treatment of the dysplastic acetabulum with Wagner spherical osteotomy: A study of patients followed for a minimum of twenty years. *J Bone Joint Surg Am* 2003;85:808-814.

The authors evaluated the long-term clinical and radiographic results of 22 Wagner spherical acetabular osteotomies done in patients with hip dysplasia. At a minimum 20-year follow-up (median follow-up, 23.9 years; maximum follow-up, 29.3 years) osteotomy was shown to have improved the mean lateral center-edge angle from $-2°$ to $+13°$, and the mean acetabulum-head index improved from 52% to 72%.

Siebenrock KA, Schoeniger R, Ganz R: Anterior femoro-acetabular impingement due to acetabular retroversion: Treatment with periacetabular osteotomy. *J Bone Joint Surg Am* 2003;85:278-286.

The authors performed 29 periacetabular osteotomies for femoroacetabular impingement, which was diagnosed by the presence of symptoms, a positive anterior impingement test result, and MRI scans in 22 patients (average age, 23 years). The radiographic diagnosis of acetabular retroversion was based on the crossover and posterior wall signs. At an average follow-up of 30 months, there was significant improvement in anterior center edge angles, range of motion, and clinical scores, with an overall good or excellent result in 26 hips.

van Bergayk AB, Garbuz DS: Quality of life and sports-specific outcomes after Bernese periacetabular osteotomy. *J Bone Joint Surg Br* 2002;84:339-343.

This prospective study of 26 consecutive patients who underwent periacetabular osteotomy demonstrated significant improvement in the pain ($P < 0.0001$) and function ($P < 0.0001$) scales of the Western Ontario and McMaster Universities Osteoarthritis Index and the Medical Outcomes Study Short Form 36-Item Health Survey physical score ($P < 0.0001$) by comparing preoperative scores and outcomes 2 years postoperatively. Mean sports activity score also improved, and there was a high mean satisfaction rating of 89.7 (range, 0 to 100).

van Hellemondt G, Sonneveld H, Schreuder M, Kooijman M, de Kleuver M: Triple osteotomy of the pelvis for

acetabular dysplasia: Results at a mean follow-up of 15 years. *J Bone Joint Surg Br* 2005;87:911-915.

The authors report the long-term results of 51 pelvic osteotomies in 43 patients with a mean 15-year follow-up (range, 13 to 20 years). The mean patient age was 28 years (age range, 14 to 46 years). Three patients were lost to follow-up, and six had undergone THA. Of 48 hips, 42 (88%) were preserved, with good to excellent clinical results in 27 (64%). The authors concluded that pelvic reorientation osteotomy for symptomatic hip dysplasia can provide satisfactory and reproducible long-term clinical results.

Proximal Femoral Osteotomy

Drescher W, Furst M, Hahne HJ, et al: Survival analysis of hips treated with flexion osteotomy for femoral head necrosis. *J Bone Joint Surg Br* 2003;85(7):969-974.

The authors of this study reported the results of 70 intertrochanteric osteotomies in 64 patients (mean follow-up, 10.4 years); 19 hips underwent THA at a mean of 8.7 years. A 5-year survivorship of 90% was reported, and hips with Ficat stage 2 and 3 disease had a higher survivorship. The arc of the necrotic region on the AP and lateral radiographs that was less than 200° (combined) had a better survival probability.

Koo KH, Song HR, Yang JW, et al: Trochanteric rotational osteotomy for osteonecrosis of the femoral head. *J Bone Joint Surg Br* 2001;83(1):83-89.

In this study, the MRI scans of 17 patients with osteonecrosis were used to determine the arc of the intact femoral head. Patients younger than 55 years with a 120° intact arc underwent a transtrochanteric osteotomy. Additional collapse of the femoral head did not occur at more than 42-month follow-up. The authors concluded that these criteria aided in the success of the procedure.

Morita S, Yamamoto H, Hasegawa S, et al: Long-term results of valgus-extension femoral osteotomy for advanced osteoarthritis of the hip. *J Bone Joint Surg Br* 2000;82(6):824-829.

In this study, 31 hips with advanced osteoarthritis from acetabular dysplasia were treated with valgus extension femoral osteotomy. At an average 12.7-year follow-up, survivorship was 82% using a pain score as a failure index. Better results were found with patients with a roof osteophyte > 5 mm in length; if not present, the authors recommended that an acetabuloplasty should be added.

Schneider W, Aigner N, Pinggera O, Knahr K: Intertrochanteric osteotomy for avascular necrosis of the head of the femur: Survival probability of two different methods. *J Bone Joint Surg Br* 2002; 84(6):817-824.

The authors of this study compared different types of intertrochanteric osteotomy for the treatment of osteonecrosis of the hip. Sixty-three flexion osteotomies (partly combined with vargus or valgus displacement), 29 rotational osteotomies, 13 varus osteotomies, 8 medializing osteotomies, and 2 extension osteotomies were performed. The mean follow-up for all

115 procedures was 7.3 years (maximum, 24.6 years). At follow-up, 27 of 29 patients in the rotational osteotomy group had already undergone THA, compared with 36 of 63 patients in the flexion osteotomy group. A high incidence of complications (55.2%) was seen early in the rotational osteotomy group, compared with 17.5% in the flexion osteotomy group. For all osteotomy groups, there was a high correlation between the size of the necrotic area and the incidence of failure, which also correlated with the preoperative Ficat and Steinberg stages of disease.

Shannon BD, Trousdale RT: Femoral osteotomies for avascular necrosis of the femoral head. *Clin Orthop Relat Res* 2004;418:34-40.

This is a symposium review of the indications, techniques, and results of proximal femoral osteotomy for osteonecrosis of the femoral head.

Conversion to Total Hip Arthroplasty

Parvizi J, Burmeister H, Ganz R: Previous Bernese periacetabular osteotomy does not compromise the results of total hip arthroplasty. *Clin Orthop Relat Res* 2004; 423:118-122.

This is a retrospective review of 41 patients who underwent THA after periacetabular osteotomy. At an average follow-up of 7 years, all patients had significant relief of pain and improvement in function. Technical issues included acetabular retroversion in 23 patients and the need for trochanteric osteotomy in 24 patients because of abnormal proximal femoral anatomy. There were two revisions in the series.

Classic Bibliography

Chiari K: Medial displacement osteotomy of the pelvis. *Clin Orthop Relat Res* 1974;98:55-71.

Detenbeck LC, Coventry MB, Kelly PJ: Intertrochanteric osteotomy for degenerative arthritis of the hip. *Clin Orthop Relat Res* 1972;86:73.

D'Souza SR, Sadiq S, New AM, et al: Proximal femoral osteotomy as the primary operation for young adults who have osteoarthrosis of the hip. *J Bone Joint Surg Am* 1998;80(10):1428-1438.

Ferguson GM, Cabanela ME, Ilstrup DM: Total hip arthroplasty following failed intertrochanteric osteotomy. *J Bone Joint Surg Br* 1994;76:252-257.

Ganz R, Klaue K, Vinh TS, Mast JW: A new periacetabular osteotomy for the treatment of hip dysplasias: Technique and preliminary results. *Clin Orthop Relat Res* 1988;232:26-36.

Harris WH, Enneking WF: Characteristics of the articular cartilage formed after intertrochanteric osteotomy: A case report. *J Bone Joint Surg Am* 1995;77(4):602-607.

Hersche O, Casillas M, Ganz R: Indications for intertrochanteric osteotomy after periacetabular osteotomy for adult hip dysplasia. *Clin Orthop Relat Res* 1998;347:19-26.

Jacobs MA, Hungerford DS, Krackow KA: Results of intertrochanteric hip osteotomies for avascular necrosis of the femoral head. *J Bone Joint Surg Br* 1989;71:200.

Mogensen BA, Zoega H, Marinko P: Late results of intertrochanteric osteotomy for advanced osteoarthritis of the hip. *Acta Orthop Scand* 1980; 51:85.

Pauwels F: *Biomechanics in the Normal and Diseased Hip*. Berlin, Germany, Springer Verlag, 1976.

Perlau R, Wilson MG, Poss R: Isolated proximal femoral osteotomy for treatment of residua of congenital dysplasia or idiopathic osteoarthrosis of the hip: Five to ten-year results. *J Bone Joint Surg Am* 1996;78(10):1462-1467.

Steel HH: Triple osteotomy of the innominate bone. *J Bone Joint Surg Am* 1973;55:343.

Sugioka Y: Intertrochanteric anterior rotational osteotomy of the femoral head in the treatment of osteonecrosis affecting the hip: A new osteotomy operation. *Clin Orthop Relat Res* 1978;130:191.

Tooke SM, Amstutz HC, Hedley AK: Results of transtrochanteric rotational osteotomy for femoral head osteonecrosis. *Clin Orthop Relat Res* 1987;224:150-157.

Wiberg G: Studies on dysplastic acetabular and congenital subluxations of the hip joint with special reference to the complications of osteoarthritis. *Acta Chir Scand* 1939;83(suppl):58.

Chapter 37

Metal-On-Metal Resurfacing Hip Arthroplasty

Michael A. Mont, MD

Phillip S. Ragland, MD

Thomas P. Schmalzreid, MD

Introduction

Hip resurfacing, which conserves the femoral head and neck, is a viable alternative to standard total hip replacement in patients with arthritis of the hip. In resurfacing hip arthroplasty, a small amount of diseased bone is removed from the femoral head to allow placement of a metal cap that is anatomically similar to the native femoral head. In limited femoral head resurfacing, the metal cap articulates with the relatively unaffected, native acetabular cartilage, whereas in total hip resurfacing (used in patients with arthritis of both sides of the joint), there is a mated acetabular component.

Although resurfacing hip arthroplasty has recently gained popularity, the procedure dates back to the mid-20th century; since then, a variety of materials such as glass, stainless steel, ivory, and Teflon (Dupont, Wilmington, DE) have been used. However, experience in the 1970s and early 1980s with femoral head resurfacing and cemented polyethylene acetabular components led to a decline in resurfacing hip arthroplasty because of high failure rates. Limited femoral head resurfacing continued to be used in the management of moderate to late-stage osteonecrosis of the femoral head (see chapter 44). Recent advances in metallurgy have brought about a resurgence in the use of metal-on-metal designs for total hip resurfacing, particularly in the management of hip arthritis.

The Rationale for the Use of Resurfacing Hip Arthroplasty

The concept of resurfacing in hip arthroplasty allows limited bony excision on the femoral side, with preservation of the femoral neck as well as the central portion of the femoral head. Previous designs required extensive bony excision on the acetabular side because of the large diameter of the femoral prosthesis; however, thinner acetabular shells now permit a more conservative preparation of the acetabulum that is similar to that required for standard total hip arthroplasty (Figure 1). The prosthesis is designed to resurface the acetabulum and cap the femoral head without the use of an in-

tramedullary device. This is an advantage over standard total hip arthroplasty in that preserving proximal femoral bone stock might allow stress transfer to the femur comparable to that of the native femoral head, thus avoiding the typical stress shielding patterns that occur with standard total hip arthroplasty. In addition, the large femoral head (typically ranging from 36 to 54 mm) may kinematically resemble a normal hip more than the standard heads (ranging in size from 22 to 32 mm) that are used in standard total hip replacements. Other theoretic advantages include lower dislocation rates because of the large diameter femoral head, fewer problems with impingement, and easier revision because the proximal femur is spared. One disadvantage to total hip resurfacing, however, is the inability to modify leg length because of the lack of modularity of the components. Femoral neck fracture and osteonecrosis are other potential concerns.

Resurfacing Hip Arthroplasty: Historical Review

Metal-on-metal resurfacing was introduced in the 1960s. The early design was a press-fit cobalt-chromium-molybdenum replacement. Other constructs allowed motion across components and between the metal and bone. These designs were abandoned in the 1970s when seizing and loosening caused by inherent high frictional torque coefficients of the components led to unacceptably high failure rates. Metal-on-polyethylene resurfacing was introduced as an alternative in the 1970s. Although early results were promising, long-term outcome studies yielded unacceptably high failure rates because of errors in patient selection, surgical techniques, and implant manufacturing and design issues. It was found that the mating of large metal femoral head components with thin diameter acetabular cups eventually induced an intense osteolytic reaction. Additionally, there were several concomitant reports of high success rates with standard metal-on-polyethylene prostheses, which contributed to loss of interest in metal-on-metal prostheses and an increase in popularity of metal-on-polyethylene

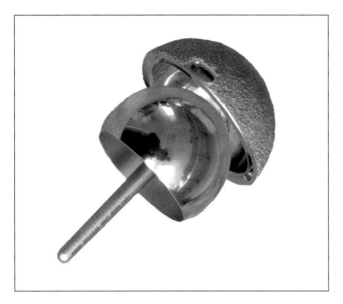

Figure 1 Photograph of a Conserve Plus implant with a thin acetabular component.

prostheses. The likely reason for the high frictional torque generated in the metal-on-metal devices was the manufacturing technique used, which at that time had variations in tolerances. These poor results caused a decline in the use of resurfacing until recent changes in prosthetic designs and manufacturing techniques.

Present-Day Devices

Modern metallurgy processes produce metal-on-metal bearings with drastically reduced tolerances (several millimeters versus < 25 μm). In the late 1980s and early 1990s, newer metal-on-metal surface replacements were developed and used in patients. Several studies showed good results with newer designs. Unfortunately, there are only a few published studies of the results of resurfacing hip arthroplasty with modern metal-on-metal designs.

One such study reported on 19 patients (21 hips) who underwent hip resurfacing using either cementless (4 hips) or cemented devices (17 hips). All patients were doing well clinically at a mean follow-up of 16 months (range, 10 to 25 months). Despite concerns with bone interface radiolucencies in 12 hips, the authors proposed this modality as a more conservative and durable treatment of hip arthritis. Another study reported on 235 resurfaced hips at a mean follow-up of 5 years. Patients were divided into four cohorts based on method of fixation: press-fit prostheses on both sides, cement fixation on both sides, hydroxyapatite-coated acetabulum prostheses, and hydroxyapatite-coated acetabulum prostheses with cemented femoral components. Success rates of 90%, 93%, 100%, and 100%, respectively, were reported, and the authors concluded that this device provides consistent fixation.

One study reported on 83 patients (94 hips) who underwent hip resurfacing using the Conserve Plus device (Wright Medical, Arlington, TN). Patients with a mean age of 34 years (range, 15 to 40 years) who had a minimum 2-year follow-up or whose implants had failed were included in the results. Based on the analysis of three hips that needed to be revised and 10 hips that had significant radiographic changes, a surface arthroplasty risk index was calculated to predict failure. Patients who had a prosthesis placed with an average femoral neck-shaft angle of 133° had an increased risk of failure compared with a normal risk group with an average femoral neck-shaft angle of 139°. Patients with a surface arthroplasty risk index score greater than 3 had a risk for fracture that was 12 times greater than patients with an index less than 3. Factors that were found to lead to increased risk included a history of prior surgery, femoral cysts larger than 1 cm, and valgus positioning of the stem.

Another study reported on the 2- to 6-year follow-up (average, 3.5 years) of the first 355 patients (400 hips) who were implanted with the Conserve Plus device. The mean age of the patients was 48 years (range, 15 to 77 years). The reported overall rate of survival at 4 years was 94.4%. For patients with a surface arthroplasty risk index score greater than 3, the rate of survival was 89% compared with a 97% rate of survival for those with a surface arthroplasty risk index score less than 3. Twelve patients had a revision to a standard total hip replacement because of loosening (N = 7), femoral neck fracture (N = 3), recurrent subluxations (N = 1), and infection (N = 1). Important risk factors for femoral component failure included large femoral head cysts, patient height, female gender, and smaller component size in male patients.

Another study used standardized radiographs to assess the biomechanical results of total hip resurfacing. Joint reactive forces of 50 resurfaced hips were compared with those of 40 hips that had a standard cementless total hip arthroplasty. The authors found that the biomechanical results of hip resurfacing were significantly associated with the preoperative anatomy of the proximal femur. Limb lengthening can be achieved, but horizontal offset is essentially unchanged by resurfacing, which increased reliably in patients who underwent standard total hip replacement. The authors concluded that arthritic hips that are more than 1 cm shorter than the contralateral limb or that have low horizontal femoral offset may be better treated using a standard total hip replacement.

In a study of postoperative gait evaluations of total resurfacing patients, the gait characteristics of patients who underwent resurfacing hip arthroplasty were compared with matched normal patients, patients with osteoarthritis, and patients who underwent standard total hip replacement. The patients who underwent resurfacing hip arthroplasty had walking speeds comparable to

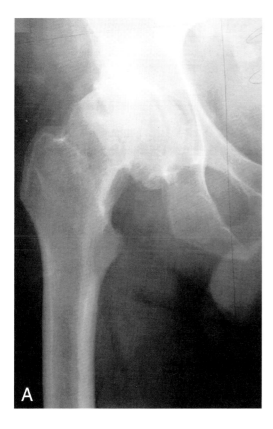

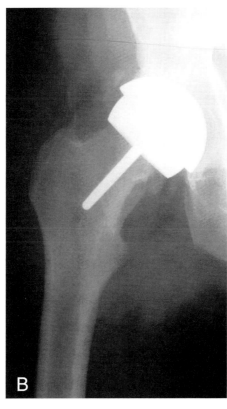

Figure 2 A, Preoperative AP radiograph of a 54-year-old patient with severe osteoarthritis of the right hip. **B,** Postoperative AP radiograph showing total joint resurfacing components in place.

those of normal patients (average, 126 m/s) and superior to those of patients who underwent standard total hip replacement and patients with osteoarthritis (99 m/s and 96 m/s, respectively). Superior hip kinematics and functionality were also identified in patients who underwent resurfacing hip arthroplasty when compared with those who underwent standard hip replacement. These findings may be the result of the effect hip surgery has on horizontal offset, as was noted in another study that compared joint reactive forces in 50 resurfaced hips compared with those of 40 hips that had a standard cementless total hip arthroplasty. The authors of this study found that horizontal offset is essentially unchanged by resurfacing and was reliably increased in patients who underwent standard total hip replacement. Standard total hip replacement, however, was recommended for patients with arthritic hips that are more than 1 cm shorter than the contralateral limb or that have low horizontal femoral offset.

Indications/Contraindications

The indications for hip resurfacing include primary osteoarthritis, osteonecrosis, developmental dysplasia of the hip, rheumatoid arthritis, and posttraumatic arthritis (Figure 2). Other potential candidates for hip resurfacing include patients with a high risk of dislocation (chronic alcoholics), those with extra-articular deformities of the hip joint that preclude placement of an intramedullary device, and those with retained hardware

in the proximal femur (such as blade plates, intramedullary rods, and cannulated screws). The most important preoperative requirement for resurfacing is adequate femoral head bone stock, which can be further assessed using preoperative dual-energy x-ray absorptiometry in elderly patients if necessary. Although patients who undergo hip resurfacing are typically younger than 60 years, there is no age limitation for these devices.

Absolute contraindications to resurfacing include patients with inadequate femoral head or neck bone stock and those with deficient acetabula. Patients with body mass indices greater than 35 have been shown to have an increased risk of femoral neck fracture and have therefore typically been excluded. Higher failure rates have also been reported in tall patients, female patients, and patients with femoral head cysts larger than 1 cm, although these are not absolute contraindications.

Resurfacing is typically performed with the various standard approaches used for conventional total hip replacements. No studies have compared the two major approaches (anterolateral and posterior). Anterior approaches have been used to try to preserve the femoral head blood supply, which preserves the lateral epiphyseal vessels. However, most surgeons performing resurfacing use posterior approaches that retain capsule; these approaches do not have any adverse effect on the blood supply or outcome of resurfacing. This is despite the fact that in these approaches there is usually much dissection involved because mobilization of the femoral head is required to visualize the acetabulum. The effect on the blood supply of the femoral head on final outcome of resurfacing has yet to be determined.

Although the exposure of the hip is comparable to that for standard hip arthroplasty, the retained femoral head and the inability to use screw fixation with most devices make preparation of the acetabulum more difficult. In preparation of the femur, it is essential to maintain the integrity of the femoral neck cortical bone and avoid notching when using the specialized reamers because this can produce a stress riser and increase the risk of fracture postoperatively. The femoral components typically vary in size from 36 to 54 mm to mimic the sizes of the native femoral head. Most devices use a small stem that allows for centralization of the components on the prepared femoral head. Newer techniques using different instrumentation permit smaller incisions and less invasive approaches.

The advantages of metal-on-metal resurfacing need to be balanced against the theoretic adverse effects of metal debris. Various authors have shown increased levels of metal ions in the blood and different tissue after these procedures. It is also possible that metal ions can lead to allergic hypersensitivity reactions. Fortunately, no direct evidence has been published that causally or directly links any metal-on-metal bearing surfaces with any adverse effects. Elevated metal ion levels have been found in patients after the implantation of these devices, but the significance of these elevations is unknown. These theoretic concerns may not be problematic, but they at least need to be mentioned to all patients, especially premenopausal women.

Summary

Resurfacing hip arthroplasty appears to be a viable treatment option in that it provides a type of hip replacement that conserves the femoral head and neck. There are now at least six commercially available devices, and the use of resurfacing hip arthroplasty is becoming more widespread throughout the world. Improvements in metallurgy and manufacturing appear to have addressed the flaws of historical designs. Although recent studies have reported promising early results, long-term results are needed to fully understand the role these devices can play in the treatment of hip arthritis.

Annotated Bibliography

The Rational for the Use of Resurfacing Hip Arthroplasty

Etienne G, Mont MA, Ragland PS: The diagnosis and treatment of nontraumatic osteonecrosis of the femoral head. *Instr Course Lect* 2004;53:67-85.

The authors of this article provide a review of the management of osteonecrosis of the hip.

Present-Day Devices

Beaule PE:, Dorey FJ, Duff M, Gruen T, Amstutz HC: Risk factors affecting outcome of metal-on-metal surface arthroplasty of the hip. *Clin Orthop* 2004;418:87-93.

The authors reported three conversions in 93 patients with metal-on-metal prostheses at a minimum 2-year follow-up.

Lieberman JR, Berry DJ, Mont MA, et al: Osteonecrosis of the hip: Management in the 21st century. *Instr Course Lect* 2003;52:337-355.

The authors provide a comprehensive review of total hip replacement treatment strategy for patients with osteonecrosis of the hip.

Mont MA, Ragland PS, Bhave A, Etienne G, Starr R: Gait analysis of metal-on-metal surface arthroplasty: A comparison study, in *Proceedings of the 72nd Annual Meeting*. Rosemont, IL, American Academy of Orthopaedic Surgeons, 2005, p 374.

The authors of this study used gain analysis to show normalized gait mechanics in patients who underwent metal-on-metal total hip resurfacing.

Silva M, Lee KH, Heisel C, Dela Rosa MA, Schmalzried TP: The biomechanical results of total hip resurfacing arthroplasty. *J Bone Joint Surg Am* 2004;86:40-46.

The authors of this study reported that patients treated with metal-on-metal resurfacing had no change in the horizontal offset after surgery compared with an average increase in patients who underwent standard total hip arthroplasty.

Classic Bibliography

Amstutz HC, Grigoris P, Safran MR, Grecula MJ, Campbell PA, Schmalzried TP: Precision-fit surface hemiarthroplasty for femoral head osteonecrosis: Long-term results. *J Bone Joint Surg Br* 1994;76:423-427.

Head WC: Total articular resurfacing arthroplasty: Analysis of component failure in sixty-seven hips. *J Bone Joint Surg Am* 1984;66:28-34.

McMinn D, Treacy R, Lin K, Pynsent P: Metal on metal surface replacement of the hip: Experience of the McMinn prothesis. *Clin Orthop Relat Res* 1996;329:S89-S98.

Muller ME: The benefits of metal-on-metal total hip replacements. *Clin Orthop* 1995;311:54-59.

Schmalzried TP, Fowble VA, Ure KJ, Amstutz HC: Metal-on-metal surface replacement of the hip. *Clin Orthop* 1996;(suppl 329):S106-S114.

Chapter 38

Hip Arthroscopy

Joseph C. McCarthy, MD

Jo-ann Lee, MS

Introduction

Arthroscopic management of hip disorders continues to evolve with the recent development of minimally invasive diagnostic and surgical procedures. Although the concept of hip arthroscopy was first introduced in 1931, the results of few studies were published until the 1980s when reports of clinical application of arthroscopic techniques in the hip joint began to appear. One such study measured and reported on hip capsule distention and distraction forces necessary to allow adequate visualization of the femur and the acetabulum. Another study first described the lateral decubitus position and peritrochanteric portal placement. The ongoing development of arthroscopy equipment and instruments designed specifically for the hip joint continue to make visualization and instrumentation of the hip efficacious.

Rationale

Hip arthroscopy provides physicians with the ability to thoroughly inspect the joint and directly identify and address labral lesions as well as any previously undiagnosed intra-articular pathology. Patients with longstanding, unresolved mechanical hip joint pain and positive physical findings may benefit from an arthroscopic evaluation for diagnostic and therapeutic reasons. The benefit of being able to document and stage any pathology within the joint with a minimally invasive procedure also has the advantage of allowing long-range treatment and recommendations.

Anatomic Constraints of the Hip Joint

Anatomically, the femoral head is deeply recessed in the bony acetabulum beneath a thick fibrocapsular and muscular envelope. Unlike the knee or shoulder joint, the curvilinear articular surfaces of the hip require substantially greater distraction force to visualize. This distraction is resisted not only by the body architecture, but also by the iliofemoral ligament and the vacuum effect of negative intra-articular pressure. Muscle relaxation and the mechanical advantage afforded by a dedicated hip distractor are necessary to overcome these factors. The rel-ative proximity of the sciatic nerve, lateral femoral cutaneous nerve, and femoral neurovascular structures place them at potential risk with portal placement.

Indications

The number of joint conditions for which hip arthroscopy has application continues to expand. Current indications are listed in Table 1.

Labral Tears

Patients with a torn acetabular labrum may report catching, locking, or a painful click in the hip joint. It has been suggested that a torn acetabular labrum may predispose a patient to subsequent degenerative changes. Labral tears may occur with or without a history of trauma. There is a high incidence of labral tears associated with acetabular dysplasia, slipped capital femoral epiphysis, and Legg-Calvé-Perthes disease. In dysplasia, repetitive torque or impingement may result in hypertrophic changes that can predispose patients to bruising, fraying, and tearing. Tears most commonly occur at the avascular labroarticular margin; therefore, healing will not occur. If left untreated, a torn labrum may progress with further intra-articular damage of the chondral surfaces of the adjacent acetabulum and femoral head. Labral tears occurring at the watershed zone may destabilize the adjacent acetabular cartilage (Figure 1). Repetitive loading of the joint pumps fluid under pressure beneath the delaminating acetabular cartilage. This process eventually forms a subchondral cyst, which may further contribute to the progression of hip osteoarthritis that begins with the delamination process. The duration of symptoms and severity of labral injury found at arthroscopy have been statistically correlated. Treatment of acetabular labral tears involves judicious mechanical débridement of the unstable labral segment back to a stable base. Overresection of the labrum should be scrupulously avoided.

Loose Bodies

The clinical presentation of locking or catching with activity can be associated with intra-articular loose bodies

Table 1 | Current Indications for Hip Arthroscopy

Loose bodies

Labral tears

Chondral lesions of the acetabular or femoral head

Osteonecrosis of the femoral head (without femoral head collapse)

Ruptured or impinging ligamentum teres

Dysplasia (with mechanical symptoms)

Synovial abnormalities

Collagen disease (such as rheumatoid arthritis and systemic lupus erythematosus with impinging synovitis)

Crystalline hip arthropathy (gout and pseudogout)

Capsular shrinkage (Ehlers-Danlos syndrome)

Synovial chondromatosis

Infection (primarily in the pediatric population)

Total hip arthroplasty (establish diagnosis or removal of intra-articular third bodies)

Trauma (dislocation, Pipkin fracture, removal of foreign body)

Osteoarthritis (early stages)

Intractable pain (with positive physical findings)

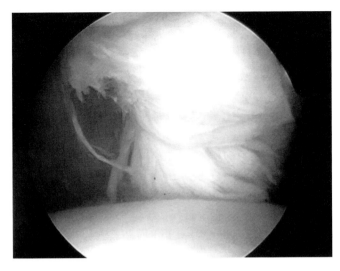

Figure 1 Arthroscopic photograph of an enlarged, frayed, and torn labrum in a patient with mild acetabular dysplasia.

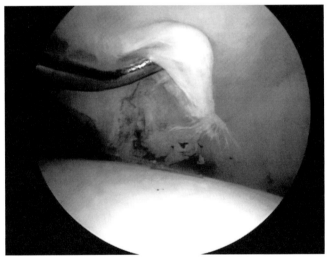

Figure 3 Arthroscopic photograph of a patient with a torn labrum that was diagnosed using magnetic resonance arthrography shows a torn labrum with a chondral lesion at the labroarticular junction (watershed zone).

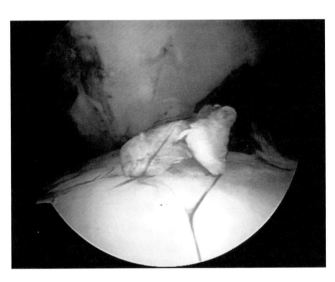

Figure 2 Arthroscopic photograph of patient with mechanical symptoms and negative radiographic workup who was found to have an intra-articular loose body.

and/or a labral tear. CT with or without contrast is more sensitive than radiography in visualizing these loose bodies, which will not appear on plain radiographs unless ossified. One study showed that up to 67% of loose bodies were not evident on conventional radiographic studies. Arthroscopy provides a method to confirm the diagnosis in a patient with mechanical symptoms and negative radiographic workup while simultaneously providing a means of treatment (Figure 2). Loose bodies may occur as an isolated fragment or they may be found in multiples (up to 300), as occurs in patients with synovial chondromatosis. In these patients, the loose bodies may aggregate in grape-like clusters that are adhered to the synovium

about the fovea. Large or aggregated loose bodies must be morcellized to be removed arthroscopically.

Chondral Lesions

Chondral lesions may occur in association with labral tears, loose bodies, dysplasia, or other hip conditions, including early degenerative arthritis. In a study of 457 patients, it was reported that chondral injuries occurred in the anterior acetabulum in 269 patients (59%), the superior acetabulum in 110 (24%), and the posterior acetabulum in 114 (25%). These lesions were most frequently associated with a labral tear and the most common location was the labrochondral junction (watershed zone) (Figure 3). Seventy percent of the anterior, 27% of the superior, and 36% of the posterior

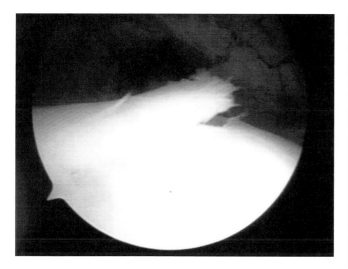

Figure 4 Arthroscopic photograph of a patient with stage 2 osteonecrosis, preservation of a spherical femoral head, and mechanical symptoms. Arthroscopy was done simultaneously with core decompression and this arthroscopic photograph shows a chondral flap lesion of the femoral head.

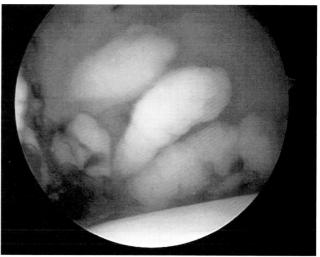

Figure 5 An arthroscopic photograph of a patient with synovial chondromatosis showing multiple loose bodies aggregated at the fovea.

chondral lesions were Outerbridge grade III or IV in severity. Poor surgical outcomes are typically associated with extensive acetabular and/or femoral chondral lesions, regardless of the joint space observed on plain radiographs. These chondral lesions are frequently missed preoperatively because of limitations of MRI and CT to thoroughly evaluate the chondral joint surfaces.

Osteonecrosis

The main goal in the treatment of osteonecrosis is to minimize pain and prevent collapse of subchondral bone. However, a loose body, labral injury, or a chondral flap lesion can be treated via the arthroscope simultaneously with a core decompression (Figure 4). Although arthroscopy has no role in the treatment of end-stage disease, it should be considered for patients with osteonecrosis who develop mechanical symptoms and have a preserved spherical femoral head.

Synovial Chondromatosis

Treatment of synovial chondromatosis consists of arthroscopic removal of loose bodies (typically between 5 to 300). They often require morcellization, especially those clustered within the fovea (Figure 5). Articular damage can be addressed and partial synovectomy performed at the same time. Although recurrence has been reported in 10% to 14% of these patients, a second arthroscopy may be beneficial in the absence of advanced chondral destruction.

Arthroscopic débridement of the synovium can be useful in the management of inflammatory conditions because it does not necessitate a prolonged rehabilitation period. Arthroscopic synovectomy has been described as an adjunct to diagnosis and treatment of pigmented villonodular synovitis. Patients with rheumatoid arthritis accompanied by intense joint pain that is unresponsive to extensive conservative treatment may benefit from arthroscopic intervention with lavage, synovial biopsy, and/or partial synovectomy and treatment of intra-articular cartilage lesions. Surgical outcomes directly depend on the stage of articular cartilage involvement.

Crystalline diseases such as gout or pseudogout can produce extreme hip joint pain that often goes undetected unless it coexists with a labral or chondral injury. Arthroscopic treatment consists of copious lavage and mechanical removal of crystals that are diffusely distributed throughout the synovium as well as embedded within the articular cartilage. A synovial biopsy done at the same time can be helpful for medical management.

Patients with Ehlers-Danlos syndrome may report pain and instability. In combination with medical diagnosis, arthroscopic treatment has consisted of skin and synovial biopsy to further define disease classification. In addition, thermal capsular shrinkage has been performed judiciously with favorable short-term results.

Total Hip Arthroplasty

A patient with pain after undergoing total hip arthroplasty can usually be diagnosed clinically (for example, limb-length discrepancy or abductor weakness), radiographically (for example, component loosening, malposition, or trochanteric nonunion), or with special studies (such as bone scanning and aspiration arthrography for patients with subtle loosening or sepsis). If a patient has a negative workup and has failed conservative treatment, arthroscopy may be warranted to establish a diagnosis. In addition, intra-articular third bodies such as broken wires or loose screws can be removed arthroscopically.

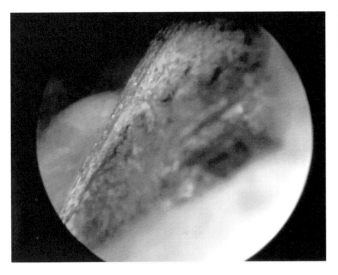

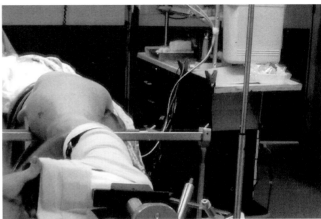

Figure 7 Photograph of the operating room setup shows a patient in the lateral decubitus position using the hip distractor.

Figure 6 An arthroscopic photograph of an intra-articular bullet fragment in a 22-year-old man who was shot at age 17 years.

Trauma

Even minor trauma involving the hip joint can result in hematomas, chondral loose bodies, and labral tears. Foreign bodies such as bullet fragments that produce intra-articular symptoms can be removed arthroscopically (Figure 6). Dislocations and fracture-dislocations can result in loose bodies, labral injuries, or shear damage to the chondral surfaces of the femoral head or acetabulum that are not often detected with MRI. Pipkin fractures can result in displaced bone or cartilage from the femoral head or a ruptured ligamentum teres.

A direct correlation between the stage of cartilage loss, especially on the acetabular side, and poor outcome following arthroscopy has been reported. Therefore, if there is radiographic evidence of advanced osteoarthritis with osteophyte formation, subchondral sclerosis, and cystic changes, arthroscopy is not indicated. However, focal degenerative chondral lesions may appear normal on AP pelvis radiographs. Débridement and chondral abrasion may have a role in the management of osteoarthritis with accompanying mechanical symptoms that is not advanced enough to justify joint arthroplasty.

Contraindications

The foremost disadvantage to hip arthroscopy is the length of the surgical learning curve because of the difficulty of the procedure. As mentioned earlier, access to the hip joint is difficult because of the resistance to distraction resulting from the large muscular envelope, the strength of the iliofemoral ligament, and negative intra-articular pressure.

Because of difficulty achieving distraction and the length of instruments necessary to access the joint, morbid obesity is a relative contraindication for hip arthroscopy. Hip arthroscopy is not appropriate for the treatment of sepsis with accompanying osteomyelitis or abscess formation, which require open surgery. Stage III or IV osteonecrosis, moderate dysplasia, and synovitis in the absence of mechanical symptoms do not warrant arthroscopy. Conditions that limit the potential for hip distraction such as joint ankylosis, dense heterotopic bone formation, or considerable protrusio are contraindications for arthroscopy, as is advanced osteoarthritis.

Surgical Approaches

Arthroscopy can be performed with the patient in either the supine or lateral position. The lateral approach requires that the patient be positioned in the lateral decubitus position and that a modified fracture table or specially modified distraction device fitted to a regular fluoroscopic table be used. The patient must be adequately padded to protect against neurapraxia and pressure. Adequate visualization requires that the femoral head is distracted from the acetabulum to achieve between 7 and 10 mm of chondral distraction. Without sufficient distraction, the femoral head prevents maneuvering of instruments into the recesses of the acetabulum. The hip is placed in slight forward flexion (approximately 10° to 20°), with the foot maintained in neutral to slightly externally rotated position. A well-padded lateral peroneal post is positioned transverse to the long axis of the torso approximately 10 to 15 cm distal to the ischial tuberosity and adjusted for the abduction force (Figure 7). Because significant variation in the force required to achieve adequate distraction, lower extremity muscles must be completely relaxed to minimize the amount of force required.

The supine approach requires that the patient is placed supine on the fracture table against a large perineal post. It is essential that the post is well padded to minimize the likelihood of pudendal nerve neurapraxia. The involved limb is secured to the traction foot stirrup, and initial gentle traction is established while the contralateral limb is abducted and restrained in a second foot stirrup so that the peroneal post rests laterally against the medial thigh of the surgical leg. A spinal needle can be advanced into the capsule under radiographic guidance. Longitudinal traction can then be increased using the C-arm image to ensure appropriate femoral head distraction, which should be between 7 and 15 mm. Considerable variability is encountered in the ease with which femoral movement can be accomplished depending on the mechanical response of the hip. A tensiometer placed on the hip distraction device may be of adjunctive value in preventing neurapraxia.

Portal Placement

Portal placement requires palpation, identification, and marking of the anatomic landmarks, including the femoral pulse with its neurovascular bundle and the trochanter. There are five portals: the direct anterior, anterolateral, and posterolateral (most commonly used with the supine approach) and the anterior and posterior paratrochanteric (most commonly used with the lateral approach). The five portals provide varying visualization of different anatomic structures. Knowledge of anatomic relationships is of utmost importance in the use of the various portals. Patient position, lower extremity positioning, and portal placement can affect these relationships.

Direct Anterior Portal

The direct anterior portal can be used with the patient in either the supine or lateral position. An 18-gauge spinal needle is advanced toward the femoral head at the intersection of a vertical line from the anterior-superior iliac spine and a horizontal line drawn from the superior aspect of the symphysis pubis and directed laterally under fluoroscopic guidance. The arthroscope is then inserted through the sartorius muscle into the anterior capsule. When placing anterior portals, caution must be taken to avoid the lateral femoral cutaneous nerve and femoral neurovascular bundle. This approach allows visualization of the anterior femoral neck, superior retinacular fold, and the ligamentum teres.

Anterolateral Portal

This anterolateral portal is placed at the anterior margin of the greater trochanter while aiming close to the femoral head and parallel to the floor to avoid puncturing the lateral labrum. The path of the spinal needle can be verified with fluoroscopic guidance. The nerve in closest proximity is the superior gluteal nerve. The cannula penetrates the gluteus medius and enters the lateral capsule at the anterior margin. This portal provides visualization of the anterior femoral neck, ligamentum teres, synovial tissues beneath the zona orbicularis, and anterior aspect of the joint.

Posterolateral Portal

The posterolateral portal is placed along the posterior aspect of the greater trochanter under arthroscopic visualization with the patient's leg in neutral position because of the proximity of the sciatic nerve. The arthroscope is advanced through the gluteus medius and gluteus minimus muscle into the lateral capsule at the posterior margin. This approach has been useful for removal of posteriorly lodged foreign bodies and for access to the posteroinferior recesses of the hip joint.

Anterior Paratrochanteric Portal

The anterior paratrochanteric portal is located at the junction of the anterior and middle one third of the superior trochanteric ridge. The arthroscope enters the anterior hip capsule by passing through the anterior musculotendinous junction of the gluteus medius while aimed toward the center of the acetabulum at the fovea. The neurovascular structure that is at potential risk with this portal is the superior gluteal nerve. Because this nerve is located 4 to 6 cm above the trochanter, the relative risk of injury to it is minimal. This portal provides excellent visualization of the femoral head, anterior neck, anterior labrum, and synovial tissues beneath the zona orbicularis. In combination with the posterior paratrochanteric portal, it is an extremely useful portal for instrumentation and treatment of anterior labral lesions and acetabular chondral lesions.

Posterior Paratrochanteric Portal

The entry point for this portal is placed at the junction of the posterior and middle one third of the superior trochanteric ridge, essentially mirroring the placement of the anterior paratrochanteric portal. The posterior trochanteric portal passes through the posterior margin of the musculotendinous junction of the gluteus medius muscle. It is placed slightly superior and slightly anterior to the trochanteric ridge, with the patient's leg placed in neutral or slight internal rotation to avoid potential injury to the sciatic nerve. The posterior paratrochanteric portal is used to view the posterior capsule, posterior labrum, and posterior femoral head. The posterolateral portal is considered a safe portal when made under direct visualization by placing the camera in the anterolateral portal first.

Hip-Specific Instrumentation

The depth of the hip joint often requires specially designed extra-long arthroscopic instruments passed through cannulae long enough to protect the soft tissues surrounding the hip. A specially designed Nitinol wire is then passed through the center of a spinal needle; once the needle is removed and the position in the joint is established, a tapered blunt cannulated trocar is inserted over the Nitinol wire for controlled penetration of the hip capsule.

Table 2 | Treatment Outcomes for Labral and Chondral Lesions

Injury Classification	No. of Patients	Treatment Outcomes, No. of Patients		
		Excellent-Good	Fair	Poor
Stage 1	10	9	1	0
Stage 2	11	8	1	2
Stage 3A	21	15	4	2 (additional surgery required)
Stage 3B	10	4	4	2 (additional surgery required)
Stage 4	9	0	2	7 (3 required additional surgery)

Table 3 | Complication Rates for Arthrotomy and Arthroscopy

	Arthrotomy (% of Patients)	Arthroscopy (% of Patients)
Infection	0.5	0
Deep venous thrombosis	10 to 24	0.05
Pulmonary embolism	1 to 2	0
Osteonecrosis	2 to 5	0
Permanent nerve injury	1 to 2	0
Heterotopic bone	8 to 15	0
Trochanteric nonunion/muscle weakness	5 to 19	0

Once the portals have been attained, the hip is distended with fluid and an arthroscopic pump is used to maintain constant pressure. A standard arthroscope with a 30° lens can be used to visualize most of the joint by varying the position and exchanging portals; however, a 70° lens is sometimes needed for complete visualization, particularly in patients with a tight hip joint. Extra-long curved shaver blades allow for surgical arthroscopy around the femoral head. Long suction punches and long graspers facilitate resection of tissues and retrieval of loose bodies. Thermal devices are useful in débriding the torn labral and chondral flaps or inflamed synovial tissue folds.

Temperature-controlled thermal energy or lasers can be used for cutting and coagulation as well as ablation and capsular shrinkage; however, these tools need to be used judiciously to avoid extensive scarring and osteonecrosis that has been reported to occur in other joints.

Classification and Outcome of Labral and Chondral Injuries

Labral and chondral injuries are typically classified as falling into one of the following stages. Stage 1 injuries have a free margin with intact cartilage. Stage 2 injuries are labral tears with subjacent femoral head chondromalacia. Stage 3A injuries are labral tears with an acetabular articular cartilage lesion smaller than 1 cm, and stage 3B injuries are labral tears with an acetabular articular cartilage lesion larger than 1 cm. Stage 4 injuries are labral tears with diffuse degenerative joint disease. Treatment outcomes for labral and chondral lesions are summarized in Table 2.

Complications

Although open arthrotomy provides excellent exposure, it has associated risks and disadvantages. The disadvantages of arthrotomy include soft-tissue scarring, muscle

effects requiring formal rehabilitation, and heterotopic ossification. The risks include osteonecrosis, deep venous thrombosis, trochanteric nonunion, and neurovascular complications. There is no disruption of muscle or tendons with hip arthroscopy; therefore, there is minimal scarring and rehabilitation is generally brief. The patient can bear full weight on the hip without support as soon as comfort permits, which is usually 3 to 5 days after surgery (Table 3).

The risks associated with hip arthroscopy are variable, depending on the experience of the surgeon and surgical approach. Comprehensive knowledge of anatomy and landmarks are crucial to prevent damage to neurovascular structures. Damage to the pudendal nerve is one of the more devastating potential complications of hip arthroscopy. Transient injury to the sciatic nerve has also been reported. Perforation of the labrum on entry to the joint is a serious complication that can be avoided by using the image intensifier to confirm instrument placement. Scuffing of the femoral head can occur to a varying extent with or without distraction. Scuffing and fluid extravasation are the most frequently reported complications, but they rarely cause permanent damage. Instruments can break intraoperatively, in which instance additional surgery may be required (Table 4). Avoiding complications involves judicious patient selection. Candidates for hip arthroscopy should include only those patients with mechanical symptoms (catching, locking, or buckling) who have failed to respond to conservative therapy.

Summary

Proper patient selection and diagnostic acumen are critical to achieving successful outcomes in hip arthroplasty. Physical examination findings can include any or all of the following: a positive McCarthy sign (with both hips fully flexed, the patient's pain is reproduced by extending the affected hip, first in external rotation, then in internal rotation), inguinal pain with flexion, adduction

Table 4 | Complication Rates Among 1,500 Patients Who Underwent Hip Arthroscopy

Complications	Of 1,500, No. Of Patients (%)
Deep venous thrombosis	1 (0.07) with factor V Leiden deficiency
Pulmonary embolism	0
Heterotopic bone	0
Osteonecrosis	0
Fluid extravasation	0
Major nerve or vessel injury	
Sciatic	0
Femoral	0
Lateral femoral cutaneous	2 (0.13) transient
Compartment syndrome	0
Broken instruments	0
Ankle strain	20 (1.33)
Transient peroneal or pudendal hypoesthesia	25 (1.67)
Mild chondral scuffing	14 (0.93)

and internal rotation of the hip, and anterior inguinal pain with ipsilateral resisted straight-leg raising. Gadolinium-enhanced MRI is much more sensitive for detecting labral tears than traditional MRI, but it is not as reliable for detecting chondral defects or nonossified loose bodies. The challenge of hip arthroscopy is that it involves a steep learning curve. Visiting medical centers in which a high volume of hip arthroscopies are performed, attending relevant instructional courses, and practicing in bioskills laboratories all can facilitate technical proficiency. Meticulous attention to positioning, distraction time and portal placement are essential. Complications are most often related to distraction. Improvements in technique and instrumentation have made hip arthroscopy an efficacious way to diagnose and treat a variety of intra-articular problems.

Annotated Bibliography

Labral Tears

Farjo LA, Glick JM, Sampson TG: Hip arthroscopy for acetabular labral tears. *Arthroscopy* 1999;15(2):132-137.

The authors reviewed the history, physical examination, and imaging findings as well as the outcomes of 290 patients who underwent hip arthroscopy and arthroscopic débridement of acetabular labral tears. Twenty-eight patients who met the study criteria were stratified into one of two groups based on the presence of significant radiographic evidence of joint arthritis. Of patients without joint arthritis, 10 of 14 (71%) had good to excellent results, and 2 underwent total hip arthroplasty at an average of 52 months after surgery. Of those with arthritis, 3 of 14 (21%) had good to excellent results, and 6 patients underwent total hip arthroplasty at an average of 14

months after surgery. Complications consisted of nerve palsies (two sciatic, one pudendal) that resolved completely without any remaining functional or sensory deficits.

McCarthy JC, Noble PC, Schuck MR, Aluisio FV, Wright J, Lee J: Acetabular and labral pathology, in McCarthy JC (ed): *Early Hip Disorders: Advances in Detection and Minimally Invasive Treatment.* New York, NY, Springer-Verlag, 2003, pp 113-134.

The authors discuss classification and treatment available for patients with acetabular labral and chondral lesions that are amenable to arthroscopic surgery.

McCarthy JC, Noble PC, Schuck MR, Wright J, Lee J: The role of labral lesions to development of early degenerative hip disease. *Clin Orthop Relat Res* 2001;393: 25-37.

This study examined the relationship between labral lesions and early degenerative hip disease by assessing 436 consecutive hip arthroscopies as well as examining 54 acetabula from human adult cadavers. Two hundred forty-one of the 436 patients (55.3%) who had arthroscopies had 261 labral tears, all of which were located at the articular and not the capsular margin of the labrum. Overall, no significant differences were identified when comparing the arthroscopic and cadaveric populations in terms of the incidence of labral tears. Arthroscopic and anatomic observations supported the concept that labral lesions are frequently part of a continuum of joint disease.

Newberg AH, Newman JS: Imaging the painful hip. *Clin Orthop Relat Res* 2003;406:19-28.

The authors of this article discuss why MRI with arthrography has become the diagnostic imaging modality of choice for patients with disorders of the acetabular labrum and for the evaluation of articular cartilage at the hip.

Osteonecrosis

Newberg AH, Newman JS: Imaging the painful hip. *Clin Orthop Relat Res* 2003;406:19-28.

MRI has become the first-line diagnostic imaging test for patients with suspected occult fracture, transient marrow edema, and osteonecrosis. CT and MRI are invaluable for the evaluation of various arthropathies, such as pigmented villonodular synovitis and synovial osteochondromatosis. Magnetic resonance arthrography with gadolinium enhancement has become the diagnostic imaging test of choice for disorders of the acetabular labrum and for the evaluation of articular cartilage at the hip.

Synovial Chondromatosis

Krebs VE: The role of hip arthroscopy in the treatment of synovial disorders and loose bodies. *Clin Orthop Relat Res* 2003;406:48-59.

This article describes arthroscopic intervention for evaluation and treatment of synovial chondromatosis and osteochondromatosis, pigmented villonodular synovitis, inflammatory arthropathies (including rheumatoid arthritis), acute septic arthritis, and conditions that result in acute and chronic synovitis within the hip. The author notes that increased awareness of the association between synovial abnormalities and cartilage degeneration has resulted in hip arthroscopy being used in early stages of disease and early in the course of symptomatic dysfunction. Outcome studies are needed to determine whether patients benefit from the procedure.

Portal Placement

Byrd JW: Hip arthroscopy: The supine position. *Clin Sports Med* 2001;20(4):703-731.

The author discusses performing hip arthroscopy with the patient in the supine position to remove loose bodies or impinging osteophytes, as well as treatment of labral tears, acute articular injuries, and damage to the ligamentum teres. The author also discusses the techniques of surgical arthroscopy for the hip with the patient in the supine position.

Glick JM: Hip arthroscopy: The lateral approach. *Clin Sports Med* 2001;20(4):733-747.

This article outlines the advantages and disadvantages of the lateral approach for arthroscopic access to the hip joint. Potential problems are detailed that can arise from traction on the branches of the pudendal nerve or the sciatic nerve. The author recommends that traction should be applied for no more than 2 hours and the amount of traction should not exceed 75 lb. In this study, the sciatic nerve was monitored using both evoked potentials and motor potentials in more than 50 patients. The author found that a well-padded peroneal post as well as a vertical post with the pelvis well supported to eliminate direct pressure on the pudendal nerve provided a safe way of performing hip arthroscopy. In addition, the author reported that the entire confines of the joint were visualized with the arthroscope and reached with surgical instruments using this approach.

Mason JB, McCarthy JC, O'Donnell J, et al: Hip arthroscopy: Surgical approach, positioning, and distraction. *Clin Orthop Relat Res* 2003;406:29-37.

This article describes seminal features of positioning and surgical approaches for arthroscopic access to the hip.

Hip-Specific Instrumentation

Dienst M, Seil R, Godde S: Effects of traction, distension, and joint position on distraction of the hip joint: An experimental study in cadavers. *Arthroscopy* 2002;18(8):865-871.

The authors of this cadaver study measured different parameters to determine optimal hip joint distraction for performing arthroscopy while minimizing soft-tissue and neurologic effects. They found that a combination of distention and

slight flexion and abduction of the hip reduced the force of traction required.

Complications

Clarke MT, Arora A, Villar RN: Hip arthroscopy: Complications in 1054 cases. *Clin Orthop* 2003;406:84-88.

The authors of this study of 1,054 consecutive hip arthroscopies reported an overall complication rate of 1.4%, which included neurapraxia, portal wound bleeding, portal hematoma, trochanteric bursitis, and instrument breakage.

Sampson TG: Complications of hip arthroscopy. *Clin Sports Med* 2001;20(4):831-835.

The author of this article reports a hip arthroscopy complication rate of 0.5%. Most of the complications were transient neurapraxias and fluid extravasations, resulting in no permanent damage. Severe scuffing of two femoral heads and one instance of osteonecrosis were considered serious and permanent.

Classic Bibliography

Burman M: Arthroscopy or the direct visualization of joints. *J Bone Joint Surg* 1931;4:669-695.

Eriksson E, Arvidsson I, Arvidsson H: Diagnostic and operative arthroscopy of the hip. *Orthopedics* 1986;9(2):169-176.

Farjo LA, Glick JM, Sampson TG: Hip arthroscopy for acetabular labral tears. *Arthroscopy* 1999;15(2):132-137.

Fitzgerald RH Jr: Acetabular labrum tears: Diagnosis and treatment. *Clin Orthop* 1995;311:60-68.

Funke EL, Munzinger U: Complications in hip arthroscopy. *Arthroscopy* 1996;12(2):156-159.

Glick JM: Hip arthroscopy using the lateral approach. *Instr Course Lect* 1988;37:223-231.

Hawkins RB: Arthroscopy of the hip. *Clin Orthop* 1989;249:44-47.

Janssens X, Van Meirhaeghe J, Verdonk R, Verjans P, Cuvelier C, Veys EM: Diagnostic arthroscopy of the hip joint in pigmented villonodular synovitis. *Arthroscopy* 1987;3(4):283-287.

McCarthy JC, Busconi B: The role of hip arthroscopy in the diagnosis and treatment of hip disease. *Orthopedics* 1995;18(8):753-756.

Villar R: Hip arthroscopy. *J Bone Joint Surg Br* 1995;77(4):517-518.

Chapter 39

Minimally Invasive Total Hip Arthroplasty

Richard A. Berger, MD

Lawrence D. Dorr, MD

Introduction

The history of total hip arthroplasty (THA) has demonstrated continuous evolution, and the relatively high complication rates associated with early prostheses and techniques led to the improvement of implants and the refinement of the surgical procedures. Gradual adoption of these improvements and their eventual diffusion into the surgical community led to improved success and increased rates of implantation. This increase in surgical experience was eventually accompanied by the development of standardized hospitalization protocols or pathways and shorter hospital stays, with more rapid rehabilitation and return to function.

Almost all surgical techniques improve over time by evolving toward less invasive approaches. The need for wide exposure diminishes as experience guides the surgeon to more accurate incision placement, more precise dissection, and more skillful mobilization of structure. Less invasiveness appears to be a hallmark of experience gained with a given procedure.

Minimally invasive THA has the potential for reducing surgical trauma, pain, and recovery. Minimally invasive procedures in THA include single-incision and two-incision techniques. These techniques are variations and refinements of existing traditional approaches as well as new approaches. Examples of variations and refinements of existing traditional approaches are the mini-incision anterolateral and mini-incision posterolateral techniques. The minimally invasive two-incision technique is an example of a new technique in which one incision is used for preparation and placement of the acetabular component, and the other incision is used for preparation and placement of the femoral component. These two incisions allow preparation and placement of the components through intermuscular planes without transecting any muscle or tendon. Unique instruments and fluoroscopic guidance aid in many steps of this procedure to ensure accurate component position and alignment.

In evaluating reports on minimally invasive techniques, it is important to note that a minimally invasive THA is not simply a standard approach done through a small incision. Instead, minimally invasive approaches avoid transecting most muscle and tendons below a small incision. There are, and will likely be, reports that claim no advantage of minimally invasive surgery over traditional surgery. However, these studies have described techniques of making a small skin incision without avoiding injury to underlying muscle and tendon; this is not minimally invasive surgery.

To achieve the potentially rapid recovery that truly minimally invasive techniques allow, the entire traditional perioperative pathway needs to be expedited. When a true minimally invasive THA is used and a new pathway expedites the entire recovery process, outpatient THA is not only possible, but it can now be routinely performed.

A Comprehensive Outpatient Clinical Pathway

A comprehensive outpatient clinical pathway should include preoperative, intraoperative, and postoperative care. This pathway should be the result of a combined effort of the surgery, anesthesia, nursing, physical therapy, and occupational therapy teams and discharge planners. At each step in the process, critical points that can delay the patient's discharge should be identified and addressed. The most common postoperative problems encountered are typically hypotension and nausea.

Preoperatively, patients attend a class taught by a nurse. In addition to explaining the potential complications of THA, the entire hospital course and postoperative care are delineated. After this class, patients have a single physical therapy session for instruction in gait training with a cane and weight bearing as tolerated. Patients are also evaluated by an internist, and donate two units of blood before surgery. The hospital discharge planner then calls the patient at home before surgery to ensure that appropriate arrangements for discharge are made, including arrangements for someone to take the patient home at the time of discharge.

On the morning of surgery, 40 mg of valdecoxib (Bextra, Pfizer, Princeton, NJ) had been administered until its recall; subsequently, 400 mg of celecoxib (Celebrex, Pfizer, Princeton, NJ) and 10 mg of oxycodone hydrochloride (OxyContin, Purdue Pharma, Stamford, CT) were administered orally. At surgery, an epidural anesthetic without narcotic additives is used unless it cannot be inserted. The use of both intravenous and epidural narcotics is avoided. Propofol (Diprivan, Astra-Zeneca Pharmaceuticals, Wilmington, DE), a short-acting sedative, is titrated during surgery for sedation. Four mg of ondansetron hydrochloride (Zofran, Glaxo SmithKline, Philadelphia, PA) is administered intravenously to decrease nausea. Patients are kept well hydrated to prevent postoperative hypotension and nausea. A Foley catheter is inserted in all patients, and prophylactic intravenous antibiotics are administered before the skin incision. One unit of autologous blood is transfused at the end of surgery.

In the recovery room, a second dose of ondansetron hydrochloride is administered, and the second unit of autologous blood is transfused. The patient is kept well hydrated to prevent postoperative hypotension and nausea. The epidural anesthetic (10 µg/mL of fentanyl and 0.1% bupivacaine) is continued in the recovery room (6 mL [1 mL every 15 minutes] with 40 mL for 4-hour lockout).

The Foley catheter is discontinued 2 hours postoperatively. At that time, 20 mg of oxycodone hydrochloride is given orally, and the epidural is removed 4 hours postoperatively. The intravenous tubing is removed just before physical therapy. Occupational therapy and physical therapy are done 4 to 6 hours postoperatively. The patients bear weight as tolerated. One additional dose of intravenous antibiotics is given after physical therapy.

Discharge is permitted when strict criteria are met. All patients must complete a formal physical therapy protocol. This protocol requires that patients can independently transfer out of bed to a standing position and into bed from the standing position, rise from a chair to a standing position and sit from a standing position, ambulate 100 feet, and ascend and descend a full flight of stairs. The patient must exhibit stable vital signs, tolerate a regular diet, and have adequate pain control from oral analgesics. Only after all of these criteria are met is the final criteria invoked: the patient must feel comfortable going home and want to be discharged. When ready, all patients are discharged to home (not to other care facilities).

Upon discharge, patients continue taking celecoxib (200 mg daily) and gradually decrease their dose of oxycodone hydrochloride as needed; hydrocodone is taken as needed for breakthrough pain. All patients receive aspirin for venous thrombosis prophylaxis for 3 weeks. Patients are encouraged to start activities as tolerated. They are allowed to drive when no longer taking any narcotics. Home physical therapy is used until the patient can drive; then outpatient physical therapy is started. Patients are evaluated clinically and radiographically in the office at 1 week, 2 weeks, 6 weeks, and 3 months.

In a prospective study, the first 100 consecutive patients enrolled in this pathway were chosen from 309 patients that met the criteria for enrollment. The average patient age was 56 years (age range, 41 to 72 years). No intraoperative complications occurred in any of the 100 patients. Ninety-two percent of patients chose to go home on the day of surgery, 8% went home the day after surgery, and all went home within 23 hours. All patients were discharged to home. One patient presented to the emergency department 2 days postoperatively with chest pain, which spontaneously resolved. Otherwise, at 3-month follow-up, no readmissions, no dislocations, and no revisions were reported.

Outpatient therapy was initiated in 9% of patients immediately, in 62% of patients by 1 week postoperatively, and in all patients by 2 weeks postoperatively. The mean time to discontinue the use of crutches, discontinue the use of narcotic pain medications, and resume driving was 6 days. The mean time to return to work was 8 days, to discontinue the use of any assistive device was 9 days, and the resumption of all activities of daily living was 10 days. The mean time to walk one half mile was 16 days.

Of the 100 patients enrolled in this outpatient protocol who underwent minimally invasive THA with two incisions, 92% were discharged on the day of surgery. Therefore, in selected patients, outpatient THA is safe with no complications requiring readmission or revision up to 3 months after discharge. Moreover, a rapid rehabilitation protocol is safe and fulfills the potential benefits of a rapid recovery with minimally invasive THA. This comprehensive pathway, which was subsequently applied to the next 200 consecutive patients who underwent minimally invasive THA with two incisions, resulted in all 200 patients going home on the day of surgery and no acute readmissions occurring as the result of early discharge.

Surgical Techniques
Anterolateral Minimally Invasive THA With Two Incisions

Two-incision THA can be performed on most patients. Notable exceptions include patients with retained hardware, such as a dynamic hip screw that must be removed via a longer incision, and patients with Crowe type 4 hip dysplasia that requires a subtrochanteric osteotomy. As with all new techniques, surgeons should first select patients who are generally smaller and less muscular, have minimal deformity, and few osteophytes. As confidence

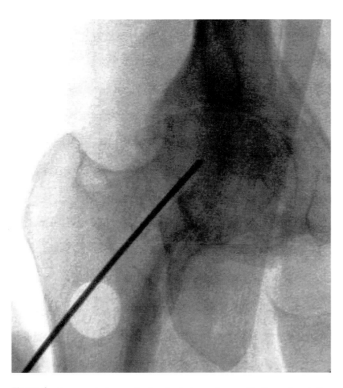

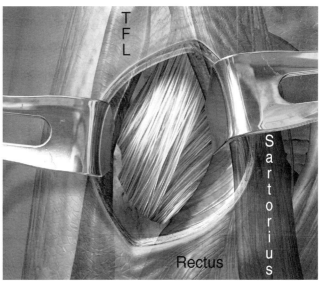

Figure 2 Illustration of the anterior dissection. The sartorius muscle and tensor fascia latae (TFL) are visible after retraction.

Figure 1 Fluoroscopic image showing the incision site over the femoral neck. The incision is made from the femoral head-neck junction distally to the intertrochanteric line (approximately 1.5 inches).

and skill level improves, this technique can be used for almost all patients.

A radiolucent operating room table is used. The patient is placed in the supine position with a small bolster under the ischium on the affected side. The leg and hip are prepared and draped. The fluoroscope is used to define the location of the femoral neck. A metal marker is used to mark the midline of the femoral neck from the junction of the head distally for 1.5 inches (Figure 1). An incision is made directly over the femoral neck from the base of the femoral head distally for 1.5 inches. The fascia of sartorius muscle is present in the proximal-medial incision, whereas the tensor fascia lata lies at the distal-lateral portion of the incision. The sartorius muscle and tensor fascia lata can be observed beneath the fascia. Just medial to the tensor fascia lata, the fascia is incised longitudinally, parallel to the sartorius muscle and tensor fascia lata. This lateral fascial incision avoids the lateral femoral cutaneous nerve, which is located superficial to the sartorius muscle. The sartorius muscle is retracted medially, and the tensor fascia lata is retracted laterally, exposing the lateral border of rectus femoris. The medial retractor is repositioned to retract the rectus muscle medially (Figure 2). This exposes the lateral circumflex vessels, which are coagulated using electrocautery. The fat pad then is retracted medially and laterally exposing the capsule over the femoral neck.

Two lighted, curved Hohmann retractors (Zimmer, Warsaw, IN) are placed extracapsularly around the femoral neck, illuminating the capsule. The capsule is incised in line with the femoral neck. This incision is made from the edge of the acetabulum distally to the intertrochanteric line. The capsule can be elevated approximately 1 cm medially and laterally along the intertrochanteric line if additional exposure of the femoral neck and head is needed. The two lighted, curved Hohmann retractors are repositioned intracapsularly to expose the femoral head and neck from the acetabulum to the intertrochanteric line (Figure 3).

The femoral head is removed in two pieces. The first neck cut is made at the equator of the femoral head with an oscillating saw, and a second cut is made 1 cm distal to this (Figure 4). The small 1 cm wafer of bone is removed using a threaded Steinmann pin. A threaded Steinmann pin is then placed into the femoral head, and the head is removed. If the ligamentum teres is intact, a curved osteotome is used to transect the ligamentum teres. Based on preoperative templating, the final femoral neck osteotomy is completed. Appropriate femoral neck resection is confirmed with fluoroscopy or by flexing and externally rotating the hip into a figure-of-4 position, which exposes the lesser trochanter.

Three lighted, curved Hohmann retractors are placed around the acetabulum, one anteriorly around the acetabulum, a second posteriorly around the acetabulum, and the third directly superiorly over the brim of the acetabulum. This retracts the capsule and allows excellent visualization of the acetabulum (Figure 5). The labrum is excised, exposing the entire peripheral bony rim of the acetabulum.

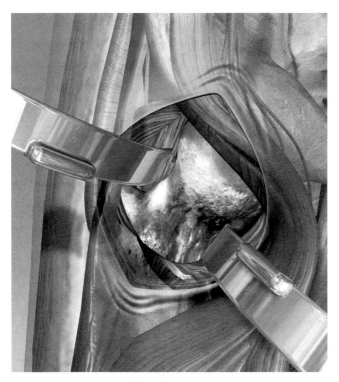

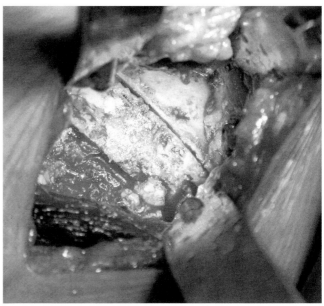

Figure 4 Intraoperative photograph of Hohmann retractors being used intracapsularly around the femoral neck, exposing the femoral head and neck. Two lines show the placement of the initial two cuts in the femoral head and neck.

Figure 3 Illustration of lighted, curved Hohmann retractors being used intracapsularly around the femoral neck, exposing the femoral head and neck.

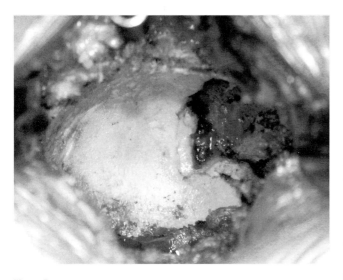

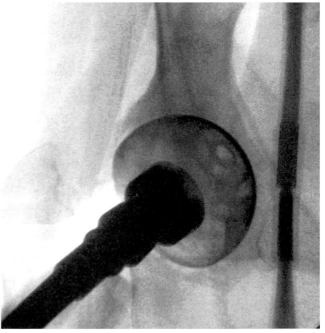

Figure 5 Intraoperative photograph a superior view of acetabulum.

Figure 6 Fluoroscopic image showing reamer seated in acetabulum while reaming. During reaming the cutout reaming appears hemispherical.

The superior retractor is removed while the anterior and posterior retractors are left in place. Specially designed, low-profile reamers that are cut out on the sides are used to ream the acetabulum. These reamers have square cutting teeth; therefore, it is possible to start with a reamer that is close in size to the intended final reamer to avoid inserting and extracting many reamers. Furthermore, the open design of these reamers allows visualization of the acetabulum during reaming. With gentle traction on the leg, the reamer is inserted in line with the femoral neck, with the cutouts of the reamer aligned with the two retractors. The acetabulum is reamed at 45° of abduction and 20° of anteversion. The fluoroscope is used for visualization as the acetabulum is reamed (Figure 6). The acetabulum is sequentially reamed until a healthy bleeding bed of cancellous bone is present throughout.

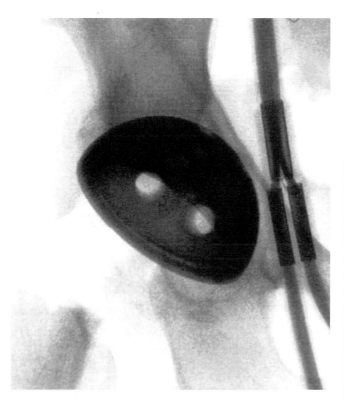

Figure 7 Fluoroscopic image showing final acetabular component placement.

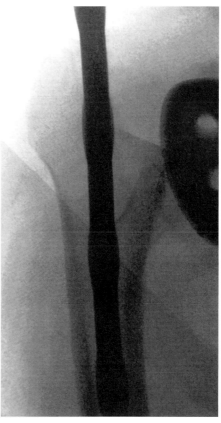

Figure 8 Fluoroscopic image showing the lateralization reamer clearing the trochanteric bed and achieving a neutral alignment.

A specially designed dogleg acetabular inserter is used to place the chosen acetabular shell. The anterior and posterior retractors are left in place as gentle traction is placed on the leg. The bolster beneath the ischium is removed so that the patient is completely supine. The acetabular component is inserted as the retractors keep the capsule from invaginating. The acetabulum is viewed with the fluoroscope as the cup is positioned in 45° of abduction and 20° of anteversion, following the native acetabulum alignment. The cup is then impacted in place and the inserter is removed (Figure 7). With the lighted, curved acetabular retractor in place around the acetabulum, the stability of the shell is assessed. Two supplemental screws are placed in the posterosuperior quadrant of the shell. Finally, a small curved osteotome is used to remove any osteophytes around the rim of the acetabulum, and the polyethylene liner is impacted into the shell. All retractors are removed from the acetabulum, and attention is turned to the femur.

The leg is adducted fully and placed in neutral rotation. A 1- to 1.5-inch incision is made in the posterior lateral buttocks, colinear with the piriformis fossa, allowing access to the femoral canal. A Charnley awl is guided through the posterior incision, posterior to the abductors, and anterior to the piriformis fossa down the femoral canal. Fluoroscopy can aid this starting point and can be used to visualize the leg in a frog-lateral po-

sition to ensure the awl is well centralized anteriorly and posteriorly. Specially designed lateralization side-cutting reamers are used to enlarge this starting hole and position the starting point laterally against the trochanteric bed. These lateralization reamers are used sequentially through the posterior incision within the same track as the Charnley awl (Figure 8). Flexible reamers are used to ream the canal until cortical chatter is obtained. Straight reamers with a tissue-protecting sleeve are then used to ream the femoral diaphysis until good cortical chatter is obtained.

After reaming to the appropriate size, broaching is done. With visualization though the anterior wound, the rasp is rotationally aligned to the calcar. This initial rasp is fully seated. Larger rasps then are sequentially introduced and seated, finishing with appropriate size (Figure 9). When the final rasp is seated, care must be taken to visualize the rotation of the rasp in the anterior wound to ensure alignment with the metaphysis.

A trial reduction is then performed. The trial femoral head and neck are placed on the broach from the anterior wound. The hip is then put through a range of motion to assess stability. The hip should be stable in full extension with 90° of external rotation and 90° of flexion with 20° of adduction and at least 50° of internal rotation. The fluoroscope can be used to assess leg lengths by comparing the level of the lesser trochanters with the obturator foramen. In addition, with the patient

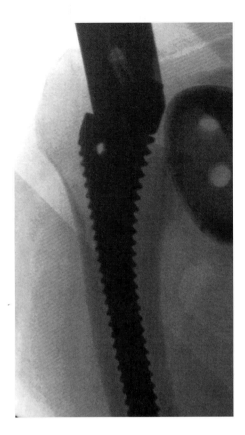

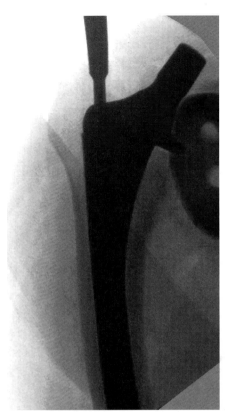

Figure 9 Fluoroscopic image showing the final femoral rasp being seated.

Figure 10 Fluoroscopic image showing the femoral component being seated into the final position.

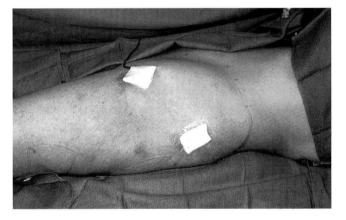

Figure 11 Photograph showing the final dressing on a patient who underwent minimally invasive two-incision THA. Two 2-inch by 2-inch bandages cover the incisions.

in the supine position, the medial malleoli may be checked to assess leg length. When the trial reduction is complete, the femoral head and neck are removed through the anterior incision, and the broach is removed through the posterior incision.

Two Hohmann retractors are placed into the posterior wound, one anterior to the femoral neck and one posterior to the femoral neck. These retract the soft tissue as the stem is placed into the femoral canal. The stem then is introduced into the femoral canal from the posterior incision and impacted into place (Figure 10). Visualization through the anterior incision ensures no soft-tissue entrapment between the calcar and the collar and ensures correct stem version.

With the actual component in place, repeat trial reduction is performed, placing the head from the anterior incision. The hip should be stable and leg lengths equal. With the hip in external rotation and the bone hook around the neck, the real femoral head is then placed on the neck and gently impacted in place. The hip is located with gentle traction and internal rotation. The capsule is then closed. The fascia between the sartorius and the tensor fascia lata is closed, followed by closure of the anterior and posterior incisions. Two 2-inch by 2-inch bandages are used to cover the incisions (Figure 11), and postoperative radiographs are obtained for comparison with radiographs obtained preoperatively (Figure 12).

Posterior Minimally Invasive THA With One Incision
Minimally invasive surgery for THA can also be done using a posterior single incision. As with the anterolateral approach, specialized tools including retractors, reamers, and implant holders are needed. Several features are required for these instruments. Long handles are a necessity for the retractors to allow retraction with little soft-tissue tension, to keep the assistant's hands and bodies clear of the wound and the operating surgeon, and to allow the assistant to hold multiple retractors and thereby minimize the number of assistants needed. The use of lighted retractors significantly en-

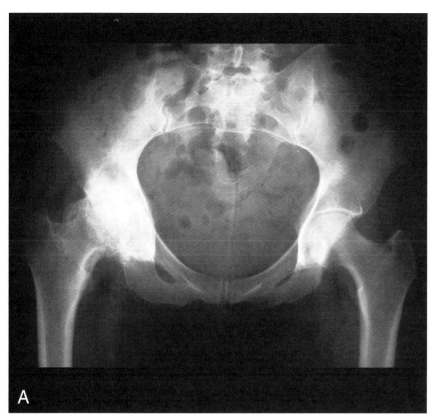
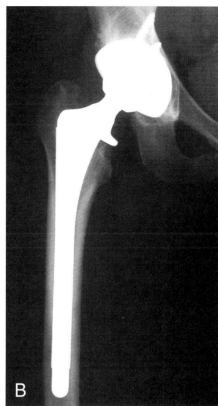

Figure 12 Preoperative **(A)** and postoperative **(B)** radiographs of a patient who underwent THA with the minimally invasive two-incision approach.

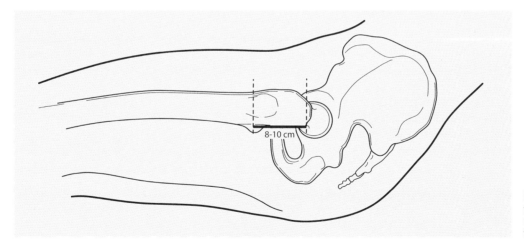

Figure 13 Schematic representation of cut 1. The incision must be made along the posterior border of the greater trochanter.

hances the surgeon's ability to visualize the acetabular cavity. The deeper the wound (the thicker the muscle or skin and fat), the more help is provided by the lighted retractors.

The patient is in the lateral decubitus position and supported at the pelvis and at the chest so that there is complete stability of the body. An incision is made posterior to the greater trochanter (Figure 13). The site of the incision is absolutely critical. This incision must be on the posterior border of the trochanter; if it is anterior

to that position, an extension of the incision will be necessary to complete the procedure. The length of the incision is proximally from the tip of the greater trochanter to distally at the level of the vastus tubercle of the femur. The preferable length of the skin incision is 8 to 10 cm because it provides the best visual exposure for the surgeon and the assistants.

Only three cuts of the hip muscle and capsule are done. The incision is made through the skin and the subcutaneous tissue and 6 cm of gluteus maximus muscle fi-

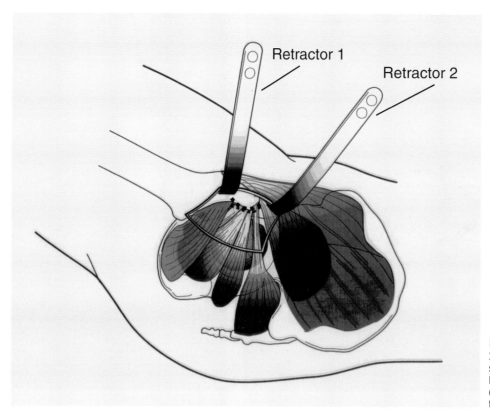

Figure 14 Schematic representation of cut 2. The incision is through the capsule and small external rotators as shown by the dotted line. The quadratus femoris muscle is not incised. This flap is closed at the completion of the operation. (Retractor 3 is not shown.)

bers adjacent to the posterior edge of the greater trochanter (cut 1). After the initial skin incision, the remainder of the exposure is done with electrocautery. The leg is then turned into internal rotation with the knee kept in the center of the table (and on top of the lower leg). It is important not to let the knee drop over the side of the table because this position puts too much tension on the soft-tissue structures in the posterior hip. With the leg in this position, the separation between the gluteus medius muscle and the gluteus minimus muscle is divided with the surgeon's finger. This can easily be found by identifying the piriformis tendon and then sliding the finger under the gluteus medius and on top of the gluteus minimus. The gluteus medius muscle is retracted by retractor 2 from the gluteus minimus muscle. The gluteus minimus muscle is then incised to the pelvic bone beginning just superior to the attachment of the piriformis tendon because the superior edge of the acetabulum is just proximal to the piriformis tendon. The incision is continued as a single flap distally for 3 cm to the proximal edge of the quadratus muscle, and then the capsule is divided beneath the quadratus muscle, leaving the quadratus muscle intact (cut 2) (Figure 14). In some patients, the most superior attachment of the quadratus muscle to the trochanter must be released for 2 to 3 mm to relax the muscle enough that the capsule underneath it can be incised. The advantage of saving the quadratus muscle is that it is the largest external rotator muscle with the greatest mechanical advantage for control of the

trochanter. By saving the quadratus muscle, the stability of the hip is improved by limiting the internal rotation to that permitted by the intact quadratus femoris muscle.

Once the hip is dislocated, a retractor is placed around the femoral neck underneath the quadratus femoris muscle to both retract the quadratus femoris muscle from the femoral neck and to protect the sciatic nerve. The level of the femoral neck cut is determined by the use of preoperative templates. Most often the level of neck cut needed to recreate the offset and leg length for a patient is 15 to 20 mm below the distal edge of the femoral head. Initially, the lesser trochanter was used to determine the level of femoral neck cut, but with retention of the quadratus femoris muscle this was not possible, and this new technique has proved to be predictable. Following removal of the femoral head, the acetabulum is visualized and retractor 4 is then placed on the posterosuperior acetabulum between the bone and the posterosuperior capsule and external rotators. This allows excellent visualization of the superior acetabular labrum and the anterior superior capsule that overhangs the acetabulum with the femur in this position. The labrum is excised. The snake retractor (retractor 5) is positioned on the ilium by pushing the point of the retractor through the anterior capsule. The third cut (cut 3) of this approach is an incision of the posterior medial capsule (which includes the ischiofemoral ligament). This capsular incision relaxes this contracted tissue, which further allows the femur to be retracted ante-

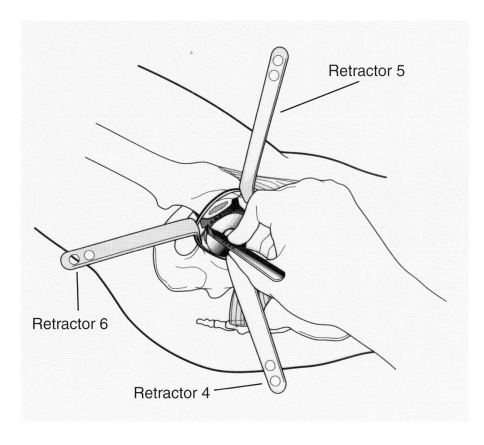

Retractor 5

Retractor 6

Retractor 4

Figure 15 Schematic representation of cut 3. This incision is made through the medial capsule to the transverse acetabular ligament. This cut allows the femur to be translated anterior to the acetabulum for the preparation of the acetabulum.

riorly as well as allows the femur to be internally rotated and flexed. It also makes easier the placement of retractor 7 against the cortical bone of the cotyloid notch. A light attached to this retractor significantly enhances the visualization of the acetabulum during preparation.

Reaming is initiated by using a straight-handled reamer transversely into the acetabulum for the purpose of reaming the acetabular ridge to the level of the cortical bone of the cotyloid notch. Using specially designed half reamers gives much better visual confirmation of the reamer position in the bony acetabulum. The anterior wall of the acetabulum is at risk for being overreamed with this preparation. The reamer must be transverse, but also anteverted between the anterior and posterior walls of the bony acetabulum so that the reamer is not pointed at the anterior wall. When this preparation is complete, there will be cancellous bone exposed beneath the now absent ridge, and the cortical bone of the medial wall will form the floor of the acetabulum.

Reaming is completed with the curved reamer (Figure 15) used to prepare a hemisphere by shaping the iliac bone of the acetabulum. If a curved reamer is not used, the superior wall of the acetabulum is at risk because a straight reamer can be levered into an adverse superior position by the handle of the reamer abutting the distal wound edge. When the surgeon becomes ex-

perienced with this reaming technique, the acetabular preparation can usually be done with two reaming steps: the use of the straight reamer once and the curved reamer once. This preparation with a curved reamer is more precise (less reaming time) for a press-fit of the cup than the singular use of straight reamers when a long incision is used.

A curved holder is necessary for ease and accuracy of cup position (Figure 16). Just as with a straight reamer, a straight implant holder can abut on the distal wound edge and promote malposition of both the inclination and anteversion of the cup. A trial acetabular component should be used for greatest accuracy of fit. Reaming the bony acetabulum 1 mm smaller than the actual implants gives even greater assurance that the fit will be secure without any adjunctive screws. A line-to-line fit with reaming is satisfactory if screws are to be used to fix the cup in every hip operation. To test the press-fit stability of the cup, an attempt should be made to life the cup out of the bony acetabulum by pulling on the handle of the cup holder. If the cup moves, screws are required to provide immediate fixation stability. The medial edge of the cup should be level with the tear drop (the edge of the cortical bone of the cotyloid notch). The anterior edge should be about 5 mm below the pubic tubercle, and preferably the metal edge of the cup is not proud above the anterior bony wall (so the iliopsoas tendon will not be irritated by the metal). Supe-

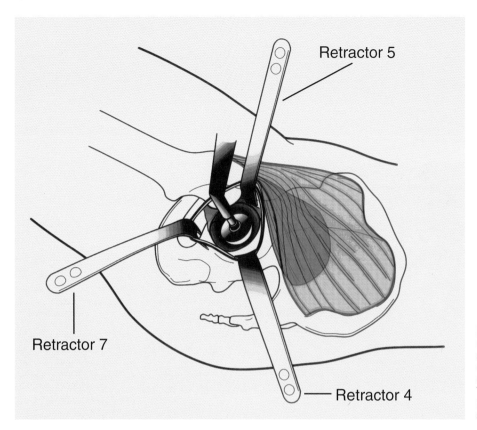

Figure 16 Schematic representation of the curved reamer being used. This technique allows safe reaming of the acetabulum without the handle of the reamer abutting against the distant edge of the wound, which can alter its direction. The curved reamer will correctly shape the acetabulum into a hemisphere with the desired anteversion.

riorly, the metal edge of the cup should be flush with the anterosuperior acetabular bone to prevent impingement of the metal femoral neck against the metal edge of the cup in flexion. Posterosuperiorly, there may be 5 mm of exposed metal that ensures that the cup inclination does not exceed 45°.

Femoral preparation is performed with only the cut surface of the femoral neck as a bony reference. The quadratus femoris muscle obscures the femoral neck and lesser trochanter, although both can be felt. The preparation of the femoral bone can be done using either reamers and/or broaches as necessary followed by insertion of the implant. Insertion of the implant sometimes results in the metal femoral neck impinging on the jaws retractor so that the leg will need to be internally rotated to avoid this impingement (Figure 17). The internal rotation of the leg for this maneuver must be done with the leg on the table (resting on the lower leg). Internal rotation of the leg when it is hanging over the side of the table can stretch the sciatic nerve. In the future, the use of modular necks with the femoral component will avoid this particular technical problem. Following implantation of the femur, the femoral head is placed onto the femoral neck using a tool that allows this to be accomplished inside the small incision.

Leg lengths are manually confirmed by the position of the lesser trochanter to the ischium inside the hip and by overlaying the leg and measuring the position of the patella and the foot of the upper leg to the lower leg. Satisfactory offset can be manually determined by taking the hip through an entire range of motion and using the index finger of the free hand to check that the femur clears the pelvis in the maximally flexed and internally rotated position and the maximally abducted and externally rotated position. The lesser trochanter should clear the ischium in the maximally extended and externally rotated position. This clearance should be just by one fingerbreadth. Two-fingerbreadth clearance means the offset is increased, and impingement of the bone against the bone means that the offset is too small. When checking the clearance of the femoral bone from the pelvis, the index finger can also be used to ensure that the metal femoral neck is not impinging against the metal edge of the acetabular cup. The extremes of the arc of motion that are used to evaluate the stability and offset are limited by the soft tissues (both static and dynamic) of the hip. When available, flexion should be taken to 100°. Adduction and internal rotation should be evaluated with the hip as near 90° as possible. With the hip in 20° of adduction, internal rotation should be stable to 40°. It is not necessary to have stability in internal rotation beyond 40° because the hip, in the awake patient, never exceeds that range. In extension, the hip should be brought with full extension to maximum external rotation, the lesser trochanter should clear the ischium, and the hip should be stable anteriorly. The hip

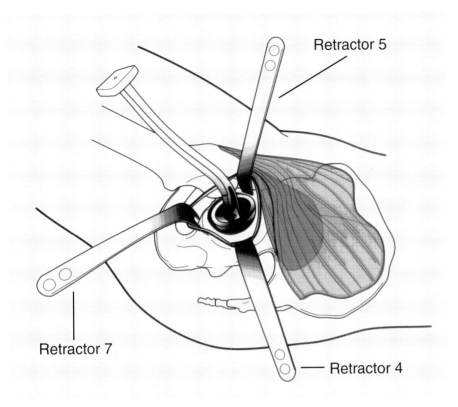

Retractor 5

Retractor 7

Retractor 4

Figure 17 Schematic representation of acetabular exposure as obtained by retractor 5 (which is into the iliac bone and retracting the femur anteriorly), retractor 4 (which is in the posterosuperior acetabulum and retracting the posterosuperior capsule), and retractor 7 (which has the long hook that is against the edge of the cotyloid notch and the paddle sits on the ischium so that the posteromedial capsule is retracted). A light in this retractor provides excellent illumination of the acetabulum. The curved acetabular cup holder allows the cup to be placed without the distal wound effecting the position of the cup by levering the cup holder.

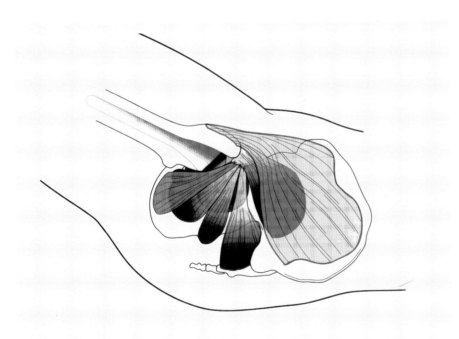

Figure 18 Schematic representation of the external rotators and capsule repaired together to the cut edge of the gluteus minimus. This provides a closure without any dead space of the hip joint and also allows the gluteus minimus to improve its function, which is to contract against the femoral head.

should also be brought with maximum external rotation into full abduction, there should not be impingement of the greater trochanter, and the hip should be stable anteriorly in this position.

Closure is done with the capsule and external rotators sutured to the cut edge of the gluteus minimus (Figure 18). This closure helps improve the function of the gluteus minimus muscle, which is to contract against the femoral head and help hold it into position; this closure provides further protection against dislocation. This closure also best eliminates any dead space between the closed capsule and external rotators and the metal femoral neck and head. Another way to help reduce the dead space in the closed hip is to use as large a femoral head as can be used in combination with the acetabular component. A large femoral head can ultimately improve the range of motion of the patient and further protection against impingement of either the metal femoral neck or the femoral bone by increasing the head-neck ratio.

Summary

Minimally invasive surgery has the potential to minimize surgical trauma and pain while improving functional recovery in patients who undergo THA. The minimally invasive two-incision total hip technique, in which no muscle or tendon is cut, appears to facilitate the early recovery benefits of less pain and functional improvement over traditional THA. Furthermore, unique instruments and fluoroscopic assistance have enabled accurate component position and alignment.

Although mini-incision techniques that transect some muscle may come close to producing some of the benefits of minimally invasive THA, minimally invasive two-incision THA may show greater promise. However, this technique requires meticulous surgical technique, specialized instrumentation, and special instruction. As such, preclinical exercises, anatomy laboratories, cadaver training, and proctoring programs are strongly recommended for surgeons interested in this new technique to minimize complications and ensure the success of this new procedure. In the future, further improvements in technique are likely to follow with advanced guidance systems that facilitate accurate surgical technique.

Annotated Bibliography

Berger RA: The technique of minimally invasive total hip arthroplasty using the two-incision approach. *Instr Course Lect* 2004;53:149-155.

The author reports that the two-incision technique for THA avoids transection of any muscle or tendon and has the potential to reduce surgical trauma, pain, and morbidity and can significantly shorten patient recovery.

Berry DJ, Berger RA, Callaghan JJ, et al: Minimally invasive total hip arthroplasty: Development, early results, and a critical analysis. *J Bone Joint Surg Am* 2003;85-A: 2235-2246.

This symposium presents the viewpoints of advocates for and those with reservations about minimally invasive THA and provides preliminary information on the results of these procedures.

Chimento GF, Pavone V, Sharrock N, Kahn B, Cahill J, Sculco TP: Minimally invasive total hip arthroplasty: A prospective randomized study. *J Arthroplasty* 2005;20(2): 139-144.

Patients were randomized to undergo minimally invasive THA with either 8-cm incisions (group A, N = 28 patients) or 15-cm incision (group B, N = 32 patients). The groups were demographically comparable. The authors found that group A had significantly less intraoperative blood loss (*P* < 0.003) and less total blood loss (*P* < 0.009). They also reported that fewer patients in group A limped at 6-week follow-up (*P* < 0.04), but at 1- and 2-year follow-up, there was no difference between the two groups.

DiGioia AM III, Plakseychuk AY, Levison TJ, Jaramaz B: Mini-incision technique for total hip arthroplasty with navigation. *J Arthroplasty* 2003;18:123-128.

This prospective study compared a mini-incision technique (group 1, N = 33 patients) and traditional posterior approach (group 2, N = 33 patients) for THA. The average length of the incisions was 11.7 cm (range, 7.3 to 13.0 cm) for group 1 and 20.2 cm (range, 14.8 to 26.0 cm) for group 2. The authors reported that at 3-month follow-up, patients in group 1 had significant improvement in limp (*P* < 0.05) and ability to climb stairs (*P* < 0.01) compared with group 2. At 6-month follow-up, group 1 was significantly better in terms of limp (*P* < 0.05), distance walked (*P* < 0.001), and stair climbing (*P* < 0.001). No significant difference between the two groups was reported for pain, function, or range of motion at 1-year follow-up.

Dorr LD: *Hip Arthroplasty: Minimally Invasive Techniques and Computer Navigation.* Philadelphia, PA, Elsevier, 2005.

This book provides detailed information on the preoperative planning, intraoperative technique, and postoperative rehabilitation for the posterior minimally invasive THA with one incision.

Sculco TP, Jordan LC: The mini-incision approach to total hip arthroplasty. *Instr Course Lect* 2004;53:141-147.

Using a surgical technique based on the classic Moore approach to the hip, the authors performed THA with incisions from 6 to 10 cm in length and reported significantly less deep soft-tissue disruption compared with longer incisions (20 to 25 cm).

Wenz JF, Gurkan I, Jibodh SR: Mini-incision total hip arthroplasty: A comparative assessment of perioperative outcomes. *Orthopedics* 2002;25:1031-1043.

The authors of this study compared patients who underwent THA via a direct lateral approach with patients who underwent THA via a mini-incision approach. They reported that the latter group of patients had significantly earlier ambulation, less transfer assistance, and more favorable discharge dispositions. The authors also reported that the mini-incision group also had decreased transfusion requirements and better functional recovery with early physical therapy and that this procedure achieved accurate and reproducible implantation, regardless of patient habitus.

Chapter 40

Primary Total Hip Arthroplasty: Cementless and Cemented

John H. Velyvis, MD

Harry E. Rubash, MD

John J. Callaghan, MD

Cementless Primary Total Hip Arthroplasty

During the early 1980s, periprosthetic osteolysis and aseptic loosening were thought to result from the use of methylmethacrylate bone cement. The prevalence of these complications following the implantation of cemented components for both primary and revision total hip arthroplasty (THA), along with the desire to fix the implant directly to host bone and to load the femur in a more physiologic manner, were the driving forces for the introduction of cementless fixation.

Numerous studies have greatly advanced the understanding of fixation by means of bone ongrowth using roughened surfaces and bone ingrowth using microporous materials. In addition, important investigations have been performed into a multitude of related factors, including the geometry of porous-coated prostheses, the biocompatibility of various metals, the surface properties and the extent of the porous coating, agents that enhance or inhibit bone ingrowth, the requirements for stable osseointegration, and the adaptation of the host bone to a cementless prosthesis. As a result, a consistent migration to the use of cementless implants in primary and revision THA has occurred.

Development of Extensively Coated Cementless Stems

The first implants to demonstrate the capacity for biologic fixation, such as the Austin-Moore prosthesis of the 1950s, used a macrointerlock with large fenestrations. In the 1960s and 1970s, reports from Europe by various authors including Judet and Lord demonstrated success with roughened surfaces that permitted bony ongrowth. The initial use of a microporous surface implant with potential for bone ingrowth occurred in 1977, in a US Food and Drug Administration (FDA) clinical trial of the extensively porous-coated Anatomic Medullary Locking (AML) implant (Johnson & Johnson/ DePuy, Warsaw, IN). This first-generation extensively coated stem (80% of the surface was coated) was approved by the FDA in 1983. In subsequent evolutions of this design, a greater variety of sizes was added for improved initial stability, the porous coating was removed

from the distal eighth of the stem, initial fixation was improved by using the scratch-fit technique, a porous-coated acetabular component was designed, and a modular head was added.

The advantage of an extensively coated stem is that osseointegration is possible along the entire length of the stem. However, the distal part of the stem most consistently contacts cortical bone and most dependably demonstrates the greatest amount of bone integration. The extensively coated implant has an advantage over proximally coated implants when the proximal femoral anatomy is distorted and for revision arthroplasty. In addition, when osseointegration fails to occur, fibrous tissue growth into the porous surface more often is able to prevent subsidence of the stem, resulting in patient satisfaction and radiographic stability.

Development of Proximally Coated Cementless Stems

Shortly after the introduction of extensively microporous-coated ingrowth stems, concerns with proximal stress shielding, early and late instability, persistent thigh pain, and osteolysis led to the introduction of proximally porous-coated femoral implants. These designs were intended to achieve biologic fixation solely in the femoral metaphysis and thereby reduce proximal stress shielding. Examples of first-generation stems include the Porous-Coated Anatomic (PCA) implant (Stryker Howmedica Osteonics, Kalamazoo, MI), which was not patch coated, but coated 360°, and the Harris-Galante Porous I (HGP-I) implant (Zimmer, Warsaw, IN), which used a patch porous coating on the anterior and posterior proximal surfaces of the stem. Although some first-generation stems performed well, the latter design often did not provide sufficient initial stability to allow bone ingrowth and stability. Other complications associated with these implant designs included persistent thigh pain and femoral osteolysis in the proximal and distal aspects of the femur.

These findings led to the development of a second generation of proximally porous-coated femoral components. Second-generation stems were designed with im-

Classification	Distal Geometry	Proximal Geometry	Overall Geometry	Examples
Tapered				
	Tapered	Two-dimensional	Coronal taper over entire length	Tri-Lock (Johnson & Johnson/DePuy) Spectron (Smith& Nephew, Memphis, TN) Accolade (Stryker) Taperloc (Biomet) M/L Taper (Zimmer)
	Tapered	Three-dimensional	Sagittal and coronal taper over entire length	Synergy (Smith &Nephew) Mallory Head (Biomet) Versys Fiber Metal Taper (Zimmer) Summit (Johnson & Johnson/DePuy) Secur-Fit (Stryker)
Cylindrical				
	Cylindrical	Two-dimensional	Metaphyseal only coronal taper and rectangular lateral border with diaphyseal cylinder	Harris-Galante (Zimmer) Versys MidCoat (Zimmer) Echelon (Smith & Nephew) Progressive (Biomet) AML (Johnson & Johnson/DePuy) Secur-Fit Plus (Stryker)
	Cylindrical	Three-dimensional	Metaphyseal only lateral and coronal taper with diaphyseal cylinder	Versys Enhanced Taper (Zimmer) Meridian (Stryker)
Anatomic				
	Cylindrical	Anatomic	Asymmetric lateral and coronal taper with anteverted neck	Image (Smith & Nephew) Profile (Johnson & Johnson/DePuy)
		Anatomic	Metaphyseal only asymmetric lateral and coronal taper with diaphyseal cylinder	Citation (Stryker) Prodigy (Johnson & Johnson/DePuy) Anatomic (Zimmer)

Classification is dependent on combination of proximal and distal geometry without reference to type of ingrowth/ongrowth surface

proved metals, multiple sizes, improved initial implant stability, and circumferential proximal porous coatings. Midterm data (10-year follow-up) from these second-generation stems have shown excellent survivorship, decreased thigh pain, and the elimination of distal femoral osteolysis.

Recently, a third generation of porous-coated stems has been developed to maximize osseointegration using bioactive and osteoconductive surface coatings, such as hydroxyapatite and tricalcium phosphate. Also, shorter stems have been designed to preserve the endosteum of the diaphysis and to facilitate removal of the stem should revision surgery be necessary.

Stem Geometry

Cementless stems are classified as tapered, cylindrical, anatomic, or combination (modular). A tapered stem narrows in two or three dimensions over its entire length, whereas a cylindrical stem has a constant diameter in the diaphyseal portion. Tapered stems achieve fix-ation solely in the metaphyseal region of the femur. By contrast, proximally coated cylindrical stems have engaging flutes or splines that improve initial rotational stability by means of an interference fit in the proximal diaphysis of the femur. Stems that taper in two dimensions (dual tapered wedge) narrow in the coronal plane and have a nontapered rectangular lateral border. Stems that taper in three dimensions (flat tapered wedge) narrow in both the coronal and sagittal planes. Anatomic stems have an asymmetric proximal segment consisting of an anteverted neck and metaphyseal portion, forming what is referred to as a metaphyseal flare (Table 1).

Femoral stems also are classified as collared or collarless. Collared stems may provide proximal stress transfer to the calcar, at least in the short term, but also may limit full wedging of the component into the proximal metaphysis. In contrast, collarless components allow for implant subsidence for possible improvement of the initial prosthetic fit but may subside excessively and lead to failure of stable ingrowth.

Table 2 | Properties of Ingrowth/Ongrowth Surfaces Commonly Used With Cementless Femoral Components in THA

Ingrowth/Ongrowth Surface	Process	Characteristics	Examples
Microporous beads (ingrowth)	Titanium or chromium-cobalt alloy beads sintered to substrate	Pore size: 150 to 400 μm Bead size: 100 to 250 μm Porosity: 30% to 35%	Tri-Lock (Johnson & Johnson/DePuy)
Fiber metal mesh (ingrowth)	Ti-GAl-4V alloy fiber diffusion bonded to substrate	Pore size: average 250 μm Porosity: 50% to 60%	Fiber Metal Taper (Zimmer) Meridian (Stryker) Citation (Stryker)
Plasma spray (ongrowth)	Heated titanium alloy powder flame-sprayed on substrate	Pore size: 100 to 1,000 μm	TaperLoc (Biomet, Warsaw, IN)
Grit-blasted (ongrowth)	Varies	Surface roughness: 4 to 6 μm	Zweymuller-Alloclassic (Sulzer, Winterthur, Switzerland)
HA, TCP* (substrate dependent)	Varies by manufacturer	Thickness: ~30 μm Minimal effect on underlying surface porosity	Accolade (Stryker)
Porous tantalum (ingrowth)	Varies by manufacturer	Dodecahedron-shaped pores Pore size: 430 to 650 μm Porosity: 75% to 80%	Trabecular Metal Cup (Zimmer)

HA = hydroxyapatite; TCP = tricalcium phosphate. HA and TCP are fixation adjuncts applied to underlying ingrowth/ongrowth surfaces

Metallurgy

The principal metals used in cementless hip arthroplasty are cobalt-chromium or titanium alloys. Cobalt-chromium alloys are used where high strength and corrosion resistance are desired. The most commonly used cobalt-chromium alloy is cobalt-chromium-molybdenum (Co-Cr-Mo). The primary titanium alloy used today is titanium-aluminum-vanadium (Ti-6Al-4V), which has high strength and fatigue resistance and is more biologically inert than cobalt-chromium, inducing less activation of local osteoblasts. Titanium is also 50% less stiff than cobalt-chromium, which improves the proximal transfer of stress in a proximally porous-coated implant.

The ultimate stiffness of an implant is a function of both its material properties and its geometry. Stems made from titanium alloy with a diameter at the distal end smaller than 14 mm have approximately the same stiffness as a normal femur. However, larger-diameter titanium alloy stems and all cobalt-chrome alloy stems are much stiffer. With increasing stiffness of the stem, more of the load is transferred to bone, and more distally. Design modifications such as slots or grooves have been added to contemporary stems to decrease the implant stiffness; however, there are structural limits to the extent an implant can be modified.

The primary drawback of titanium is that it functions poorly as a bearing surface. Titanium has poor wear resistance and high notch sensitivity, and it is susceptible to third-body abrasive wear. By contrast, cobalt-chromium alloys have greater hardness and wear resistance, which makes them ideally suited for articulating surfaces. For these reasons, cobalt-chromium femoral heads are often combined with titanium femoral

stems. Corrosion as a result of the battery effect of approximating the two different metal types has not been shown to be a serious problem, probably because of the relative inertness of both alloys.

New prosthetic biomaterials such as porous tantalum are actively being studied (Table 2). Conventional implants of solid metal are rigid, which may result in stress shielding or thigh pain. The porous coatings that must be bonded to these solid metal substrates have relatively low volumetric porosity for biologic ingrowth and low frictional characteristics for initial implant stability. New porous structural biomaterials may help to advance the current generation of prostheses and address unresolved clinical applications. For instance, the trabecular structure of porous tantalum offers several potential advantages over conventional porous coatings. Although further study is needed, its greater porosity (two to three times that of conventional porous coatings) may improve tissue ingrowth. The higher coefficient of friction can provide greater scratch fit and initial stability, and the high compressive and shear strength, combined with a relatively low modulus of elasticity that is comparable to that of cancellous bone, produces more normal physiologic loading and reduces stress shielding.

Another example of the use of a novel biomaterial in THA prosthetic design is the EPOCH composite stem (Zimmer). Developed to address modulus mismatch between the femur and the prosthetic stem, this extensively coated low-modulus stem consists of a core of cobalt-chromium alloy, an outer ingrowth surface of titanium fiber mesh, and an intervening layer of polyaryletherketone polymer matrix that is injection-molded onto the metallic core. The composite stem is

Table 3 | Long-Term Results of Extensively Coated Femoral Components

Stem	Author (Year)	Design	No. of Hips	Patient Age in Years	Mean Follow-up (Range)	Stable on Radiographs	Distal Lysis	Thigh Pain	Rate of Survival
AML (Johnson & Johnson/DePuy)	Engh (2001)	Chromium-cobalt, beads, collar, cylindrical	129	55	15.5 years (15-17.6)	96.6%	None	Not reported	98.9% at 15 years
Prodigy (Johnson & Johnson/DePuy) AML (Johnson & Johnson/ DePuy)	Della Valle (2002)	Chromium-cobalt, beads, collar, cylindrical	348	53	14.2 years (10-17)	99.4%	None	6%	96% at 15 years
Lord (Benoist Girard)	Grant (2004)	Chromium-cobalt, cast beads, collar, cylindrical	116	62	17.5 years (15-20)	98%	None	Not reported	98% at 17.5 years

currently available only in larger sizes (14 mm to 18 mm); implants of this size that are made of conventional materials have a stiffness exceeding that of native bone. Smaller sizes are made of solid metal without the interposed polymer matrix layer. The bending stiffness of the composite stem is 75% less than that of a comparable cobalt-chromium alloy stem and 50% less than that of a titanium alloy stem. At mean follow-up of 4 years (range, 2 to 7 years) of 400 hips, 100% had survived. In a randomized comparison study of the EPOCH stem and a stiffer stem (Anatomic, Zimmer) for implant sizes greater than 14 mm, significantly less proximal loss of bone mineral density occurred in the EPOCH group after 2 years, with no differences in clinical outcomes. Excellent primary fixation also was documented for the composite stem, with no failures after 2 years. Longer term studies of the performance of this stem are needed, however.

Biology of Ingrowth

The physiologic response to a porous-coated implant resembles the healing cascade of a cancellous bone defect, with newly formed bone occupying the voids of the porous surface material. The optimal interface contact is with cortical bone. Direct contact between the porous implant surface and the host bone correlates with bone ingrowth and strength of fixation. Gaps > 0.5 mm result in decreased bone ingrowth, decreased strength of fixation, and a greater proportion of cancellous rather than cortical ingrowth. Circumferentially porous-coated femoral implants create a proximal bone–implant seal that protects against the migration of wear particles into the femoral diaphysis and provides a large surface area for bone ingrowth and initial component stability.

The porous surfaces most commonly used in the clinical setting are sintered beads, fiber metal, plasma spray, grit blasting, and chemical etching (Table 2). Bioresorbable calcium phosphate ceramic coatings such

as hydroxyapatite and tricalcium phosphate were introduced to implants to enhance osseointegration by accelerating the adherence of bone to the implant and to promote the filling of gaps between implant and bone. Recent evidence confirms that these coatings help to compensate for an imperfect fit between bone and prosthesis by filling in larger gaps.

Clinical Outcomes

To evaluate the clinical performance of a particular THA component, objective end points are used, such as revision for aseptic loosening and definite radiographic loosening, because the end point of revision for any reason is inconsistently reported. Rates for revisions for any reason will be higher, and in some cases substantially higher, when factors are included such as sepsis, septic loosening, severe polyethylene wear (with exchange of the liner only or revision of both the shell and liner), and osteolysis and mechanical failures such as locking mechanism failure or liner spin-out are taken into account.

Results for Extensively Coated Stems

Long-term follow-up after THA using extensively coated stems is now available. The first porous-coated stem to become available and the most studied is the AML stem, a cast cobalt-chromium design with a Co-Cr alloy beaded surface. Survival rates at 15-year follow-up ranged from 96% to 98.9% for mechanical failure of the stem (Table 3). In one long-term study of 129 hips using the AML stem at 13.9-year follow-up, the rate of loosening of the stem was 3.4%, which compares favorably with other long-term series. The overall rate of revision for any reason, however, was much higher (18%). Most of the revision operations (22 of 39) were performed proactively, with no loosening present, for progressive femoral osteolysis and acetabular wear. A large increase in osteolysis and wear occurred after 10 years. For this

Table 4 | Midterm and Long-Term Results for Proximally Porous-Coated Tapered Stems

Stem	Author (Year)	Design	Patient Age in Years	Follow-up (Range)	Stable on Radiographs	Distal Osteolysis	Thigh Pain	Rate of Survival
Tri-Lock (Johnson & Johnson/DePuy)	Teloken (2002)	Chromium-cobalt, beads, collarless, 2-D tapered	50	12 years (10-15)	96%	None	2%	96% at 15years
Omnifit (Stryker Howmedica Osteonics)	Hellman (1999)	Chromium-cobalt, beads collarless, two-dimensional tapered	45	10 years (5-12.5)	97.4%	None	4.1%	95.9% at 10 years
Taperloc (Biomet)	Parvizi (2004)	Titanium plasma, collarless, two-dimensional tapered	61	11 years (6-15)	100%	None	3.6%	99.1% at 11 years
Mallory Head (Biomet)	Park (2003)	Titanium, collarless, plasma spray, three-dimensional tapered	50	10.1 years (9-13)	97.3%	None	4.4%	97.3% at 13 years
Integral (Biomet)	Marshall (2004)	Titanium, collared, plasma spray, three-dimensional tapered	56	11.6 years (10-15)	99%	None	2.3%	98% at 10 years
Profile (Johnson & Johnson/DePuy)	Kim (2003)	Titanium, beads, collarless, anatomic tapered	46.8	9.8 years (8-11)	100%	None	10% initially, 0% at 2 years	99% at 10 years
IPS (Johnson & Johnson/DePuy)	Kim (2003)	Titanium, beads, collarless, anatomic tapered	45.3	6.6 years (5-7)	100%	None	4%	100% at 6.6 years

series, the polyethylene liners were sterilized by gamma irradiation in air. The incidence of periprosthetic osteolysis was 40%. Larger osteolytic lesions were associated with revision surgery, younger patients, and longer follow-up, highlighting the importance of regular (both early and long-term) follow-up with such patients. For all loose stems, failure of bony ingrowth was indicated on the radiographs obtained by the 2-year follow-up visit.

A major concern with the use of extensively coated stems is a pathologic fracture of the greater trochanter associated with trochanteric osteolysis. A long-term study of 208 consecutive THAs demonstrated a 4.3% rate of greater trochanteric fracture associated with proximal osteolysis occurring at a mean follow-up of 10.7 years. The risk of sustaining a fracture was independent of the size of the osteolytic lesion; however, the risk increased significantly when the lysis eroded the cortical bone of the greater trochanter. Seven of 9 fractures healed in situ without major displacement; one resulted in a nonunion of the tip of the greater trochanter.

In support of the use of extensively coated stems, one study compared bone loss and bone density between extensively coated and proximally coated stems in comparison to the contralateral normal femur of each patient. Dual-energy x-ray absorptiometry demonstrated marked loss of bone mineral content in both groups of patients, but the extensively coated group had less bone loss on average than did the proximally coated

group (18.4% versus 38.6%) and also less decrease in bone density than did the proximally coated group (14.3% versus 28.4%).

A long-term (17.5-year) follow-up on a macrotextured ongrowth implant, the Lord prosthesis (Benoist Girard, Bagneux, France), was reported. Used from 1981 to 1985, the Lord prosthesis demonstrates the excellent long-term outcomes possible with extensively coated femoral ongrowth components (Table 3). The device has a straight Co-Cr alloy stem with an extensively roughened macroporous coating created by direct casting of 1-mm balls. Only four stem sizes were available for the series, and a modular 32-mm Co-Cr head with a threaded Co-Cr cup and a polyethylene liner sterilized in air was used in all patients. The stem had a 98% cumulative survival rate for revision because of mechanical loosening, stem fracture, or radiographic loosening. With "revision for any reason" as the end point, the rate of survival of the stem was 92% at 17.5 years.

Results of Proximally Coated Stems
Many types of proximally coated implant designs are in use, giving rise to a large number of midterm follow-up reports and a few long-term follow-up reports on stems of varying geometries and ingrowth/ongrowth surfaces. These results are summarized in Tables 4 through 6.

A study of one of the earliest proximally coated designs, the patch-porous–coated titanium HGP-I stem, identified several shortcomings with first-generation cementless proximal fixation technology and served as an

Table 5 | Midterm and Long-Term Results for Proximally Porous-Coated Cylindrical and Anatomic Stems

Stem	Author (Year)	Design	Patient Age (Years)	Mean Follow-up (Range)	Stable on Radiographs	Distal Osteolysis	Thigh Pain	Rate of Survival
HGP-I (Zimmer)	Parvizi (2004)	Titanium fiber metal, collar, two-dimensional cylindrical	57	14.9 years (12-18)	96%	NR	4%	82% at 15 years
Multilock (Zimmer)	Sinha (2004)	Titanium, fiber metal, collar, distal flutes, three-dimensional cylindrical	54	6.5 years (5-10)	99%	0	10%	97% at 10 years
PCA (Stryker Howmedica Osteonics)	Bojescul (2003)	Chromium-cobalt, beads, collarless, anatomic	58	15.6 years (15-17)	95%	4%	13%	93% at 17 years
Anatomic Hip (Zimmer)	Archibeck (2001)	Titanium, fiber metal, collarless, anatomic cylindrical	52	10 years (8-11)	100%	None	9%	100% at 10 years

NR = not reported

Table 6 | Midterm Results for Proximally Porous-Coated Stems With Hydroxyapatite

Stem	Author (Year)	Design	Patient Age (Years)	Mean Follow-up (Range)	Stable on Radiographs	Distal Osteolysis	Thigh Pain	Rate of Survival
Freeman (Finsbury Instruments)	Skinner (2004)	Titanium and chromium-cobalt, collarless, roughened shot-blasted with ridges and stipples, proximal one third HA, tapered	57	10 years	100%	None	NR	100% at 10 years
JRI-Furlong (JRI Instrumentation)	Singh (2004)	Titanium, smooth surface, collared, fully coated HA, cylindrical	42	10 years (5-14)	100%	None	None	100% at 12 years
ABG (Stryker Howmedica Osteonics)	Herrera (2004)	Titanium, roughened proximal one third, anatomic, collarless, proximal HA, tapered	65	8.5 years (7-10)	98.7%	None	17.7%	98.7% at 8.5 years
Omnifit (Stryker Howmedica Osteonics)	Capello (2003)	Chromium-cobalt, proximal one third porous-coated, collarless, proximally coated HA, two-dimensional tapered	39	11 years (10-14)	99.1%	None	3%	98.9% at 14 years
IPS (Johnson & Johnson/DePuy)	Kim (2003)	Titanium, proximal one third porous-coated, collarless, proximal one third HA, anatomic tapered	45.3	6.6 years (5-7)	100%	None	4%	100% at 6.6 years

NR = not reported; HA = hydroxyapatite

important transition point in the development of more successful second-generation stems. Early short-term reports demonstrated high rates of aseptic loosening (9% to 25%) and distal endosteal osteolysis (up to 60%).

In one study of the HGP-I stem, the rate of survival at 15 years for the femoral component was 86.8% free of revision and 82.0% free of mechanical failure. In another study at 13 years, survival rate was 76.3%, and in a third study, after 10 years, 25% of the stems were revised or loose. Femoral osteolysis ranged from 25.8% to 52%.

The Anatomic Porous Replacement system (APR-I) (Intermedics Orthopaedics, Austin, TX) femoral component was another first-generation proximal patch-porous–coated stem. The femoral component had an anatomic shape with a proximal rectangular double wedge. One study reported a revision rate of 16% with a mechanical failure rate of 11% at an average of 6.7 years. Seventy percent of hips had progressive loss of fixation. Loss of femoral component fixation was correlated with younger patient age, higher patient activity level, metaphyseal fill of less than 90%, and increased polyethylene wear and osteolysis.

The HGP-I and APR-I results demonstrated early failure caused by instability and intermediate and late failure because of progressive osteolysis. The smooth surfaces between the patch porous coatings served as channels for particulate debris migration and resultant high levels of distal endosteal osteolysis. Proximal patch coating has been replaced by circumferential coatings in the more successful second-generation stems that aim to create a seal of the proximal femur. Stems that use circumferential proximal porous coating are rarely associated with distal endosteal osteolysis. Second-generation stems are available in a multitude of sizes, as well as varying combinations of metaphyseal and diaphyseal sizing. The result is a greater ability to achieve critically important initial implant stability, eliminate micromotion, and create an environment that is amenable to bony ingrowth/ongrowth. Midterm results with second-generation stems indicate a high rate of radiographic stability (Tables 4 and 5).

The PCA stem was a first-generation circumferentially proximally coated collarless implant released in the early 1980s. Reported long-term survival rates of the stem range from 90.7% to 96.8% at follow-up of 12.4 to 17 years. For these early designs, thigh pain occurred in 9% to 26% of patients and osteolysis, often seen with stem loosening, in 0 to 19% of patients (Table 5). The excellent survival with this first-generation stem is comparable to that of many second-generation stems (Tables 4 and 5).

The Harris-Galante Multilock (Zimmer) experience clearly illustrates the improved fixation and the elimination of distal osteolysis achievable with second-generation stems. This cylindrical, collared titanium implant shared a similar geometry to the HGP-I, but with improved sizing and a circumferential, proximal one third, fiber metal ingrowth surface. Midterm results demonstrated a 10-year survivorship of 97% and no detected distal osteolysis (Table 5).

A large variety of cementless proximally porous-coated implants currently are available. The vast number of implant design variables and study parameters makes meaningful comparison difficult. What is certain

is that second-generation proximally coated implants enjoy universally good survivorship at midterm and long-term follow-up. The problem of distal femoral osteolysis has been eliminated by the use of circumferentially proximally coated implants. Thigh pain, which is attributed to instability and a rigid distal stem, continues to be a source of concern, with rates ranging from 0 to 36%. Although there is little agreement as to what implant design best reduces thigh pain, better initial stability and the use of more biocompatible titanium implants has decreased its incidence.

Results of Ceramic Coated Stems

Midterm (10- to 11-year) results are available for cementless stems with calcium phosphate ceramic coatings such as hydroxyapatite and calcium triphosphate (Table 6). These bioactive, osteoconductive coatings are applied to either roughened or porous-coated surfaces because the ceramic coating itself is not a substitute for initial stability. For stems with sufficient ongrowth or ingrowth capability and a ceramic coating, the outcomes have been excellent, with survivorships of more than 98% reported after 10 years for both roughened and porous designs (Table 6).

Several studies have compared hydroxyapatite-coated stems with identical noncoated stems. In one recent prospective, randomized study with a mean follow-up of 6.6 years, the clinical and radiographic results of a proximal one third porous-coated femoral prosthesis (IPS, DePuy) with identical geometries, differing only with regard to the presence or absence of hydroxyapatite coating, were similar. Other comparative reports have demonstrated similar findings with both roughened and porous stems, suggesting that the addition of osteoconductive coatings to a stem with sufficient capacity for ongrowth or ingrowth may not be necessary to achieve a sufficient volume of osseous fixation for clinically satisfactory and durable results.

Some concerns remain, however, with the long-term outcomes of hydroxyapatite coatings on femoral prostheses, such as occlusion of the underlying ongrowth or ingrowth surface, coating resorption and delamination causing formation of additional particulate debris with resultant premature wear and osteolysis, formation of heterotopic bone around the hip joint, and accelerated proximal femoral bone loss. Although the survival of the ABG stem (Stryker Howmedica Osteonics) was 98.7% after a mean follow-up of 8.5 years, one study of more than 230 patients reported a 55% rate of proximal femoral stress shielding, a 62% rate of substantial polyethylene wear, a 17% rate of femoral and periacetabular osteolytic lesions, and a high rate of heterotopic ossification (81% of patients with Brooker grade 0 or 1 and 6.5% with grade 3) (Table 7). Further long-term assessment will be required to confirm that the excellent midterm results of coated femoral stems are maintained.

Table 7 | Long-Term Results of Early First-Generation Hemispherical Cups With Line-To-Line Reaming and Screw Fixation

Cup	Author (Year)	Design	Head Size	No. of Hips	Patient Age (Years) (Range)	Follow-Up (Range)	Definite Loosening	Periacetabular Osteolysis	Shell Survivorship
HGP-I (Zimmer)	Della Valle (2004)	Titanium mesh, modular, locking tines, 5.1-mm screws	28 mm	142	52 (20-84)	16.3 years (15-18)	3%	25%	99%
PCA (Stryker Howmedica Osteonics)	Callaghan (2004)	Chromium-cobalt, Beads, two peripheral lugs, monoblock	32 mm	100	58 (22-81)	Minimum 15 years	21%	29.6%	83%
HGP-1 (Zimmer)	Callaghan (2004)	Titanium mesh, modular, locking tines, 5.1-mm screws	28 mm	120	62 (26-86)	Minimum 13 years	0	7.1%	97.5%
PCA (Stryker Howmedica Osteonics)	Moskal (2004)	Chromium-cobalt, Beads, two peripheral lugs, monoblock	32 mm	107	69 (27-95)	12.4 years (11-13)	0	7.5%	87.7%
HGP-I (Zimmer)	Duffy (2004)	Titanium mesh, modular, locking tines, 5.1-mm screws	22-32 mm	84	38 (16-50)	Median 10 years	0	9.5%	97.3%

Development of Porous-Coated Acetabular Components

One of the most important advances in THA has been the development of cementless acetabular components. Cemented acetabular components were the main mode of fixation for approximately 20 years, beginning with the development of the low-friction arthroplasty by Charnley. Initial clinical results were excellent for 10 years, but after the first decade, cemented sockets demonstrated increasing rates of radiographic loosening and revision, despite attempts to improve cementing technique. Although some cementless designs have failed, cementless hemispheric cups with a porous exterior surface have been adopted widely, fixed either by press-fit or with screws.

First-generation cementless designs, such as the Acetabular Reconstruction Component (ARC, Howmedica), the PCA, and the HGP-I, reproducibly achieved stable initial fixation to bone but were associated with unacceptable rates of pelvic osteolysis and increasing rates of mechanical failure for the ARC and PCA cups. First-generation design locking mechanisms often allowed micromotion between the liner and the shell, with a resultant increase in the generation of wear debris through backside wear. Early locking mechanisms were not designed with sufficient mechanical properties to withstand the forces generated about the hip with long-term use, resulting in fatigue failure, breakage of the tines for the HGP-I cup, and reports of liner dissociation. Lack of conformity between the liner and shell, along with a rough inner surface of the shell, also contributed to increased generation of backside wear debris (as in the Acetabular Cup System [DePuy]).

Early implantation techniques with line-to-line fit did not maximize the initial stability of the shell. Multiple screw holes in some cups, such as the HGP-I, permitted wear debris to gain access to the pelvis with resultant balloon-type periprosthetic osteolysis. Concerns with fixation via screws through the cup included fretting at the screw-cup junction, screw penetration into the back of the liner, and screw breakage because of undersized screws. Finally, in certain instances, suboptimal sintering of the ingrowth surface contributed to shedding of beads or the porous surface and accelerated third-body wear.

Recognition and increased understanding of these problems and modes of failure led to the development of second-generation cups. Manufacturing processes improved and complication rates were reduced by the development of shells with a limited number of holes (or no holes), improved locking mechanisms, a polished inner surface of the shell, and increased conformity of the liner and shell. Other advancements included the addition of osteoconductive coatings such as hydroxyapatite and tricalcium phosphate. New metals such as porous tantalum were introduced to enhance fixation, especially in the difficult revision situation, and may decrease periacetabular stress shielding from the shell.

Currently, the greatest difficulty with modern cementless cups is wear and periprosthetic osteolysis. It is clear that wear, ingrowth, and osteolysis are all interrelated. It has not yet been determined which combination of design and fixation method achieves the best compromise to maximize the long-term outcomes of hemispherical press-fit cups.

Results of Porous-Coated Acetabular Components

Long-term clinical outcomes of porous-coated cementless acetabular components are available now with more than 15 years of follow-up. One of the most studied designs is the first generation HGP-I cup. This component, introduced in 1984, has a hemispheric tivanium (titanium-aluminum-vanadium) metal shell with a titanium fiber mesh coating, multiple screw holes, and a modular liner that is held in place with multiple pairs of titanium tines along the shell rim. Initially, most HGP-I cups were implanted with line-to-line reaming and screw fixation using two to three titanium 5.1-mm screws.

For the first-generation HGP-I cup, reported survival rates of the shell at 10- to 16-year follow-up range from 97% to 99% for aseptic or radiographic loosening, with conventional polyethylene sterilized by gamma irradiation in air and various head sizes (22 to 32 mm) (Table 7). Survival for any reason, including exchange of the polyethylene liner, decreases the survival rate to 88% to 93%. Periacetabular osteolysis has been reported in 7% to 25% of patients, with an increasing incidence as patients are followed for longer terms. Definite radiographic loosening or loosening at revision surgery ranged from 0 to 3%.

The PCA is another first-generation design with long-term follow-up. In contrast to the HGP-I cup, this cup has had higher reported failure rates that are affected by multiple factors, including the routine use of 32-mm femoral heads with increased volumetric wear and relatively thin polyethylene liners that are heat-pressed to polish the outer surface. The PCA acetabular component was a chromium-cobalt shell with a porous surface of sintered chromium-cobalt beads. Two peripheral lugs were used for additional fixation, which frequently led to final alignment of the shell in increased abduction. The liner had low conformity with the shell, and at the outer rim of the metal shell, the liner undergoes a sharp decrease in thickness. This led to increased wear, rim fractures of conventional polyethylene, and inferior outcomes for this design.

Recent reports on survival of the PCA shell for aseptic or radiographic loosening range from 83% to 87% at 12- to 15-year follow-up, with conventional polyethylene sterilized by gamma irradiation in air and 32-mm femoral head sizes (Table 7). Periacetabular osteolysis has been reported in 7% to 29% of patients. The rate of definite radiographic loosening or loosening at revision surgery has been reported to be as high as 21%.

In a study of retrieved PCA acetabular components, all cups had substantial evidence of backside and articular surface wear of the polyethylene. All but one of the retrieved acetabular failures in this series occurred in cups with diameters smaller than 55 mm. The smaller diameter shells used in conjunction with 32-mm femoral heads resulted in the use of thin polyethylene liners, especially at the rim of the shell, where the liner dramatically thins to approximately 2 mm for 46-mm cups and to 3 mm for 55-mm cups. It has been shown that conventional polyethylene thickness should not be less than 6 to 8 mm.

Intermediate follow-up is now available for second-generation acetabular component designs. The second generation Harris-Galante Porous II (HGP-II, Zimmer) socket was introduced in 1988 with several design modifications, including a locking mechanism with an increased number of tines, increased thickness of the shell, and larger 6.5-mm cancellous bone screws.

The results of the second-generation HGP-II cups generally have been inferior to the previous HGP-I model because the updated design was manufactured with an increased shell thickness that resulted in thinner polyethylene liners and led to increased failures. Recent reports with intermediate follow-up after 10 years have demonstrated survivorships of the shell ranging from 88% to 96%, with conventional polyethylene sterilized by gamma irradiation in air and 28-mm femoral head sizes.

A major issue with both HGP-I and HGP-II cup designs was locking mechanism failure and liner dislodgement. A recent study reported a 2.6% incidence of liner dislodgement over a 4-year period with the HGP-II cup. Another report found up to 20% of the revisions of HGP cups were caused by locking mechanism failure resulting from fatigue failure of the locking tines. In a series assessing both HGP-I and HGP-II cups, of 18 locking mechanism failures, 17 occurred with the second-generation design. The average time of locking mechanism failure was 7 years, and all shells remained well fixed.

In a long-term study with 15 years of follow-up from a single institution, the outcomes of 4,289 primary THAs with multiple first- and second-generation hemispherical porous-coated cementless cups were documented. Overall, 203 cups (4.7%) were revised. Of these, 139 (3.2%) were exchanged with a modular polyethylene liner, and 64 (1.5%) were revisions of the shell. Only 18 of the 64 revised shells were loose (0.2%) at the time of surgery. The 15-year survivorship for aseptic loosening was 94.7% for the spiked cups, 98.4% for press-fit cups with screws, and 100% for press-fit cups without additional screws. Using revision for any reason as an end point, the 15-year survivorship was 82.9% for the spiked cups, 71.6% for press-fit cups with screws, and 72% for press-fit components. There were no statistical differences among the cup designs. Cumulatively, survivorship in the first 7 years declined at a rate of 0.5%, whereas between 7 and 15 years, survivorship declined at a rate of about 2% per year. Overall, loosening of the cup remained low at long-term follow-up despite an increasing incidence of osteolysis.

Several other second-generation cementless acetabular designs are now available that use a hemispheric geometry and provide supplemental fixation with either screws or other augmentation methods (Table 8). Many of these designs have had excellent midterm outcomes.

Table 8 | Second-Generation Results of Hemispherical Cups

Cup	Author (Year)	Design	Head Size	No. of Hips	Age (Years) (Range)	Follow-Up (Years) (Range)	Fixation	Definite Loosening	Peri-acetabular Osteolysis	Shell Survivor-ship
Multiple Types	Engh (2004)	Multiple types	NR	4,289	61 (16-92)	2-15	Line-to-line and 1 mm PF	0.3%	0.6%	> 90% for all designs
APR (Sulzer)	Udomkiat (2002)	Titanium alloy, cancellous structured Titanium coating	26-32 mm	110	61 (23-86)	10.2 (7-11.9)	1-3 mm PF	0.9%	3.6%	99.1%
Duraloc (J&J DePuy)	Kim (2003)	Porocoat titanium beads	22 mm	118	46 (21-49)	9.8 (8-11)	2 mm PF	0	9%	99%
HG-II (Zimmer)	Archibeck (2001)	Titanium mesh Locking tines	28 mm	92	52 (32-69)	10 (8-11)	Line-to-line	2%	16%	96.4%
Mallory Head (Biomet)	Jiranek (2004)	Titanium alloy, rim fins, titanium alloy heads	28-32 mm (titanium alloy head)	67	57 (23-80)	10.4 (9-12.5)	1 mm PF	18%	30%	72%
Zweymuller CSF (Sulzer)	Grubl (2002)	Titanium alloy Threaded	28-32 mm	208	61 (22-84)	10	Line-to-line	0	0	93%
Trilogy (Zimmer)	Gonzalez Della Valle (2004)	Titanium mesh, modular, locking ring, 6.2 mm screws	22-32 mm	308	64 (23-86)	4-7	2 mm PF	0.4%	5%	98%

NR = not reported. PF = press fit

For the Duraloc (DePuy) cup, survivorships at a mean 5- to 9.8-year follow-up have ranged from 98% to 100% with head sizes of 22 to 28 mm and polyethylene liners sterilized by gamma irradiation in both air and vacuum. Enhanced highly crystalline polyethylene (Hylamer, DePuy) had reported wear rates of 5 times the rate of conventional (Enduron, DePuy) liners sterilized by gamma irradiation in air with increasing shelf storage time. Periacetabular osteolysis has ranged from 9% to 41% in recent studies. Osteolysis occurred much more frequently in patients with greater than or equal to 0.2 mm/yr of linear wear, confirming the need for closer monitoring of patients with higher rates of wear. For Duraloc cups placed before 1995, reports have revealed an incidence of up to 3.5% of advancement or complete separation of the apex hole eliminator, which is best visualized on iliac oblique radiographs. The hole eliminator was redesigned in 1995 to prevent this complication.

The APR cup is a hemispheric titanium alloy shell with a porous coating of cancellous structured titanium. A report on cups that were press-fit by 1 to 3 mm without the use of supplementary screws, polyethylene liners sterilized by gamma irradiation in air, and with femoral head sizes of 26 mm to 32 mm demonstrated a 12-year

survival rate of 99.1% for aseptic loosening, 95.3% for revision for any reason, and 79.6% for polyethylene liner exchange as the end point. Overall, 30 of 110 hips had a polyethylene liner exchange, including 4 that had a liner dissociation. Wear was observed to be highest with cup abduction angles greater than 50°.

Overall, the literature indicates that revision for aseptic loosening of a hemispheric porous-coated cup is a rare complication. The rate of cup loosening remains low at long-term follow-up despite an increasing incidence of osteolysis. Ongoing research will help to better quantify the size, location, and progression of these generally asymptomatic osteolytic lesions and to define those lesions that jeopardize cup stability to guide the need for surgical intervention.

Results of Ceramic Coated Cups
Intermediate term results are available for cups coated with osteoconductive ceramics. Overall, hydroxyapatite-coated grit-blasted cups that lack a porous coating have performed suboptimally. One grit blasted hydroxyapatite-coated cup (Kyocera, Kyoto, Japan) had a 14-year survivorship of 62% for radiologic evidence of acetabular loosening and a rate of stable fixation with

Table 9 | Midterm Results of Proximally Porous-Coated Stems With HA (HA-Coated Cups)

Cup	Author (Year)	Design	Head Size	No. of Hips	Age (Years)	Follow-Up	Fixation	Definite Loosening	Peri-acetabular Osteolysis	Shell Survivor-ship
Landos Corail (Landos Corail)	Reikeras (2002)	Grit-blasted smooth titanium, HA plasma spray	28 mm	191	47	7 to 10 years	1-2 mm PF	20.4%	1%	79.5%
Kyocera (Kyocera)	Miyakawa (2004)	Grit-blasted smooth titanium, HA flame spray	22 mm	35	61	12.6 years	Line-to-line	31%	27%	62.3%
Reflection (Smith and Nephew)	Rohrl (2004)	Porous titanium, HA plasma spray	28 mm	22	59	5 years	1-2 mm PF	0	9%	100%
ABG (Stryker Howmedica Osteonics)	Herrera (2004)	Porous titanium, HA plasma spray	28 mm	312	65	8.5 years	Line-to-line	1.3%	NR	96.8%
JRI-Furlong (JRI Instrumentation)	Robertson (2005)	Threaded titanium, HA plasma spray	28 mm	68	48	8.8 years	Line-to-line	0	NR	98%

NR = not reported; HA = hydroxyapatite

bony ongrowth of only 46%. Another study of a smooth hydroxyapatite-coated cup (Landos Corail, Landanger, Chaumont, France) had a 20.4% mechanical loosening rate at 7- to 10-year follow-up.

In contrast, cups with a fully porous-coated surface and a ceramic coating have performed well, with survivorships of 96% to 100% at short- to intermediate-term follow-up (Table 9). Few studies have demonstrated that hydroxyapatite-coated cups have a clear clinical superiority over nonceramic coated hemispheric cups with a porous coating. With reports of aseptic loosening of 0 to 2% for hemispheric porous-coated shells, an improvement in initial stability with the use of hydroxyapatite coating may be unnecessary for the uncomplicated primary THA. One randomized prospective study with a 5-year follow-up compared different methods of fixation and found no difference among cups inserted with a press-fit technique, press-fit augmented with screws or pegs, and press-fit with hydroxyapatite coating. The only statistical difference after 5 years was fewer radiolucent lines for the hydroxyapatite-coated cups. Longer-term follow-up and further study is needed to demonstrate whether the potential benefits of an hydroxyapatite-coated interface, such as improvements in sealing effect, bone-implant contact, gap healing, and better tolerance to instability, will be clinically significant.

The goal for the future is to improve long-term acetabular fixation and to reduce the incidence of osteolysis. This may be achieved by a variety of methods, such as decreasing wear debris through improved bearing surfaces (such as improved cross-linked polyethylenes,

ceramics, and metal-on-metal articulations), inhibiting bone resorption (with bisphosphonate therapy), or improving bone ingrowth into the cup with new materials (such as porous tantalum) or growth factors (such as osteogenic protein-1, transforming growth factor-β, and bone morphogenetic protein-2).

In primary THA, the choice of fixation with modern implants depends greatly on the surgeon's philosophical outlook on design. There are a large number of acceptable cementless femoral component designs that have shown excellent intermediate- and long-term results. Most modern implants develop a proximal ingrowth seal to inhibit the distal migration of particulate debris, as demonstrated by the development and success of circumferentially proximally porous-coated implants. Unresolved questions regarding the optimal porous coating, stem geometry, stem stiffness, and material composition continue to be studied.

For the bearing surface, investigations on wear and oxidation resistance are ongoing. The use of alternative couplings continues, including ceramic-on-polyethylene and hard-on-hard bearing surfaces. Research also continues into innovative coatings such as diamond and oxidized zirconium. The use of first-generation highly cross-linked polyethylenes of various manufacturing techniques is in the early stages of clinical evaluation. Currently, second-generation highly cross-linked polyethylenes are in development or ready for release, including those that use cross-linking by chemical means and compressive techniques.

For the acetabular component, the choice is relatively straightforward. Although cemented cups have shown good longevity at intermediate- and long-term follow-up, most surgeons are now using a cementless porous-coated hemispheric modular shell with a polyethylene liner, which may incorporate different offset, extended lips, and other features to maximize the stability of the hip. Current controversies regarding fixation techniques with the socket continue, such as the degree of press fit, use of adjuvant screws, and the use of enhanced ingrowth surfaces such as porous tantalum and surface coatings such as hydroxyapatite/calcium phosphate. Other areas of continued concern include the cup locking mechanism and backside wear.

Overall, for primary cementless THA, the most concerning and prevalent issue is particulate wear debris around the effective joint space and osteolysis. The consensus is that continued close observation of the patient is mandatory to evaluate the performance of these implants in the long term. Despite the concern with osteolysis and the problems with first-generation designs, the evidence supports the use of modern cementless components in primary THA.

Cemented Primary Total Hip Arthroplasty

Cemented THA was introduced in Europe in the early 1960s and in the United States in the late 1960s and early 1970s. The functional results have now been reported for younger patients (younger than 50 years) who have had 25 years of service from their hip implants. The functional outcome of patients was excellent with Medical Outcomes Study Short Form 36-Item survey scores that were comparable with normative values of healthy age-matched subjects. The 6-minute walk distance and Western Ontario and McMaster Universities Osteoarthritis Index scores were slightly lower than healthy normatives, but were thought to be influenced by the medical comorbidities. Although comorbid medical and musculoskeletal conditions significantly hindered most measures of function, revision surgery or radiographic loosening of components had no significant influence on function. The mortality rates of this cohort of patients were similar to normative values at both 10 and 25 years after surgery. These findings corroborate those of other studies regarding the need to consider comorbidities when assessing long-term function.

Long-Term Outcomes

Long-term follow-up reports of THA with Charnley flatback polished prosthesis have now been published. In a minimum 30-year follow-up, 7% of acetabular components and 3% of femoral components were revised, and the total radiographic loosening prevalence (including revisions) was 16% on the acetabular side and 8% on the femoral side. For patients living 30 years after

undergoing THA, the revision prevalence was 26% on the acetabular side and 10% on the femoral side. Using the same prosthesis in patients younger than 50 years the radiographic loosening prevalence was 34% on the acetabular side and 13% on the femoral side at minimum 25-year follow-up. Acetabular revision prevalence was twice that of older patients undergoing THA (14%). In a study of the original Charnley prosthesis in patients younger than 30 years (most of whom had rheumatoid arthritis), the 25-year acetabular component survivorship was 68% and the femoral component survivorship was 73%. There are no long-term follow-up studies of cemented or cementless THA in patients younger than 20 or 30 years in which patients with rheumatoid arthritis are excluded. In all long-term studies, patients with rheumatoid arthritis have performed better than patients with osteoarthritis presumably because of their lower activity level.

The relatively high failure rate of cemented acetabular components, especially when compared with cemented femoral components, has led most surgeons in the United States to abandon this form of acetabular fixation. However, some surgeons continue to perform the procedure based on issues of increasing wear and osteolysis reported with cementless acetabular components. The procedure is typically recommended for patients older than 60 years. Hypotensive epidural anesthesia allows for a dry surgical field. Requirements for optimal results include a dry cancellous bone bed, perforation and removal of peripheral sclerotic areas, pressurization of the entire cement mantle, and complete capture of the acetabular component by the acetabulum. These recommendations are based on a decrease in cemented acetabular component survival rates in studies in which zone 1 (superolateral) radiolucencies were present on initial postoperative radiographs. Under these conditions, acetabular component survival rates of 99% have been reported at 15-year follow-up. In one long-term study (with an average follow-up of 9 years) of patients older than 75 years at the time of surgery, no revisions for loosening were reported in patients with a cemented all-polyethylene acetabular component.

Over the past several years, the greatest controversies concerning cemented femoral components have been concerning which patient is the more optimal candidate for a cemented versus a cementless femoral component and which design and surface finish is optimal for the cemented femoral construct. As previously stated, there are data to support the use of cemented femoral fixation in elderly and younger patients, but no substantial data are available to support the use of cemented femoral fixation in patients younger than 20 or 30 years who do not have rheumatoid arthritis. Some studies report inferior results with cemented femoral fixation in younger patients with osteonecrosis. Although these findings may only be related to patient age, they may also be related to poor bone quality in this patient population. Recent mechanical studies have suggested that an increase in cement stresses occurs when higher offset is used and in heavier patients. Although there are no substantial data to support it, many surgeons now recommend cemented femoral fixation only for older, lighter, less active patients with less optimal bone quality.

Cemented femoral design has evolved into two basic positions. One position is to use a component that optimally resists torsion, is made of a stiff material (such as chromium-cobalt or stainless steel), and incorporates a collar. Multiple studies have demonstrated that cemented stems made of a less stiff material (titanium) have inferior results when compared with chromium-cobalt stems. This design philosophy should decrease stresses in the cement. The second position is to use a collarless, tapered component that allows for microsubsidence and places all cement stresses in compression. There is consensus that this second position is optimized by the use of a stem with a polished surface finish. For torsionally stable components, both relatively smooth (5- to 50-microinch roughness arithmetic average [Ra] and relatively rough (50- to 250-microinch Ra) surface finishes have been used. A component with a rough surface finish provides better adherence of the cement to the prosthesis and thus decreases cement stresses. However, if the component loosens within the cement mantle, there is greater abrasion and cement particle generation. A component with a smooth surface finish does not adhere well to cement, so there is potential for an increase in cement stresses. However, if the component loosens, abrasion of the cement is minimized. Three independent studies of rough surface (80-microinch Ra) femoral components with relatively high offsets that were precoated with methylmethacrylate had failure rates approaching 10% at 5- to 10-year follow-up. Osteolysis occurred rapidly around most of these cement mantles. However, there are at least two prospective randomized studies demonstrating no differences in loosening rates between identical femoral stems with smooth versus rough surface finish at an average 4.8-year and a minimum 5-year follow-up in relatively older patients. There is one other prospective randomized study of newer cobra-shaped, matte-finished Charnley and a rougher surface Spectron (Smith & Nephew) prosthesis that showed higher failure rates with the Charnley prosthesis. A recent prospective randomized report of a collared versus collarless torsionally stable, low-offset, matte-finish, HDII cemented stem (Hypertension Diagnostics, Eagen, MN) showed no differences in loosening at an average 9.6-year follow-up.

Although there are no recent reports of the original Exeter double-tapered collarless polished cemented stem, there is a recent 7-year follow-up report of a polished collarless triple-tapered stem. At a 3.5-year aver-

age follow-up, 0 of 500 stems were revised for femoral loosening.

Other findings concerning cemented femoral fixation include a joint registry study finding that infection rates have been reduced by using antibiotic-impregnated cement, that cement porosity is reduced by heating the femoral stem, and that optimizing cement mantles (2 to 3 mm circumferentially if the canal geometry allows), especially when rough surface femoral stems are used, has reduced mechanical failure. In addition, broach only versus reaming and broaching of the canal prior to inserting cement has been reported to provide better interdigitation of the cement into bone.

Annotated Bibliography

Cementless Primary Total Hip Arthroplasty

Archibeck MJ, Berger RA, Jacobs JJ, et al: Second-generation cementless total hip arthroplasty: Eight to eleven-year results. *J Bone Joint Surg Am* 2001;83-A(11):1666-1673.

In this study, 78 primary THAs in 74 patients from a consecutive series were evaluated; patients received the cementless, anatomically designed, circumferential proximal porous-coated hip component and a cementless hemispheric porous-coated acetabular component. The patients were followed for a mean of 10 years (range, 8 to 11 years). The mean age at the time of the arthroplasty was 52 years. The mean preoperative Harris Hip Score of 51 points improved to 94 points at the time of final follow-up; 86% of the hips had a good or excellent result.

Bojescul JA, Xenos JS, Callaghan JJ, Savory CG: Results of porous-coated anatomic total hip arthroplasty without cement at fifteen years: A concise follow-up of a previous report. *J Bone Joint Surg Am* 2003;85-A(6):1079-1083.

This study updates the results of a prospective series of primary cementless THAs at an average 15.6-year follow-up (range, 15 to 17 years). One hundred consecutive THAs were performed using the PCA system; 55 patients (64 hips) were alive at 15-year follow-up. The authors reported that 17% of the entire cohort (17 hips) and 23% of the living cohort (15 hips) had undergone revision because of loosening of the acetabular component or osteolysis. Seven percent of the entire cohort (7 hips) and 6% of the living cohort (4 hips) had undergone revision for loosening of the femoral component or osteolysis. Only 4 femoral stems had been revised for isolated loosening (without osteolysis).

Callaghan JJ, Savory CG, O'Rourke MR, Johnston RC: Are all cementless acetabular components created equal? *J Arthroplasty* 2004;19(4, suppl 1)95-98.

The authors of this study evaluated 15-year follow-up results of two cementless acetabular components (the HG-I and the PCA) in terms of revision and radiographic evidence of loosening. Three of 120 HG-I acetabular components were revised for wear and osteolysis without loosening. Seventeen of 100 PCA components were revised for aseptic loosening (with or without osteolysis). Including revisions, 21 PCA acetabular components had radiographic evidence of loosening, and no HG-I components had radiographic evidence of loosening.

Capello WN, D'Antonio JA, Feinberg JR, Manley MT: Ten-year results with hydroxyapatite-coated total hip femoral components in patients less than fifty years old: A concise follow-up of a previous report. *J Bone Joint Surg Am* 2003;85-A(5):885-889.

The authors reported the results of a proximally HA-coated femoral component at a minimum follow-up of 10 years in a group of patients who were younger than 50 years at the time of the primary procedure. In the 5 years since the publication of the preliminary results of this study, two additional stems have undergone revision. Therefore, a total of six stems have been revised. A small amount of erosive scalloping of the proximal part of the femur was seen in approximately one half of the hips; however, all unrevised stems were radiographically stable and no hip had intramedullary osteolysis. The revision rate because of aseptic loosening of the stem was 0.9%, which compares favorably with that for other stems and other fixation methods in young patients.

Claus AM, Hopper RH Jr, Engh CA: Fractures of the greater trochanter induced by osteolysis with the anatomic medullary locking prosthesis. *J Arthroplasty* 2002; 17(6):706-712.

In this study of 208 consecutive THAs with mean 12.2-year radiographic follow-up, the authors reviewed the incidence, presentation, treatment, and outcome of fractures of the greater trochanter. They reported that 9 fractures of the greater trochanter were induced by osteolysis at a mean follow-up of 129 months. Five of these fractures were diagnosed at the time of their radiographic appearance. Four were treated without surgical fixation (crutches and limited weight bearing for 4 to 6 weeks). Seven fractures healed in situ without major displacement. The authors concluded that the risk of fracture was independent of the size of the osteolytic lesion; however, the risk increased significantly when the lysis eroded the cortical bone of the greater trochanter.

Crowther JD, Lachiewicz PF: Survival and polyethylene wear of porous-coated acetabular components in patients less than fifty years old: Results at nine to fourteen years. *J Bone Joint Surg Am* 2002;84-A(5):729-735.

In this study, 71 primary THAs were performed in 56 patients who were younger than 50 years; the HG-I porous-coated acetabular component was placed in all patients with a line-to-line fit and fixed with a mean of four screws. The authors reported that 56 of the 71 hips were available for radiographic and clinical analysis at a mean follow-up of 11 years (range, 9 to 14 years). No metal shell was revised because of aseptic loosening, and no shell was loose at the time of the latest follow-up. A nonprogressive radiolucent line was seen in one zone in 10 hips (18%) and in two zones in 6 hips (11%).

No hip had a radiolucent line in all three zones. Pelvic osteolysis was noted in 13 hips (23%); the osteolysis was observed in the ischium in 11 hips and around the screws in 2 hips. Survivorship analysis revealed that the probability of survival of the metal shell was 98% at 10 years.

Duffy GP, Prpa B, Rowland CM, Berry DJ: Primary uncemented Harris-Galante acetabular components in patients 50 years old or younger: Results at 10 to 12 years. *Clin Orthop* 2004;427:157-161.

In this study, 73 patients (84 hips) who were 50 years or younger were treated with primary THA using the HGP-I cementless acetabular component. At a median follow-up of 10 years, seven acetabular metal shell revisions were reported (5 because of osteolysis, one because of aseptic loosening, and one because of dislocation). Ten polyethylene exchanges without metal acetabular shell removal were performed. None of the unrevised acetabular components had radiographic evidence of loosening, but eight had pelvic osteolysis. The 10-year survival rate without revision of the acetabular metal shell was 87.9%. The 10-year survival rate without revision for aseptic acetabular component loosening was 97.3%.

Dumbleton J, Manley MT: Hydroxyapatite-coated prostheses in total hip and knee arthroplasty. *J Bone Joint Surg Am* 2004;86-A(11):2526-2540.

At 15-year follow-up after THA, the authors reported that hydroxyapatite-coated femoral stems perform as well as, and possibly better than, other types of cementless devices, with the added benefit of providing a seal against wear debris.

Engh CA, Hopper RH Jr, Engh CA Jr: Long-term porous-coated cup survivorship using spikes, screws, and press-fitting for initial fixation. *J Arthroplasty* 2004;19 (7 suppl 2)54-60.

This study examined the long-term outcomes of a single institution's experience with 4,289 primary THAs using hemispheric porous-coated cups. Of 203 revised hips, only 18 cups were found to be loose at the time of revision. Using revision for any reason as an end point, 15-year survivorship was 82.9% ± 5.6% for spiked components, 71.6% ± 8.5% for press-fit cups with adjunctive rim screws, and 72.0% ± 12.6% for press-fit components. Using revision for aseptic loosening as an end point, 15-year survivorship was 94.7% ± 3.4% for spiked cups, 98.4% ± 1.9% for press-fit cups with screws, and 100% ± 0.1% for press-fit cups.

Epinette JA, Manley MT, D'Antonio JA, Edidin AA, Capello WN: A 10-year minimum follow-up of hydroxyapatite-coated threaded cups: Clinical, radiographic and survivorship analyses with comparison to the literature. *J Arthroplasty* 2003;18(2):140-148.

In this study, 418 threaded HA-coated acetabular cups (Arc2f, Osteonics, Allendale, NJ) implanted in a consecutive series of 384 patients undergoing primary THA were evaluated. In all patients, the cup was screwed into the prepared acetabulum. Bone screws were used to provide secondary fixation. At a minimum 10-year follow-up, 304 cups were available for analysis. The authors reported that the cumulative survivorship (with mechanical failure as end point) was 99.43%.

Gaffey JL, Callaghan JJ, Pedersen DR, Goetz DD, Sullivan PM, Johnston RC: Cementless acetabular fixation at fifteen years: A comparison with the same surgeon's results following acetabular fixation with cement. *J Bone Joint Surg Am* 2004;86-A(2):257-261.

In this study, 120 consecutive, nonselected primary THAs were performed in 108 patients with a HG-I cementless acetabular component and a cemented femoral component with a 28-mm head. At 13- to 15-year follow-up, 66 patients (72 hips) were living and 42 patients (48 hips) had died. No acetabular component had been revised because of aseptic loosening, and no acetabular component had migrated. With revision of the acetabular component for any reason as the end point, the survival rate was 81% ± 8% at 15-year follow-up. With revision of the acetabular component for clinical failure (osteolysis, wear, loosening, or dislocation) as the end point, the survival rate was 94% ± 8% at 15-year follow-up.

Grant P, Nordsletten L: Total hip arthroplasty with the Lord prosthesis: A long-term follow-up study. *J Bone Joint Surg Am* 2004;86-A(12):2636-2641.

The authors reported the results at a mean follow-up of 17.5 years (range, 15 to 20 years) with the Lord prosthesis (102 patients, 116 hips; mean patient age, 62 years). One femoral component was revised because of mechanical loosening, and one was revised because of a stem fracture. One stem appeared to be have radiographic evidence of loosening. Kaplan-Meier survivorship analysis with revision of the femoral component because of mechanical loosening, stem fracture, or radiographic evidence of loosening as the end point revealed a cumulative survival rate of 98% (with 28 hips at risk) at 17.5 years.

Grubl A, Chiari C, Gruber M, Kaider A, Gottsauner-Wolf F: Cementless total hip arthroplasty with a tapered, rectangular titanium stem and a threaded cup: A minimum ten-year follow-up. *J Bone Joint Surg Am* 2002;84-A(3):425-431.

In this study, 208 THAs were performed in 200 consecutive patients (average age, 61 years; range, 22 to 84 years); a tapered, rectangular titanium stem and a threaded cup without cement were used in all patients. At a median 120.7-month follow-up, there were 123 living patients who had not undergone revision. The probability of survival of both the femoral and the acetabular component at 10 years with any revision as the end point was 92%. The probability of survival was 93% for the cup and 99% for the stem.

Kim YH, Kim JS, Oh SH, Kim JM: Comparison of porous-coated titanium femoral stems with and without hydroxyapatite coating. *J Bone Joint Surg Am* 2003;85-A(9):1682-1688.

This prospective, randomized study evaluated the clinical and radiographic results associated with proximally porous-coated titanium stems that were identical in geometry but differed with regard to proximal surface treatment (with or without hydroxyapatite coating). Fifty patients (100 hips) had sequential bilateral primary THAs. A proximally porous-coated titanium stem with hydroxyapatite coating was implanted on one side and a proximally porous-coated titanium stem without hydroxyapatite coating was implanted on the other side during the same surgical setting in all 50 patients. A cementless acetabular component made of titanium was used in all hips. The mean age at the time of the surgery was 45.3 years. The mean duration of follow-up was 6.6 years. The Harris Hip Scores in the hydroxyapatite-coated group (mean, 94 points) and non–hydroxyapatite-coated group (mean, 92 points) were similar at the final follow-up examination. The prevalence of transient pain in the thigh was 4% in each group. No acetabular or femoral component demonstrated aseptic loosening.

Kim YH, Oh SH, Kim JS: Primary total hip arthroplasty with a second-generation cementless total hip prosthesis in patients younger than fifty years of age. *J Bone Joint Surg Am* 2003;85-A(1):109-114.

The authors performed a prospective study of primary THA in young patients (mean age, 46.8 years; range, 21 to 49 years) who had been followed for a minimum of 8 years with a second-generation cementless prosthesis. Eighty patients (118 hips) were included in the study. At an average follow-up of 9.8 years (range, 8 to 11 years), the average Harris Hip Score improved from 48.8 points preoperatively to 92 points at the final follow-up examination. The prevalence of transitory thigh pain was 10% (12 of 118 hips). There was no aseptic loosening. One hip was revised because of recurrent dislocation. The average amount of linear wear was 1.18 mm, and the average wear rate was 0.12 mm/yr. Fourteen hips (12%) had osteolysis in the calcar femorale, and 11 hips (9%) had acetabular osteolysis, but all of the osteolytic lesions were less than 1 cm.

Marshall AD, Mokris JG, Reitman RD, Dandar A, Mauerhan DR: Cementless titanium tapered-wedge femoral stem: 10- to 15-year follow-up. *J Arthroplasty* 2004;19(5):546-552.

The authors assessed the use of a titanium, biplanar tapered-wedge, collared femoral component with a circumferential proximal plasma-spray porous coating in 200 hips (186 patients). Nineteen patients died before the 10-year follow-up, and 50 patients were lost to follow-up. The mean follow-up of the remaining 129 hips was 11.6 years. Harris Hip Scores improved from 58 to 93. The incidence of thigh pain was 2.3%. Radiographic analysis revealed adaptive distal remodeling in zones 2, 3, 5, 6, and 13, with no evidence of osteolysis below the level of the calcar and the greater trochanteric region. Only two femoral stems were revised: one with suspected fibrous fixation at 7 years postoperatively and another with a broken trunion at 10 years postoperatively.

McAuley JP, Szuszczewicz ES, Young A, Engh CA Sr: Total hip arthroplasty in patients 50 years and younger. *Clin Orthop* 2004;418:119-125.

This study reviewed the long-term results of patients who were age 50 years and younger who had extensively porous-coated cobalt-chromium femoral components matched with various beaded, press-fit acetabular components of cobalt-chrome or titanium. During the past 20 years, 561 hip replacements were done on 488 patients in this age group. At 15-year follow-up, the survivorship of the stems was 96% for patients 50 years and younger and 94.7% for patients 40 years of younger. For the cups, at 15-year follow-up, the survival rate of the shells minus polyethylene liner exchanges was 86% and 60% when liner exchanges were included. The survival rates for femoral and acetabular components, using any revision as an end point (including liner exchanges), were 89% at 10-year follow-up and 60% at 15-year follow-up.

Meding JB, Keating EM, Ritter MA, Faris PM, Berend ME: Minimum ten-year follow-up of a straight-stemmed, plasma-sprayed, titanium-alloy, uncemented femoral component in primary total hip arthroplasty. *J Bone Joint Surg Am* 2004;86-A(1):92-97.

The study evaluated the 10-year results of primary THA performed with use of a proximally porous-coated, plasma-sprayed, straight-stemmed, titanium-alloy femoral component. A consecutive series of 105 total hip replacements in 95 patients was reviewed 10 to 12 years postoperatively. The average Harris Hip Score improved from 46 points preoperatively to 92 points postoperatively. The average pain score at the time of the most recent follow-up was 42 points, with 83 hips (79%) rated as pain-free. Thigh pain was identified in only two patients. All radiolucent lines were seen around the tip of the stem. All hips had some degree of femoral remodeling consistent with osseous ingrowth. No femoral component was revised, and no femoral component had evidence of loosening. The 12-year survival rate was 100%. Eight acetabular components were revised because of loosening and wear, and one was revised because of recurrent dislocation. One focal femoral osteolytic lesion was seen.

Nercessian OA, Wu WH, Sarkissian H: Clinical and radiographic results of cementless AML total hip arthroplasty in young patients. *J Arthroplasty* 2001;16(3):312-316.

This retrospective study assessed 52 cementless THAs in 52 patients (mean age, 48.3 years). The follow-up ranged from 9 to 12 years (mean, 10.5 years). The authors reported that 88% of patients had good or excellent results; 81% reported anterior thigh pain 3 months after surgery when weight bearing was allowed. The pain continued for a mean period of 4.3 months. In four patients (8%), this pain persisted after the first postoperative year. Calcar resorption was seen in 21 patients (40%), and 16 patients (31%) showed clinically insignificant heterotopic ossification. Four patients required revisions: one for acetabular loosening, one for persistent thigh pain, and two for massive osteolysis of the proximal femur. There were no dislocations, infections, thromboembolic events, or neurologic injuries.

Park MS, Choi BW, Kim SJ, Park JH: Plasma spray-coated Ti femoral component for cementless total hip arthroplasty. *J Arthroplasty* 2003;18(5):626-630.

This retrospective study of tapered, proximal plasma-spray coated titanium components included 67 patients (76 hips) with a mean age of 50.1 years. The mean follow-up was 10.1 years (range, 9 to 13 years). The authors reported excellent or good clinical results in 64 patients. Minimal thigh pain was found in 3 patients (4.4%). Seventy-one hips (93.4%) showed fixation by bony ingrowth, and 3 (3.9%) showed stable fibrous fixation. Bony ongrowth and ingrowth were also seen in 16 hips (21%) at distal smooth and grit-blast areas. Two femoral components were revised (survival rate, 97.3%), one for subsidence and other for recurrent infection.

Park YS, Lee JY, Yun SH, Jung MW, Oh I: Comparison of hydroxyapatite- and porous-coated stems in total hip replacement. *Acta Orthop Scand* 2003;74(3):259-263.

In this study, 24 patients underwent bilateral THA using a modular system; a porous-coated sleeve was used in one hip and an HA-coated sleeve was used in the other. Of the 20 patients who were followed for at least 4 years with clinical and radiographic evaluations, the authors found no difference between the two sides regarding the time of disappearance of thigh pain and hip scores. Radiographs showed a buttress sign in 18 HA-coated and 15 porous-coated stems.

Parvizi J, Keisu KS, Hozack WJ, Sharkey PF, Rothman RH: Primary total hip arthroplasty with an uncemented femoral component: A long-term study of the Taperloc stem. *J Arthroplasty* 2004;19(2):151-156.

This study evaluated the long-term result of a tapered, cementless femoral component in 121 patients (129 hips) who underwent primary THA. At an average follow-up of 11 years (range, 6 to 15 years), the mean Harris Hip Score was 92.1. The authors reported thigh pain in five patients (3.6%); one stem was revised at 6 years to treat severe proximal femoral osteolysis. No evidence of radiographic subsidence or loosening around any stems was noted.

Parvizi J, Sharkey PF, Hozack WJ, Orzoco F, Bissett GA, Rothman RH: Prospective matched-pair analysis of hydroxyapatite-coated and uncoated femoral stems in total hip arthroplasty: A concise follow-up of a previous report. *J Bone Joint Surg Am* 2004;86-A(4):783-786.

The authors of this prospective study reported that a mean clinical and radiographic follow-up of 9.8 years, all femoral components were stable with no evidence of progressive radiolucency or osteolysis and that 10 acetabular components were revised because of aseptic loosening and wear.

Parvizi J, Sullivan T, Duffy G, Cabanela ME: Fifteen-year clinical survivorship of Harris-Galante total hip arthroplasty. *J Arthroplasty* 2004;19(6):672-677.

The authors assessed the long-term outcome of cementless THA using HG-I components in 90 hips (80 patients; average age, 57.5 years). At a mean 14.9-year follow-up, hip scores improved significantly, and there was clinical and radiographic evidence of bony ingrowth on the acetabular components in all patients. The survivorship free of revision and free of mechanical failure for the acetabular component at 15 years was 95.7% and 91.9%, respectively. The survivorship at 15 years for the femoral component was 86.8% free of revision and 82.0% free of mechanical failure.

Radl R, Aigner C, Hungerford M, Pascher A, Windhager R: Proximal femoral bone loss and increased rate of fracture with a proximally hydroxyapatite-coated femoral component. *J Bone Joint Surg Br* 2000;82(8):1151-1155.

This study reviewed the outcomes of 118 patients (124 hips; mean patient age, 66.5 years; age range, 19 to 90 7years) who underwent THA with a cementless femoral component proximally coated with hydroxyapatite. The authors reported that at mean 5.6-year follow-up (range, 4.25 to 7.25 years) the mean Harris Hip score was 92 (range, 47.7 to 100).

Reikeras O, Gunderson RB: Failure of HA coating on a gritblasted acetabular cup: 155 patients followed for 7-10 years. *Acta Orthop Scand* 2002;73(1):104-108.

The authors assessed the 7- to 10-year outcome of 191 acetabular grit-blasted titanium cups with a hemispherical design for press-fit insertion and coated with hydroxyapatite and report that this particular design of hydroxyapatite-coated cups had a high rate of debonding and failure.

Singh S, Trikha SP, Edge AJ: Hydroxyapatite ceramic-coated femoral stems in young patients: A prospective ten-year study. *J Bone Joint Surg Br* 2004;86(8):1118-1123.

The authors of this study assessed the outcomes of 38 THAs with hydroxyapatite-ceramic coated femoral component in patients younger than 50 years (mean age, 42 years; age range, 22 to 49 years). At mean follow-up of 10 years (range, 63 to 170 months), mean Harris Hip Scores improved from 44 to 92 at the last follow-up. At 12-year follow-up, the cumulative survival for the stem was 100%. No femoral components were revised.

Sinha RK, Dungy DS, Yeon HB: Primary total hip arthroplasty with a proximally porous-coated femoral stem. *J Bone Joint Surg Am* 2004;86-A(6):1254-1261.

In this study of 123 second-generation circumferentially proximally porous-coated titanium-alloy femoral stems that were implanted in 101 patients (average age, 53.8 years), patients were followed prospectively and evaluated clinically and radiographically at a minimum of 5 years postoperatively. At an average follow-up of 6.5 years, the average Harris Hip Score was 95.

Valle AG, Zoppi A, Peterson MG, Salvati EA: Clinical and radiographic results associated with a modern, ce-

mentless modular cup design in total hip arthroplasty. *J Bone Joint Surg Am* 2004;86-A(9):1998-2004.

Of 271 patients (308 hips) available for clinical and radiographic follow-up at 4 to 7 years, one cup was revised because of aseptic loosening, and there were seven additional revisions (five because of aseptic loosening of the stem with a well-fixed cup, and two because of deep infection). The authors also reported that 266 (98%) had retention of the cup and 264 (97%) had retention of both components with a good or excellent clinical result.

Cemented Primary Total Hip Arthroplasty

Callaghan JJ, Templeton JE, Liu SS, et al: Results of Charnley total hip arthroplasty at a minimum of thirty years. *J Bone Joint Surg Am* 2004;86-A(4):690-695.

In this study, 330 Charnley THAs were evaluated at minimum 30-year follow-up. Ten percent of patients were still alive. Revision for acetabular loosening was performed in 7.3% of hips and for femoral loosening in 3.2% of hips.

Crites BM, Berend ME, Ritter MA: Technical considerations of cemented acetabular components: A 30-year evaluation. *Clin Orthop Relat Res* 2000;381:114-119.

The authors evaluated 2,237 consecutive cemented acetabular components. Radiolucencies in zone 1 correlated with increase loosening rates. For the acetabular side of a THA, the biology of the bone and the techniques of cement insertion that include a dry cancellous bone bed, perforation and removal of peripheral sclerotic areas, pressurization of the entire cement mantle in the socket at one time, and complete burying of the acetabular component within the boundary of the bony acetabulum were shown to be the essential factors for success, but not porosity reduction in the cement.

Harrington MA Jr, O'Connor DO, Lozynsky AJ, Kovach I, Harris WH: Effects of femoral neck length, stem size, and body weight on strains in the proximal cement mantle. *J Bone Joint Surg Am* 2002;84-A:573-579.

A mechanical stair climbing simulation was used to evaluate the effects of femoral neck length, stem size, and body weight on proximal cement mantle strains. Strains were shown to be increased most by increases in body weight, followed by decreases in stem size and less so by increase in femoral neck length; however, all three increased the strains.

Keener JD, Callaghan JJ, Goetz DD, Pedersen D, Sullivan P, Johnston RC: Long-term function after Charnley total hip arthroplasty. *Clin Orthop Relat Res* 2003;417:148-156.

The authors evaluated outcomes scores, 6-minute walk results, and mortality rates at a minimum 25-year follow-up in patients younger than 50 years at the time of Charnley THA. Results were comparable with normative populations, especially when factoring in medical comorbidity.

Keener JD, Callaghan JJ, Goetz DD, Pedersen DR, Sullivan PM, Johnston RC: Twenty-five-year results after Charnley total hip arthroplasty in patients less than fifty years old: A concise follow-up of a previous report. *J Bone Joint Surg Am* 2003;85-A(6):1066-1072.

In this study, 93 Charnley THAs in patients younger than 50 years were followed for a minimum of 25 years. The authors reported that 18 acetabular and 5 femoral components were revised for loosening. Including the revised components, 34% of acetabular components and 13% of femoral components were radiographically loose.

Kleemann RU, Heller MO, Stoeckle U, Taylor WR, Duda GN: THA loading arising from increased femoral anteversion and offset may lead to critical cement stresses. *J Orthop Res* 2003;21(5):767-774.

The authors evaluated the variables of femoral anteversion and stem offset on cement stresses in a musculoskeletal in vitro model. They reported that increasing anteversion (52% increase) and offset (5% increase) both increased cement stresses with anteversion having the greatest effect.

Levy BA, Berry DJ, Pagnano MW: Long-term survivorship of cemented all-polyethylene acetabular components in patients greater than 75 years of age. *J Arthroplasty* 2000;15(4):461-467.

In this study, 132 consecutive cemented acetabular components were placed in patients age 75 years or older. At average follow-up of 8.9 years (14.6 years for living patients), no acetabular component had been revised for aseptic loosening.

Li C, Schmid S, Mason J: Effects of pre-cooling and pre-heating procedures on cement polymerization and thermal osteonecrosis in cemented hip replacements. *Med Eng Phys* 2003;25(7):559-564.

The authors of this study demonstrated heating the femoral prosthesis resulted in fewer cement prosthesis voids and had no effect on bone-cement interface temperatures.

Meneghini RM, Feinberg JR, Capello WM: Primary hybrid total hip arthroplasty with a roughened femoral stem: Integrity of the stem-cement interface. *J Arthroplasty* 2003;18(3):299-307.

In this study, 102 cemented 40-microinch Ra stems were evaluated at a minimum 5-year and average 9-year follow-up. The aseptic femoral loosening prevalence was 2%.

Ong A, Wong KL, Lai M, Garino JP, Steinberg ME: Early failure of precoated femoral components in primary total hip arthroplasty. *J Bone Joint Surg Am* 2002; 84-A(5):786-792.

The authors of this study compared 514 rough surface stems with uncoated matte finish stems at 8.4- and 13.5-year follow-up, respectively. They reported that 9.5% of precoated stems and 3.9% of uncoated stems were revised for mechanical failure.

Rasquinha VJ, Ranawat CS, Dua V, Ranawat AS, Rodriguez JA: A Prospective, randomized, double-blind study of smooth versus rough stems using cement fixation: minimum 5-year follow-up. *J Arthroplasty* 2004; 19(7):2-9.

In this study, 244 cemented femoral stems with identical geometry were randomized to one of two surface finishes (17-microinch Ra and 170-microinch Ra). At a minimum 5-year follow-up, there were no differences in femoral failure between the two groups.

Settecerri JJ, Kelley SS, Rand JA, Fitzgerald RH Jr: Collar versus collarless cemented HD-II femoral prostheses. *Clin Orthop Relat Res* 2002;398:146-152.

In this study, 84 THAs were randomized into collared or collarless groups. At an average 9.6-year follow-up, no significant differences in loosening rates were reported.

Vail TP, Goetz D, Tanzer M, Fisher DA, Mohler CG, Callaghan JJ: A prospective randomized trial of cemented femoral components with polished versus grit-blasted surface finish and identical stem geometry. *J Arthroplasty* 2003;18(7):95-102.

In this study, 226 hybrid THAs were randomized into two groups of femoral stems of identical stem geometry but different (polished versus grit blasted) surface finish. At an average 4.8-year follow-up, no differences in femoral failure rates were reported.

Wroblewski BM, Siney PD, Fleming PA: Triple taper polished cemented stem in total hip arthroplasty: Rationale for the design, surgical technique, and 7 years of clinical experience. *J Arthroplasty* 2001;16(8):37-41.

In this study, 500 polished triple tapered collarless cemented stems were evaluated at an average follow-up of 3.5 years. No stems were revised for aseptic loosening.

Zimmerma S, Hawkes WG, Hudson JI, et al: Outcomes of surgical management of total hip replacement in patients aged 65 years and older: Cemented versus cementless femoral components and lateral or anterolateral versus posterior anatomical approach. *J Orthop Res* 2002;20(2):182-191.

In this study, 271 hips in patients (age, ≥ 65 years) with primary osteoarthritis underwent cemented or cementless THA at 12 community hospitals. No differences in revision rates between cemented and cementless fixation were reported.

Classic Bibliography

Clohisy JC, Harris WH: The Harris-Galante uncemented femoral component in primary total hip replacement at 10 years. *J Arthroplasty* 1999;14(8):915-917.

Chapter 41

Hip Revision

Scott M. Sporer, MD, MS

Wayne G. Paprosky, MD, FACS

Daniel J. Berry, MD

Femoral Revision

The current surgical techniques and implants used in primary total hip arthroplasty (THA) provide predictable long-term results. However, revision THAs account for 18% of hip procedures performed on patients receiving Medicare. The number of revision hip surgeries is expected to increase as the indications for THA broaden and as the average life expectancy of patients continues to increase.

Surgeons who elect to perform revision THA may be faced with many preoperative, intraoperative, and postoperative challenges. As a result, preoperative planning is crucial and includes forming a surgical team with knowledge of revision surgery, having access to appropriate surgical instrumentation and implants, and acquiring knowledge on various surgical approaches and methods of reconstruction.

Preoperative Assessment
Differential Diagnosis
Patients requiring revision hip surgery most often present to the orthopaedic surgeon with reports of pain. The surgeon should identify the cause of pain so that a successful outcome can be achieved. Hip pain that is localized over the greater trochanter is often found in patients with trochanteric bursitis. This pain can be diagnosed and quickly relieved through the administration of a subcutaneous injection of a local anesthetic. Low back pain must also be ruled out as an etiology of hip pain after THA. Patients with hip pain that is caused by low back pain frequently describe isolated lumbar pain or pain that radiates down the posterior aspect of the leg. A loose femoral component often causes anterior thigh pain or knee pain that is significantly worse when the patient first begins to ambulate. The "start-up" pain may subside as the component settles and obtains a stable position. Patients also may have a sense of hip instability during participation in activities. A limb-length discrepancy can be identified if the component subsides and a progressive external rotation contracture frequently occurs as the component rotates into retroversion. Occult

infection must always be considered as an etiology for hip pain. A thorough patient history may help identify red flags, including reports of pain while at rest, night pain, night sweating, a recent dental procedure, or prolonged wound healing following the index procedure.

A patient's gait patterns also can help identify the etiology of hip pain. Patients with a loose femoral component may have an antalgic gait pattern caused by the micromotion of the femoral stem within the femoral canal during load application. An abductor lurch may be present in patients who have undergone previous surgery for the treatment of deficient abductors. If the biomechanics of the hip are altered, the abductors may be placed in a mechanically disadvantaged position. Stem subsidence will effectively shorten the length of the abductors. Consequently, patients will shift their weight over the affected hip in the stance phase to minimize the abductor moment needed to prevent lowering of the contralateral hemipelvis.

Surgical Indications
Indications for femoral revision include aseptic loosening, progressive femoral osteolysis, septic loosening, and recurrent dislocation with component malposition or inadequate offset. Additional relative indications include the inability to obtain stability following an acetabular revision, difficulty visualizing the acetabulum with a monoblock stem, or the presence of an implant with a poor performance record including a cementless stem that is noncircumferentially coated.

Radiographic Studies
Evaluations including a standard AP pelvic radiograph and AP and lateral radiographs of the affected hip are required for all patients with hip pain. These radiographs must be of sufficient quality that the interface between the bone and prosthesis, bone and cement, or the cement and prosthesis can be delineated. The current radiographs should be compared with previous radiographs to assess component migration, progressive osteolysis, and polyethylene wear. Radiographic signs of

failure of a cemented component include fracture of the cement mantle, a circumferential radiolucency between the implant and cement, fracture of the stem, progressive osteolysis, or component subsidence.

Cementless femoral implants can be categorized as either ingrown, stable fibrous, or unstable. A component that is bone ingrown will show no radiolucency between the porous surface and the host bone. Proximal stress shielding may be seen and spot welds (areas of radiodensity between the endosteum and femoral component) are frequently observed at the distal extent of the porous coating. Stable fibrous components show radiolucency between the porous surface and host bone that is parallel to the endosteum. A small pedestal may be observed but the component has not subsided. An unstable component shows a nonlinear radiolucency between the porous surface and the host bone. The component frequently has subsided and a distal pedestal is generally observed. The distal femur also may show signs of remodeling into both varus and/or retroversion in patients with unstable fibrous fixation.

Femoral Bone Deficiency Classification

The ability to achieve stable prosthetic fixation is highly dependent on the type of fixation chosen and the amount of remaining host bone. Femoral defect classifications have been developed to assist surgeons in formulating an intraoperative plan of action. Ideally, these classifications should be reproducible (intraobserver and interobserver reliability), descriptive (quantitate the degree of bone loss), and should guide treatment options. The three most frequently used classification systems are those from the American Academy of Orthopaedic Surgeons (AAOS) Committee on the Hip, the Mallory classification, and the Paprosky classification. According to the AAOS system, type I defects are segmental, type II are cavitary, type III include combined segmental and cavitary defects, type IV are characterized by malalignment, type V by femoral stenosis, and type VI by femoral discontinuity. There are subclasses of defects based on the location of the defect and the quality of remaining bone.

Both the Mallory and Paprosky classification systems attempt to guide treatment. The Mallory classification of femoral bone stock deficiency is based on the integrity of the cortical bone. Type I and type II defects have an intact cortical tube. Cancellous bone is present in type I defects and absent in type II defects. Type III defects have cortical bone loss. In type IIIA defects, the bone loss extends to the lesser trochanter; in type IIIB the loss extends between the lesser trochanter and isthmus; and type IIIC defects are characterized by bone loss extending to the level of the isthmus.

The Paprosky femoral defect system classifies the remaining host bone into one of four defect types. Type I defects have minimal damage to the proximal metaphysis and can be reconstructed with techniques similar to those used in primary THA. Type II defects have mild metadiaphyseal bone damage with an intact diaphysis. Type III defects have significant metadiaphyseal damage. Type IIIA defects allow more than 5 cm of "scratch fit" at the isthmus and type IIIB allow less than 5 cm. Type IV defects are characterized by extensive metadiaphyseal damage with thin cortices and a widened femoral canal. Most femoral revisions observed in clinical practice have moderate proximal bone deficiency with an intact isthmus (type II or IIIA defects).

Preoperative radiographs may result in an underestimate of the degree of bone loss that is encountered intraoperatively. The host bone stock also can be damaged during attempts at extracting well-fixed implants such that the intraoperative femoral defect classification may be upgraded when compared with the preoperative defect classification. Therefore, surgeons electing to perform revision hip surgery must be comfortable with alternative methods of fixation and must have appropriate implants and instrumentation available.

Surgical Treatment
Preoperative Planning

Preoperative planning is of paramount importance when performing a revision THA. If the surgery was performed at another hospital, an attempt should be made to obtain all previous records and radiographs to determine the initial surgical indication, postoperative complications, prior surgical approaches used, and the type of implant used. Many implant manufacturers have dedicated instrumentation to help facilitate component extraction. Knowledge of the acetabular component used is crucial to determine possible head sizes as well as options to exchange the polyethylene liner if an isolated femoral revision is to be performed. Cementing a liner into a well-fixed component may be an alternative when polyethylene options are limited or locking mechanisms are poorly constructed.

Preoperative templating is the cornerstone of a successful femoral reconstruction. The amount of host bone remaining after component extraction will ultimately dictate options for femoral reconstruction. Therefore, preoperative templating must consider both preoperative radiographic areas of bone loss as well as anticipated areas of bone loss during component explantation. Appropriate templates, adjusted for radiographic magnification, should be used to plan the reconstruction. If an extensively coated stem is chosen for the reconstruction, a minimum of 4 to 5 cm of cortical bone at the isthmus must be available. If this amount of cortical bone cannot be obtained with a standard implant, either a longer stem must be used or alternative methods of fixation should be chosen.

Surgical Exposure

The surgical approach chosen for a femoral revision is dependent on the anticipated complexity of the revision, the surgeon's experience, and the prior surgical approaches used. Previous skin incisions should be used if possible to avoid complications from wound healing. An anterolateral or a direct lateral approach can be used if the amount of femoral bone loss is minor and the anticipated complexity of the revision is low. However, most surgeons elect to use a posterolateral approach during more extensive femoral revision surgery. This approach allows excellent visualization of both the femur and the acetabulum and will allow easy conversion to a more extensive approach.

When using a posterolateral approach, a surgical skin incision is made based on the location of the posterior one third of the greater trochanter and is extended distally in line with the femur. The tensor fascia lata and the fascia of the gluteus maximus are then split in line with the surgical incision and retracted with a Charnley bow. The posterior pseudocapsule and the short external rotators are then elevated as a flap. A portion of the gluteus maximus insertion may be released to allow further mobilization of the femur. The femoral head is then dislocated and the hip is placed in internal rotation.

Component Extraction

The removal of a femoral component during revision surgery remains challenging. Successful explantation of the prosthesis with minimal bone loss is as important as successful component reimplantation. Flexible osteotomes and a motorized high-speed burr should be available in the operating room to disrupt the proximal interface between the implant/host bone or cement/host bone junction. Bone from trochanteric remodeling also can be removed with these tools. Ultrasonic cement removal instrumentation can facilitate the removal of retained cement and the distal cement plug. Stem-specific component extractors that attach to the neck of the prosthesis can be helpful. If the implant manufacturer does not provide explantation equipment, the medial aspect of the prosthetic neck can be notched to allow the attachment of universal explant instrumentation. Several techniques such as the trochanteric slide, the vastus slide, and making controlled perforations in the femur have been described to facilitate stem removal with the intent of minimizing bone loss, limiting soft-tissue dissection, and decreasing surgical time. These approaches are beneficial when removing a loose stem with a prominent greater trochanter, a distal cement plug, or retained cement.

The use of an extended trochanteric osteotomy is an efficient, safe, and reliable technique to remove well-fixed implants. The advantages of this technique include easier access to the fixation surface of the failed prosthesis without further compromising the remaining bone stock, easier removal of retained cement, the ability to concentrically ream a femur with proximal remodeling, predictable healing of the osteotomized fragment, proper tensioning of the abductors with distal advancement, a potential decrease in surgical time, and enhanced exposure of the acetabulum. Although an extended trochanteric osteotomy appears to be an aggressive surgical procedure, intraoperative complications (including fracture, eccentric reaming, and femoral perforation) with rates of more than 50% have been observed in femoral revisions in which an extended trochanteric osteotomy was not used during attempts at either removing a well-fixed stem or during insertion of a stem into a patient with proximal femoral remodeling.

Preoperative radiographs are used to determine the optimal length of the osteotomy from the tip of the greater trochanter. When removing a well-fixed, extensively coated femoral component, the osteotomy should be positioned at the junction between the taper and the cylindrical portion of the stem. For cemented stems, the osteotomy site should ideally be positioned at or slightly beyond the tip of the implant. Proximally coated implants can be removed with a shorter osteotomy fragment. However, most extended trochanteric osteotomies should be at least 12 cm in length to provide adequate bone distal to the lesser trochanter for later reattachment.

Extended trochanteric osteotomy can provide predictable clinical results during revision femoral surgery. One study evaluated 142 consecutive hip revisions performed with an extended trochanteric osteotomy. Of the 122 patients available for a mean 2.6-year follow-up, there were no nonunions of the osteotomized fragments and no instances of proximal migration greater than 2 mm. Radiographically, all patients demonstrated bone union by 3-month follow-up. Other surgeons have reported similar results with the use of an extended trochanteric osteotomy. One study reported a 98% rate of union in 46 patients when an extended trochanteric osteotomy was used during revision surgery. Another study reported a 96% rate of union in 45 patients when an extended trochanteric osteotomy was performed through an anterolateral approach at an average 3.8-year follow-up. The incidence of trochanteric escape and trochanteric fracture, however, was higher than previous reports through a posterolateral approach. The amount of migration depended on the method of fixation, with trochanteric cables demonstrating less migration than cerclage wires.

Femoral Reconstruction

After the previous femoral component is removed, the remaining bone stock should be assessed for areas of unsuspected bone loss as well as for the quality of the remaining host bone. This assessment is easily accom-

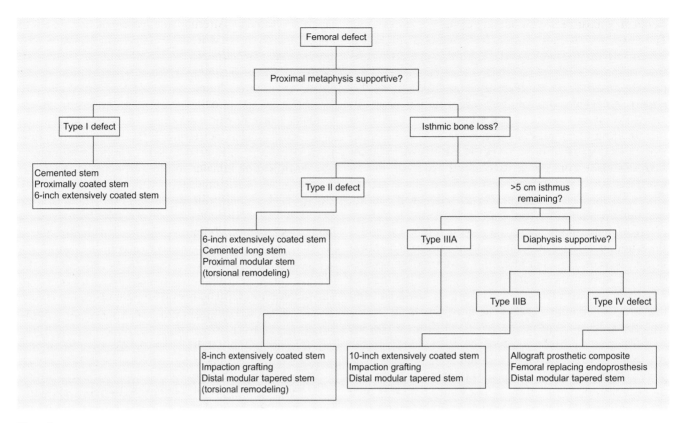

Figure 1 An algorithmic approach to femoral revision based on the Paprosky femoral defect classification.

plished through the use of a reverse hook curett placed into the medullary canal. Intramedullary palpation with these instruments also will allow removal of all fibrous pseudomembrane and can be used to verify and complete the removal of previously used cement. The most important factors to consider when evaluating the remaining host bone are the remaining length of intact isthmus, the quality of the remaining cortex, and whether the remaining metaphysis is supportive (Figure 1).

Intraoperatively, the surgeon must consider goals such as restoration of limb length, offset, and range of motion. Although these goals are not mutually exclusive, patients must understand that the first priority in revision surgery is to obtain intraoperative stability of the femoral component in the remaining host bone. Maintaining hip stability throughout a functional range of motion is the next priority; in some instances, a limb-length discrepancy may be accepted. Many surgeons find the Paprosky femoral defect classification system helpful to guide reconstructive options. In the type I defect, the metaphysis is supportive with minimal bone loss, the isthmus is intact, and the diaphyseal cortex is intact. Bone loss with this pattern is found in undersized, cementless implants or in a painful press-fit hemiarthroplasty. Although this type of defect is uncommon, patients with a type I defect can undergo reconstruction with methods similar to those used in primary THA. If a cemented implant is chosen, the "neocortex" should first

be removed to allow appropriate cement interdigitation. A proximally coated implant also can be used if intraoperative stability to axial and rotational loads can be achieved.

Type II femoral defects show an unsupportive metaphysis with an intact isthmus and diaphyseal cortex. Because patients with this type of defect have minimal remaining cancellous bone, a cemented revision stem is less likely to achieve long-term fixation. In these circumstances, the use of an extensively coated stem will allow distal fixation, which bypasses the proximal defect. In most patients with type II defects, a standard 6-inch stem can be used. The femoral canal is progressively reamed with circumferential reamers until the endosteal cortex is engaged. To obtain stable fixation, 4 to 5 cm of "scratch-fit" is required. The canal is generally underreamed by 0.5 mm to allow intraoperative axial and rotational stability. A hole gauge can be used to verify appropriate implant dimensions.

Type III femoral defects have a severely deficient proximal femur with an unsupportive metaphysis. The isthmus is intact with more than 5 cm of "scratch-fit" available in a type IIIA defect and less than 5 cm in a type IIIB defect. These deformities are most commonly observed following the removal of a loose cemented femoral stem, during a second-stage reimplantation, following an extended trochanteric osteotomy, or in association with a periprosthetic femoral fracture. These patients may have varus remodeling of the proximal femur and also may have torsional remodeling of the proximal femur into retroversion. Most type IIIA defects can be treated successfully with the use of an extensively porous-coated stem. Eight-inch stems are frequently chosen to achieve adequate distal fixation. Care must be taken to avoid anterior femoral perforation during reaming and component insertion because of the anterior bow of the femur. Curved implants are available and should be considered to minimize the risk of this complication. An intraoperative radiograph following trial insertion and/or component insertion will confirm the final intramedullary position.

Torsional remodeling of the proximal femur presents the surgeon with additional considerations when choosing an implant. A monoblock curved stem will not allow the independent adjustment of anteversion because of the conflict of the bowed stem against the anterior femoral bow. A modular femoral stem, which has the ability to independently adjust the femoral anteversion, can be useful in these patients. Uncemented stems such as the S-ROM (DePuy/Johnson & Johnson, Warsaw, IN) use a porous-coated sleeve that is placed into the remaining metaphyseal bone. An appropriately sized stem is then impacted through the sleeve and locked through the use of a Morse taper. Because the distal portion of the stem is slotted, it will engage the remaining endosteal bone and is fluted to provide rotational stability. Unfortunately, many type III defects have an unsupportive metaphysis and initial stability is difficult to achieve without the use of an allograft. An alternative method to obtain independent adjustment of anteversion is through the use of a distally based modular stem such as the ZMR (Zimmer, Warsaw, IN), LINK (Link Orthopaedics, Pine Brook, NJ), or the T3 stem (Stryker Orthopaedics, Mahwah, NJ). Modular tapered stems allow independent fitting of the remaining host bone both proximally and distally. These modular tapered prostheses use a titanium corundum-blasted distal taper to achieve initial axial and rotational stability. After this portion of the component is firmly seated, various proximal body segments can be added to allow alteration in offset and limb length. The proximal segment also can be rotated independently of the distal segment to adjust the amount of femoral anteversion. This type of implant can be used in conjunction with an extended trochanteric osteotomy or in patients with severe proximal bone loss. An implant with a large proximal taper should be chosen if severe metaphyseal bone loss is encountered and the taper is unsupported.

More extensive bone loss is observed in a type IIIB defect such that less than 5 cm of isthmic bone is available for fixation. Ten-inch long extensively porous-coated implants are an option for use in these patients. However, immediate fixation may be difficult to achieve with this type of device, especially in patients with larger

femoral canals. Alternative reconstructive options should be considered if immediate intraoperative fixation cannot be achieved or torsional remodeling is present. A modular tapered stem can be used to obtain stable distal fixation and can avoid the use of allograft bone. No long-term data exist on the use of this type of reconstruction in North America. Grafting of the proximal femur is rarely performed if this method of fixation is chosen. Impaction grafting also can be considered if the cortical tube remains intact. This surgical technique uses a polished, tapered implant that is cemented into firmly packed morcellized allograft. Potential advantages of this technique include the ability to restore bone stock (especially in a young patient) and the ability to recreate a cancellous bed to accept cement.

Type IV defects are characterized by extensive metadiaphyseal damage with thin cortices and a widened ectatic femoral canal. The reconstruction of a severely deficient femur can be performed with either a modular tapered stem or an allograft prosthetic composite (APC). At times, a reduction or collapsing osteotomy with cerclage wiring is advantageous. The type of reconstruction chosen is dependent on the patient's comorbidities and activity level, and the philosophy of the surgeon. An APC can potentially restore bone stock and may provide proximal support for the implant. This technique also allows reattachment of the greater trochanter and soft tissue. Reconstruction with an APC is usually performed by initially cementing the proximal portion of the implant to the allograft. The allograft is then secured to the remaining host bone. The method of fixation at the host/graft junction is highly dependent on the amount of remaining host bone and the diameter of the APC. If the host bone and APC have a similar diameter, the stem can either be press fit or cemented into the remaining host bone. Some surgeons believe applying cement distally is unnecessary, may increase the risk of nonunion, and may make further revisions more difficult. The proximal allograft/host bone junction is joined through either a step cut or oblique osteotomy. However, most cadaveric femurs have a smaller cortical diameter than the host bone and an intussusception technique may be required. If this reconstructive option is chosen, a strut graft and/or plate can be used to minimize the risk of subsidence. A femoral-replacing endoprosthesis can be used if the proximal femur cannot be reconstructed. This option is useful in elderly patients with low physical demands and in patients who cannot tolerate a more extensive procedure.

A well-fixed cemented femoral stem must be removed in some instances including those in which improved acetabular exposure is needed, when limb length or offset adjustment is required, or if damage to a monoblock femoral head is present. If the retained cement mantle is intact, recementing a new stem into the existing cement is an option. This procedure is performed by either adding monomer to the existing cement and reinserting the explanted stem or by selecting a smaller-sized implant and using a thin cement mantle.

Rehabilitation

The rehabilitation protocol following femoral revision is highly dependent on the degree of bone loss and the extent of the reconstruction. Ideally, patients should be mobilized as quickly as possible after surgery to minimize cardiovascular, pulmonary, and skin complications. Patients with mild to moderate bone loss who were treated with a cementless implant generally participate in toe-touch weight bearing for 6 weeks to minimize micromotion and encourage bone ingrowth. Restricted weight bearing for 6 to 12 weeks may be recommended if either a structural allograft or an impaction bone grafting procedure was used to facilitate bone consolidation. Active abduction should not be performed for a minimum of 6 weeks following an extended trochanteric osteotomy to avoid trochanteric escape. An abduction orthosis may be used if there are concerns about patient compliance with total hip precautions or postoperative hip stability.

Results

Cemented Stems

The results of femoral revision are dependent on the degree of bone loss and the method of fixation. Cemented femoral revisions have shown less reliable long-term fixation. It is postulated that the loss of cancellous bone in a revision setting results in a decrease in the shear strength at the host/cement junction. First-generation cement techniques consist of hand packing the cement without the use of a distal cement restrictor. Several authors have shown a high rate of early mechanical failure along with an alarmingly high rate of progressive radiolucencies (Table 1). Longer follow-up of these same patients demonstrated an escalating number of revisions for aseptic loosening. Second-generation cement techniques include the use of a cement gun to allow retrograde filling of the femoral canal along with the use of a distal cement restrictor. This surgical technique provided improved clinical results compared with those found in earlier studies.

Cementless Stems

The increasing failure rates of cemented femoral revision after 10 years prompted many surgeons to adopt alternative methods of fixation. The results of cementless fixation are mainly dependent on the degree of bone loss and the type of stem used. Monoblock, proximally porous-coated implants have demonstrated poor long-term results in most revision situations. These implants rely on proximal bone stock, which is frequently deficient at the time of revision. Several series have shown a high rate of stem subsidence and aseptic loosening. Extensively porous-coated stems were used to obtain distal fixation and bypass the deficient proximal bone. The results from this type of implant have been encouraging. Several surgeons have shown component survival rates greater than 95% at a minimum follow-up of 10 years for patients with type II and type IIIA defects. The successful results found with the use of extensively coated stems have prompted many surgeons to extend the surgical indications of this type of implant to patients with severe femoral bone loss (for example, type IIIB and IV defects). The intermediate clinical results with these stems have been mixed. The ability to obtain immediate stable fixation is compromised in patients with a large ectatic femoral canal, poor quality cortical bone, and in those with minimal remaining isthmus. Extensively coated stems have a high rate of failure when used in this subset of patients.

Modular Stems

Modularity was introduced to allow independent filling of the proximal and distal bone. The midterm results of the S-ROM implant remain encouraging. A recent 7-year follow-up of 320 hips showed a revision rate of only 1.4% for aseptic loosening. When used in patients with severe proximal femoral deficiency, the proximal sleeve must be cemented into an allograft, and distal fixation must be achieved through the slotted distal stem.

Impaction Grafting

Impaction grafting of the proximal femur may allow the restoration of femoral bone stock and may be indicated in younger patients with severe femoral deficiencies. Several authors, however, have shown high rates of intraoperative and postoperative complications, including femoral fracture and component subsidence leading to subsequent instability. The variable short-term results have caused impaction grafting to lose favor in comparison with alternative methods of fixation.

Conical Implants

Nonmodular, tapered titanium implants such as the Wagner SL (Sulzer Medica, Baar, Switzerland) obtain distal fixation through the tapered design and axial stability through splines. These implants can be used successfully in patients with severe proximal femoral deficiencies. Several studies have shown the potential for proximal bone remodeling because of the lower modulus of elasticity of titanium. Unfortunately, the monoblock design of this implant has resulted in a high rate of subsidence. Modular tapered stems are now available to address the concerns of subsidence and facilitate intraoperative placement. However, long-term follow-up of these second-generation implants is currently unavailable.

Table 1 | Femoral Revision

Author(s) Year	Hips	Follow-up	Surgical Variables	Outcome	Conclusion
Extensively Coated Revision Femoral Components					
Weeden and Paprosky (2002)	170 hips	14.2 years (11 to 16 years)		3.5% revision for aseptic femoral loosening 4.1% mechanical failure rate	Extensively coated stems should be used during revision femoral surgery
Sporer and Paprosky (2003)	51 hips	6 years (2 to 11 years)	Type IIIB or IV defects treated with 9 - or 10-inch stem	0% failure in type IIIB with canal < 19 mm 18% failure in type IIIB with canal > 19 mm 37.5% failure in type IV	Consider alternative methods of fixation in type IIIB defects with a canal >19 mm or a type IV defect
Engh et al (2002)	26 hips	13.3 years	Bone loss > 10 cm below lesser trochanter	89% survival at 10 years for aseptic femoral revision 15% aseptic femoral loosening rate	Extensively coated stems can be used to bypass severe proximal bone loss
Moreland and Moreno (2001)	137 hips 134 patients	9.3 years (5 to 16 years)		4% revision rate of aseptic femoral loosening 83% radiographic bone ingrowth	Extensively coated stems provide durable fixation
Krishnamurthy et al (1997)	297 hips 297 patients	8.3 years (5 to 14 years)		1.7% femoral revision for aseptic loosening 2.4% mechanical failure rate	Diaphyseal fixation should be used in femoral revisions to avoid bone loss in the proximal metaphysis
Moreland and Bernstein (1995)	175 patients	5 years		96% component survival 83% bone ingrown	Extensively coated stems provide durable fixation
Lawrence et al (1994)	83 hips 81 patients	9 years (5 to 13 years)		10% femoral re-revision 11% mechanical failure of femoral component	Extensively coated stems can provide reliable fixation during femoral revision
Cemented Revision Femoral Components					
McLaughlin and Harris (1996)	35 hips 38 patients	10.8 years (5.8 to 16.6 years)	Calcar replacing component	18% rate of aseptic femoral revision 32% rate of mechanical failure	
Mulroy and Harris (1996)	43 hips 41 patients	15.1 years (14.2 to 17.5 years)	Second-generation cement technique	20% rate of aseptic femoral revision 26% rate of aseptic femoral loosening	Second-generation cement technique decreases the prevalence of aseptic femoral loosening
Katz et al (1995)	79 hips 73 patients	47 hips with minimum 10-year follow-up	Second-generation cement technique	9.5% rate of femoral revision for aseptic loosening at 10 years 26.1% rate of radiographic femoral failure at 10 years	Second-generation cement technique improves clinical and radiographic results Cemented femoral revision demonstrates high rate of mechanical failure
Kavanagh and Fitzgerald (1987)	45 hips 45 patients	41 months	First-generation cement technique	16% rate of femoral revision 28% rate of radiographic loosening	Cemented re-revision shows poor clinical and radiographic results
Pellicci et al (1985)	99 hips	8.1 years (5 to 12.5 years)	First-generation cement technique	29% rate of mechanical failure	Increased failure rate with longer follow-up of cemented stems
Kavanagh et al (1985)	166 hips 162 patients	4.5 years	First-generation cement technique	44% radiographic aseptic loosening 9% rate of femoral revision	The high incidence of radiographic signs of loosening is a concern
Callaghan et al (1985)	139 hips	3.6 years (2 to 5 years)	First-generation cement technique	15.8% definite mechanical failure 8.6% femoral revision caused by aseptic loosening	Mechanical failure and progressive radiolucencies were associated with poor quality of bone

Table 1 | Femoral Revision (cont)

Author(s) Year	Hips	Follow-up	Surgical Variables	Outcome	Conclusion
Proximally Coated Revision Femoral Components					
Mulliken et al (1996)	52 hips 51 patients	4.6 years	Monoblock titanium stem	10% femoral revision for aseptic loosening; additional 14% radiographically loose 40% intraoperative fracture	Proximally porous-coated stems in revisions with femoral bone loss show inadequate fixation
Malkani et al (1996)	69 hips 69 patients	3 years	Monoblock stem	8.7% femoral revision 29% mechanical failure 82% 5 year survival	Proximally coated stems do not provide reliable fixation during revision surgery
Berry et al (1995)	375 hips	4.7 years	Monoblock stems	58% survivorship at 8 years for aseptic femoral revision 20% survivorship for aseptic femoral loosening	Stable fixation with proximally coated femoral components cannot be reliably achieved
Woolson and Delaney (1995)	25 hips	5.5 years	Monoblock titanium stem	20% rate of femoral re-revision 45% mechanical failure	Proximally porous-coated femoral components should not be used in revision surgery
Proximal Modular Femoral Components					
Cameron (2002)	320 hips	7 years (2 to 12 years)	S-ROM stem 109 primary stems, 211 revision stems	No primary stem revisions for aseptic loosening 1.4% revision for aseptic loosening with revision stem	A proximal ingrowth, proximally modular stem can be used in revision hip surgery
Christie et al (2000)	163 hips	(4 to 7 years)	Type II and III defects S-ROM stem	2.9% rate of aseptic failure	A proximal ingrowth, proximally modular stem can be used in revision hip surgery
Chandler et al (1995)	52 hips 48 patients	3 years	S-ROM stem 22 patients required structural allograft	Mechanical loosening occurred in 5 hips	A proximal ingrowth, proximally modular stem is versatile can be used in difficult revision hip surgery
Cameron (1994)	91 hips	(2-6 years)	S-ROM stem 29 primary stems, 62 revision stems	86% excellent/good results with primary stem—1 revision 80% excellent/good results with revision stem—10 revisions	Modularity is an option for femoral revision
Modular Tapered Revision Femoral Components					
Kwong et al (2003)	143 hips	40 months (2 to 6 years)	Link MP stem	97.2% component survival 2.1 mm average subsidence	The Link MP hip stem allows successful revision THA reconstruction of the proximally compromised femur
Nonmodular Tapered Revision Femoral Components					
Isacson et al (2000)	43 hips	25 months	Wagner SL stem	5 patients with subsidence > 20 mm 9 recurrent dislocations requiring 8 revisions	High rate of component subsidence and dislocation
Grunig et al (1997)	40 hips	47 months (3 to 7 years)	Wagner SL stem	3 hips revised for aseptic femoral loosening	The authors recommend the Wagner SL femoral revision stem, not as a routine procedure to treat loosening, but for patients with severe femoral bone resorption after THA
Proximal Femoral Allograft					
Blackley et al (2001)	63 hips 60 patients	11 years (9 to 15 years)	Long stem implant cemented into allograft	77% with a successful clinical result 25% allograft complications	Viable option for patients with severe proximal deficiency

Table 1 | Femoral Revision (cont)

Author(s) Year	Hips	Follow-up	Surgical Variables	Outcome	Conclusion
			Impaction Grafting		
Ornstein el al (2002)	144 hips	1 year	Polished tapered stem	39 femoral fractures	Intraoperative complication rate high with impaction grafting
van Biezen et al (2000)	21 hips	5 years (41 to 85 months)	Polished tapered stem	19% subsidence > 10 mm No femoral re-revision	Impaction grafting may be useful in severely damaged femora
Meding et al (1997)	34 hips	30 months (24 to 42 months)	Polished tapered stem	6% revision for aseptic loosening 38% subsidence, average = 10 mm	Impaction bone-grafting recommended only when proximal femoral osteopenia is so severe that stability cannot be obtained with insertion of a long-stemmed femoral component without cement
Eldridge et al (1997)	79 patients		Polished tapered stem	11% subsidence > 10 mm	High rate of subsidence causes concern
Gie et al (1993)	58 hips	30 month	Polished tapered stem	No revision for aseptic loosening 79% subsidence > 1 mm	Impaction bone grafting is a viable option in femoral reconstruction

Allograft Prosthetic Composite

Femoral reconstruction with an APC is reserved for severe femoral deficiency. A recent study of 63 hips at an average 11-year follow-up showed a 77% rate of successful clinical outcomes. These results are encouraging given this challenging patient population. Similar to other femoral reconstructions, the ability to obtain intraoperative stability of the APC is mandatory for a successful outcome.

Acetabular Revision

Introduction

Historically, the most common indication for acetabular revision has been loosening of the acetabular component. Recently, revision for the combined problems of polyethylene wear and osteolysis has increased in frequency and importance. For implant loosening or periprosthetic osteolysis the clinical indication for revision may be hip pain, progressive acetabular bone loss, or a combination of both. Other frequent indications for acetabular revision include recurrent hip dislocation and treatment of the infected THA (as a one-stage or two-stage procedure).

Goals

The main goals of acetabular revision are (1) to extract failed implants with minimal bone and soft-tissue damage, (2) to implant a new acetabular component that provides long-term pain relief and good function, and (3) to manage bone deficiencies effectively and when

possible to restore bone stock. As with any revision procedure, stable implant fixation is essential to a good long-term clinical result. Optimal implant position also is essential, especially for acetabular revision, to provide the best likelihood of hip stability. The choice of an optimal bearing surface improves the likelihood of long-term durability of the arthroplasty.

Classification

Several different acetabular classification systems have been devised to aid in evaluating a failed acetabular component that requires revision. The two most commonly used systems are those of the AAOS and Paprosky. The AAOS classification system divides bone loss into four main categories relevant to acetabular revision: type I (segmental deficiencies), type II (cavitary deficiencies), type III (combined segmental and cavitary deficiencies), and type IV (pelvic discontinuity) (Figure 2). The Paprosky system was devised after the introduction of cementless hemispherical acetabular components, and it is designed to provide guidance about when such implants can be used successfully (Table 2). Despite the practical value of acetabular bone loss classification systems, a recent study demonstrated moderate to poor intraobserver and interobserver consistency in defect classification using these systems.

Preoperative Planning and Diagnostic Imaging

Preoperative planning is an important aspect of most reconstructive hip surgeries and is particularly valuable for revision surgery. Preoperative planning helps the

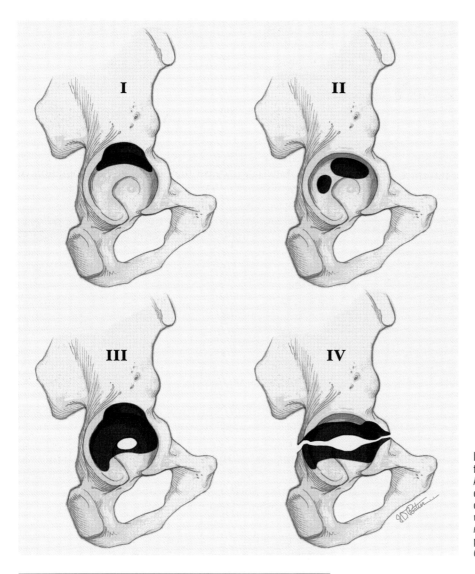

Figure 2 Classification of acetabular bone defects encountered in revision THA according to the AAOS. Type I: segmental. Type II: cavitary. Type III: combined cavitary and segmental. Type IV: pelvic discontinuity. *(Reproduced with permission from Lewallen DG, Berry DJ: Acetabular revision: techniques and results, in Morrey BG (ed): Joint Replacement Arthroplasty, ed 3. Philadelphia, PA, Churchill Livingstone, 2003, pp 824-843.)*

Table 2	Paprosky Classification of Acetabular Bone Deficiencies
Type I	Acetabular rim intact and undistorted
	Acetabulum hemispherical in shape with supportive dome
Type II	Acetabular rim distorted or has minor deficiencies but fully supportive of hemispherical shell
	At least 50% of hemispherical component in contact with host bone
	Hip center migration less than 3 cm superior to superior obturator line
	Minimal ischial bone loss
	The defects are subcategorized as Type IIA, IIB, or IIC according to bone loss pattern and location
Type IIIA	Marked superolateral acetabular bone loss with greater than one third of acetabular rim circumference deficient
	Hemispherical cup does not have inherent stability on host bone
Type IIIB	Marked superomedial (± lateral) acetabular bone loss
	Failed implant migration medial to Kohler's line; migration greater than 3 cm superior to superior obturator line
	Extensive ischial osteolysis

surgeon anticipate instrument, bone graft, and implant needs for revision surgery. Furthermore, good preoperative planning helps the surgeon consider reconstruction alternatives that may be needed based on possible intraoperative finding scenarios.

In addition to a careful history and physical examination that focus on the etiology of implant failure and the preoperative status of muscle, bone, and neurovascular structures, the surgeon needs to determine whether there is evidence of infection, which is usually done by obtaining a screening erythrocyte sedimentation rate and C-reactive protein level and, when indicated, performing hip aspiration. Standard preoperative imaging before surgery includes an AP pelvis film and a true lateral radiograph of the affected hip. Judet oblique pelvic views are indicated when pelvic discontinuity is suspected. Although three-dimensional imaging modalities such as CT usually are not required, they occasionally can be helpful to more accurately determine the pattern of an unusual acetabular bone deficiency.

Rarely, an acetabular component may migrate sufficiently medially to potentially be entangled with, or adherent to, intrapelvic neurovascular structures. Use of arteriography, venography, and CT with contrast have been recommended to assess this concern. In patients with severe migration of the acetabular component, these preoperative studies may be helpful, but in most patients, gradual medial migration of the acetabular component occurs in association with a fibrous membrane and bony tissues that create an interface between the implant and intrapelvic structures.

Exposures and Failed Implant Removal

The surgical exposure used for acetabular revision surgery is determined by a combination of surgeon preference, anticipated exposure needs for implant removal, and anticipated exposure needs for component implantation.

For most straightforward revisions, a conventional anterolateral or posterior approach may be used depending on surgeon preference. For more complex revisions, a conventional or extended trochanteric osteotomy may be considered. Although conventional greater trochanteric osteotomy provides maximum acetabular exposure with minimum risk of damage to the superior gluteal nerve and vessels, it is associated with a risk of greater trochanteric nonunion. For a more detailed discussion of exposures to the hip see chapter 30.

Implant removal is an important and sometimes overlooked aspect of revision surgery. Substantial bone loss at the time of component removal is undesirable because it makes the subsequent reconstruction more difficult and potentially less successful.

The well-fixed, cemented acetabular component usually is removed by first freeing the component from the cement mantle followed by piecemeal removal of the cement. Care should be taken to avoid damage to intrapelvic structures if cement is extruded intrapelvically through medial wall deficiencies. Well-fixed cementless sockets traditionally have been considered difficult to remove; however, new instrumentation has made the process more straightforward. Modular, size-specific, curved osteotomes that follow the radius of the outside diameter of the socket are now available and help spare bone.

Reconstruction Methods

Although many different methods have been used for acetabular revision, with time the number of methods commonly in use has diminished. One method is currently predominant in North America: hemispherical porous-coated cementless implants fixed with screws. Outside of North America, impaction bone grafting of the acetabulum followed by insertion of a cemented implant is also a common method of acetabular revision. Other specialized methods now are used primarily to treat patients with the most severe acetabular deficiencies, including antiprotrusio cages, modular acetabular components with additional flanges or augmentation devices, and custom acetabular components.

Hemispherical Porous-Coated Cementless Acetabular Component

Hemispherical porous-coated cementless acetabular components are used for most acetabular revisions in North America because they provide a combination of good results and a straightforward surgical technique that is applicable to most acetabular revisions.

After the failed component is removed, the acetabulum is reamed until a hemisphere of supportive acetabular bone is established. In most instances, this involves recontouring of the peripheral rim of the acetabulum and the dome of the acetabulum. A new cementless socket, usually 1 to 2 mm larger than the last reamer, is then inserted. In addition to an interference fixation, typically the revision socket also is fixed with screws (Figure 3).

Results of hemispherical porous-coated cementless acetabular components have been favorable, and recently several reports have provided information at more than 10 years of follow-up. One series of 138 revision THAs that were followed for 15 to 19 years reported that only one cup was re-revised for aseptic loosening, resulting in a 15-year survivorship (free of revision for aseptic loosening) of 97%. Notably, however, a total of 20 metal shells were re-revised (7 at the time of femoral revision, 7 for recurrent dislocation, and 6 for infection). In another report of 61 consecutive revisions of failed cemented cups, none of the cementless hemispherical revision cups were re-revised for loosening, but two cups were radiographically loose. A series of 48 revision THAs performed with cementless hemispherical cups followed for 7.4 years demonstrated no cup re-revisions for loosening. A review of 4,726 revision THAs from the Norwegian Arthroplasty Registry recently demonstrated that cementless acetabular components significantly reduced the risk of re-revision compared with cemented acetabular revision (either with or without bone grafting in association with the cementation).

Jumbo cementless cups and cementless cups placed at a high hip center increase the spectrum of acetabular revision problems that can be solved with cementless hemispherical components. Both methods rely on the concept that the surgeon "chases the good bone." The high hip center method involves placing a socket more superiorly on the ilium where good bone remains (usually using a small outside diameter socket). The jumbo cup method involves reaming the socket to a larger diameter to gain contact of the large socket against the remaining rim of acetabular bone (Figure 4). Most surgeons prefer the jumbo cup method because it helps restore the hip center

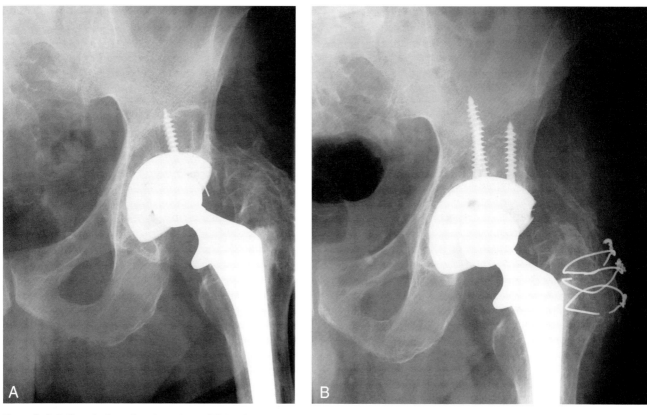

Figure 3 **A,** Radiograph of a patient who underwent THA that failed because of acetabular loosening and osteolysis. **B,** Radiograph of the same patient after revision with uncemented porous-coated hemispherical cup fixed with screws.

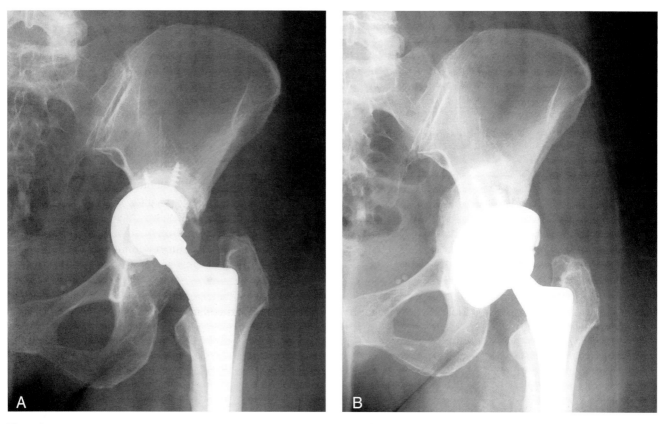

Figure 4 **A,** Radiograph of a patient who underwent THA that failed because of acetabular loosening. **B,** Radiograph of same patient after revision with jumbo uncemented porous-coated hemispherical cup fixed with screws.

of rotation, improves soft-tissue tension about the hip, and limits the risk of femoral-pelvic impingement. A series of 89 revisions using extra large cementless hemispherical cups resulted in only 4 loose cups at a minimum 5-year follow-up. In another series of 43 jumbo cups, only 2 cups were re-revised for loosening at a minimum 5-year follow-up (mean, 10 years).

The amount of contact between the cementless hemispherical component and bone necessary to provide long-term biologic fixation is uncertain. For many years, a rule of thumb of approximately 50% implant-host bone contact has been advocated. However, it has become apparent that location of bone contact is as important as contact area. If host bone provides implant support in critical areas, biologic fixation may be possible in many instances. Recently, manufacturers have developed implant surfaces that provide a high-friction surface in combination with high potential for bone ingrowth that may allow successful biologic fixation, even with smaller areas of implant surface-host bone contact.

Impaction Grafting and Cement
This method involves impacting cancellous bone graft densely into the bone deficiencies in the acetabulum, followed by cementing a component into the impacted bone graft. Peripheral segmental deficiencies are reconstructed with metal mesh before bone impaction. A recent report of the technique in 173 acetabular revisions demonstrated that 97.2% of implants were unrevised at 4-year follow-up. More severe acetabular bone deficiency was associated with a greater risk of cup migration.

Antiprotrusio Cages
Antiprotrusio cages have been used for reconstruction in patients with severe acetabular bone loss. These devices provide a large surface area that distributes load, bridges bone defects, protects bone grafts, and resists migration. Cages are fixed with multiple screws and provide a mechanical fixation construct. Most of these devices are not fixed biologically, however, and therefore are at risk for mechanical loosening or breakage with time. A recent report demonstrated a high failure rate when more than 60% of an acetabular reconstruction ring or cage was supported only by cement or particulate bone graft. Nevertheless, a recent article reported a 92% 21-year survivorship free of revision of Burch-Schneider cages in 38 acetabular revisions. One unrevised cage was radiographically loose. An average 10-year follow-up study of massive structural grafts in association with an antiprotrusio cage demonstrated satisfactory results in 10 of 13 patients, attesting to the value of cage protection of certain large bulk grafts. As methods of cementless acetabular reconstruction have improved, the indications for antiprotrusio cages have concomitantly diminished. Use of these devices now is relegated to patients with the most severe deficiencies

in which hemispherical cementless acetabular components have a low chance of success.

Bilobed and Nonhemispherical Cementless Porous-Coated Implants
Monoblock, bilobed, and nonhemispherical cementless implants that fill bone defects with metal have been used to treat patients with selected segmental bone deficiency patterns. Variable results have been reported in several midterm reports. Modular implants also have been devised that allow bone deficiencies to be filled with metallic augments attached to cementless implants. In a recent short-term report on 16 tantalum trabecular metal cups with modular metal augments, there were no mechanical failures at a mean 32-month follow-up.

Custom Acetabular Components
Custom porous-coated implants can be manufactured that combine large porous-coated surfaces with large phalanges that rest against the ilium, ischium, and pubis. Preoperative CT is used to generate a model of the pelvis, following which a custom implant is fabricated according to specific design criteria. The implant is fixed to the pelvis with screws. Favorable results have been reported from a few relatively small series; in one recent report of 26 hips with severe bone loss (Paprosky type IIIB), 23 hip reconstructions performed with this method were successful at a mean 4.5-year follow-up. All three failures occurred in patients with pelvic discontinuity.

Bipolar Implants
Bipolar implants have generally been abandoned for use in acetabular revision based on the high rate of component migration and inguinal pain.

Acetabular Bone Grafts
Bone deficiencies may be managed by filling them with bone graft, bone substitutes, or metal. Particulate allograft is most commonly used for cavitary (or medial segmental) acetabular bone loss. Particulate grafts appear to provide the best potential for bone stock restoration.

Bulk bone grafts generally are used for large segmental bone deficiencies, most commonly of the superolateral acetabulum or posterior wall and column. These grafts appear to have a high rate of union to the pelvis. The main concerns with large bulk allograft include risk of resorption and collapse with time. Notably, however, according to a recent study on 23 hips with Paprosky type IIIA bone defects that were treated with a cementless hemispherical cup and laterally placed bulk distal femoral allograft, success in 17 hips at a minimum 10-year follow-up was reported. Allograft resorption occurred in 2 of 5 revised hips and was observed in 6 of the remaining 17 cups, only 1 of which was radiographically loose.

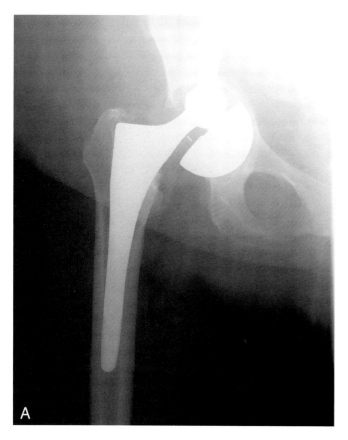
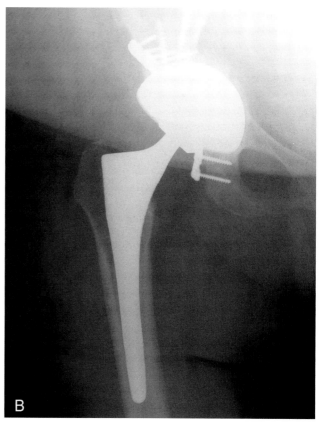

Figure 5 **A,** Radiograph of a patient with pelvic discontinuity. Note the visible fracture line, the break on Kohler's line (with offset of superior and inferior pelvis relative to one another) and rotation of the obturator ring. **B,** Radiograph of the same patient after stabilization of the pelvis with posterior column plating and acetabular reconstruction with an uncemented hemispherical cup.

Reconstruction Based on Bone Loss

Most AAOS and Paprosky type I and II bone deficiencies and many AAOS type III bone deficiencies can be managed with a hemispherical cementless socket fixed to the bone with screws in conjunction with limited particulate grafting of the remaining bone defects. These defect patterns also may be managed by impaction bone grafting with cement. Severe AAOS type III bone deficiencies and Paprosky type III bone deficiencies sometimes require alternative techniques. Large segmental superolateral or posterior column deficiencies may be managed with a bulk bone graft and cementless socket, bilobed cups, or antiprotrusio cages. Modular metal augments combined with cementless cups may assume a role in treatment of these deficiencies if preliminary favorable experience is corroborated. Large AAOS type III bone deficiencies with severe medial bone loss (Paprosky type IIIB deficiencies) sometimes may be managed with a cementless socket that gains support on a remaining peripheral rim of the acetabulum in conjunction with bone grafting. For some such deficiencies, however, reconstruction with hemispherical cups is not possible. In these patients, a structural graft with an antiprotrusio cage or a custom triflange porous-coated component may be considered.

Management of Pelvic Discontinuity

Pelvic discontinuity is a condition in which the superior pelvis and inferior pelvis are separated, typically through a transverse nonunited acetabular fracture through weak and deficient bone. The identifying features of pelvic discontinuity on preoperative radiographs include a visible fracture line, a break in Kohler's line such that the superior pelvis and inferior pelvis are offset relative to one another, or a rotation of the inferior aspect of the hemipelvis relative to the superior aspect of the hemipelvis visible as a rotation of the obturator ring (Figure 5, *A*).

Pelvic discontinuity usually is managed with stabilization of the pelvis followed by reconstruction with a cementless hemispherical component (when bone loss allows) or a bulkier device such as an antiprotrusio cage or custom triflange implant when bone loss is severe enough to preclude use of an hemispherical implant (Figure 5, *B*).

Acetabular Revision for Osteolysis

Since the widespread use of cementless sockets, osteolysis increasingly occurs in association with a bone ingrown cup. When revision is indicated, the surgeon must decide whether to retain or remove the socket. Advantages of removing the socket include a more thorough débridement of retroacetabular osteolytic lesions and the opportunity to place a new socket of modern design in optimal position. Drawbacks of removing the cementless socket include the time required for removal of the implant, the potential for bone loss during implant removal, and the potential for failure of fixation of a new implant. Most surgeons prefer to maintain a well-fixed cementless porous-coated socket if it is in good position and of sufficient diameter to allow a new polyethylene liner of sufficient thickness and diameter to provide satisfactory hip stability.

A recent series of isolated liner exchanges in 24 hips through an anterolateral surgical approach reported only 2 re-revisions at a mean follow-up of 36 months. Accessible osteolytic lesions were grafted, and in 18 patients for whom CT scans were obtained, the lytic lesion regressed or resolved. Notably, the dislocation rate in that series was zero, as opposed to several early series of head and liner exchange that reported higher dislocation rates.

If cup retention is planned, the socket should be rigorously tested at the time of surgery to ensure it is ingrown and not just partially stabilized with fibrous tissue. Peripheral osteolytic lesions can be débrided under direct vision. Retroacetabular lesions can be débrided through holes in the acetabular component; care should be taken to avoid damage to pelvic contents. Cavitary deficiencies may be filled with particulate allograft bone or bone substitutes. A new polyethylene liner then is inserted into the shell. When a modern liner is available that matches the shell, and if the shell has a good locking mechanism, the liner may be snapped into place. When a matching modern liner is not available or the locking mechanism is not deemed adequate, laboratory and clinical studies have demonstrated that a new polyethylene liner may be cemented into the shell. If the shell has screw holes, additional contouring of the interior metal shell surface is not necessary; however, if it is smooth, roughening with a metal cutting instrument provides better interface strength. If the backside of the polyethylene liner is smooth and not designed for cementation, a spider web-shaped pattern of scoring with a high-speed, approximately 4 mm burr provides a rough surface that resists failure at the polyethylene-cement interface. One recent report of this method showed no cemented acetabular liner loosening in 16 hips at a minimum 2-year follow-up after revision.

Summary

Femoral reconstruction is a technically demanding and equipment-intensive procedure. Preoperative planning is essential to develop a strategy to safely extract the retained component, prepare the remaining host bone, and implant a new component. Preoperative radio-

graphs can be used to estimate the degree of host bone deficiency. However, alternative methods of reconstruction should always be available if greater bone loss is unexpectedly encountered. The amount of remaining host bone will ultimately determine the method of reconstruction. Extensively coated stems can be used in most femoral revisions. If torsional remodeling is present, implants that allow independent adjustment of anteversion may be beneficial. Patients with severe proximal bone loss may require a device that obtains distal fixation in the remaining bone, a femoral replacing endoprosthesis, or an APC. Regardless of the reconstructive option selected, a successful long-term result can be expected only if immediate intraoperative stability of the implant can be achieved.

In the past decade, improvements in technology and surgical technique have made acetabular revision more straightforward in most cases and more successful in difficult cases. The severity and location of bone loss, which can be predicted from preoperative radiographs, determines the best methods of reconstruction and likelihood of success. Intermediate to long-term results demonstrate that revision of most failed implants with mild to moderate bone loss can be performed with uncemented porous-coated hemispherical cups. Severe bone loss may be managed with new uncemented hemispherical cups, antiprotrusio cages, custom uncemented implants, and structural bone grafts.

Annotated Bibliography

Femoral Revision

Blackley HR, Davis AM, Hutchison CR, Gross AE: Proximal femoral allografts for reconstruction of bone stock in revision arthroplasty of the hip: A nine to fifteen-year follow-up. *J Bone Joint Surg Am* 2001;83-A: 346-354.

The results of 63 femoral revisions in 60 patients with an average 11-year follow-up were reported using a proximal femoral allograft prosthesis construct. Successful outcomes were found in 77% of patients. Allograft complications, including five hips with deep infection, three hips with aseptic loosening, two hips with recurrent dislocation, and one allograft-host nonunion, were seen in 25% of patients.

Bohm P, Bischel O: Femoral revision with the Wagner SL revision stem: Evaluation of one hundred and twenty-nine revisions followed for a mean of 4.8 years. *J Bone Joint Surg Am* 2001;83-A:1023-1031.

The results of 129 femoral revisions in 123 patients with an average 4.8-year follow-up were reported using a Wagner SL monoblock revision stem. Repeat revision was needed for 6 hips; 113 hips (88%) demonstrated restoration of proximal bone stock.

Cameron HU: The long-term success of modular proximal fixation stems in revision total hip arthroplasty. *J Arthroplasty* 2002;17(4, suppl 1)138-141.

At an average follow-up of 7 years, the results of 320 femoral revision surgeries using a proximally modular, proximal ingrowth noncemented stem were reported. In 109 patients treated with short stems, no revisions for aseptic loosening were needed; however, 3 of 211 long stems (1.4%) required revision.

Christie MJ, DeBoer DK, Tingstad EM, Capps M, Brinson MF, Trick LW: Clinical experience with a modular noncemented femoral component in revision total hip arthroplasty: 4- to 7-year results. *J Arthroplasty* 2000;15: 840-848.

The results of 129 femoral revisions in Paprosky type II or III defects were reported at a minimum 4-year follow-up. The aseptic failure rate was 2.9% and the prevalence of osteolytic lesions less than 5 mm was 2.3%.

Engh CA Jr, Ellis TJ, Koralewicz LM, McAuley JP, Engh CA: Extensively porous-coated femoral revision for severe femoral bone loss: Minimum 10-year follow-up. *J Arthroplasty* 2002;17:955-960.

The authors of this study evaluated 25 patients (26 hips) who underwent revision with fully porous-coated femoral components ≥ 190 mm. At a minimum 10-year follow-up (mean, 13.3 years) with femoral revision as the end point, survivorship was 89%.

Isacson J, Stark A, Wallensten R: The Wagner revision prosthesis consistently restores femoral bone structure. *Int Orthop* 2000;24:139-142.

The authors report the short-term results for 43 hip revision procedures using the long-stemmed Wagner prosthesis. At an average 25-month follow-up, Charnley scores for pain, movement, and walking were 5.2, 4.0, 4.0, respectively. All patients except one showed abundant new bone formation.

Kwong LM, Miller AJ, Lubinus P: A modular distal fixation option for proximal bone loss in revision total hip arthroplasty: A 2- to 6-year follow-up study. *J Arthroplasty* 2003; 18(3,suppl 1)94-97.

The results of 143 femoral revisions treated with a modular tapered stem with distal fixation at an average 40-month follow-up were reported. The component survival rate was 97.2% with an average femoral subsidence of 2.1 mm.

Moreland JR, Moreno MA: Cementless femoral revision arthroplasty of the hip: Minimum 5 years followup. *Clin Orthop Relat Res* 2001;393:194-201.

The authors report on 134 patients (137 hips) who underwent cementless femoral revision arthroplasty of the hip. At a mean 9.3-year follow-up (range, 5 to 16 years), 10 (7%) of the stems had been removed. Five (4%) were removed for fixation problems and five (4%) for infection.

Ornstein E, Atroshi I, Franzen H, Johnsson R, Sandquist P, Sundberg M: Early complications after 144 consecutive hip revisions with impacted morselized allograft bone and cement. *J Bone Joint Surg Am* 2002;84:1323-1328.

The authors of this study report the early complications that occurred in 144 consecutive hip revision arthroplasties (108 stems and 130 sockets) performed with impacted morcellized allograft bone and cement. Thirty-nine femoral fractures occurred in 37 hips; 29 of the fractures occurred during surgery and 10 occurred within 5 months after surgery. Of the intraoperative femoral fractures, 12 were proximal, 9 were diaphyseal, and 8 involved the greater trochanter. Of the postoperative femoral fractures, one was proximal and nine were diaphyseal.

Sporer SM, Paprosky WG: Revision total hip arthroplasty: The limits of fully coated stems. *Clin Orthop* 2003; 417:203-209.

At an average follow-up of 6 years, the results of 51 patients treated with either a 9- or 10-inch fully porous-coated stem were reported. The mechanical failure rate among the 9-inch and 10-inch fully porous-coated stems was 0% in type IIIB defects with femoral canals less than 19 mm (15 patients), 18% in type IIIB defects with femoral canals greater than 19 mm (2 of 11 patients), and 37.5% in type IV defects (3 of 8 patients).

van Biezen FC, ten Have BL, Verhaar JA: Impaction bone-grafting of severely defective femora in revision total hip surgery: 21 hips followed for 41-85 months. *Acta Orthop Scand* 2000;71:135-142.

The authors conducted a prospective study to evaluate the application of impacted allograft bone particles during revision surgery of severely defective femora. At a mean follow-up of 60 months (range, 41 to 85 months), the authors reported that the mean Harris Hip Score improved by 39 points to 78 points. They concluded that in patients who undergo total hip revision surgery, even severely damaged femora can be successfully treated using impaction allografting.

Weeden SH, Paprosky WG: Minimal 11-year follow-up of extensively porous-coated stems in femoral revision total hip arthroplasty. *J Arthroplasty* 2002; 17(4 suppl 1)134-137.

The results of 188 femoral revision surgeries using an extensively coated stem with an average follow-up of 14.2 years were reported. Bone ingrowth was found on 82% of stems and the overall mechanical failure rate was 4.1%

Acetabular Revision

Hallstrom BR, Golladay GJ, Vittetoe DA, Harris WH: Cementless acetabular revision with the Harris-Galante porous prosthesis: Results after a minimum of ten years of follow-up. *J Bone Joint Surg Am* 2004;86:1007-1011.

In this study, 122 hips revised with an uncemented porous-coated acetabular component were followed for at least

10 years. The rate of repeat revision for aseptic loosening of the acetabular component was 4%, but the rate of repeat revision for the acetabular shell for any reason was 15%. The total aseptic loosening rate was 11%.

Jamali AA, Dungy DS, Mark A, Schule S, Harris WH: Isolated acetabular revision with use of the Harris-Galante cementless component: Study with intermediate-term follow-up. *J Bone Joint Surg Am* 2004;86:1690-1697.

In this study, 63 acetabular component revisions with uncemented porous-coated hemispherical socket were followed for a minimum of 60 months. Only four cups were revised because of aseptic loosening; however, the authors reported a high rate of complications, particularly dislocation.

Jones CP, Lachiewicz PF: Factors influencing the longer-term survival of uncemented acetabular components used in total hip revisions. *J Bone Joint Surg Am* 2004;86:342-347.

In this study, 135 hips were followed for a minimum of 5 years after acetabular revision using an uncemented hemispherical socket fixed with screws. Three cups were removed for mechanical loosening, three for infection, and one for recurrent dislocation. The total rate of aseptic loosening including radiographic evidence of loosening was 2%. The rate of dislocation was significantly higher in hips treated with isolated acetabular component revision (20%) than in those in which both components were revised (8%).

Lie SA, Havelin LI, Furnes ON, Engesaeter LB, Vollset SE: Failure rates for 4762 revision total hip arthroplasties in the Norwegian Arthroplasty Register. *J Bone Joint Surg Br* 2004;86:504-509.

Data from the Norwegian Arthroplasty Registry from 1987 to 2003 were analyzed. Uncemented acetabular components significantly reduced the risk of acetabular failure when compared with cemented acetabular components. Relative risk of re-revision of uncemented acetabular components without allograft compared with cemented acetabular components was 0.66 and for uncemented acetabular components with allograft was 0.37 when compared with cemented acetabular components.

Sporer SM, Paprosky WG, O'Rourke M: Managing bone loss in acetabular revision. *J Bone Joint Surg Am* 2005;87:1620-1630.

The authors discuss their classification system and treatment algorithm for acetabular bone defects.

Taek RY, Jong KS, Eun KS, Jae YC, Hyoung YS, Yu BP: Cementation of a metal-inlay polyethylene liner into a stable metal shell in revision total hip arthroplasty. *J Arthroplasty* 2005;20:652-657.

In this study, a polyethylene liner was cemented into a well-fixed shell in 39 revision THAs. At a mean 2.8-year follow-up, no metal shells had failed, and only one liner had dislodged from the metal shell.

Templeton JE, Callaghan JJ, Goetz DD, Sullivan PM, Johnston RC: Revision of a cemented acetabular component to a cementless acetabular component: A ten to fourteen-year follow-up study. *J Bone Joint Surg Am* 2001;83:1706-1711.

Revision of a cemented acetabular component to an uncemented acetabular component was performed in 61 hips. No acetabular revisions were performed for aseptic loosening. Two acetabular components had radiographic evidence of loosening.

Whaley AL, Berry DJ, Harmsen WS: Extra-large uncemented hemispherical acetabular components for revision total hip arthroplasty. *J Bone Joint Surg Am* 2001;83:1352-1357.

In this study, the results of 89 extra-large uncemented hemispherical acetabular components (outside diameter ≥ 66 mm in men and ≥ 62 mm in women) were reported at a mean follow-up of 7.2 years. Only four cups were revised (two for loosening). Two other acetabular components had radiographic evidence of loosening. The authors reported that the probability of survival of the acetabular component at 8 years was 93% with removal for any reason as the end point and 95% with revision for aseptic loosening as the end point.

Classic Bibliography

Berry DJ, Harmsen WS, Ilstrup D, Lewallen DG, Cabanela ME: Survivorship of uncemented proximally porous-coated femoral components. *Clin Orthop* 1995;319:168-177.

Berry DJ, Lewallen DG, Hanssen AD, Cabanela ME: Pelvic discontinuity in revision total hip arthroplasty. *J Bone Joint Surg Am* 1999;81:1692-1702.

Berry DJ, Muller MM: Revision arthroplasty using an anti-protrusio cage for massive acetabular bone deficiency. *J Bone Joint Surg Br* 1992;74:711-715.

Callaghan JJ, Salvati EA, Pellicci PM, Wilson PD Jr, Ranawat CS: Results of revision for mechanical failure after cemented total hip replacement, 1979 to 1982: A two to five-year follow-up. *J Bone Joint Surg Am* 1985;67:1074-1085.

Cameron HU: The two- to six-year results with a proximally modular noncemented total hip replacement used in hip revisions. *Clin Orthop Relat Res* 1994;298:47-53.

Chandler HP, Ayres DK, Tan RC, Anderson LC, Varma AK: Revision total hip replacement using the S-ROM femoral component. *Clin Orthop Relat Res* 1995;319:130-140.

Dohmae Y, Bechtold JE, Sherman RE, Puno RM, Gustilo RB: Reduction in cement-bone interface shear strength between primary and revision arthroplasty. *Clin Orthop* 1988;236:214-220.

Eldridge JD, Smith EJ, Hubble MJ, Whitehouse SL, Learmonth ID: Massive early subsidence following femoral impaction grafting. *J Arthroplasty* 1997;12:535-540.

Gie GA, Linder L, Ling RS, Simon JP, Slooff TJ, Timperley AJ: Impacted cancellous allografts and cement for revision total hip arthroplasty. *J Bone Joint Surg Br* 1993;75:14-21.

Gill TJ, Sledge JB, Muller ME: The Burch-Schneider anti-protrusio cage in revision total hip arthroplasty: Indications, principles, and long-term results. *J Bone Joint Surg Br* 1998;80:946-953.

Grunig R, Morscher E, Ochsner PE: Three- to 7-year results with the uncemented SL femoral revision prosthesis. *Arch Orthop Trauma Surg* 1997;116:187-197.

Katz RP, Callaghan JJ, Sullivan PM, Johnston RC: Results of cemented femoral revision total hip arthroplasty using improved cementing techniques. *Clin Orthop* 1995;319:178-183.

Kavanagh BF, Fitzgerald RH Jr: Multiple revisions for failed total hip arthroplasty not associated with infection. *J Bone Joint Surg Am* 1987;69:1144-1149.

Kavanagh BF, Ilstrup DM, Fitzgerald RH Jr: Revision total hip arthroplasty. *J Bone Joint Surg Am* 1985;67:517-526.

Krishnamurthy AB, MacDonald SJ, Paprosky WG: 5- to 13-year follow-up study on cementless femoral components in revision surgery. *J Arthroplasty* 1997;12:839-847.

Lawrence JM, Engh CA, Macalino GE, Lauro GR: Outcome of revision hip arthroplasty done without cement. *J Bone Joint Surg Am* 1994;76:965-973.

Malkani AL, Lewallen DG, Cabanela ME, Wallrichs SL: Femoral component revision using an uncemented, proximally coated, long-stem prosthesis. *J Arthroplasty* 1996;11:411-418.

McLaughlin JR, Harris WH: Revision of the femoral component of a total hip arthroplasty with the calcar-replacement femoral component: Results after a mean of 10.8 years postoperatively. *J Bone Joint Surg Am* 1996;78:331-339.

Meding JB, Ritter MA, Keating EM, Faris PM: Impaction bone-grafting before insertion of a femoral stem with cement in revision total hip arthroplasty: A minimum two-year follow-up study. *J Bone Joint Surg Am* 1997;79:1834-1841.

Moreland JR, Bernstein ML: Femoral revision hip arthroplasty with uncemented, porous-coated stems. *Clin Orthop Relat Res* 1995;319:141-150.

Mulliken BD, Rorabeck CH, Bourne RB: Uncemented revision total hip arthroplasty: A 4-to-6-year review. *Clin Orthop* 1996;325:156-162.

Mulroy WF, Harris WH: Revision total hip arthroplasty with use of so-called second-generation cementing techniques for aseptic loosening of the femoral component: A fifteen-year-average follow-up study. *J Bone Joint Surg Am* 1996;78:325-330.

Paprosky WG, Perona PG, Lawrence JM: Acetabular defect classification and surgical reconstruction in revision arthroplasty: A 6-year follow-up evaluation. *J Arthroplasty* 1994;9:33-44.

Pellicci PM, Wilson PD Jr, Sledge CB, et al: Long-term results of revision total hip replacement: A follow-up report. *J Bone Joint Surg Am* 1985;67:513-516.

Slooff TJ, Buma P, Schreurs BW, Schimmel JW, Huiskes R, Gardeniers J: Acetabular and femoral reconstruction with impacted graft and cement. *Clin Orthop Relat Res* 1996;324:108-115.

Woolson ST, Delaney TJ: Failure of a proximally porous-coated femoral prosthesis in revision total hip arthroplasty. *J Arthroplasty* 1995;10(suppl):S22-S28.

Chapter 42

Total Hip Arthroplasty Complications

Bassam A. Masri, MD, FRCSC

Darin Davidson, MD

Clive P. Duncan, MD, FRCSC

David G. Lewallen, MD

Nicolas O. Noiseux, MD, FRCSC

Chitranjan S. Ranawat, MD

Vijay J. Rasquinha, MD

James B. Stiehl, MD

Infection

Infection of total hip arthroplasty (THA) is a devastating complication, requiring prolonged management and, in most instances, at least one additional surgical procedure. Because of the associated morbidity, prevention of infection is of paramount importance.

Epidemiology

The first reported rates of infection following THA were unacceptably high (9% to 12% of patients in some series). Infection rates decreased with the use of prophylactic antibiotics, improved surgical sterility, and the evolution of surgical technique. A recent large, American review of Medicare data revealed an incidence less than 1% for primary procedures and 1.1% for revisions. The risk was most significant within the first postoperative month and reached a plateau at 4 to 6 weeks in patients who underwent primary THA and 6 to 8 weeks in those who underwent revision. Infection remains a common etiology for revision THA, comprising 7% to 11% of revisions in Scandinavian arthroplasty registries.

Classification

Traditional classification systems have included three stages based on chronology. Acute infection occurs within 4 weeks of THA, hematogenous infection occurs by seeding within 4 weeks of infection at another site, and chronic infection occurs more than 4 weeks postoperatively. Additional factors that should be included in this classification system are whether the infection occurs in the setting of a primary or revision THA, loss of bone stock, use of allograft, and the presence of drug-resistant organisms. The chronologic classification has been used with the addition of the two categories of medical status and state of the affected extremity, each with three subgroups of increasing severity. This system was found, retrospectively, to correlate significantly with outcome, as determined by infection eradication and complications. This system is yet to be prospectively studied and will not be discussed in detail in this chapter.

Risk Factors

Risk factors for infection can be divided into patient factors, technical factors, hospital and operating room factors, and perioperative management. The latter two have received significant recent attention in the literature.

Hospital factors have generally been studied as a function of the annual volume of THAs performed. In a review of more than 5,000 Medicare patients, a 69% reduction in the rate of deep infection and dislocation was correlated with hospitals in which more than 100 THAs were performed annually. Factors associated with decreased complication rates included private hospitals, academic institutions, dedicated orthopaedic nursing teams, and laminar airflow in the operating room, with the most significant determinant being increased surgeon caseload.

Several strategies have been implemented in the operating room environment to decrease the risk of contamination and subsequent infection. The use of body exhaust suits and sterile helmets has been associated with an infection rate of 0.3%. Although a significant risk reduction has not been consistently reported with this strategy, separation of the anesthesiologist from the surgical team via Plexiglas was found to significantly decrease bacterial colonization on settle plates positioned in the surgical field. The impact of contamination on infection rates was assessed in a study in which contamination of surgical instruments, surgeons' gloves, and light handles was reported in 63% of patients, with the risk of infection among these patients being no higher than the general risk of 1%.

Hematoma formation and profuse postoperative wound drainage have been shown to be risk factors for the development of a superficial wound infection, with an odds ratio of 11.8 and 1.32, respectively. Prolonged wound drainage was the only risk factor found to increase the incidence of infection in a study in which 12% of those with wound drainage developed infection, whereas none with a dry wound developed infection. The risk of deep infection subsequent to superficial infection is 10%, with the same organism being isolated from both sites in most instances. One study compared 86 surgical procedures in which a postoperative suction drain was used with 120 surgical procedures in which no postoperative drain was used and found no increased risk of hematoma or wound exudate at 48 hours. It is recommended, therefore, that drains should be removed by the second postoperative day.

Postoperative urinary tract infection has been shown to be a risk factor for deep infection; however, the significance of preoperative urinary tract infection and asymptomatic bacteriuria is unknown. Current recommendations are for organism-specific antibiotic treatment of preoperative bacteriuria because there is no evidence supporting delaying THA because of preoperative bacteriuria if appropriate antibiotic coverage is implemented. Intermittent urinary catheterization has been shown to result in decreased bacteriuria when compared with indwelling catheterization. In one study, 24% of patients with an indwelling catheter and 6% of patients with intermittent catheterization developed bacteriuria. The rates of THA infection were not reported in these patients.

The role of blood transfusion in the risk of infection has been investigated. Homologous transfusion is associated with suppression of cell-mediated immunity, leading to a potential risk of increased infection. In a series of 1,200 patients, 14% of those who received homologous transfusion developed infection, whereas those who received autologous transfusion did not develop deep infection. Others have reported no significant difference in infection rates between groups receiving homologous, autologous, combined, or no transfusion. This area remains controversial, and additional data are required.

Etiology

The majority of offending organisms produce a biofilm glycocalyx, including *Staphylococcus aureus* and *Staphylococcus epidermidis*. Infection with *S aureus* typically produces early infection, whereas *S epidermidis* and other epidermal flora result in delayed infection. Recently, a shift toward an increased prevalence of coagulase negative staphylococcal species and decreased gram-negative species has been encountered. The most commonly identified organisms remain *S aureus* and *S epidermidis* (27% and 28% of instances of infection, respectively). Typically virulent organisms, such as gram-negative species, *S aureus*, and β-hemolytic *Streptococcus* are the most difficult to eradicate because of the production of the glycocalyx and evolving antibiotic-resistant strains. There is increasing concern regarding emerging vancomycin resistance, particularly among enterococcal species and *S aureus*. Conditions that weaken the immune system, such as diabetes, human immunode-

ficiency virus, acquired immune deficiency syndrome, transplantation, liver failure, and steroid use, have also been associated with a high risk of infection.

Prevention

Perioperative parenteral antibiotics are widely used and have been proved to dramatically decrease the risk of perioperative infection in placebo, randomized controlled trials. The ideal timing of the first dose is 30 to 60 minutes before skin incision to allow for peak serum and bone concentrations. A recent, large retrospective review of 1,367 primary total joint arthroplasties demonstrated an equivalent effect of a single preoperative dose of cefazolin compared with a total of three doses of cefuroxime. Because of concerns regarding the increasing prevalence of methicillin-resistant bacteria, a single preoperative dose of teicoplanin has also shown to be effective.

A review of 10,905 patients revealed a decreased revision rate among those treated with parenteral antibiotics and antibiotic cement. Effective antibiotic elution with adequate bactericidal local levels when tobramycin and vancomycin are combined has been demonstrated. Review of the Swedish Hip Registry revealed the use of cement without antibiotics to be a risk factor for infection. Despite its demonstrated effectiveness, antibiotic cement is not routinely used in primary THA as a means of prophylaxis. One theoretic concern limiting its use is evolution of antibiotic-resistant organisms, although there has been no evidence in the literature to support this concern. Other concerns such as weakening of the cement have not been proved. The primary disadvantages to the routine use of antibiotic-loaded cement are cost and the inability to use reinfusion drains when antibiotic-loaded cement is used.

Clinical Evaluation

A high index of suspicion is required to make a timely diagnosis, allowing for the best opportunity to eradicate the infection. The diagnosis may be apparent, particularly in patients with acute, fulminating infection. However, the signs and symptoms in a chronic infection may be subtle. Fever is a classic indicator of infection; however, there is a normal postoperative febrile response that must be distinguished from fever associated with infection. A recent study of 100 patients undergoing total knee arthroplasty and 100 patients undergoing THA revealed that the normal postoperative febrile response peaked on the first postoperative day and normalized by the fifth day. Each patient was treated with a 48-hour course of prophylactic antibiotics, and none developed infection over a 2-year follow-up. In 19% of patients, the maximum body temperature was between 39°C and 39.8°C. There was a trend toward increased postoperative fever when three or more units of blood were transfused. Initiation of a septic workup is not indicated if based solely on the presence of fever, and any investigations should be directed by the clinical assessment. In the acutely infected hip, swelling, erythema, and drainage are common findings. In the chronically infected hip, the clinical findings are sparse and are often indistinguishable from failure for other causes.

Radiographic Evaluation

Plain radiographs have limited usefulness in the diagnosis of infection, except in chronic infection that may manifest radiographic changes, such as lacy periostitis, osteopenia, endosteal resorption, loosening of the prosthesis, and rapid progression of osteolysis. MRI is not widely used because of decreased scan definition resulting from scatter from the metallic implants. MRI can, in some instances, reveal the presence of an abscess and delineate the extent of osteolysis when special so-called metal artifact reduction sequences are used. They may also be useful to define the extent of distal cement when radiolucent cement is used. Untrasound has been used to detect deep abscesses, particularly around the psoas tendon. Similarly, CT may be used, although artifacts from the prosthesis, unless dedicated sequences are used, may limit its utility.

Bone Scanning

Technetium Tc 99m (^{99m}Tc) bone scanning has high sensitivity but low specificity for the diagnosis of infection after THA, making it an effective tool for excluding the diagnosis of infection. Therefore, a positive ^{99m}Tc scan must be interpreted with caution, particularly because the scan can be abnormal for up to 1 year after uncomplicated THA. Indium-111-labeled white blood cell scans have been investigated, for which authors have reported a 77% sensitivity, 86% specificity, 54% positive predictive value, and 95% negative predictive value. The sensitivity and specificity are further improved by performing these two scans in sequence; however, this method cannot distinguish occult infection from mechanical failure. Extending the time frame for the imaging of ^{99m}Tc-labeled white blood cells to 24 hours after injection has been evaluated, and 100% specificity, 100% positive predictive value, and 98% accuracy have been reported. Radioactive labeled immunoglobulin G scans have been investigated, but were found to have a sensitivity and specificity equivalent to that of laboratory investigations and consequently are not widely used. Monoclonal antibody fragment (Fab) scintigraphy has been investigated in the diagnosis of occult infection. The overall sensitivity is 100%, specificity 58%, positive predictive value 57%, and negative predictive value 100%, with 81% accuracy. Its use is limited in those with a Girdlestone arthroplasty because the accuracy decreased to 43% in this patient population. The

clinical usefulness of radionuclide scanning is primarily for exclusion of infection. Delayed imaging may be used in conjunction with three-phase scanning to improve the specificity and thereby increase its ability to make the diagnosis of infection.

Positron Emission Tomography

Positron emission tomography using fluorine-18-fluoro-2-deoxy-D-glucose (FDG-PET) has been investigated. A recent study reported nonspecific increased FDG-PET uptake in the region of the femoral head and neck persisting for an average of 71 months postoperatively in patients with uncomplicated THA. A classification system was developed in which increased FDG-PET uptake in the area of the femoral head and neck or distal to the prosthesis tip was considered nonspecific and increased uptake localized to the proximal femur adjacent to the stem was indicative of infection. An additional study of the same technique reported the location of increased uptake to be more significant than the intensity of the uptake. The sensitivity was 91.7% and the specificity was 96.6% with this classification. The limitations of this study included a small patient population of 41 hips. Additional investigation of this technology is required to establish its role in the diagnosis of infection, although the findings of initial studies appear promising.

Laboratory Evaluation
Serologic Tests

Initial investigation consists of measurement of the erythrocyte sedimentation rate (ESR), C-reactive protein (CRP) level, and white blood cell (WBC) count. An ESR greater than 30 mm/hr has an 82% sensitivity, 85% specificity, 58% positive predictive value, and 95% negative predictive value for THA infection. The ESR has been found to increase postoperatively, reaching an average peak value of 74 mm/hr on the fifth postoperative day. Noninfectious etiologies for an elevated ESR must be considered. Among patients with low-grade infections, there is a more subtle increase in the ESR, which has led some authors to advocate the use of preoperative measurement to allow for postoperative comparison.

The CRP level is a more sensitive indicator of infection. An elevated CRP level greater than 10 mg/L has a sensitivity of 96%, specificity of 92%, positive predictive value of 74%, and negative predictive value of 99% for infection of THA. It reaches a peak level on the second to third postoperative day and subsequently normalizes by 2 to 3 weeks. After the eradication of infection, the CRP level returns to normal more rapidly than the ESR. An increasing CRP level after the third postoperative day is highly suggestive of infection.

The WBC count is not useful in the diagnosis of infection because it is rarely increased. The sensitivity is 20% and the specificity is 96% for THA infection.

Gram Stain Culture and Sensitivity

Hip joint synovial fluid Gram stain and culture should, ideally, be performed after the patient has been off antibiotics for at least 2 weeks. Using the criteria of two out of three positive culture results as indicative of infection, the sensitivity has recently been shown to be 86%, with 94% specificity, 67% positive predictive value, and 98% negative predictive value. Another study reported the sensitivity and specificity compared with intraoperative cultures to be 50% and 88%, respectively. There has been variability of reported sensitivity and specificity in the literature, and discrepancies may be related to technique, method of transportation of the sample to the laboratory, and the criteria used to define a positive result. Current recommendations are for preoperative aspiration, using ultrasound or arthrography to confirm position, with Gram stain and culture, in all patients in whom infection is suspected based on clinical or laboratory criteria. Preoperative aspiration is not required in patients in whom history and physical examination do not suggest infection and both the ESR and CRP level are within the normal range.

The use of ultrasonication of removed THA components to disrupt the bacterial glycocalyx biofilm and thereby improve detection of colonizing bacteria by standard culture techniques has been evaluated. Identification of bacteria in 26 of 120 patients (22%) in whom infection was not suspected has been reported and led to the recommendation of this technique to diagnose occult infection. The most commonly isolated organisms were *Propionibacterium acnes* in 12 patients, followed by staphylococcal species in 10 patients. A more recent study using similar techniques suggested that occult bacterial colonization may occur, but more uncommonly than previously thought. In this study, organisms were identified in only two of 21 implants. Further study of this technique is required, and it currently does not have a role in routine clinical practice.

Molecular Biologic Techniques

Polymerase chain reaction (PCR) has been used to identify the presence of bacteria through isolation of DNA. This technique depends on the availability of bacterial DNA and is unable to distinguish between infecting organisms and dead pathogens, thereby preventing distinction between active and eradicated infection. Standard culture techniques have been found to underestimate the incidence of bacterial colonization compared with that detected using immunofluorescence microscopy and PCR. Immunologic methods documented a 63% incidence of colonized explanted prostheses, whereas PCR detected colonization in 72%. Tissue culture revealed infection in 4%, and combined tissue and implant culture increased the detection rate to 22%. The lack of information regarding organism susceptibility to antibiotics significantly limits the use of these evolving techniques.

Another method of identification of bacteria is the use of enzyme-linked immunosorbent assay (ELISA), which has been associated with a 93.3% sensitivity and 96.9% specificity using immunoglobulin G levels specific to the offending organisms. The limitations of this technique include its specificity to a particular organism and the requirement for repeat testing for additional organisms. This technology continues to evolve, and further refinement may allow for more widespread use of ELISA testing. At present, these are investigational techniques with no role in routine clinical practice.

Intraoperative Gram Stain

Intraoperative Gram stain was prospectively investigated in 202 THAs; using tissue culture as the gold standard, the sensitivity was 19%, the specificity was 98%, the positive predictive value was 89%, and the negative predictive value was 89%. A retrospective review of intraoperative Gram stain reported the sensitivity to be 14.7% with a specificity of 98.8%. Another study reported the sensitivity of intraoperative Gram stain to be 19% with 98% specificity, and positive and negative predictive values of 63% and 89%, respectively. A prospective study of 297 revision total joint arthroplasties was performed with the recommendation that five to six specimens be analyzed and at least three positive surgical specimens be used for the definition of infection, resulting in a sensitivity of 65% and a specificity of 99.6%. The role of intraoperative Gram stain is controversial, given the variability of results.

Intraoperative Culture

Intraoperative cultures have been considered to be the gold standard for the diagnosis of infection. At least three tissue samples are taken from the most affected areas before antibiotic administration. Using the criteria of a positive culture result in two or more samples, the sensitivity is 94%, specificity is 97%, positive predictive value is 77%, and negative predictive value is 99%. An earlier study reported 42 of 138 revision THAs to have a positive intraoperative culture result, of which only one developed infection over the course of an average 4-year follow-up.

A retrospective review of 34 patients with infected total joint arthroplasties revealed that intraoperative synovial fluid analysis inoculated in blood culture vials had a sensitivity of 92%, a specificity of 100%, and an accuracy of 94%. This technique was more sensitive than swab stick cultures and tissue biopsy, particularly in the setting of anaerobic infection, as it reduces exposure of the specimen to air.

Frozen Section and Histology

The criterion value for the histologic diagnosis of infection has been reported to be either 5 or 10 neutrophils per high power field. The sensitivity for the cutoff of

5 neutrophils has been 100%, with a specificity of 96%. Other studies using this criterion have reported a sensitivity of 43% to 80%, specificity of 94% to 100%, and positive and negative predictive values of 74% to 100% and 96% to 98%, respectively, with 98% accuracy. Using the cutoff criterion of 10 neutrophils per high power field, the sensitivity and negative predictive value of this method have not changed; however, the specificity increased to 99% and the positive predictive value increased to 89%.

At the time of the second stage of a two-stage revision, intraoperative frozen section has been investigated using the criterion for infection of 10 neutrophils per high power field. The sensitivity was 25%, with 98% specificity, 50% positive predictive value, and 95% negative predictive value. The authors advocated that in this setting, intraoperative frozen section is effective in excluding the presence of persistent infection. A recent, prospective study investigated the utility of intraoperative frozen section compared with intraoperative culture at the time of revision THA. The sensitivity was 45%, with a specificity of 92%, positive predictive value of 55%, and negative predictive value of 88%, using the cutoff of 10 neutrophils per high power field. These results led the authors to question the usefulness of routine frozen section as a diagnostic test.

Both microbiologic and histologic investigations have been recommended in all patients undergoing revision THA. In 11% of those in whom infection was diagnosed on clinical grounds and by frozen section, microbiologic techniques failed to make the diagnosis, leading to the implication that clinical, histologic, and microscopic findings may need to be combined.

Diagnostic Approach

In conjunction with a detailed history and physical examination and the overall clinical impression, the sensitivity and specificity of investigations can be used to establish a diagnostic approach. In a prospective study of 202 patients, the probability of infection when both the ESR and CRP level were negative was zero; when both were positive, the probability was 83%. These results indicate that if both are negative, it is highly suggestive against infection and further evaluation can be discontinued. When a negative hip aspiration was added to normal ESR and CRP level findings, the probability of infection remained zero. When all three test results were positive, the probability of infection increased to 89%. If the ESR and CRP levels were elevated and intraoperative cultures were positive, there was a 93% probability of infection; if the results of a preoperative aspiration was also positive, the probability of infection was 100%.

The current recommendations are for measurement of the ESR and CRP level initially, with a hip aspiration being performed if these values indicate infection. Radio-nuclide scans should be reserved for patients in whom there is high clinical suspicion in the setting of negative initial test results. Intraoperative tests may, in some instances, be required for definitive diagnosis.

Treatment
Antibiotic Suppression

In one study, 16% of positive intraoperative cultures at the time of revision THA treated with a 6-week course of intravenous antibiotics resulted in reinfection at 2-year follow-up. The course of 19 patients treated with long-term antibiotic suppression was reviewed, and 37% required revision at an average of 4.1 years. The authors suggested that although two-stage exchange revision was preferred, infection could be managed with antibiotic suppression in patients refusing revision or those with medical contraindications. Another study reported 100% eradication of streptococcal infection of orthopaedic implants with a 3- to 6-month course of ciprofloxacin and rifampin. The study included 8 THAs among 31 patients. The addition of rifampin increased the eradication rate from 58% to 100%.

Long-term antibiotic suppression following incision and drainage of total joint arthroplasty was investigated in 36 patients, including 15 THAs. The infection was acute in 47% of patients; however, the results were not stratified on the basis of infection classification. Intravenous cefazolin or oxacillin was used for methicillin-sensitive organisms, and vancomycin was used for resistant organisms with oral rifampin in all instances. The average duration of antibiotics was 52 months; at an average 5-year follow-up, the success rate was 69%, with implant retention in 86.2%. Of the five treatment failures, three were the result of methicillin-sensitive and two the result of methicillin-resistant *S aureus*.

The findings of a retrospective review of nine acute and nine chronic infected total joint arthroplasties, including six THAs, have been reported. Each patient was treated with incision and drainage, intravenous antibiotics for 6 to 8 weeks, and long-term oral antibiotics for an average of 48.9 months. In four patients, including one THA, there was recurrence of infection at an average of 9 months after stopping antibiotic therapy. These recurrent infections occurred in one of the nine early and three of the nine late infections. Two patients with chronic methicillin-resistant *S aureus* infection who were treated with a 2-month course of linezolid were reported to have no recurrence of infection at 9- and 8-month follow-up, respectively.

The usefulness of the CRP level as a determinant of when to discontinue antibiotics was retrospectively investigated in 28 patients treated with a variety of incision and drainage or one- or two-stage exchange. Antibiotics were stopped when the CRP level decreased to less than 10 mg/L and there was suggestion of clinical improvement. The average duration of intravenous antibiotics was 4.6 weeks, with 6.8 weeks of oral antibiotics, and there were no recurrent or persistent infections.

Incision and Drainage
Successful outcomes have been reported in 71% of acute postoperative and 50% of acute hematogenous infections. Others have documented successful results in only 26% of acute infections. The time from onset of symptoms to treatment has been investigated, with a 56% reported success rate among patients treated within 2 days compared with 13% treated more than 2 days after onset of symptoms and no successful outcomes after 2 weeks. Poor results have been consistently reported with chronic infections, with a failure rate of 96% in one study and 94% in another.

At average 6.3-year follow-up, according to a retrospective study of 42 patients composed of 19 acute, 19 chronic, and 4 hematogenous infections, only six patients (14%) were treated successfully, each of whom presented with an acute or hematogenous infection and were treated at an average of 6 days after onset of symptoms. The average time to treatment after symptom onset was 23 days among the remaining patients. The indication for incision and drainage and prosthesis retention was suggested to be an acute infection with less than 2 weeks duration of symptoms.

The outcomes of seven patients with acute postoperative infection who were treated with incision and drainage within 2 weeks of symptom onset were reported at an average 30-month follow-up. There were four acute, two acute hematogenous, and one chronic infection. There were only two instances of persistent infection. Using a Markov statistical model, two-stage exchange revision was compared with incision and drainage. The results revealed improved quality-adjusted life expectancy and cost-effectiveness for revision in younger, healthy patients, whereas incision and drainage was more beneficial in patients with decreased life expectancy.

Arthroscopic débridement of late infection (at an average of 9 days after onset of symptoms) was investigated in eight consecutive patients. Intravenous antibiotics were initiated for 2 to 6 weeks postoperatively, followed by long-term oral antibiotics. At an average 70-month follow-up, no reinfections were reported. The authors emphasized that prompt treatment of infections with sensitive organisms is required for success. The limitation of a small patient group was acknowledged. An additional four patients have been reported, for a total of 12, with one recurrence at an average 6-year follow-up.

Resection Arthroplasty
Although resection arthroplasty is a reliable method by which to eradicate infection, it limits functional outcome

and, therefore, is most appropriate in patients with limited functional demands or extensive medical comorbidities. The results of 78 resections for infection were reported at an average 5-year follow-up, with infection eradication reported in 86% of patients and adequate pain relief in 83%. The authors advocated the use of resection for salvage of infection. The outcome of reimplantation following Girdlestone arthroplasty for treatment of infection in 44 patients with a minimum 2-year follow-up was reported. The average Harris Hip Score increased from 40 to 78 points; however, there was dislocation in 11.4% of patients, reinfection in 2.3%, and substantial limp in 39%, leading the authors to suggest alternative treatment strategies to decrease the complication rate.

Single-Stage Revision
Single-stage exchange revision using antibiotic-loaded cement has been associated with a success rate between 78% and 90%. In a study of 24 patients who were followed for an average of 9.1 years, a recurrence rate of 8.3% was reported. Only 12 of the original 24 patients were included in the final analysis, thus limiting the validity of the results. Exclusion criteria included presence of a draining sinus, inability to adequately débride necrotic tissue, immunocompromised state, or poor bone stock. In a series of 162 single-stage exchange revisions with an average follow-up of 12.3 years, a success rate of 85.2% was reported, with 12.3% requiring a second revision for reinfection. An additional 2.5% of patients had ongoing infection, but their prostheses were retained.

A meta-analysis of single-stage revision included 12 studies with a total of 1,299 patients and an average 4.8-year follow-up. The success rate was 83%. The authors reported that the indications for single-stage revision included a healthy patient with susceptible organisms, good soft tissue and bone stock, no need for extensive reconstruction, and the use of antibiotic cement. They concluded that because few patients meet these requirements, single-stage revision has a limited role. The outcome of 20 consecutive patients, including 3 with an actively draining sinus, was reported at an average 9.9-year follow-up. Antibiotic cement was used, and the average duration of parenteral antibiotics was 5 weeks followed by 4.7 weeks of oral antibiotic therapy. There were no instances of recurrent or persistent infection. All studies have advocated removal of all necrotic tissue and foreign material, use of antibiotic cement, prolonged antibiotics initiated intraoperatively, and patient selection. There have been no studies, to date, directly comparing single- and two-stage exchange revision.

Two-Stage Exchange Revision
The time between stages remains controversial. In one study, 22% of patients who underwent reimplantation

more than 22 weeks after the first stage became reinfected compared with 14% of those treated within 6 weeks. A study of 50 consecutive two-stage revisions reported a 92% success rate with performance of the second stage at 3 weeks, although the authors advocated delaying reimplantation if there were signs of persistent infection, wound healing complications, or poor bone stock. Another series reported 82% success without the use of antibiotic cement compared with 90% success with antibiotic cement and 92% success when antibiotic-loaded cement was left in situ between stages. Poorer results have been consistently reported when antibiotic cement is not used, with reinfection rates ranging between 11% and 18%.

Another issue of debate is the use of allograft at the second stage, which can act as a sequestrum with increased infection rate, as has been reported in between 9% and 11% in some series. One review of 11 patients, with an average 47.8-month follow-up, reported no reinfection. The average time between stages was 5.5 months. Another series of 53 patients undergoing two-stage revision that required femoral impaction grafting reported 4 patients with reinfection (7.5%) at an average 53-month follow-up; 5 patients died within 2 years of the second stage. Factors associated with reinfection included positive intraoperative culture results and radiographic evidence of lucencies between graft and host bone. Combining antibiotics with morcellized allograft bone has been investigated in a porcine model with vancomycin, and good osteogenic activity was reported in healing a tibial defect.

Two-stage revision after 6 weeks of intravenous antibiotics was investigated in 26 patients with antibiotic-resistant organisms and 20 with antibiotic-sensitive organisms. At an average 5-year follow-up, reinfection occurred in 4.8% with antibiotic-sensitive organisms and in 8% with antibiotic-resistant organisms, which was not statistically significant. The results of 19 THAs infected with susceptible organisms and 16 antibiotic-resistant organisms treated with incision and drainage, intravenous antibiotics, and various combinations of repeat incision and drainage or exchange arthroplasty were reported. Infection eradication occurred in 81% with susceptible organisms compared with 48% with resistant strains, which was statistically significant.

The use of oral rifampin between stages, in which an antibiotic-loaded cement spacer was used, was investigated in 10 patients with an average 23.4-month follow-up. There were no instances of reinfection, and the addition of rifampin was believed to assist with the interruption of the biofilm.

Recent studies have called into question earlier reports of poor results with cementless revision at the second stage. The results of 50 consecutive patients were reported at an average 5.8-year follow-up. The reinfection rate was 8%. Antibiotic spacers were used between stages, and the reimplantation was performed at 3 weeks, but delayed in 16% of patients because of wound healing concerns or medical comorbidities. Following reimplantation, antibiotics were continued for a minimum of 3 months. This study included 18 patients in whom morcellized allograft was used with no reinfection. Cementless reconstruction was reported in another 25 patients at an average 41-month follow-up, with recurrence in 8%. Six weeks of antibiotic therapy were completed between stages. The results of cementless revision THA following two-stage exchange using an antibiotic cement spacer was reported in nine patients at an average 35.7-month follow-up. There was a successful outcome in eight patients, and one patient experienced recurrent infection. All series reported no adverse outcomes because of a lack of locally delivered antibiotics or use of allograft and emphasized the potential for improved long-term fixation with cementless revision.

Articulated Spacers

The past 5 years have seen an increased use of articulated spacers between stages. The prosthesis with antibiotic-loaded acrylic cement (PROSTALAC, DePuy, Warsaw, IN) has been the most extensively studied spacer. The most commonly used combination of antibiotics is 3.6 g of tobramycin and 1.5 g of vancomycin for each package of polymethylmethacrylate cement. If a drain is to be used postoperatively, there should be no suction used because it will decrease the local antibiotic concentration. A review of 48 patients revealed infection eradication in 94%, with 80% having a Harris Hip Score of greater than 80 or a greater than 30-point increase postoperatively. The Harris Hip Scores increased, on average, from 34 to 55 points between stages. The improved functional results were the result of increased mobility and limb-length preservation between stages. There were two periprosthetic fractures, one of which required fixation, and seven dislocations, none of which required revision. There were 43 patients satisfied with function, 3 were dissatisfied, and 2 were uncertain. The prosthesis with antibiotic-loaded acrylic cement has also been investigated in 30 patients with major proximal femoral bone loss at an average 47-month follow-up. Infection eradication was documented in 96% of patients. Weight bearing was restricted because of the large degree of bone loss. There were five dislocations; during the latter course of the study, four patients were treated with a snap-fit cup, which was designed to decrease the risk of dislocation. None of these patients experience dislocation, although additional study is required to determine the effectiveness of this design.

Several other devices based on principles similar to those used in prostheses with antibiotic-loaded acrylic cement have been suggested. The results in 21 patients treated with a variation acrylic antibiotic-loaded cement spacer (Spacer-G, Tecres, Sommacampagna, Italy) were evaluated at an average 33-month follow-up, and three instances of dislocation and one recurrence of infection were reported. Seventeen patients had infection eradication with no complications. The antibiotic-loaded cement hemiarthroplasty device consists of a Teflon block cast around an Austin-Moore femoral prosthesis that includes a site for insertion of antibiotic cement. Two Steinmann pins are used as the stem; however, full weight bearing is restricted because of mechanical weakness.

In another study, the removed femoral component and antibiotic cement with a cup-shaped cement spacer was used in 26 patients with an average 63-month follow-up. The antibiotic combination consisted of 1 g of tobramycin for each package of cement. The success rate was 96%. Another method used a central flexible rod with antibiotic cement molded around it in 20 patients with an average 38-month follow-up. There was a 10% rate of spacer fracture and dislocation, but no instances of reinfection were reported, and 17 patients underwent successful second-stage reconstruction. The spacer was retained in situ in three patients with no complications.

A single Rush pin has been used as the stem around which antibiotic cement with 3.6 g of tobramycin and 1 g of vancomycin per package was molded. The results were evaluated in 18 patients, of whom 12 had been followed for a minimum of 2 years. Each patient was able to ambulate with assistive devices, and there were no instances of reinfection. The use of a spacer with 2 g each of vancomycin, gentamicin, and cefotaxime was reported in 22 patients. Custom acetabular molds were used to construct the femoral head component, and the stem was molded by hand. Eradication of infection occurred in 95% of patients, and there were no dislocations. Of the 22 patients, 18 were able to ambulate between stages.

The outcome of 12 patients treated with manually molded antibiotic cement spacers using gentamicin was reported. A variety of methods were used to reinforce the cement, including a blade plate, dynamic hip screw, and cannulated screws. The average follow-up was 27 months, and no instances of reinfection were reported; however, complications included dislocation in five patients and cement fracture in one patient because of mechanical weakness.

The results of using either the removed femoral component after being autoclaved or an inexpensive modular component with a cemented polyethylene acetabular liner were investigated in 32 consecutive patients at an average 1.7-year follow-up. Antibiotic cement containing 1 g of vancomycin and 1.2 g of tobramycin per package of cement was used. There were three instances of reinfection (9%).

With the PROSTALAC articulated spacer system, an all-polyethylene snap-in constrained one-size-fits-all

component is cemented into the acetabular defect using highly antibiotic-loaded cement at a late stage of polymerization to allow easy removal at the second stage. A series of molds of variable lengths and sizes are used to manufacture a temporary femoral component. Antibiotic-loaded cement is inserted into the mold, and a metal endoskeleton is then inserted. After cement hardening, the mold is removed, and the final construct is press fit into the femur. The second stage procedure is performed at 3 months, and intravenous antibiotics are given for 6 weeks after the first stage procedure.

Antibiotic Cement

The peak concentration and elution of vancomycin and tobramycin from cement occurs between 3 and 18 hours after implantation, with no substantial increase 5 days postoperatively. At an average of 4 months postoperatively, 47 of 48 joints have measurable levels of tobramycin, and 44 of 48 had measurable levels of vancomycin with the joint. A total of 3.6 g of tobramycin maintains the antibiotic concentration above the breakpoint sensitivity limit for the organism, and less than 2.4 g may allow for development of antibiotic resistance. The standard combination of 1.2 g of tobramycin and 1 g of vancomycin per package of cement may be inadequate for the management of infection.

The pharmacokinetics of 2.5 g of gentamicin and 5 g of vancomycin impregnated in 100 g of cement were studied with the use of microbiologic methods and fluorescence polarization immunoassay. There was synergistic activity against *Escherichia coli* and *Enterococcus faecalis*. The elution of gentamicin was independent of vancomycin, whereas the vancomycin release decreased (from 1.16% of the total amount to 0.51%) when the two were combined. An initial high release of both antibiotics with sustained release from the third until tenth day was reported, at which time the concentration of each drug alone was less than the susceptibility limit of commonly infecting organisms. Gentamicin demonstrated good stability after 10 days at core body temperature, whereas vancomycin demonstrated 15.4% decreased activity at 3 days and 34.1% decreased activity at 10 days.

The effect of different methods of sterilization on the antimicrobial activity of 50-mg and 100-mg doses of gentamicin and 1 g of cefazolin per 40 g of cement molded into blocks was studied. The method of sterilization (gas or steam) did not affect activity. The concentration decreased after 24 hours, but remained greater than the minimum inhibitory concentration for 9 days at the conclusion of the study. A decrease in the strength of gentamicin cement was noted regardless of the dose or method of sterilization, whereas unsterilized and steam-sterilized cefazolin cement both maintained strength compared with plain cement.

The combination of tobramycin and vancomycin has been reported to result in a synergistic increase in elution, with a 68% increase for tobramycin and a 103% increase for vancomycin. One report documented a significant decrease in fatigue strength and a trend toward decreased compressive strength with addition of either tobramycin or vancomycin. In contrast, others studies have reported a minimal decrease in bending strength (between 1% to 6%) and fatigue strength of this combination. The decrease in mechanical strength can be decreased by reducing porosity, with the consequent effect of decreasing elution.

In an animal model, vancomycin levels in bone were greater than threefold the break point of organism susceptibility in 92% of specimens and fivefold the break point in 50%. A decrease in concentration was encountered after 6 months. In vivo studies of vancomycin levels in wound drainage revealed greater than fivefold the break point at 24 hours, but by 4 days the level was equivalent to the break point. Because of the rapid decrease in concentration, there may be an increased risk of development of resistance to vancomycin. The effect of combining vancomycin with other antibiotics was not studied.

The combination of 1.5 g of gentamicin and 40 g of cement has been shown to exceed the 90% minimum inhibitory concentration of *S aureus* and *S epidermidis* for at least 28 days. When 2 g of vancomycin was mixed with 40 g of cement, the 90% minimum inhibitory concentration for methicillin-resistant *S aureus* was exceeded for 6 days.

From the evidence that is available in the literature, it seems unwise to use vancomycin in isolation in bone cement, and the current practice of combining tobramycin with vancomycin is justified.

Treatment of Recurrent Infection

The results of treatment of reinfection are poor. One study of 34 patients with an average 5-year follow-up reported a 38% rate of reinfection, which occurred at an average of 2.2 years. Most patients were subsequently treated with long-term antibiotics or resection arthroplasty. The authors concluded that reinfection is a contraindication to direct exchange, but two-stage exchange may be considered if the reinfection was caused by the same organism.

Early postoperative or acute hematogenous infections that occur within a relatively short period after the onset of symptoms may be treated with débridement and irrigation followed by 6 weeks of intravenous antibiotics and a prolonged course of oral antibiotics until the inflammatory markers are back to normal. A substantial number of patients will not respond to this form of treatment and will have a chronically infected hip replacement. The treatment of choice for a chronic infection at the site of a hip replacement is a two-stage ex-

change arthroplasty. With this technique, treatment is expected to be successful in more than 90% of patients.

Dislocation

Dislocation continues to be one of the most common and frustrating complications of THA. It has even been found to be associated with a higher mortality rate than in patients who never sustain a dislocation. Early dislocation is usually considered to occur within 3 months of the procedure and is more often attributed to soft-tissue laxity. However, 6 weeks and even 1 month have also been used as this transition point based on the presumed time of periarticular soft-tissue healing. Overall, instability is the second most common reason for revision arthroplasty after aseptic loosening. Seventy-five percent to 90% of all dislocations are in a posterior direction. Even among hip replacements done through an anterolateral, direct lateral, or transtrochanteric approach, more than 60% of dislocations are posterior. Sixty percent of dislocations are single events and do not recur. In various studies, 63% to 83% of dislocations are treated successfully with conservative measures. These constitute mainly first and second episodes of instability.

Epidemiology

Most clinical series report a rate of dislocation that varies from 0.4% to 7% following primary THA, with an average of 2% to 3%. A comprehensive review including 16 series and nearly 36,000 hips found an incidence of 2.24% for primary THAs. A more recent review of 6,623 THAs with long-term follow-up described a cumulative risk of 1% at 1 month, 1.9% at 1 year, and an additional 1% cumulative risk per 5 years up to 7% at 25 years (if not revised by that time). The overall incidence of dislocation in this cohort was 4.8%. In revision surgery, the dislocation rate more commonly approaches 10%, and it has been noted to be as high as 26.6% in a series of multiple THA revisions. One study reported an incidence of 7.4% dislocation in more than 1,500 revision THAs that were followed for a mean of 8 years, excluding those done for recurrent instability.

There has been little recent change in the overall rates of instability, which is likely attributable to factors that may balance each other. Conversely, increased surgeon experience, newer implants focused on maximizing range of motion, and improved techniques may actually be decreasing the dislocation rate. THA, however, is now more widely available to patient populations with worse comorbidities, and certain aspects of modularity that actually increase impingement may be increasing the dislocation rate.

Approximately 60% to 70% of dislocations occur in the first 6 weeks after surgery. These are accompanied by a lower rate of recurrence than later first episodes, particularly if they happen in the first month. A first dislocation that occurs later than 3 months has a significantly higher risk of recurrence. Less than 1% of first dislocations occur after 5 years, but these have the highest rate of recurrence (44% to 55%).

Risk Factors

Most studies have found a 2:1 to 3:1 higher risk of dislocation in women, with the greatest discrepancies in first-time dislocators after 5 years. One large review found an overall relative risk of 2.1 for women. Unfortunately, no specific factor in women such as soft-tissue laxity, muscle mass, or bone density has been pinpointed as a possible explanation for this phenomenon.

Patient age greater than 75 years is often referred to as a known risk factor for dislocation. Generally, however, the evidence for age as an independent risk factor for instability is rather weak. The relative risk for patients older than 70 years was 1.3 in another large series compared with those younger than 70 years. The increased number of dislocations in older patients may be confounded by increasing rates of cognitive dysfunction, medical comorbidities, primary diagnoses of femoral neck fracture, and poorer overall health.

It has been speculated that obese patients may develop soft-tissue impingement sooner in movements such as flexion because of the increased limb girth contacting the prominent abdomen, leading to greater ease of dislocation. Tall patients with longer limbs have a greater lever arm that tends to increase forces at the hip, which theoretically might affect the tendency to dislocate. Although one study has found an association between tall male patients and instability, height and weight have not otherwise emerged as major factors influencing hip stability.

Dislocations are more common in hip replacements done for developmental dysplasia of the hip, osteonecrosis, fracture, and inflammatory arthritis when compared with a primary diagnosis of osteoarthritis. This is most likely related to the amount of hypertrophy and fibrosis the capsule has undergone in patients with osteoarthritis, which limits preoperative and postoperative hip motion and contributes to joint stability. Among these, acute fracture is the most strongly linked to dislocation, whether treated with a hemiarthroplasty or a THA and regardless of the approach. Without the stabilizing effect of a thickened capsule, a wider arc of hip motion is attainable, thereby increasing the risk of instability. The dislocation rate may also be influenced in some patients by neurogenic weakness of the hip abductors related to the initial injury or subsequent surgery (such as superior gluteal nerve injury associated with acetabular fracture). A recent prospective cohort study of primary THA done in patients with inflammatory arthritis versus patients with osteoarthritis showed dislocation rates of 10% and 3%, respectively, at a minimum 2-year follow-up.

The most significant preexisting risk factor for dislocation is prior hip surgery. History of surgery on the same hip, for any indication, has been shown to increase the rate of dislocation twofold or more. Probable explanations include impaired muscle strength or dysfunction, damaged soft-tissue attachments to the proximal femur, and the adverse impact these factors have on resting soft-tissue tension and dynamic control of the joint.

Impaired mental status reduces the ability of patients to comply with precautions regarding hip positioning and may make falling more likely. Neurologic disorders such as Parkinson's disease or spasticity caused by a prior stroke can reduce the ability of patients to control their limb position and also increase the frequency of falls. Dislocation rates after THA and endoprosthetic replacement of the hip in patients with Parkinson's disease have been reported to be as high as 37%. In a series of 52 patients with a history of Parkinson's disease who underwent 56 elective THAs, an overall dislocation rate of 10.7% was found (7% with an anterolateral approach and 16% with a posterior approach). An anterolateral approach is recommended, with an adjunctive adductor tenotomy to reduce dislocation risk, in patients with any form of spasticity and a flexion or adduction contracture.

Subclinical neurologic compromise may play a role in an even larger number of dislocations. A prospective, matched-control study found balance and vibration sense to be impaired in patients with dislocations. The presence of neurologic or cognitive dysfunction, including cerebral palsy, muscular dystrophy, psychosis, dementia, or alcohol dependency, has been reported in 22% of one-time dislocators and in 75% of recurrent dislocators compared with 14% in THA patients without a dislocation. Another series found a 13% rate of dislocation in patients with similar neurologic or cognitive diagnoses versus 3% in those without. One large study also found a significant increase in the rate of dislocation among chronic alcohol abusers.

Previous femoral osteotomy can alter the abductor moment, and hip arthrodesis can lead to significant abductor weakness, if not complete atrophy. Beyond the effects of previous surgery, these patients are at particular risk for instability. In other situations, multifactorial causes of poor soft-tissue quality, such as smoking or radiation exposure, can also lead to increased risk of abductor dysfunction, although this is as yet poorly defined in the literature.

Surgical Technique

In one study, a 5.8% dislocation rate was documented using a posterior approach compared with 2.3% with an anterior approach in 10,500 hips. The loss of most posterior soft-tissue restraints was undoubtedly the main culprit, but there also seems to be a tendency to overestimate the anteversion of the cup, and therefore place it in less actual anteversion. This is often because of the pelvis rolling forward when the leg is in the dislocated position and a strong force is applied to the anterior retractors. Recent studies have found dramatically reduced rates of instability when posterior soft-tissue structures are specifically repaired during closure. One group reduced dislocations from 7.5% of patients to 1% by repairing the short external rotators to the greater trochanter. Others found decreased rates of 4% to 0.2% and 6.2% to 0.8% in two different series when reattaching the external rotators and performing a formal capsulorrhaphy. Various other capsulorrhaphy reports found reduced rates of 2.8% to 0.6% in 1,000 patients and 4.8% to 0.7% in more than 1,500 patients. Overall, however, most recent studies that directly compare approaches still find lower dislocation rates with anterolateral or direct lateral approaches. A recent meta-analysis reviewing 14 studies and 13,203 hips found the following rates: 3.23% for posterior (3.95% without soft-tissue repair, 2.03% with posterior repair), 2.18% for anterolateral, 1.27% for transtrochanteric, and 0.55% for direct lateral approaches. This study also compared the incidence of limp and found rates to be comparable (4% to 20% for lateral versus 0 to 16% for posterior approaches). Nonetheless, others believe that larger femoral heads close the gap even more. For example, the subgroup with 32-mm heads in the large 10,500 patient cohort had similar dislocation rates regardless of approach. Although it is difficult to imagine the argument over optimal approach ever being conclusively resolved, when the presurgical risk of dislocation is clearly elevated, it is perhaps wisest to consider an approach other than the posterior approach. Furthermore, if trochanteric osteotomy is performed, ultimate union of the trochanter is the key factor for hip stability. In the same large series, a rate of instability of 2.8% was seen if union of the trochanter occurred versus 17.6% when the trochanter remained ununited with displacement greater than 1 cm. A recent investigation also noted that abductor avulsion or poor healing after a lateral approach may have a similar impact.

Component Orientation

Many orthopaedic surgeons consider acetabular orientation to be the most sensitive factor for predisposing patients to dislocation. A classic article described a safe zone of 40° ± 10° of abduction and 15° ± 10° of anteversion. Outside of this safe range, the rate of dislocation increased fourfold, from 1.5% to 6%. More recently, a revised safe zone of 45° ± 10° of abduction and 20° ± 10° of anteversion has been suggested based on computer

models, with greater anteversion recommended for posterior approaches. Interestingly, although anteversion is consistently linked to the risk of instability, some studies have found little association between abduction angle and dislocation. Rather, it is more commonly recognized that vertical cups cause higher amounts of eccentric wear because of altered loading and because horizontal cups impinge early and decrease range of motion. It is more likely that a given acetabular abduction angle has an associated optimal amount of combined anteversion for the cup and the stem. This has been demonstrated in three-dimensional models in which a smaller abduction angle required greater anteversion of both components to sit, stoop, and tie shoelaces.

The most common implant malposition is believed to be excessive anteversion of the femoral stem. Studies have found that 44% of dislocators have femoral implant malposition compared with only 6% in patients without a dislocation. Although improper stem version has been called a rare isolated cause of instability, it appears that more than 20° of anteversion or less than 0° of retroversion in combination with other factors increases the risk. It is important to recognize that anteversion of both components is additive in preventing posterior instability, but it can risk anterior dislocation if excessive. The interaction of cup and stem position on motion to impingement and dislocation has also been studied using a computer model, and it was shown that femoral position can compensate for or aggravate cup malposition. Combined femoral and acetabular anteversion of 40° has been suggested as optimal. The ideal orientation for components likely depends not only on established guidelines of angulation, but also on the choice of approach, the relative position of the cup and the stem, and patient-related factors. The potential pitfalls of proper implant positioning are listed in Table 1.

Component Location

It has been reported that cups placed in a higher position in the ilium have an increased rate of dislocation. Another study showed that lower acetabular placement (nearer to or at the true hip center) is associated with less instability. Proximal cup positioning may predispose patients to impingement of the bony femur on the ilium. Extended liners and longer femoral neck lengths can somewhat compensate for this problem.

Soft-Tissue Tension

A complex, multifactorial predictor of dislocation, tension in the myofascial sleeve surrounding a THA depends on the position of the hip center, femoral offset, periarticular muscle tone, compliance of the soft-tissue envelope, and the quality of the posterior soft-tissue repair or the relative damage to the abductors and trochanter, depending on the approach. Any factor that ad-

Table 1 | Potential Pitfalls in Proper Implant Positioning

Poor exposure	Lack of visualization of internal landmarks, especially on the acetabular side
Anatomic variations	For example, excessive anteversion seen in dysplastic hips
Peripheral osteophytes	Obscuring the true acetabular rim and orientation
Patient positioning errors	Rolling the pelvis and torso forward, thereby reducing the true anteversion of a cup placed in the "usual" position
Surgical approach	A posterior approach tends to facilitate retroversion of components, especially the acetabulum; the anterolateral approach facilitates proper cup positioning but encourages stem malposition, especially in varus and flexion, and can cause damage to the hip abductors or trochanter that may facilitate dislocation

versely affects the quality of soft-tissue attachments to the proximal femur will tend to increase the dislocation rate. Other examples include double-digit dislocation rates that have been reported in patients who underwent THA and had markedly deficient or absent proximal femoral bone stock. In evaluation of proximal femoral allograft-prosthetic composite replacements, dislocation rates have ranged from 9% to 25%. Similar rates have been reported with proximal femoral replacement stems, which are an alternative surgical technique in many of these patients. They are similarly plagued by dislocation rates ranging from 10% to 25% when combined with conventional acetabular components. These results have led some authors to recommend the prophylactic use of either bipolar heads or constrained acetabular components in these patients to reduce the risk of dislocation.

Implant Design

Femoral Head Size

It has long been postulated that large femoral heads should decrease the rate of dislocation. A large femoral head increases the primary arc range before impingement as well as the excursion distance the head must travel to exit the acetabulum. Moreover, a large femoral head will many times eliminate the need for a skirt when using longer neck lengths, thereby further reducing early impingement. The displacement required of large femoral heads should also cause greater tension in the restraining soft tissues, which tends to prevent dislo-

cation. In spite of these theories, most historical clinical studies have been unable to demonstrate an advantage to using large femoral heads. Even the review of 10,500 primary THAs showed no clinical correlation between femoral head size and dislocation rates. With the evidence that femoral heads larger than 32 mm produced more volumetric polyethylene wear, the practice became unpopular. More recently, however, alternate bearings and improved polyethylene wear characteristics have brought about a second wave of enthusiasm for large femoral heads. Clinical studies have shown more promise, particularly in the revision setting, where the use of large femoral heads has long been believed to be beneficial. A recent series demonstrated decreased rates of instability using 28- and 32-mm femoral heads compared with a 22-mm femoral head in revision THA. A 1999 study showed statistically significant improvements in stability for 32-mm versus 26-mm femoral heads in 2,728 hips, including primary and revision THAs. As yet, there is still a dearth of data on the use of femoral heads larger than 32 mm, but femoral heads this large may show an even more profound effect on the rates of instability. Highly cross-linked polyethylene and other new bearings have made the use of such large heads possible, but early studies on their effectiveness are just now beginning to emerge. One study that assessed metal-on-metal THA found no dislocations in 616 patients with 38-mm femoral heads and a 2.5% dislocation rate in 78 patients with 28-mm heads at 3-month follow-up. In vitro, femoral heads larger than 32 mm were found to have significantly more range of motion, virtually eliminated impingement, and provided a significant increase in both flexion before dislocation and excursion distance. Another in vitro study found excursion distance to increase by 5 mm when a 22-mm femoral head replaced a 40-mm femoral head. More time will be needed to make valid conclusions about the advantages of extra large femoral heads.

Femoral Head-to-Neck Ratio

Probably more important than pure head size, the head-neck ratio is the actual factor that determines the arc range of motion. Modular femoral heads require larger necks for stability compared with older monoblock stems, and longer neck lengths, when required, often need to be supplemented by a skirt. Both these factors lead to a decreased femoral head-neck ratio and thus a smaller effective range of motion before impingement. This has been proved to cause more wear, but should logically also increase the rate of dislocation. Once again, experimental evidence has corroborated these findings, but clinical studies have so far been inconclusive or underpowered.

Femoral Head-to-Acetabulum Ratio

This relationship, on the other hand, has been proved to be clinically relevant. In a prospective randomized trial, it was found that 22-mm femoral heads (versus 28-mm femoral heads) dislocated more frequently when matched with a cup that was 56 mm or larger (versus cups ≤ 54 mm). In a larger retrospective cohort, the same group found that 28-mm femoral heads dislocated more often if the acetabulum was greater than 60 mm. The proposed explanations are that such a large femoral head-acetabular ratio causes the pseudocapsule to reattach more than 1 cm away from the head, basically eliminating its role as a checkrein to head escape or that it causes the bony femur to impinge on the cup rim even before the neck impinges on the liner, limiting range of motion significantly.

Femoral Offset

Reestablishing femoral offset to properly tension the abductor musculature and to avoid bony femoropelvic impingement is a well-recognized tool in limiting instability. Clinical studies have demonstrated a strong correlation between decreased offset and higher rates of dislocation. Surgeons must be vigilant, however, to avoid the temptation of excessively lengthening the leg just so that offset can be recreated. Other methods, such as stems with more medial takeoff of the femoral neck or a more varus neck angle, are available to achieve offset goals without adding to leg length. When a longer femoral neck length does seem necessary, surgeons are cautioned against the use of skirted heads and should perhaps consider offset liners to reach the same end result with less risks of impingement. Both of these methods do, however, lengthen the leg. It is important to remember that although offset is associated with dislocation, stability has not been shown to be related to leg length itself. Diligently removing periarticular osteophytes is another way to minimize impingement risks.

Femoral Neck Geometry

Experimental and small clinical studies have shown that trapezoidal femoral necks provide greater range of motion before impingement and result in fewer dislocations than circular necks.

Liner Profile

Acetabular liners with an elevated rim, usually placed posteriorly, increase the amount of contact with the femoral head in the area at risk for dislocation, thereby locally increasing jump distance. They also, however, decrease effective range of motion in extension and external rotation, causing earlier impingement. A 2.19% versus 3.7% rate of dislocation was found when 10° elevated rimmed liners were compared with standard liners in 5,100 Charnley THAs. The effect was significant at 2-year follow-up but not at 5-year follow-up be-

cause of smaller numbers, and despite a later report that no increase in loosening was seen with the elevated liners, their routine use in primary THA was not recommended. Twenty degree liners have been called excessive and risky for opposite direction dislocation. Various newer modifications to liner profiles have broadened the applications for their use, and other modifications have attempted to keep the benefits of traditional elevated liners while minimizing the disadvantages. So-called oblique liners with built-in version can reorient the arc of motion without decreasing it, which is especially useful in a well-fixed but slightly malpositioned cup. Offset or lateralized liners move the hip center away from the midline, increasing offset and leg length as mentioned. Elevated liners with a smaller-angled and wider chamfer zone have been shown to have a comparable ability to withstand dislocation while maintaining greater range of motion. Although this is another tool with some efficacy that can be considered for selective use in patients with high risk, this type of liner has not been recommended for routine use.

Late Dislocation

When dislocations first occur more than 5 years after THA, a slightly different set of risk factors and outcomes seems to apply. Historically, late dislocations are thought to constitute fewer than 1% of instances of instability, recur at higher rates (> 50%), and require revision surgery more often (45% versus 33% overall). In this subset, no association to prior hip surgery, surgical approach, or trochanteric union status was found. The patients with dislocation did tend to have a greater range of motion, especially in flexion. One theory purports that in this subset of patients, the pseudocapsule stretches over time and leads to decreased soft-tissue restraints. Others believe that polyethylene wear and cold flow lead to deeper seating of the head in the cup, sooner impingement, and increased instability. In terms of treatment, equal success rates have been reported for surgical correction of dislocations occurring more than 5 years after THA compared with those of dislocations first occurring at less than 5 years after THA. A study of 19,680 primary THAs has recently shed some more light on the circumstances surrounding late dislocators. The authors of this study found a significantly higher incidence than previously reported, with 32% (165 of 513) of the dislocations occurring more than 5 years after THA. The entire cohort had a dislocation rate of 2.6%. The authors also detected several separate processes, some distinct from those associated with early dislocation, that seem to be predictors of late instability. These include female gender, younger age at primary THA (63 years versus 67 years), history of subluxation without dislocation, a substantial episode of trauma, and recent decline in cognitive or neurologic function. Associated

Table 2 | Principles of Dislocation Prevention

All Patients

Careful preoperative plan using the normal hip as a reference	Note the center of rotation to guide cup placement Plan for adequate medialization Attempt to recreate normal length and offset
Careful intraoperative visualization	Adequate exposure: it is important to see the entire acetabular rim and on the femoral side expose down to the level of the top of the lesser trochanter Remove periarticular osteophytes Prepare the cup from the abdominal side of the patient, regardless of the approach Identify the sciatic notch, ischium, both walls, rim, and transverse ligament
Rely primarily on internal anatomic landmarks	Edge of the sciatic notch equates to 25° of anteversion for the cup Use the tip of the greater trochanter as a marker for the center of rotation of the femoral head to verify correct length Beware of external alignment guides
Carefully check and recheck	Motion Impingement Stability in extension and 90° flexion with and without internal and external rotation and abduction and adduction
If it does not feel right intraoperatively, better to fix it than hope for the best	
Careful repair of the muscle attachments for all surgical approaches, but especially for the posterior approach	

High-Risk Patients

Consider the anterior approaches for some high-risk conditions (such as cerebral palsy parkinsonism)

Check for an adduction contracture intraoperatively and consider a tenotomy if present

Consider increasing the offset or length (up to 1 cm) for improved stability

Consider the use of an extra large diameter femoral head if it is available for the implant being used

Consider an elevated rim liner in a revision on well-fixed cup and suboptimal intraoperative stability or cup position

Consider trochanteric advancement in isolated acetabular cup revisions with retained femoral components and lax soft tissues

Consider prophylactic postoperative bracing or, less frequently, casting

Consider the use of a constrained insert or tripolar design for extremely high-risk patients (such as takedown of a hip fusion, paralysis of hip musculature, proximal femoral resection and/or replacement, revision of a multiply operated patient, recurrently unstable hip). Remember all constrained acetabular inserts are not the same. Mechanical failures and disassemblies have been reported. Use of a validated design is strongly encouraged

Consider the use of computer navigation; although proponents claim this should reduce dislocation risk by improving the precision of implant position and reducing outliers, no data from large clinical series are yet available to document this advantage

radiographic findings were acetabular implant malposition, polyethylene wear of greater than 2 mm, and some loose implants with migration. The recurrence rate was 55%, and revision THA was performed in 33% of patients. It has also been shown that marked weight loss in a relatively short time, particularly if related to a chronic illness but also if voluntary, is an important risk factor for late dislocation.

Risk of Recurrent Instability

Thirty-three percent of dislocations recur. Men have a higher overall rate of chronic instability. There is also a higher likelihood of recurring dislocation if the first episode occurs more than 3 months postoperatively. As with a first episode, prior hip surgery is the number one risk factor for dislocation recurrence. The two most common causes of dislocation recurrence are component malposition and failure of the abductor mechanism. The principles of dislocation prevention are listed in Table 2.

Acute Management

After performing a thorough history and physical examination, including limb neurovascular status, AP pelvis, AP hip, and cross-table lateral hip radiographs should be obtained to confirm the direction of the dislocation. These radiographs may also display other rare but potentially important findings, such as liner dissociation, femoral head-neck dissociation, greater trochanter migration, or fracture. If no indications for emergent open reduction are found, a gentle closed reduction can be attempted and is typically successful in more than 90% of patients. It is preferable to perform this procedure with the patient under general anesthesia in the operating room, but if this is not imminently available, monitored conscious sedation in the emergency department is acceptable. For posterior dislocations, the Allis maneuver or some variation should be attempted first. In-line traction is applied to the femur through the lower leg while being ever mindful of the knee, particularly if a total knee replacement is present. The hip is then gently flexed toward 90°. An assistant should apply downward pressure on the anterior-superior iliac spine. A second assistant, if available, should push or milk the femoral head back into the acetabulum from the affected side. The leg is rocked back and forth from internal rotation to external rotation. Finally, progressive adduction is added to optimize the femoral head location for reduction. Alternatively, the Stimson position can be used. The patient is placed in the prone position, however, which complicates monitoring and ventilation if needed. The legs are allowed to dangle off the distal edge of the bed at the hips. The hips and knees are brought to 90°. Downward in-line traction is applied to the hip through the calf, and again a rocking motion is performed between internal and external rotation. If these are unsuccessful, closed reduction under general anesthesia may be necessary, and open reduction is necessary if the latter procedure fails. On reduction, stability should be verified with gentle physiologic ranging of the hip. If open reduction is required, the current radiograph (as well as older radiographs if available) should be scrutinized for identifiable and correctable sources of instability. It is also imperative to rule out any suspicion of infection because infection can be a rare cause of spontaneous dislocation after THA.

Postreduction radiographs should include an AP pelvis, AP hip, and cross-table (true or groin) lateral view of the hip. In addition to confirming reduction, the first two radiographs should be used to assess the abduction angle, limb-length discrepancy, and offset. On the lateral radiograph, the amount of anteversion (or retroversion) should be estimated by comparing the inclination of the cup to a vertical line drawn perpendicular to the radiograph, keeping the ischial tuberosity posterior (Figure 1). Physicians should be aware, however, that pelvic rotation (whether the patient was flat on the table) can alter the apparent anteversion. CT is the diagnostic imaging modality of choice to accurately measure anteversion.

Definitive Treatment

Once acute reduction is achieved, if surgery was not required, many options are available. For a first or second episode of dislocation, observation can be used for a re-

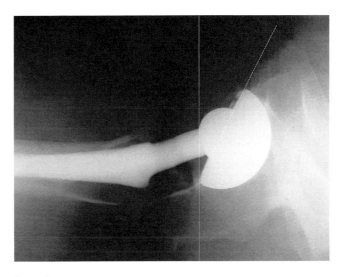

Figure 1 Lateral radiograph showing the amount of anteversion estimated by comparing the inclination of the cup to a vertical line drawn perpendicular to the radiograph.

liable patient who clearly recalls accidentally violating the prescribed hip precautions via a slip or minor fall, but this should only be done if the patient's neurologic or cognitive function is not in question. Otherwise, conservative measures may consist of an abduction brace that limits adduction to −15° and flexion to 60° for 6 weeks to 3 months. A spica cast can also be used in unreliable or noncompliant patients. Spica casts tend to have the highest success in the treatment of early dislocations because they allow soft-tissue healing that had not yet occurred to take place without additional assault. Of note, a recent randomized study has shown bracing to be ineffective in preventing the recurrence of dislocation. Protected weight bearing, physiotherapy for muscle strengthening, and patient reeducation should be part of any treatment protocol for patients with dislocations. At the first postreduction office visit, radiographs should be carefully examined for obvious sources of instability such as component malposition, grossly deficient offset, or trochanter deficiency. These sources of instability, however, will typically be detected only in a small number of patients with first or second dislocations.

Capsulorrhaphy or trochanteric advancement can be considered in patients with recurrent instability in whom all of the components appear well positioned and no obvious cause can be detected. These techniques are even more successful in patients in whom soft-tissue tension is judged to be inadequate. Modular or so-called bloodless revision has become increasingly popular and can be successful with the proper indications. With presumed abductor laxity or an offset deficit, revision to a longer neck length or an offset liner restores more offset and lengthens the leg, thereby improving abductor function. Again, these strategies should only be used in patients with well-fixed, well-positioned components. Studies have found that modular revision is effective for treating dislocation after primary THA, but much less so for dislocations after THA revisions. Exchange to a large femoral head may be considered for patients with wide range of motion who have a high suspicion of impingement and a small current femoral head-neck ratio. On revision, signs of impingement on the liner and on the femoral neck or obvious osteophytes should be sought to confirm impingement as the correct etiology. If none are found, additive measures such as an offset liner may improve chances of success.

Loose components should obviously be revised. It is also recommended that well-fixed components that are malpositioned undergo revision, particularly those with retroverted acetabuli or excessive combined anteversion with resultant anterior dislocation. In this scenario, simply removing presumed sources of impingement has shown a much lower success rate than repositioning a maloriented implant (33% versus 69%). When multiple revisions have failed or in recurrences with causes that cannot be identified or corrected, such as severely deficient abductors, the most extreme alternatives must be entertained. Ring-locked or tripolar constrained liners, conversion to a bipolar head, soft-tissue grafts or slings, and resection arthroplasty constitute the salvage procedures for chronic instability.

Constrained acetabular cups or locking liners may be necessary when significant intraoperative laxity remains despite using a large femoral head, offset liner, elevated rim liner, or otherwise maximizing the offset. Different models have had acceptable success rates in short- and medium-term studies. One study on constrained liners reported a 97.6% success rate (83 of 85 hips were stable) at 4.8-year follow-up, with an 8.2% reoperation rate. Others studies have noted a 96% success rate at 51-month follow-up with the same implant. Another type of locking liner was found to be successful in 91% of patients at 30-month follow-up and successful in 71% of patients at 31-month follow-up in two separate studies. A 10-year follow-up of tripolar constrained cups noted a 6% failure rate by repeat dislocation in 101 patients. It must be recognized, however, and carefully explained to the patient, that although these implants may significantly reduce the risk of instability, complications such as wear, early loosening, decreased range of motion, and disengagement are potential risks associated with their use. All methods of disassembly have been reported, ranging from the femoral head coming off the neck to the entire cup escaping the pelvis (Figure 2). Furthermore, repeat dislocation is virtually impossible to reduce closed, and when it can be done, it is highly suggested that revision be performed to check the locking mechanism. A Girdlestone resection arthroplasty is probably a more judicious choice in noncompliant or debilitated patients as well as for chronic alcohol

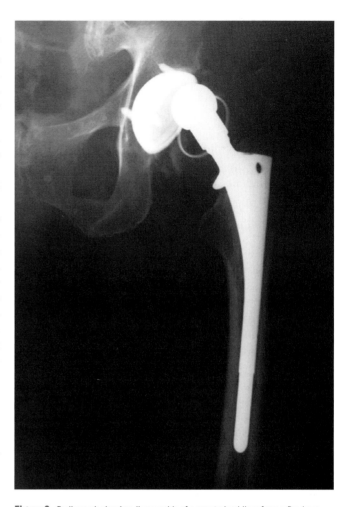

Figure 2 Radiograph showing disassembly of a constrained liner from a fixed cup.

abusers and patients with failed constrained cups or liners.

When approaching the problem of recurrent dislocation, many follow the three strikes rule. It has been shown that second dislocations still have a favorable treatment rate with conservative measures. Once the decision for revision is made, often after the third dislocation, a fervent effort should be made to find the underlying source. A thorough history should be taken, including position at the time of dislocation, alcohol use, and signs of low-grade infection. Reexamining the original and subsequent radiographs and CT scans may detect offset or orientation problems. These steps are important because reported success rates are more than 70% when the underlying cause is known and corrected, whereas if the etiology is not known success rates tend to fall below 50%. Trochanteric advancement, however, in the face of recurrent instability without obvious cause, has been shown to be 75% to 84% successful.

Instability after THA is a multifactorial problem. Certain factors clearly predispose patients to dislocation, such as major component malposition and greater trochanter migration, whereas other more subtle characteristics combine to increase the risk. No patient can be told they will or will not experience dislocation. However, meticulous surgical technique can minimize the sources of instability that are under the surgeon's control. The choice of approach and subsequent repair, femoral head sizes, optimal positioning, and methods for guiding implantation should continue to be studied to decrease the dislocation rates even further. A later first episode raises the likelihood of recurrence. Overall, about two thirds of these events will respond to nonsurgical management. Once the instability has become chronic, the key to successful surgical correction is finding and treating the underlying cause.

Limb-Length Inequality

Limb-length inequality is one of the most annoying complications and a leading cause of patient dissatisfaction and subsequent litigation after THA. The primary goals of THA are restoration of limb length, femoral offset, and center of rotation that results in a stable hip with normal gait and function. However, clinical recognition of limb-length inequality before surgery facilitates appropriate treatment during surgery. There are two essential components of limb-length inequality. The first is the actual limb-length discrepancy at the hip joint or anatomic component, which is the result of an alteration of the geometry of the hip joint itself. The second component is the apparent or functional component that is secondary to a tilt of the pelvis resulting from periarticular hip joint soft-tissue flexion-abduction contractures or fixed degenerative spinal abnormality.

A review of the early literature has confirmed an incidence of limb-length inequality in up to 50% of patients after THA. Of these patients, approximately 15% to 20% will require contralateral shoe correction to provide equalization of limb lengths. In addition, it is important to emphasize the relationship between limb length, offset, and the incidence of dislocation. A slight increase in the limb length, offset, or both can markedly improve the stability of the hip.

The goal of surgery is to avoid limb-length inequality after THA and achieve normal anatomic geometry of the hip. Thus, there are three important technical aims: restoration of the center of rotation of the socket; restoration of the offset, which in turn governs the abductor function and soft-tissue balance/stability; and restoration of the distance between the center of the femoral head and the lesser trochanter. Hence, the location of the socket should match the opposite side on the postoperative radiograph. The offset is the distance between the center of the femoral head and the central axis of the medullary canal, which along with the distance from the lesser trochanter to the center of the femoral head, determines the limb length and the soft-tissue tension, provided the center of rotation of the ac-

etabular socket or the hip is in the normal position. As mentioned previously, both of these factors contribute to limb-length inequality after THA.

Apparent or functional limb-length inequality is a discrepancy that is attributable to tightness of the anterolateral soft tissues about the hip or lumbar spine pathology, which usually includes degenerative disease with scoliosis resulting in pelvic obliquity. The apparent limb length can be estimated in the supine patient by measurement of the distance between the umbilicus and the medial malleolus or with the use of progressively thicker blocks under the contralateral foot until a sense of balance is confirmed by the standing patient. It is important to recognize that functional limb-length inequality may be present before THA because of soft-tissue contractures around the hip or lumbar spine deformity, resulting in fixed or nonfixed pelvic obliquity, depending on the chronicity of the etiology. Moreover, it is possible for the diseased hip to be shorter in terms of true limb-length measurement and functionally longer secondary to either an ipsilateral hip abduction contracture or fixed pelvic obliquity because of lumbar spine degenerative disease. Recognition of lumbar spine disease as the cause of functional limb-length inequality before surgery allows the surgeon to inform patients that THA will not correct the limb-length problem and may sometimes necessitate an additional shoe lift. In addition, attempts to correct functional limb-length inequality by increasing true leg length may increase the risk of nerve injury, whereas decreasing true leg length can affect hip stability.

Pelvic obliquity may also result from soft-tissue tightness in the hip periarticular structures, including the anterior hip capsule, rectus femoris muscle, psoas muscle and tendon, tensor fascia lata, and gluteus medius and minimus muscles. Hip disease can result in flexion and abduction or adduction contracture of the involved side with or without associated pelvic obliquity. In some patients, hip arthritis with an adduction contracture results in a short leg because of the additive effect of both anatomic and functional components. Correction of the true limb-length discrepancy is the only component required to address the pelvic obliquity and functional length component in this situation. In contrast, functional leg lengthening could result from an abduction contracture of the ipsilateral hip or adduction contracture of the contralateral hip without soft-tissue contracture on the affected side. Hence, careful preoperative recognition and clinical evaluation of the cause of functional limb-length inequality allows surgeons to counsel patients regarding expectations of limb-length correction after THA as well as to facilitate surgical plans to optimize limb length during and after surgery.

The evaluation of functional limb-length inequality after THA is usually evident when the patient stands. The complaints are typically leg lengthening and imbalance with pain in the groin or outer aspect of the hip. Sometimes low back or iliac crest pain may be present. The pelvis is tilted downward on the affected side because of tight anterior and/or lateral structures, and the ipsilateral knee attitude is either flexion or results in valgus deformity of the knee because of a tight iliotibial band. The patient's description of the magnitude of inequality typically far exceeds the radiographic measurements or true limb lengths, and the gait is usually awkward. In most of these patients, the natural history of postoperative functional limb-length inequality is a self-limited course, with a small number of patients having persistent symptoms. Most of these patients respond to soft-tissue stretching of tight abductors and iliotibial band, with physical therapy focused on lumbar spine extension and pelvic tilt exercises for 6 to 8 months after surgery. Persistent functional limb-length inequality is uncommon if hip soft-tissue tightness is the cause. It is usually observed in patients with short stature with varus femoral neck or hip protrusio deformity and is often associated with lumbar spine disease with a minor degree of fixed pelvic obliquity. Rarely, if pain is a significant complaint, soft-tissue release or exchange with a reduced offset femoral component at revision surgery may be needed.

There are various methods to restore anatomic limb length during THA. One method involves the use of radiographic templates to estimate femoral neck resection, whereas other described caliper methods include the use of fixed points on the pelvis (ilium) and greater trochanter during surgery (before and after THA) to measure the limb-length inequality and alterations made at surgery. These points are usually located away from the center of rotation of the hip, and the position of the limb in terms of abduction, flexion, and rotation has the potential for significant error in measurement. Other methods of determining limb length have included the shuck test, palpation of the knees and medial malleoli during trial reduction, intraoperative radiographs, and computer-assisted surgery.

Recently, a method for assessing limb length has been described and validated in terms of accuracy and predictability. This method comprises the placement of a Steinmann pin in the vertical orientation in the infracotyloid notch of the acetabulum (Figures 3 and 4). A mark is made with the diathermy on the greater trochanter that corresponds to the position of the pin before the dislocation of the hip, and the position of the limb is marked. The hip is dislocated, and the offset and the distance between the lesser trochanter and the center of the head are measured. These measurements are used after implantation of the femoral component to confirm the reconstruction of the anatomic geometry of the hip joint. After the socket is implanted, the femur is prepared and trial components are used. An attempt is made to match the offset and the lesser trochanter to

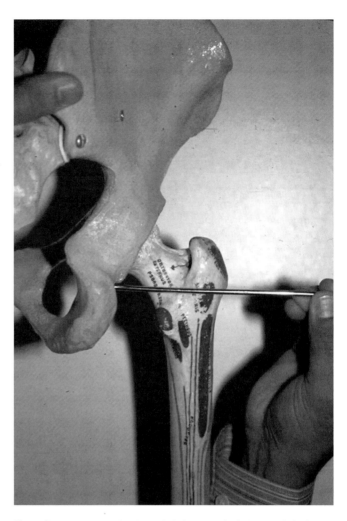

Figure 3 Photograph showing the vertical placement of a Steinmann pin in the acetabular infracotyloid groove.

the center of the femoral head distance with the previously measured dimensions. The hip is relocated at this stage, and the Steinmann pin is reinserted in the same orientation into the infracotyloid groove of the acetabulum, with the limb in the same position as before initial hip dislocation. The prior reference mark on the greater trochanter facilitates an evaluation of the amount of lengthening or shortening of the limb that has occurred. After preparation of the femur and implantation of the femoral component, the offset and distance of the lesser trochanter to the center of the femoral head is measured once again to confirm the dimensions attained with the trial implants. The hip is now reduced, and two important facets (soft-tissue contracture and combined anteversion) are assessed at this stage. The combined anteversion is evaluated with the hip in a position of neutral abduction/adduction and slight flexion (10°). The femur is internally rotated to approximately 45°. The socket and the femoral head should be coplanar or concentrically aligned at this stage. This position confirms that a good relationship and appropriate antever-

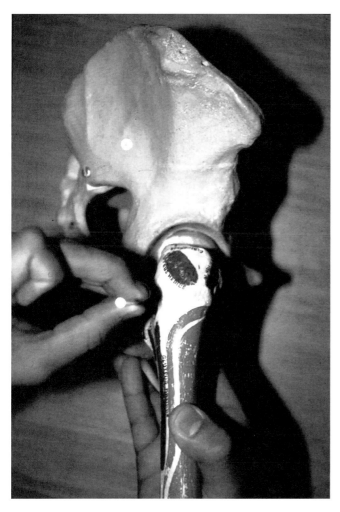

Figure 4 Photograph of a lateral view of a hip joint demonstrating the placement of a vertical Steinmann pin in the infracotyloid groove of the acetabulum.

sion has been attained between the socket and the femoral component. The soft tissues assessed for tightness include the anterior capsule, iliotibial band, iliopsoas, and rectus femoris. Tightness of the tensor fascia lata and anterolateral soft tissues is assessed using the Ober test, with palpation of the fascia lata as the leg is adducted and the knee is flexed. Tightness of the anterior capsule is evaluated with the hip in full extension and maximal passive external rotation when the posterior aspect of the greater trochanter should come within one fingerbreadth of the ischial tuberosity without making contact.

The advantages of the infracotyloid Steinmann pin technique are simplicity, accuracy, predictability, and proximity to the center of hip rotation, thereby reducing magnification of measurement errors. Shortcomings include a learning curve and inaccurate pin placement or limb position. The magnitude of limb lengthening that is appropriate after THA in most patients is 0 to 5 mm, with a maximum of 10 mm in taller patients. Patients shorter than 5 feet need particular attention because

even 5 mm of lengthening may be objectionable. It is, however, worth bearing in mind that in an average patient, 3 to 5 mm of femoral head-neck lengthening and a slight increase in the offset makes for a marked improvement in the stability of the THA.

As discussed previously, functional limb-length inequality after hip disease is secondary to pelvic tilt that in turn is usually the result of the tightness of the anterolateral structures crossing the hip, causing an abduction contracture. Tightness of the anterolateral structures may be caused by an increase in the anatomic limb length, and an additional increase in the offset may result in tightness of the iliotibial band. Pelvic obliquity may be the result of an adduction contracture of the contralateral hip or the result of spinal deformity caused by degenerative spine disease. In addition, excessive advancement of the greater trochanter after osteotomy may cause an abduction contracture. Patients who are at risk for limb-length inequality include those of short stature and those with hip dysplasia, protrusio deformity, hyperlaxity, preoperative longer lower limb, increased offset and/or limb length resulting in tight anterolateral structures, cementless fixation, and fixed pelvic obliquity secondary to lumbosacral spinal deformity.

The problem of anatomic limb lengthening after THA may result in an unhappy patient, especially in the face of a concomitant abduction contracture. The treatment of the anatomic limb-length discrepancy may necessitate the use of a shoe lift in the contralateral limb. In rare instances, surgery in the form of offset reduction is required to correct the limb-length discrepancy. In addition, the effects of limb lengthening are unpredictable and may not necessarily correlate with the magnitude of the length discrepancy. It is thus vital to be aware of the functional limb-length inequality before surgery. The surgeon must avoid increasing the anatomic limb length and offset that may result in a soft-tissue contracture, and secondary pelvic tilt that further accentuates the magnitude of the anatomic limb-length inequality. In the event that increased anatomic limb length, offset, or both are necessary to attain hip joint stability, appropriate documentation and discussion with the patient should follow.

The problems of limb-length inequality after THA may be avoided if attention is paid to preoperative clinical and radiographic planning. Additionally, patient education is as important as restoration of the anatomic and functional geometry of the hip. It should be emphasized that a small increase in the limb length and offset will significantly improve hip stability. It is advisable to evaluate soft-tissue contractures, component orientation at the time of implantation, and attempt to recreate the anatomic dimensions of the hip joint during THA. It is worth mentioning that functional limb length usually improves with time, although rarely surgical correction may be warranted.

Periprosthetic Fractures

Fracture associated with THA is a serious, multifactorial problem that requires an in-depth knowledge for prevention, recognition, and management. Fractures may be categorized as those that occur intraoperatively and those that occur postoperatively. Fractures about the acetabulum are rare, but the incidence may be rising because of the volume of patients requiring primary and revision arthroplasty, the increasing number of elderly patients with osteoporosis, the preference of cementless fixation methods that emphasize use of an oversized press-fit implant, and recent evolutionary techniques that minimize surgical exposure. Femoral fractures are more common than acetabular fractures. According to the Mayo Clinic Joint Registry, the incidence of intraoperative fractures was 0.3% of patients with cemented and 5.4% of those with cementless prostheses after primary arthroplasty and 3.6% of patients with cemented and 20.9% of those with cementless prostheses after revision arthroplasty. For postoperative fractures, the incidence is estimated to be 0.1% to 2.5% of patients over the life of the implant. Data from the Swedish National Joint Registry emphasize the severity of postoperative femoral periprosthetic fractures, with over 70% of patients having a loose femoral component at the time of fracture, 30% requiring at least one revision, and 39% reporting no pain at follow-up after surgical attempt of revision arthroplasty.

In patients with no prior surgery, intraoperative risk factors include increased bone fragility and osteopenia, rheumatoid arthritis compared with osteoarthritis, female gender, and deformity of the bone that may result from conditions such as developmental dysplasia. In the later instance, the intramedullary canal may be small in addition to anatomic variation of the proximal femur. For the acetabulum, those underreamed by more than 2 mm, patients with smaller pelves, females older than 60 years, and patients with irradiated pelves appear to be at greatest risk. With larger acetabulae, fractures tend to involve the rim, but with smaller acetabulae, major column fractures are more likely. Preservation of the subchondral plate of the anterior, posterior, and medial walls during reaming is important to maintain a strong foundation for component stability.

Several authors have cited an elevated risk of fracture during revision arthroplasty. Factors that increase the risk of fracture include diminished bone stock, altered bone morphology, the presence of bone defects, and in certain patients, prior hardware placement. Following femoral osteotomy or fracture fixation, hardware placement can lead to dense sclerotic bone or stress risers from screw removal that may, in turn, lead to subsequent fracture. Cortical perforation of the femoral canal, which can be associated with cement extrusion, has been cited as a substantial risk for late fracture. This

problem must be identified early and treated with cement removal and bone grafting to correct the mechanical weakness. Certain prosthetic constructs are prone to fracture and ultimate failure. Large femoral components have a higher risk of fracture when used in the revision setting. Weakened segments of bone from failed prior implant placement may lead to fracture if not supported by a new revision implant or an impaction grafting method that bypasses the defect. Abnormal segments of bone should be bypassed by the revision prosthesis by at least 5 cm or two diaphyseal cortical diameters. Acetabular and femoral fractures have been reported after the removal of well-fixed implants. This is especially true with extensively porous-coated devices, and specialized methods are needed to remove these implants. On the femoral side, sectioning the femoral stem and using sized trephines allows distal stem removal. For ingrown acetabular devices, careful interface exposure is needed. Sectioning the cup with a diamond-tip drill and using specialized tools such as the Explant cup osteotome (Zimmer, Warsaw, IN) can aid in difficult instances where the medial wall has incorporated into the implant.

Osteolysis in THA causes progressive nonlinear bone loss and must be identified on serial radiographs for timely intervention. In the acetabulum, bone loss may be extensive, leading to catastrophic component failure. Osteolytic bone defects and small fractures are not always apparent on routine plain radiographs and are typically underestimated. Specialized pelvic radiographs, such as Judet internal and external oblique views, and spiral CT can help identify the magnitude of these defects and major column fractures. Pelvic discontinuity must be recognized to allow for appropriate surgical planning. Radiographic indicators include the presence of a transverse fracture line involving the quadrilateral plate with a break of the iliopectineal and ilioischial lines, medial migration of the inferior portion of the hemipelvis, and apparent asymmetry of the pelvic ring. The acetabular component often migrates medial to the ilioischial (Kohler's) line and fracture of the posterior column may also be apparent.

Acetabular Fracture Classification and Treatment

A comprehensive classification has been proposed that encompasses varying treatment options (Table 3). Major groupings include intraoperative fractures resulting from acetabular component insertion, intraoperative fractures caused by acetabular component removal, traumatic fractures, spontaneous fractures, and pelvic discontinuity. For intraoperative fractures, early recognition is critical for satisfactory outcome. If the fracture is nondisplaced and the component is stable, the component may be left in place. If the component is unstable, the integrity of the major columns must be assessed and the possibility of allowing fixation of a line-to-line placed cup with multiple screws should be determined. Bone grafting is warranted and protected weight bearing for up to 12 weeks should be considered (Figure 5).

Periprosthetic acetabular fractures may occur after removal of well-fixed and osseointegrated implants at the time of revision THA. Two conditions must be met to determine component stability after reinserting a new hemispherical porous-coated cup. The remaining host bone bed must have at least 50% intact structure remaining, and the areas of primary seating for the cup (the anterior column under the anterior-inferior iliac spine and the posterior column about the ischium) must have enough integrity to mechanically support the prosthesis. As long as these criteria are met, bone coverage of the component may be lacking in certain areas (such as superior or posterior). The jumbo revision acetabular component with multiple holes for adjunct screw fixation can be used in most of these situations.

Spontaneous acetabular fractures without a prior history trauma are associated with progressive osteolytic lesions. Plain radiographs are unreliable for measuring bony integrity if more than 50% of the host bone remains for implant seating. Intraoperative assessment may be the best determinant of subsequent treatment. Severe bone loss is demonstrated by more than 2 cm of superior component migration, the presence of ischial lysis is indicative of posterior column deficiency, and a break in the ilioischial (Kohler's) line is associated with anterior column deficiency. If less than 50% of the host bone remains for fixation, consideration must be given to bulk allograft substitution of the defect. This may consist of a matched pelvic allograft or a figure-7 distal femoral graft prepared to reconstitute the defect. In such instances, an acetabular reconstruction cage may be added for additional stability and support of the ace-

tabular component (which is cemented into the cage). For fractures that lack major column stability, pelvic bone plate and screw fixation is needed to reestablish pelvic integrity. Fixation of the pelvic fracture should not be done by spanning the gap with an acetabular component that has screws placed into both pelvic segments alone because high failure rates are reported.

Table 3 | Classification of Periprosthetic Fractures of the Acetabulum Associated With THA

Type I: Intraoperative fractures secondary to acetabular component insertion

  IA: Fracture of an acetabular wall recognized intraoperatively; fracture nondisplaced and component stable

  IB: Fracture recognized intraoperatively and displaced

  IC: Fracture not recognized intraoperatively

Type II: Intraoperative fracture secondary to acetabular component removal

  IIA: Associated with loss of < 50% of acetabular bone stock

  IIB: Associated with loss of > 50% of acetabular bone stock

Type III: Traumatic fracture

  IIIA: Component stable

  IIIB: Component unstable

Type IV: Spontaneous fracture

  IVA: Associated with < 50% of acetabular bone stock

  IVB: Associated with > 50% of acetabular bone stock

Type V: Pelvic discontinuity

  VA: Associated with loss of < 50% of acetabular bone stock

  VB: Associated with loss of > 50% of acetabular bone stock

  VC: Associated with prior pelvic radiation

(Reproduced from Della Valle DJ, Momberger NG, Paprosky WG: Periprosthetic fractures of the acetabulum associated with total hip arthroplasty. Instr Course Lect 2003;52:281-290.)

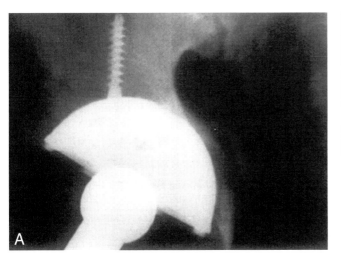 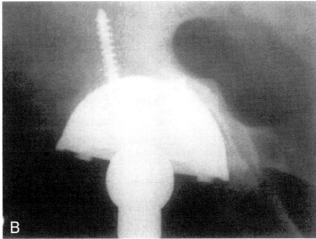

Figure 5 **A,** Intraoperative radiograph of a periprosthetic acetabular fracture with unstable fixation of the implant. **B,** Radiograph obtained at 1-year follow-up after treatment with additional screws and autologous bone graft. *(Reproduced with permission from Sharkey PF, Hozack WJ, Callaghan JJ, et al: Acetabular fracture associated with cementless acetabular component insertion: A report of 13 cases. J Arthroplasty 1999;14:426-431.)*

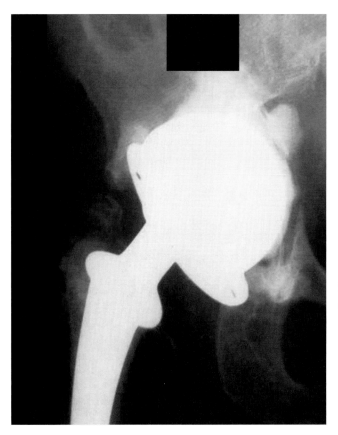

Figure 6 Pelvic discontinuity was identified on this AP radiograph with apparent disruption of the iliopectineal and ilioischial lines and obvious medial displacement of the inferior pelvic segment (consisting of the anterior column, pubic ramus, and ischium).

Table 4 | Vancouver Classification System for Intraoperative Periprosthetic Fractures

Type A: Proximal metaphyseal
   1: Cortical perforation
   2: Nondisplaced crack
   3: Unstable fracture
Type B: Diaphyseal
   1: Cortical perforation
   2: Nondisplaced crack
   3: Displaced fracture
Type C: Distal diaphyseal/metaphyseal
   1: Cortical perforation
   2: Nondisplaced crack extending into distal metaphysis
   3: Displaced distal fracture

(Adapted from Greidanus NV, Mitchell PA, Masri BA, Garbuz DS, Duncan CP. Principles of management and results of treating the fractured femur during and after total hip arthroplasty. Instr Course Lect 2003;52:309-322.)

Pelvic discontinuity represents a unique form of acetabular periprosthetic fracture in which a transverse pelvic fracture has occurred (Figure 6). In patients with adequate host bone, after an intraoperative fracture or following a posttraumatic injury, treatment consists of reconstructing the posterior column disruption with a pelvic plate and screws followed by placing a porous acetabular component with multiple adjunctive screws and bone grafting the fracture site. A high degree of success can be expected if rigid stability can be achieved and adequate postoperative weight bearing restriction is accomplished. In patients with pelvic discontinuity and poor bone stock or in patients in whom radiation has violated the biologic potential for recovery, expectations of treatment may be limited and high complication rates prevail. In general, the primary focus of reconstruction must be eliminating the pelvic discontinuity, which is best accomplished using pelvic reconstruction plates. The addition of rigidly fixed bulk acetabular allografts can be helpful in building up bone stock and stimulating healing of the discontinuity. In addition, the potential for easing the complexity of a later reconstruction is significant. The acetabular component should be either fixed with cement into a bulk allograft or into an acetabular reconstruction cage that spans the ischium to

the ilium and overlies the graft. Screw placement can be critical in these patients, and the surgeon must be aware of the screw direction to avoid damage to vital intrapelvic structures.

Femoral Fracture Classification and Treatment

According to the Vancouver classification, intraoperative fractures are grouped as proximal metaphyseal, diaphyseal, or distal diaphyseal (including the distal metaphysis) (Table 4). Each category is then subclassified into simple cortical perforation, nondisplaced linear crack, or displaced unstable fracture. Because most fractures are recognized at the time of surgery, outcome generally is satisfactory if stability of the fracture and implant are achieved. For proximal cracks or splits, if the stem is stable, a proximal cerclage cable with local morcellized bone graft has a high degree of success in preventing crack propagation and allowing healing. For the diaphyseal group, determining component stability hinges on whether there is enough distal stem fixation to allow the fracture to heal over time. If uncertainty exists, an allograft strut with cerclage cable may be added or a different longer implant designed to achieve distal stem fixation with either porous coating or flutes may be chosen. This distal fixation should extend at least two cortical diameters below the end of the fracture site. An important consideration is protected weight bearing for an extended period (6 to 12 weeks) because of the prolonged healing of diaphyseal fractures. Cortical perforations should not be ignored because the diaphyseal structural integrity can be significantly compromised. Morcellized bone graft should be applied if the area is proximal to the stem tip, but allograft struts with cerclage cable or a longer prosthesis should be considered if the perforation is distal to the prosthetic stem tip.

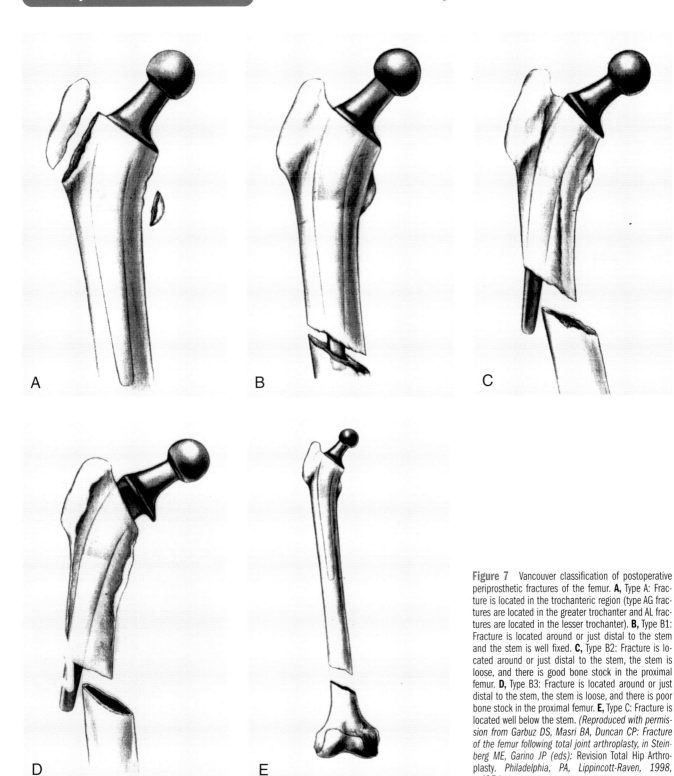

A

B

C

D

E

Figure 7   Vancouver classification of postoperative periprosthetic fractures of the femur. **A,** Type A: Fracture is located in the trochanteric region (type AG fractures are located in the greater trochanter and AL fractures are located in the lesser trochanter). **B,** Type B1: Fracture is located around or just distal to the stem and the stem is well fixed. **C,** Type B2: Fracture is located around or just distal to the stem, the stem is loose, and there is good bone stock in the proximal femur. **D,** Type B3: Fracture is located around or just distal to the stem, the stem is loose, and there is poor bone stock in the proximal femur. **E,** Type C: Fracture is located well below the stem. *(Reproduced with permission from Garbuz DS, Masri BA, Duncan CP: Fracture of the femur following total joint arthroplasty, in Steinberg ME, Garino JP (eds): Revision Total Hip Arthroplasty. Philadelphia, PA, Lippincott-Raven, 1998, p 497.)*

The Vancouver classification for postoperative periprosthetic fractures determines the site of the fracture, stability of the implant, and quality of surrounding bone (Figure 7) and (Table 5). The levels of the fracture are defined as type A (those occurring in the trochanteric region), type B (those occurring in the area about and just distal to the preexisting stem), and type C (those occurring far below the femoral stem. The most proximal fractures may involve the trochanters or loss of the integrity of the medial buttress. Type B fractures are subdivided into three groups: femoral implant solidly fixed (subtype 1), femoral implant loose but the sur-

Table 5 | Vancouver Classification of Postoperative Periprosthetic Fractures of the Femur

Type A: Fractures in the trochanteric region
  AG: At greater trochanter
  AL: At lesser trochanter
Type B: Fracture is located around or just distal to the stem
  B1: Around or just below stem, stem well fixed
  B2: At or just below stem, stem loose
  B3: At or just below stem, stem loose, poor bone stock in proximal femur
Type C: Fracture well below stem

(Adapted from Greidanus NV, Mitchell PA, Masri BA, Garbuz DS, Duncan CP. Principles of management and results of treating the fractured femur during and after total hip arthroplasty. Instr Course Lect 2003;52:309-322.)

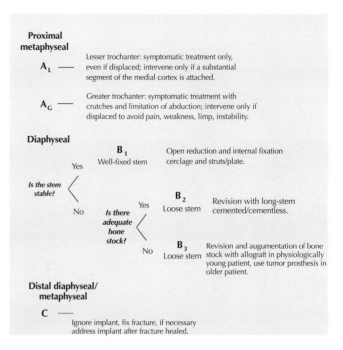

Figure 8 Management algorithm using the Vancouver classification system for postoperative fractures. *(Reproduced from Greidanus NV, Mitchell PA, Masri BA, Garbuz DS, Duncan CP: Principles of management and results of treating the fractured femur during and after total hip arthroplasty. Instr Course Lect 2003;52:309-322.)*

rounding bone stock remains good (subtype 2), and femoral implant loose with severe bone stock loss (subtype 3). In general, treatment of most type B fractures will be surgical and experience with extensile lateral exposures and fixation methods is warranted (Figure 8).

Type B1 fractures may be treated with recently developed cable-plate systems and strut allografts or two strut allografts with cerclage cable. Recent biomechanical studies demonstrate that cables are superior to wires for maintaining tension and friction on the allograft struts. Placement of allograft struts on the anterior and lateral surfaces are usually adequate and placement of struts on the medial femoral surface does not improve stability, with the added disadvantage of soft-tissue devitalization. Strut length should be a minimum of 12 cm and should be taken from a matching femoral allograft from the same region and side such that surface fit may be optimized. At least three fixation points above and below the fracture should be established. Morcellized bone graft should be applied to all healing sites to enhance bone union. As with any traumatic femoral fracture, patients must not bear weight for a minimum of 3 months. One study that reported the results of 39 patients with this type of fracture showed that union occurred in 97.5%.

Type B2 and B3 fractures are notorious for high nonunion rates when treated with cable plate combinations and conventional implants for revision. Factors leading to early failure include incremental bone loss and atrophy from the prior arthroplasty, higher rates of infection resulting in part to devascularization of soft tissues, and relatively limited methods of proximal internal fixation. Screw placement across the intramedullary canal is blocked by the presence of cement or prosthesis. Results have improved with the use of long intramedullary revision stems that offer rigid distal implant stability. One study showed fracture healing and implant stability achieved in 14 of 14 patients with the use of a fully porous-coated femoral component with

enough length to bypass the fracture site and engage the diaphyseal isthmus. The proximally coated implant could be removed with an extended osteotomy, essentially opening the fracture site like a clam shell, and then rebuilding the proximal metaphysis around the well-fixed implant.

These longer diaphyseal engaging implants required several adjustments in awareness and technique to achieve predictable results. Impingement on the femoral shaft bow occurs at or beyond the tip of a straight 8-inch femoral stem. Rounding the tip of the straight stem and using longer curved stems have reduced this problem. Meticulous preparation of the remaining distal femoral canal is essential for fixation success. For fully porous stems, at least 5 cm of isthmus prosthetic contact must be present for frictional fixation of the implant. Extended transfemoral osteotomy allows exposure of the distal canal for cement removal and orientation of reamers down the center axis of the canal. The use of fluoroscopy with cannulated flexible canal reamers avoids distal anterolateral impingement and identifies areas where cement or bone bridges may deflect the reamer out of the canal. Careful assessment with reverse hooks also allows identification of canal perforations that may jeopardize distal fixation. Finally, one or two prophylactic cerclage braided cables around the distal femoral canal prevent splitting and increase stability of the distal press-fit implant. Implant trialing assesses distal canal fixation and determines the length of prosthesis needed for suitable hip prosthetic stability.

For type B3 fractures that have a limited diaphyseal isthmus remaining for fixation, the use of fully porous femoral stems becomes problematic. In this situation, recent studies have demonstrated clinical success with fluted, rough-surfaced tapered stems. These devices may obtain press-fit stability in the subisthmus area, and because of the tapered geometry, they are less prone to distal canal impingement. Treatment of the proximal fractured area requires that bone fragments are cable wired around the distally stabilized stem. To avoid poor healing and infection, stripping of soft tissues over these fragments must be minimized. The construct may be optimized by adding allograft femoral struts adjacent to the prosthesis and then wiring the remaining host fragments over these struts. Other prosthetic options, especially in elderly patients, have included distally cemented diaphyseal tumor implants and proximal femoral allografts used with cemented or press-fit implants (allograft prosthetic constructs). The application of biologic materials that enhance fracture healing may prove beneficial in the treatment of these fractures, but current knowledge is limited.

Type C fractures are distal to the level of the prosthesis and may be treated by more conventional methods. Fractures near the knee may be suitably managed with plates and screws or retrograde intramedullary nailing systems. Those located in the diaphysis but below the prosthesis may be treated with a combination of plates and allograft struts. Some plating systems incorporate cerclage wires that may allow fixation in areas near the distal stem of the prosthesis.

Periprosthetic fractures following THA are difficult to treat. Most importantly, the biologic potential for healing is typically compromised by the previous surgical procedure. The surgeon must recognize that the bone quality may be poor, which limits the use of more conventional modes of fracture fixation. Radiographs will often underestimate the extent of this bone loss. Surgical technique should rely on sound biomechanical principles, and the surgeon should readily consider the use of autograft, allograft, or bone substitutes to enhance fracture union in patients with periprosthetic fractures.

Annotated Bibliography

Infection

English H, Timperley AJ, Dunlop D, Gie G: Impaction grafting of the femur in two-stage revision for infected total hip replacement. *J Bone Joint Surg Br* 2002;84:700-705.

A large retrospective review of femoral impaction grafting at the time of the second stage revision for infection is reported. Good results are documented and the indications for this procedure discussed. Poor prognostic factors associated with this technique are outlined.

Haddad FS, Masri BA, Garbuz DS, Duncan CP: The treatment of the infected hip replacement: The complex case. *Clin Orthop* 1999;369:144-156.

The authors provide an in-depth review of the indications, technique, and evidence for the use of articulated spacers in two-stage revision for infection. A detailed review of the authors' experience with the PROSTALAC is described, including its use in patients with substantial loss of bone stock. Good clinical outcomes are reported.

Haddad FS, Muirhead-Allwood SK, Manktelow ARJ, Bacarese-Hamilton I: Two-stage uncemented revision hip arthroplasty for infection. *J Bone Joint Surg Br* 2000; 82:689-694.

A large retrospective review of cementless two-stage revision for infection is presented. Discussion of the use of morcellized allograft in this setting is included. Good outcomes are reported and the indications for the use of this method are described.

Jackson WO, Schmalzried TP: Limited role of direct exchange arthroplasty in the treatment of infected total hip replacements. *Clin Orthop* 2000;381:101-105.

A meta-analysis of reports of one-stage revision for infected THA is presented. The review focuses on analysis of indications, poor prognostic factors, and outcome associated with this treatment method. This study describes the largest series investigating this topic.

Joseph TN, Chen AL, Di Cesare PE: Use of antibiotic-impregnated cement in total joint arthroplasty. *J Am Acad Orthop Surg* 2003;11:38-47.

This review provides an in-depth discussion of the basic science and clinical uses of antibiotic-impregnated cement. An emphasis is placed on the evaluation of the evidence regarding various clinical applications and techniques.

Kilgus DJ, Howe DJ, Strang AS: Results of periprosthetic hip and knee infections caused by resistant bacteria. *Clin Orthop* 2002;404:116-124.

This series consists of a retrospective study investigating the outcome of infection with antibiotic-sensitive and antibiotic-resistant organisms. Results were reported on the basis of type of treatment. The results of patients infected with resistant organisms were significantly less successful than those of patients infected with susceptible organisms.

Phillips CB, Barrett JA, Losina E, et al: Incidence rates of dislocation, pulmonary embolism, and deep infection during the first six months after elective total hip replacement. *J Bone Joint Surg Am* 2003;85:20-26.

A review of a large number of Medicare patients treated with primary THA is presented. The complications are emphasized, with a focus on the incidence as a function of time from the index procedure. The results are used to suggest strategies for prevention of complications.

Salvati EA, Della Valle AG, Masri BA, Duncan CP: The infected total hip arthroplasty. *Instr Course Lect* 2003; 52:223-245.

The authors present an in-depth review of the basic science, clinical, radiologic, and laboratory evaluation of infection in patients who have undergone THA. A thorough discussion of treatment options with up-to-date evidence is presented. The authors' preferred method of evaluation and treatment is described.

Spangehl MJ, Masri BA, O'Connell JX, Duncan CP: Prospective analysis of preoperative and intraoperative investigations for the diagnosis of infection at the sites of two hundred and two revision total hip arthroplasties. *J Bone Joint Surg Am* 1999;81:672-683.

This study consists of a large, prospective investigation of various diagnostic tests for infection of THA. The epidemiologic characteristics of each test are reported, allowing for formulation of an evidence-based approach for diagnosis of infection. The rationale for a proposed diagnostic algorithm is discussed.

Tang WM, Chiu KY, Ng TP, Yau WP, Ching PT, Seto WH: Efficacy of a single dose of cefazolin as a prophylactic antibiotic in primary arthroplasty. *J Arthroplasty* 2003;18:714-718.

The authors conducted a large, case-control study comparing single-dose prophylactic cefazolin with a standard three-dose regimen of cefuroxime. The results of this study provide initial evidence for the use of a single dose of preoperative antibiotics to prevent infection.

Zhuang H, Chacko TK, Hickeson M, et al: Persistent non-specific FDG uptake on PET imaging following hip arthroplasty. *Eur J Nucl Med Mol Imaging* 2002;29:1328-1333.

The authors present an analysis of positron emission tomography for diagnosis of THA infection using a prospective patient group and a retrospective cohort. They provide a classification on the basis of location of increased uptake, which relates to the likelihood of infection. The findings in uncomplicated THA are reviewed and compared with infection to provide a rationale for interpretation of results.

Dislocation

Alberton GM, High WA, Morrey BF: Dislocation after revision total hip arthroplasty: An analysis of risk factors and treatment options. *J Bone Joint Surg Am* 2002; 84(10):1788-1792.

In this study, 1,405 patients undergoing 1,548 revision THAs for reasons other than chronic instability were followed for a mean of 8.1 years with an end point of dislocation. One hundred and fifteen hips (7.4%) dislocated at least once. Elevated rim liners and large femoral heads (28- and 32-mm versus 22-mm) were found to decrease the rates of dislocation significantly. Trochanteric nonunion was a strong risk factor for subsequent dislocation. Correcting instability in revision

THAs was found to be significantly less successful than in primary THAs. Fifty of the 115 hips underwent re-revision. Whether reoperated or not, at final assessment only 57% of the 115 hips that dislocated were stable, 36% remained unstable, and 8% were unknown. The authors concluded that different risk factors make revision hip instability a much more challenging problem, particularly because of the extent of periarticular soft-tissue dissection and subsequent dysfunction.

Berry DJ, von Knoch M, Schleck CD, Harmsen WS: The cumulative long-term risk of dislocation after primary Charnley total hip arthroplasty. *J Bone Joint Surg Am* 2004;86(1):9-14.

This is a large cohort study that followed 6,623 patients who underwent primary THA (Charnley hips with 22-mm heads) for 20 to 35 years with an end point of dislocation. Survivorship analysis revealed an overall dislocation prevalence of 4.8%, with a cumulative risk of 1% in the first month, 1.9% in the first year, then an additional 1% per 5 years up to 7% at 25 years (if the patients were still alive and had not undergone revision for other reasons). Multivariate analysis revealed a relative risk of 2.1 for female gender, 1.3 for age greater than 70 years, and significantly higher risk in patients with osteonecrosis, femoral neck fracture or nonunion, and inflammatory arthritis versus those with primary osteoarthritis.

Boucher HR, Lynch C, Young AM, Engh CA Jr, Engh C Sr: Dislocation after polyethylene liner exchange in total hip arthroplasty. *J Arthroplasty* 2003;18:654-657.

The authors reported an unexpectedly high rate of dislocation (25%) in 24 patients who underwent polyethylene liner exchange for wear or osteolysis but not for instability. Of these patients (N = 6), two underwent revision for recurrent instability, one had three dislocations, two had two dislocations, and two had one dislocation at a mean 56 month follow-up.

Callaghan JJ, O'Rourke MR, Goetz DD, Lewallen DG, Johnston RC, Capello WN: Use of a constrained tripolar acetabular liner to treat intraoperative instability and postoperative dislocation after total hip arthroplasty: A review of our experience. *Clin Orthop Relat Res* 2004; 429:117-123.

The authors reported the results of using a constrained tripolar component to treat intraoperative instability or recurrent postoperative dislocation. Three groups of patients were studied: group one included patients with intraoperative instability (45 hips in 43 patients, 4 primary THAs and 41 revisions), group two included patients with recurrent dislocation who underwent full acetabular revision (56 revision hips in 55 patients), and group three included patients with intraoperative instability or recurrent dislocation with a tripolar liner cemented into a well-fixed (nonrevised) cup (31 hips in 30 patients). Group one and group two were followed for a mean of 10 years and group three was followed for 3.9 years. The authors reported eight total failures in seven patients (two in group one, four in group two, and two in group three), which represents a global failure rate of 6%. They reported no increased rate of osteolysis or aseptic loosening and concluded that these are good results for the use of this implant.

Cuckler JM, Moore KD, Lombardi AV Jr, McPherson E, Emerson R: Large versus small femoral heads in metal-on-metal total hip arthroplasty. *J Arthroplasty* 2004; 19(suppl 3):41-44.

The authors compared the early results of 616 THAs with a 38-mm head and 78 THAs with a 28-mm head; all other factors and components were identical. At 3-month follow-up, no dislocations occurred in the 38-mm femoral head group and the dislocation rate was 2.5% in the 28-mm femoral head group. Of note, these were nonrandomized consecutive cohorts (28-mm femoral heads, then 38-mm femoral heads), and 42.5% of the patients in the 38-mm femoral head group had a posterior approach compared with 55% in the 28-mm femoral head group who had more dislocations.

Dewal H, Maurer SL, Tsai P, Su E, Hiebert R, Di Cesare PE: Efficacy of abduction bracing in the management of total hip arthroplasty dislocation. *J Arthroplasty* 2004;19: 733-738.

A retrospective assessment of the effectiveness of abduction bracing after dislocation was performed. The patients were categorized as first-time (N = 91) and recurrent (N = 58) dislocations and whether they received a brace. Mean follow-up was 4.0 and 3.7 years for the two groups, and re-dislocation was defined as treatment failure. In the first-time dislocation group, 61% failed with a brace and 64% failed without a brace. In the recurrent dislocation group, 55% failed with a brace and 56% failed without a brace. Chi-squared analysis revealed no statistically significant difference. The authors concluded that the data do not support the use of abduction bracing for instability.

Lachiewicz PF, Soileau E, Ellis J: Modular revision for recurrent dislocation of primary or revision total hip arthroplasty. *J Arthroplasty* 2004;19:424-429.

Seventeen primary and six revision THAs, revised for instability with retention of components and modular exchange, were followed for a mean of 3 years. Among primary THAs, 15 had a liner exchange, 13 were given a longer femoral neck length, and 5 received a larger femoral head. Three hips redislocated, two of them recurrently and underwent subsequent component revision (11.7% re-revision rate). In six revision THAs, four had liner exchanges, three had femoral neck elongation, and two received a larger femoral head. Three of the six re-dislocated, two of which required re-revision (33%). The authors concluded that the so-called bloodless revision is acceptable after dislocation of primary THA, but much less successful for revision THA.

Lawton RL, Morrey BF: Dislocation after long-necked total hip arthroplasty. *Clin Orthop Relat Res* 2004;422: 164-166.

A matched cohort study of long-necked (skirted) implants was performed to detect the relative incidence of dislocation (125 primary and 125 revision THAs with long-necked femoral heads were matched with 250 controls with standard necks). Limb-length discrepancies were not statistically different between the two groups. Dislocation rates were 10.6% and 18% for primary and revision THAs with long skirted necks, respectively, compared with 1.6% and 10% with standard necks, respectively. The authors concluded that long skirted neck implants were strongly associated with a higher risk of dislocation.

Masonis JL, Bourne RB: Surgical approach, abductor function, and total hip arthroplasty dislocation. *Clin Orthop Relat Res* 2002;405:46-53.

This is a meta-analysis of 14 studies with 13,203 patients who met the inclusion criteria for a systematic review of surgical approach as a risk factor for dislocation in primary THA; the studies were chosen from among 260 clinical studies on the topic. The combined dislocation rates for the various approaches were 1.27% for transtrochanteric, 3.23% for posterior (3.95% without repair and 2.03% with repair/capsulorrhaphy), 2.18% for anterolateral (Watson-Jones), and 0.55% for direct lateral (Hardinge). Eight studies with 2,455 primary THAs evaluated postoperative limp, and rates of 4% to 20% for the lateral approach versus 0 to 16% for the posterior approach were found.

Sultan PG, Tan V, Lai M, Garino JP: Independent contribution of elevated-rim acetabular liner and femoral head size to the stability of total hip implants. *J Arthroplasty* 2002;17:289-292.

The authors of this study reported on increased intraoperative stability provided independently by large femoral heads and by elevated rim liners in patients who have undergone THA. In 20 primary THAs, the femoral and acetabular components were fixed, then different combinations of trial components were compared for stability (28-mm heads with both flat and 15° elevated liners and 32-mm heads with both liners). The authors reported that using 32-mm femoral heads provided an additional 8.1° of internal rotation compared with 28-mm femoral heads when intraoperative range of motion was tested to the point of instability. They also reported that 15° elevated rim liners independently provided another 8.9° of internal rotation when tested the same way and compared with flat liners. The best results were achieved with the pairing of a 32-mm head and an elevated liner; furthermore, this combination did not cause more anterior instability when tested intraoperatively.

von Knoch M, Berry DJ, Harmsen WS, Morrey BF: Late dislocation after total hip arthroplasty. *J Bone Joint Surg Am* 2002;84(11):1949-1953.

This is a report of 19,680 primary THAs that were followed for at least 5 years for the incidence of late instability (first dislocation occurred more than 5 years postoperatively). A total of 2.6% of the hips dislocated overall, with 0.8% occurring more than 5 years (median, 11.3 years) after surgery. Thus, 32% of the dislocations were late, which is much higher than previously thought. These late dislocations were found more likely to recur (55%), but equally likely to require revision surgery (approximately 33%). They were also found to have some distinct risk factors from dislocations that occurred less than 5 years postoperatively, such as neurologic decline, polyethylene wear, and episodes of trauma.

Zwartele RE, Brand R, Doets HC: Increased risk of dislocation after primary total hip arthroplasty in inflammatory arthritis: A prospective observational study of 410 hips. *Acta Orthop Scand* 2004;75:684-690.

The authors conducted a prospective comparison of dislocation rates in primary THAs done for a diagnosis of inflammatory arthritis versus osteoarthritis; 70 THAs in the inflammatory arthritis group and 340 THAs in the osteoarthritis group were followed for a minimum of 2 years. All were done through a lateral approach. The authors reported a significantly higher rate of dislocation in the inflammatory arthritis group (10% versus 3%). No differences were found in any other risk factor between the groups. Inflammatory arthritis was shown to be an independent risk factor for dislocation.

Limb-Length Inequality

Ranawat CS, Rao RR, Rodriguez JA, Bhende HS: Correction of limb-length inequality during total hip arthroplasty. *J Arthroplasty* 2001;16:715-720.

This study describes a new technique of measuring intraoperative limb length using a vertical Steinmann pin placed at the infracotyloid groove of the acetabulum. The authors evaluated this technique in 100 consecutive primary THAs and correlated the results with postoperative radiographs. The accuracy and reproducibility of this technique along with the shortcomings and advantages of this simple intraoperative technique are discussed.

Periprosthetic Fractures

Brady OH, Garbuz DS, Masri BA, Duncan CP: The reliability and validity of the Vancouver classification of femoral fractures after hip replacement. *J Arthroplasty* 2000;15:59-62.

The Vancouver classification has a high degree of reliability for interobserver radiographic assessment and with comparison to intraoperative findings. Important differences in treatment and outcome have been demonstrated for the various subtypes of this classification.

Haddad FS, Duncan CP, Berry DJ, Lewallen DG, Gross AE, Chandler HP: Periprosthetic femoral fractures around well-fixed implants: Use of cortical onlay allografts with or without a plate. *J Bone Joint Surg Am* 2002;84:945-950.

For Vancouver type B1 fractures around a stable implant in 40 patients, 98% had fracture union when cortical allograft struts were applied either alone or in conjunction with a metal bone plate without revision of the femoral stem.

Ko PS, Lam JJ, Tio MK, Lee OB, Ip FK: Distal fixation with Wagner revision stem in treating Vancouver type B2 periprosthetic femur fractures in geriatric patients. *J Arthroplasty* 2003;18:446-452.

In this series, 12 patients with Vancouver type B2 periprosthetic fractures underwent revision with a long lateral osteotomy for removal of the implant and distal fixation with the Wagner fluted taper titanium alloy stem with grit-blasted surface. All patients had a stable implant with fracture healing at follow-up, and stem subsidence occurred in two patients.

Kwong LM, Miller AJ, Lubinus P: A modular distal fixation option for proximal bone loss in revision total hip arthroplasty. *J Arthroplasty* 2003;18(suppl 1):94-97.

In this large series, 14 periprosthetic fractures were treated with a modular distal tapered titanium alloy stem. At 2- to 6-year follow-up, no apparent treatment failures were noted, and the overall group survivorship (with revision as end point) was 97.2%.

MacDonald SJ, Paprosky WG, Jablonsky WS, Magnus RG: Periprosthetic femoral fractures treated with a long-stem cementless component. *J Arthroplasty* 2001; 16:379-383.

In this study, 14 periprosthetic fractures were treated with a long porous stem of 8 or 10 inches; four of these fractures were Vancouver type B fractures about a loose stem. At average 8.2-year follow-up (minimum follow-up, 5 years), all patients had satisfactory fracture healing, and the stem achieved stability without loosening or subsidence.

Warren PJ, Thompson P, Fletcher MD: Transfemoral implantation of the Wagner SL stem: The abolition of subsidence and enhancement of osteotomy union rate using Dall-Miles cables. *Arch Orthop Trauma Surg* 2002;122: 557-560.

In 17 patients, the use of 2.0-mm cerclage Dall-Miles cables placed on the distal femur was compared with heavy wire. No subsidence of the tapered femoral stem was noted with Dall-Miles cables compared with average subsidence of 6 mm with the heavy wires ($P = 0.001$).

Classic Bibliography

Ali Khan MA, Brakenbury PH, Reynolds IS: Dislocation following total hip replacement. *J Bone Joint Surg Br* 1981;63(2):214-218.

Berry DJ, Lewallen DG, Hanssen AD, Cabanela ME: Pelvic discontinuity in revision total hip arthroplasty. *J Bone Joint Surg Am* 1999;81(12):1692-1702.

Chandler HP, Tigges RG: The tole of allografts in the treatment of periprosthetic femoral fractures. *Instr Course Lect* 1998;47:257-264.

Cobb TK, Morrey BF, Ilstrup DM: The elevated-rim acetabular liner in total hip arthroplasty: Relationship to postoperative dislocation. *J Bone Joint Surg Am* 1996; 78(1):80-86.

Coventry MB: Late dislocations in patients with Charnley total hip arthroplasty. *J Bone Joint Surg Am* 1985; 67(6):832-841.

Crockarell JR Jr, Berry DJ, Lewallen DG: Nonunion after periprosthetic femoral fractures associated with total hip arthroplasty. *J Bone Joint Surg Am* 1999;81:1073-1079.

Daly PJ, Morrey BF: Operative correction of an unstable total hip arthroplasty. *J Bone Joint Surg Am* 1992; 74(9):1334-1343.

Dorr LD, Wan Z: Causes of and treatment protocol for instability of total hip replacement. *Clin Orthop Relat Res* 1998;355:144-151.

Dorr LD, Wolf AW, Chandler R, Conaty JP: Classification and treatment of dislocations of total hip arthroplasty. *Clin Orthop Relat Res* 1983;173:151-158.

Ekelund A: Trochanteric osteotomy for recurrent dislocation of total hip arthroplasty. *J Arthroplasty* 1993;8(6): 629-632.

Fackler CD, Poss R: Dislocation in total hip arthroplasties. *Clin Orthop Relat Res* 1980;151:169-178.

Lewinnek GE Lewis JL, Tarr R, Compere CL, Zimmerman JR: Dislocations after total hip-replacement arthroplasties. *J Bone Joint Surg Am* 1978;60(2):217-220.

Ranawat CS, Rodriguez JA: Functional leg-length inequality following total hip arthroplasty. *J Arthroplasty* 1997;12:359-364.

Sharkey PF, Hozack WJ, Callaghan JJ, et al: Acetabular fracture associated with cementless acetabular component insertion: A report of 13 cases. *J Arthroplasty* 1999; 14(4):426-431.

Woo RY, Morrey BF: Dislocations after total hip arthroplasty. *J Bone Joint Surg Am* 1982;64(9):1295-1306.

Chapter 43

Pearls and Tips for Total Hip Arthroplasty

Steven A. Stuchin, MD

Pearls

Limb Length and Offset

Limb-length inequality is among the most common causes of dissatisfaction in otherwise successful total hip replacements. With 20 mm of discrepancy, patients will experience functional scoliosis, pelvic tilt, and asymmetric loads on the lower extremities. Opinions about acceptable limb-length discrepancies have varied over the years. Studies have shown that most patients can accommodate a 7-mm discrepancy. With discrepancy greater than 7 mm, the incidence of pain, limp, and need for a shoe lift rises markedly. Improved understanding of hip biomechanics and newer techniques have led to improved limb-length accuracy. Equalization within an average of 3 mm has been reported using current manual surgical techniques. The accuracy that can be achieved using electronic navigation systems remains to be realized in a broad application base, but electronic navigation systems offer the promise of greater accuracy and reproducibility in many aspects of hip replacement.

Readily available techniques include preoperative templating and measuring techniques, intraoperative jigs and calipers, and direct contralateral limb comparison.

Preoperative template techniques require intraoperative verification of known anatomic landmarks, usually the greater or lesser trochanter. These sites serve as reference points to measure femoral neck resection. On occasion, these landmarks may be distorted or absent, thereby complicating this technique.

Intraoperative jigs measure the distance between two points created before femoral neck resection. A pin is usually driven into the wing of the ilium, and a second marking point is created on the femur. With trial components in place, the distance between the fixed points must equal the expected preresection calculation. There may be several difficulties with this technique. Secure fixation of the pin in the ilium is critical. With poor fixation, the pin may wobble, leading to a change in the determined length. In the lateral position, the retroperitoneal contents may shift away from the iliac wing; nonetheless, care must be taken not to drive the pin too deeply. Additionally, the limb position must be constant at all measuring determinations. Minor shifts in abduction of the hip will cause changes of several millimeters in the position of any marking point on the femur (Figure 1).

The greatest accuracy in limb-length restoration has been reported using a method in which the calculated resection height is determined by measuring from the apex of the curve of the femoral head on radiographs to the calculated resection level on the femoral neck and determining this distance intraoperatively using a caliper. When combined with preoperative templating, limb-length discrepancies within 6 mm are achieved in 86% of patients (Figure 2).

Direct palpation methods have been advanced as the most obvious means of assessing limb-length equalization. This technique may be applicable with the patient in the supine position, but is unwieldy at best with the patient in the lateral position (Figure 3).

Offset and Stability

Increased understanding of hip and total hip biomechanics and stability issues has led to greater sophistication in soft-tissue balancing techniques and technology. Femoral neck offset is an anatomic variable that cannot be addressed with a single implant. Without restoration of offset, abductor power is diminished, thereby resulting in increased joint reaction forces. Furthermore, with decreased offset there is limitation of hip motion and increased bony impingement of the trochanter on the pelvis, which can lead to dislocation. Historically, this complication was resolved by osteotomy and advancement of the greater trochanter; however, this clearly adds to the morbidity of and recovery from the procedure.

Modular femoral heads allow for greater flexibility in femoral neck resection and offset adjustment without the need for trochanteric advancement. Limb length may be maintained and offset increased by increasing the depth of the femoral neck resection and increasing the length of the modular head.

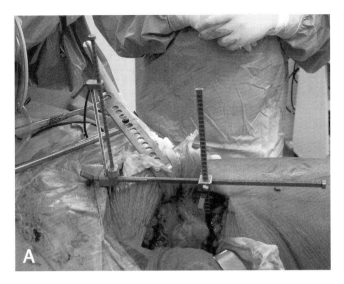
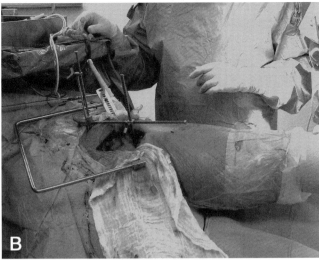

Figure 1 **A,** Intraoperative photograph shows a caliper set to mark the preresection length between the pin in the wing of the ilium and a site marked on the femur. **B,** Intraoperative photograph that shows how abducting or adducting the leg moves the femoral point closer or further from the marker on the caliper, falsely changing leg length. A spirit level has been taped to the tibia so that hip abduction can be reliably reproduced with placement of a trial implant.

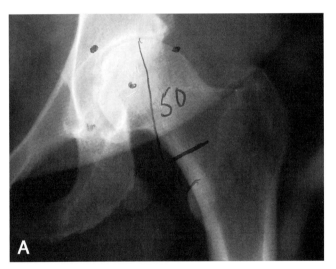
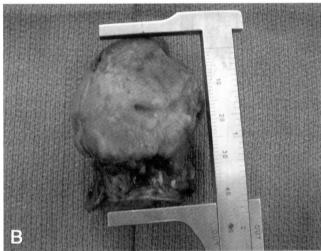

Figure 2 **A,** Radiograph markings show that increased accuracy may be attained by calculating the expected amount of femoral head/neck resection and confirming with a caliper at the time of surgery. In this instance, 11 mm of femoral neck will be preserved and 50 mm of femoral head/neck will be resected. **B,** Photograph showing how the calculated resection is confirmed with a caliper.

Unfortunately, modular femoral head technology has some drawbacks. For most hip replacement systems, extending neck lengths requires the addition of a skirt at the base of the modular head. Paradoxically, this skirt may decrease stability and increase polyethylene wear while increasing femoral neck length and offset. The diameter of the skirt adds to the femoral neck diameter, leading to impingement of the neck at the end points of internal or external rotation. The use of polyethylene liners with raised posterior lips may lead to anterior dislocation or polyethylene wear as the neck abuts this lip. Also, some anatomically varus neck femurs may still not have sufficient offset to adequately restore the preoperative trochanteric position.

Enhanced offset neck options may resolve some of these problems. Many hip replacement systems now offer both standard and increased offset choices. Increasing femoral neck offset allows for a higher level of neck resection. Shorter modular heads without skirts may then be used. Bone stock is preserved; stability and soft-tissue balance may be enhanced or at least reproduced in most patients.

With the recent interest in hard bearing surfaces such as ceramic-on-ceramic and metal-on-metal implants, these enhanced offset devices add a special advantage. Neck length options are limited with these devices, usually to no more than three neck length options. On occasion, restoration of appropriate hip mechanics cannot be achieved without enhanced offset options.

The long-term biomechanical consequences of enhanced offset femoral components are not known. Increased forces are clearly generated at the junction of the neck and body of the prosthesis, resulting in possible material failure. Additionally, an increased moment is created along the calcar, which possibly affects long-term fixation.

Balancing these possible negative consequences are some compelling positive biomechanical effects. Lateral offset of 8 mm is equivalent to advancing the greater trochanter almost 2 cm in a standard 132° femoral neck-shaft angled stem. This is equivalent to increasing neck length 10 mm in the same 132° neck angle stem without enhanced offset.

Hip implant manufacturers have chosen one of two different strategies for offset enhancement. One design maintains a 132° femoral neck angle, but moves the neck medially on the body of the prosthesis. This approach has the advantage of maintaining femoral neck height when moving from a standard to an offset design. Additionally, this strategy offers the greatest amount of offset. The alternate approach is to maintain the position of the femoral neck relative to the body of the prosthesis, and decrease the neck angle to a more varus position. Femoral neck height is lost this way, and offset is not as great, but forces on the implant and calcar may not be not raised as much. The long-term outcomes of using either of these designs is not yet known, nor has the concept of enhanced offset been scientifically established (Figure 4).

Another strategy for enhancing offset addresses the problem from the acetabular side. Some implant designs offer sockets with modular polyethylene bearings that displace the center of motion several millimeters laterally. Originally designed to restore the center of motion in hips with protrusio deformities, these inserts can be used to lateralize the center of motion in sockets placed anatomically. Even less is known about the long-term consequences of using this strategy than is known about using enhanced offset. Theoretically, joint lateralization should increase joint reaction forces, but again, this technique also lateralizes the greater trochanter, possibly enhancing abductor mechanics.

Recent interest in alternate and enhanced bearing technology has led to the development of large diameter modular femoral heads. Head sizes from 36 mm to as much as 54 mm are now commercially available as metal-on-metal and metal-on-cross-linked polyethylene bearings. These implants offer the theoretical advantage of increased hip stability. Clinical information from large series is not yet available.

The classic solution to the problem of offset adjustment remains advancement of the greater trochanter. When successful, the results are predictable and time

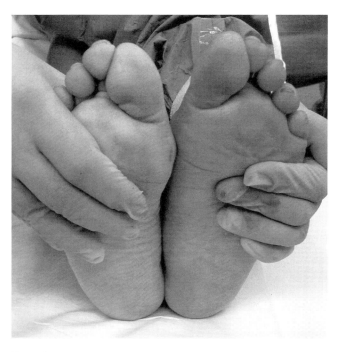

Figure 3 Photograph showing limb length being assessed directly with the patient in the supine position. Direct palpation is logical and straightforward but applicable only with the patient in the supine position and limited by draping.

tested. The disadvantages associated with trochanteric advancement include increased surgical time, increased blood loss, failure of fixation, and late complications of fixation, all of which make this treatment option less attractive given the newer alternatives.

Surgical Tips
Partial Trochanteric Osteotomy
Polyethylene failure accounts for an increasing number of late aseptic problems in patients who undergo total hip replacement. It is often necessary to create a very generous exposure to bring about isolated modular polyethylene exchange while contending with a femoral component that will be preserved. If the surgeon elects the posterior approach, exposure may require extensive dissection and resection of stabilizing soft-tissue structures. The immediate morbidity associated with increased tissue resection is obvious. The long-term consequences, however, may include chronic instability despite well-aligned components, which is difficult to explain to a patient with a previously successful arthroplasty who experiences recurrent dislocation after a simple polyethylene exchange.

A useful modification of the posterior approach that both enhances exposure and preserves stabilizing posterior structures has been described in which an osteotomy of the posterior one third of the greater trochanter is performed with soft-tissue extension into the posterior gluteus medius and superior joint capsule. With this technique, proximal dissection must be limited to no more

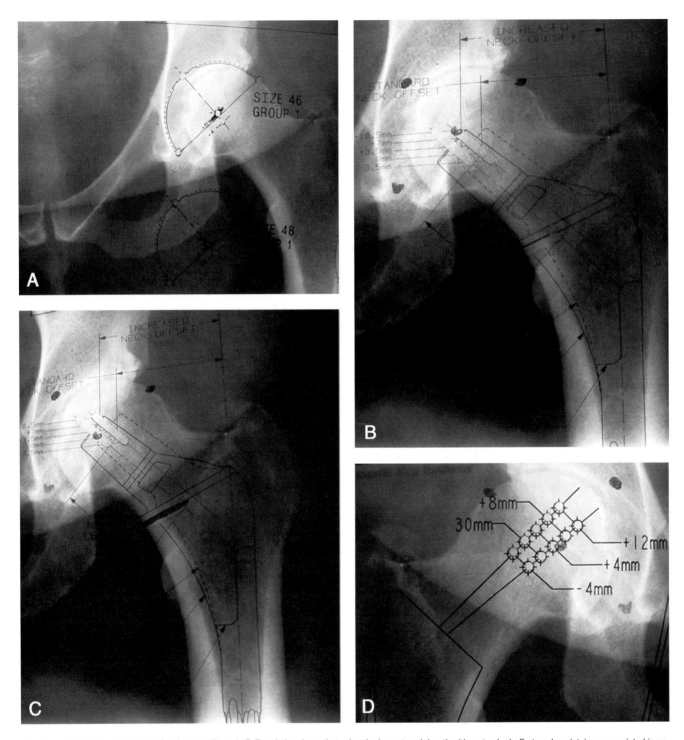

Figure 4 **A,** Socket position is templated on a radiograph. **B,** Templating shows that using the longest neck length with a standard offset neck maintains appropriate biomechanics at the expense of proximal femoral bone stock (low neck cut). **C,** Templating shows that using increased offset, hip mechanics are maintained with a much higher neck cut and a prosthetic neck length that will not require a skirted component and will allow for ceramic or metal-on-metal bearings, if desired. **D,** Templating with a stem that relies more on neck variation than medialization to enhance offset shows that neck length is lost using an offset stem. In this instance, a + 4-mm modular head is required with an offset stem to equal the leg length of a + 0-mm modular head used with a standard offset stem.

than 4 cm from the superior edge of the acetabulum to avoid possible injury to the superior gluteal nerve and artery.

By eliminating this proximal extension into the gluteus medius, concerns about the superior gluteal struc-

tures can be eliminated. The approach then becomes a posterior approach in which the posterior soft-tissue elements are detached from the greater trochanter with a bone fragment. These structures can be anatomically reattached to the greater trochanter, resulting in a sealed

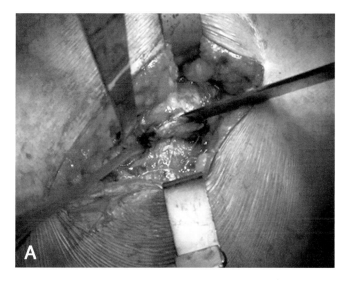

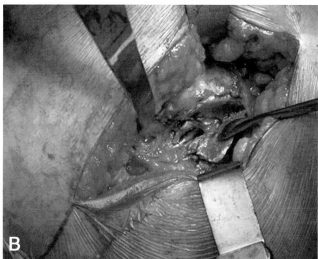

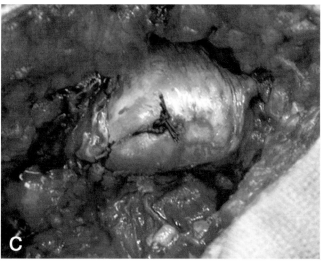

Figure 5 **A,** Intraoperative photograph shows the posterior one third of the greater trochanter outlined by the osteotome. The sucker indicates the border of the external rotators, and the overlying abductors are retracted anteriorly. **B,** Intraoperative photograph shows the osteotomized segment retracted posteriorly. The posterior stabilizing structures are preserved with this fragment, and the exposure of the socket may be better than with a standard posterior approach. **C,** Intraoperative photograph shows the fragment reattached, bringing with it the posterior structures, bone-to-bone apposition, and enhanced soft-tissue stability.

water-tight closure that preserves posterior stability (Figure 5).

Removal of Well-Fixed Cementless Sockets

Removal of well-fixed cementless sockets because of malposition or locking mechanism damage is challenging. With the exception of patients with osteolysis, there may be no readily accessible channel for a curved gouge. Furthermore, some shells are designed with spikes that impede the course of a curved gouge. Spikes can be separated from a curved shell using a high-speed metal-cutting burr and a template that fits into the shell to indicate the location of the spikes. New thin curved osteotomes that cause minimal bone destruction are now also commercially available.

On occasion, even with the use of curved gouges, there are small areas of bony fixation that have not been disrupted. A carbide punch can be used to break the cup free. A small stab incision is made in the skin

superior to the socket. The punch is pushed to the wing of the ilium. The punch is then tapped through the iliac wing to contact the superior aspect of the cup, forcing it out from the inside. Care must be taken to disrupt as much ingrowth fixation with curved gouges as possible before performing this technique; otherwise, the force of disengaging the shell may fracture the acetabulum either in the floor or across the columns.

Annotated Bibliography

Bourne RB, Rorabeck CH: Soft tissue balancing: The hip. *J Arthroplasty* 2002; 17(4 suppl 1)17-22.

The authors of this study reported that femoral offset is restored in only 40% of patients who undergo total hip replacement. They suggested that preoperative planning, obtaining intraoperative limb-length measurements, and using lateral offset femoral necks may improve this outcome to 90% of patients.

Della Valle CJ, Stuchin SA: A novel technique for the removal of well-fixed, porous-coated acetabular components with spike fixation. *J Arthroplasty* 2001;16:1081-1083.

The authors describe using a jig for positioning a high-speed burr to transect spikes in well-fixed porous cups that use spikes for adjuvant fixation, thereby allowing the cup to be removed with curved gouges.

Incavo SJ, Havener T, Benson E, McGrory BJ, Coughlin KM, Beynnon BD: Efforts to improve cementless femoral stems in THR: 2- to 5-year follow-up of a high-offset femoral stem with distal modification (Secur-Fit Plus). *J Arthroplasty* 2004;19:61-67.

The authors reviewed 81 primary femoral stems with lateral offset. All stems were stable. Limb length was clinically equal in 85% of patients. The authors concluded that lateral offset potentially improves joint stability and limb-length equalization.

Kleemann RU, Heller MO, Stoeckle U, Taylor WR, Duda GN: THA loading arising from increased femoral anteversion and offset may lead to critical cement stresses. *J Orthop Res* 2003;21(5):767-774.

The authors of this study reported that in a cemented total hip arthroplasty finite element model, variations in offset and femoral anteversion led to changes in loading, bone strain, and cement stresses. Increased anteversion and offset resulted in as much as a 67% increase in cement stresses. The authors suggested that these stresses put an implant at risk for loosening.

Classic Bibliography

Davey JR, O'Connor DO, Burke DW, Harris WH: Femoral component offset: Its effect on strain in bone-cement. *J Arthroplasty* 1993;8:23-26.

Shaw JA: Experience with a modified posterior approach to the hip joint: A technical note. *J Arthroplasty* 1991;6:11-18.

Woolson ST, Harris WH: A method of intraoperative limb length measurement in total hip arthroplasty. *Clin Orthop* 1985;194:207-210.

Woolson ST, Hartford JM, Sawyer A: Results of a method of leg-length equalization for patients undergoing primary total hip replacement. *J Arthroplasty* 1999;14(2):159-164.

Chapter 44

Osteonecrosis of the Hip

Michael A. Mont, MD

Jess H. Lonner, MD

Phillip S. Ragland, MD

Introduction

Osteonecrosis of the hip occurs in a young patient population (mean age, 35 to 40 years) and affects approximately 20,000 patients per year in the United States. Although this incidence appears relatively small, population studies have shown that patients with osteonecrosis of the hip account for approximately 10% of the total hip replacements performed in the United States.

When left untreated, patients with osteonecrosis of the hip will invariably develop an area of the femoral head that weakens, resulting in femoral head collapse and eventual joint destruction. Consequently, many patients will eventually need to undergo total joint arthroplasty to treat this arthritic condition. Unfortunately, the long-term results of total hip replacements in this patient population are poorer than those for total hip replacements for other more common arthritides. This may be a result of the younger mean age of this patient population or possibly other factors, such as the high percentage of patients with osteonecrosis who require chronic corticosteroid use. It is recommended, therefore, that attempts should be made to save these patients' hips and preserve femoral bone stock whenever possible. Because this requires early diagnosis and treatment, preferably before femoral head collapse has occurred, it is important that orthopaedic surgeons have a thorough understanding of the associated risk factors as well as different diagnostic methods for osteonecrosis of the hip. Staging patients appropriately so that the most optimal treatment methods can be used is also important, as is an understanding of the different surgical treatment methods available.

Pathophysiology, Pathology, and Associated Risk Factors

Osteonecrosis of the hip typically affects the weight-bearing superolateral portion of the femoral head. In the early stages, ischemia leads to bone death, and the dead trabeculae are then replaced by granulation tissue. It is postulated that the body's attempt to repair this dead bone through creeping substitution weakens the subchondral bone. As the lesion increases in size, bone resorption outpaces bone formation, which results in collapse of the femoral head. In the early stage of collapse, the contour of the femoral head is preserved, and fluid fills the underlying space below. This is seen radiographically as the crescent sign (Figure 1). In later stages, as the femoral head collapses, the overlying articular cartilage develops irregularities that eventually affect the adjoining acetabular cartilage, causing arthritic changes on both sides of the joint (late stage osteonecrosis/osteoarthritis).

There are several different pathophysiologic mechanisms and causes of osteonecrosis of the hip. It is useful to divide the associated risk factors into two groups: direct causes and indirect causes (Table 1). Direct causes are factors that specifically result in osteonecrosis. For example, in a traumatic dislocation of the femoral head or a fractured femoral neck, the tearing of the lateral epiphyseal vessels leads to infarction or ischemia of the femoral head and directly causes osteonecrosis. Other direct causes include intravascular decompression of nitrogen gas, resulting in bubbles that clog circulation in the femoral head of scuba divers (caisson disease). Patients with sickle cell anemia may have sickled red blood cells that sludge the circulation leading to osteonecrosis. Myeloproliferative disorders, in which the marrow of the femoral head is crowded out by tumors such as leukemia, lymphomas, and Gaucher's disease, can also be direct causes. Direct radiation to the femoral head can lead to necrosis. Other risk factors are associated indirectly with osteonecrosis in which there is not a one-to-one correlation between the risk factor and the disease. For example, corticosteroids have been associated with osteonecrosis, but in most patients (85% to 90%), those taking high-dose corticosteroids do not develop osteonecrosis. It has been postulated that there is a genetic predisposition in these patients, and corticosteroids may serve as a secondary insult that potentially initiates the disease process. Other risk factors such as alcohol and tobacco use have also shown a three- to ten-fold increase in the risk for developing osteonecrosis when compared with the general population. Genetic

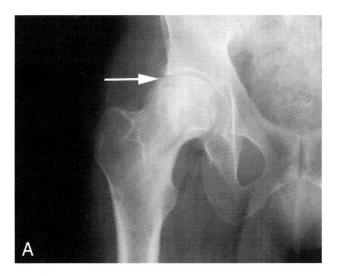
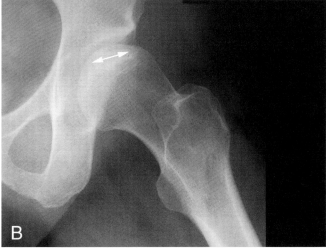

Figure 1 AP **(A)** and lateral **(B)** radiographs showing crescent sign (*arrows*). (Reproduced from Lieberman JR, Berry DJ: *Advanced Reconstruction: Hip*. Rosemont, IL, American Academy of Orthopaedic Surgeons, 2005.)

Table 1 | Etiologies and Risk Factors Associated With Osteonecrosis of the Femoral Head

Direct Causes	Indirect Causes	Less Common Risk Factors
Trauma	Corticosteroids	Polyarteritis
Irradiation	Alcohol abuse	Thalassemia
Hematologic disorders (leukemias, lymphomas)	Systemic lupus erythematosus	Carbon tetrachloride poisoning
Cytotoxins	Renal failure	Hyperlipidemia/hyperlipoproteinemia
Dysbaric osteonecrosis (caisson disease)	Organ transplant (steroids/other immunosuppressives)	Cushing disease
Gaucher's disease	Idiopathic osteonecrosis	Pregnancy/oral contraceptives
Sickle cell disease or trait	Hemophilia	Pancreatitis
	Thrombophilia	Gout/hyperuricemia
	Hypofibrinolysis	Hyperparathyroidism
		Venous occlusion
		Thermal injuries

predisposition for osteonecrosis is more readily seen in patients with inherited coagulation disorders. Studies have shown a higher incidence of thrombophilia (increased likelihood of blood clots) and hypofibrinolysis (decreased ability to lyse blood clots) in patients with osteonecrosis.

The pathophysiology of osteonecrosis has yet to be completely elucidated. Although the pathophysiology is clear in the direct causes of osteonecrosis, in the patient population with indirect causes or associated risk factors (the patients who comprise most treated instances of osteonecrosis), the pathophysiology is uncertain. Vascular theories, neurologic theories, sick bone cells, and various other theories have been proposed. Many of these theories are not mutually exclusive. Recent work has shown that inherited coagulation defects, in combination with other factors, may lead to osteonecrosis.

Diagnosis

To treat patients successfully with head-preserving procedures, early diagnosis is essential. Unfortunately, many patients do not receive definitive treatment until well beyond 6 months and often more than 1 year from the time symptoms begin. A key to diagnosis is appreciating that patients (younger and older) with groin pain and associated risk factors should be evaluated carefully to rule out osteonecrosis. The most common presenting symptom is typically groin pain, but in less than 10% of patients, other symptoms such as knee pain or posterior buttock pain may be reported. Symptoms can often be alleviated by not bearing weight, but when patients resume full weight bearing, the groin pain will typically recur. Surgeons should also understand that this osteonecrosis of the hip has been shown to occur bilaterally in more than 80% of patients in large series.

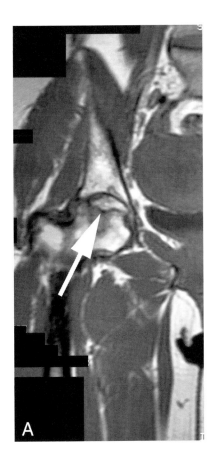
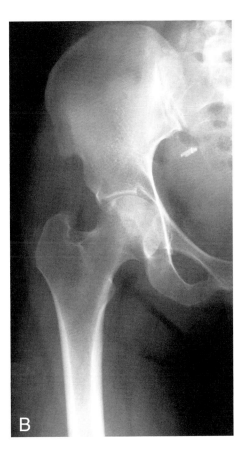

Figure 2 MRI scan **(A)** showing small necrotic segment (*arrow*) that is not visible on standard radiograph **(B)**. (Reproduced from Lieberman JR, Berry DJ: *Advanced Reconstruction: Hip*. Rosemont, IL, American Academy of Orthopaedic Surgeons, 2005.)

Radiographic Analysis

Standard radiography is the diagnostic method of choice for the initial evaluation of a patient with suspected osteonecrosis. However, because plain radiography can only detect alterations in bone density, as seen when remodeling occurs in the middle to late stages, it may not detect the early stage of the disease process when the necrotic foci is present. Standard AP and cross-table lateral radiographs are helpful to show the extent of collapse, if present. If the radiographs are pathognomonic for osteonecrosis (crescent sign) or severe collapse is present, no other further imaging modalities may be necessary. In patients with suspected osteonecrosis for whom standard radiography is inconclusive, MRI is indicated to rule out the presence of disease.

Magnetic Resonance Imaging

The most appropriate ancillary diagnostic imaging modality is MRI, which has been shown in multiple studies to be 99% sensitive and 99% specific for osteonecrosis. In the past, these studies have been very costly; however, recent advances in diagnostic imaging have considerably reduced the expense. Focal increases in signal intensity on T2-weighted images or the presence of a low intensity band on T1-weighted images are pathognomonic for osteonecrosis (Figure 2).

Other Diagnostic Modalities

Other methods have been advocated for screening for osteonecrosis. Bone scanning has been used commonly in the past, but it has been shown to miss lesions in 10% to 40% of patients. It is nonspecific and should not typically be used as a screening test because of the high sensitivity and specificity of MRI. CT was also formerly used to screen for osteonecrosis, but is no longer necessary for the diagnosis of this condition. Occasionally, CT can be used to detect whether collapse is present or to follow disease progression after treatment because CT delineates the bony contour better than MRI. In patients with mechanical symptoms and precollapse disease, hip arthroscopy can be useful because it allows the surgeon to assess the articular cartilage intraoperatively while simultaneously performing any necessary procedures. Recently, the use of positron emission tomography has been investigated for analysis of subchondral blood flow and may be useful in the near future. Other invasive testing such as core biopsy and venography are no longer recommended because of the high sensitivity of MRI.

Staging

Multiple staging systems have been described for osteonecrosis. Most of these staging systems have evolved from the Ficat and Arlet four-tier system for radiographic analysis, which is still the most commonly used system. Most systems are similar for early stage precollapse disease (stages I and II). In the Steinberg classification system, size was added as a significant prognostic factor. Other systems included considerations such as type and location of the necrotic lesion.

Treatment

Four factors should be considered to determine the appropriate treatment of patients with osteonecrosis: (1) the presence of collapse, (2) the size of the lesion, (3) the amount of head depression, and (4) acetabular involvement. Precollapse disease confers the best prognosis for patients and requires less invasive modalities for treatment. If collapse is present, more invasive procedures are likely necessary. As previously stated, CT may be more helpful in assessing the contour of the femoral head when standard radiography is equivocal. Smaller lesions fare better than larger lesions in bone-preserving procedures. Larger lesions may require prosthetic replacement if subchondral bone is affected. Lesions with less than 2 mm of depression typically have a better prognosis. Acetabular changes signify late-stage disease; thus, total joint arthroplasty is usually necessary.

Nonsurgical Treatment

Several nonsurgical treatment methods have been used. These procedures have typically been recommended for patients with early stage, precollapse disease. The most common method uses partial weight bearing with a single crutch or cane, or no weight bearing. The rationale for this treatment is to relieve weight from the femoral head to allow necrotic bone to heal. In a recent report, some necrotic lesions were shown to heal without surgical intervention; however, this occurred in a small percentage of patients (< 5%). Although no weight bearing is described as a conservative treatment method, it is actually radical in nature because it will lead to certain collapse of the femoral head and likely total hip replacement. It is therefore recommended that this nonsurgical method be used only in patients who cannot undergo a surgical procedure because of medical or physical limitations, those who wish to delay a joint preserving procedure for a short period, and those with small lesions that are asymptomatic.

The multifactorial aspect of osteonecrosis makes the use of pharmacologic agents difficult because these agents typically affect one component of the etiologic mechanism. Use of pharmacologic agents is based on the multiple hypotheses regarding the pathophysiology of this disease (such as venous stasis, cellular hypertrophy, lipid emboli, thrombosis, and elevated intraosseous pressure). These agents include lipid lowering agents, vasodilators, and anticoagulants. Although there is no consensus on the efficacy of these modalities, it is possible that

they may be used in the future in conjunction with surgical procedures to save the femoral head. One class of agents that has shown promise in foreign studies is the bisphosphonates. These agents inhibit osteoclast activity, curtail bone resorption, and can theoretically slow the progression of disease based on the hypothesis that increased resorption causes collapse of the femoral head. The use of bisphosphonates is still investigational, however, and larger studies are necessary to show their efficacy in the treatment of osteonecrosis. Surgeons should note, however, that the use of these noninvasive modalities is controversial and should never be used in patients who are biomechanically compromised.

Surgical Treatment

Surgical procedures for treating osteonecrosis of the hip can be classified as either joint preserving procedures (core decompression, bone grafting, and osteotomy) or joint arthroplasty procedures (limited femoral resurfacing, total hip arthroplasty, and total joint resurfacing).

Joint-Preserving Procedures
Core Decompression

Core decompression is an evolution of the core biopsy used by Ficat and Arlet to diagnose osteonecrosis in the 1970s. Core decompression reduces intraosseous pressure, promotes neovascularization, and provides immediate pain relief. This method of treatment is commonly used in patients with small to medium precollapse lesions. However, its use is still considered controversial because several studies have also shown high failure rates (up to 86% of patient) and/or no difference in long-term outcome when using this procedure when compared with other surgical procedures. One study compared the use of core decompression to nonsurgical management and reported successful results in 741 of 1,166 hips (63.5%) that were treated with core decompression compared with 182 of 819 hips (22.7%) that were treated nonsurgically. A more recent study reported on the use of multiple small-diameter (3.2-mm) drilling to perform core decompression (Figure 3). The authors reported an 80% success rate in patients with stage I lesions and a 57% success rate in those with stage II lesions at a mean follow-up of 2 years (range, 20 to 39 months). These results were comparable to those reported in another study that compared 30 hips treated with core decompression using the standard (8- to 10-mm trephine) drilling method to 35 hips treated with multiple small drillings. The authors reported a 55% rate of collapse in the group of patients who underwent the standard drilling method and a 14.3% rate of collapse in the group of patients who underwent multiple drilling at a mean follow-up of 60.3 months.

The most common method of core decompression uses an 8- to 10-mm trephine inserted through the fem-

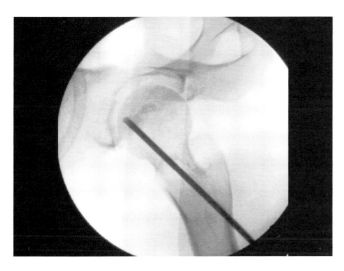

Figure 3 Intraoperative fluoroscopic image of the small pin (3.2-mm) technique.

oral neck under fluoroscopic guidance to the site of the lesion in the femoral head. Subtrochanteric fractures can occur if the entry point to the femoral neck is too far distally (in the diaphysis). When using the multiple small drilling technique described previously, the potential for fracture is essentially eliminated, and the percutaneous approach further reduces morbidity because it is less invasive.

The key to using core decompression to successfully manage patients with osteonecrosis of the hip is early diagnosis and treatment before collapse of the femoral head. This modality has been shown to be an effective treatment option in symptomatic patients with small to medium precollapse lesions.

Vascularized Bone Grafting

Vascularized bone grafting introduces a vascular supply into the ischemic bone while simultaneously bolstering the necrotic segment. The rationale for this procedure is that it may allow decompression of the femoral head, removal of the necrotic segment, mechanical support of weakened subchondral bone, autogenous substrate, and revascularization of the femoral head. The technique typically involves the use of a pedicle from the fibula, with the peroneal vessels inserted into a core tract through the femoral neck. The peroneal vessels are then anastomosed to the ascending branches of the lateral femoral circumflex artery. Several studies have shown this to be an effective modality for small to medium lesions. Some authors have compared the outcomes with other modalities such as core decompression. One such study compared the outcomes of free vascularized bone grafting to core decompression and reported successful outcome in 8 of 19 patients (42%) in the core decompression group compared with 16 of 20 (80%) in the vascularized bone grafting group. The superiority of vascularized grafting in this cohort could be because of

larger lesions and late-stage disease in the hips that failed and for which the results of core decompression are historically poor. These results were similar to those reported in another study that compared the two modalities in patients with stage II lesions (postcollapse) and found superior results with vascularized fibular grafting.

In another study, only 29 of 63 stage I, II, and III hips were successful treated using vascularized fibular grafting at a minimum 4-year follow-up. The high failure rate may be in part the result of the inclusion of patients with late-stage postcollapse lesions. Regarding placement of the strut, the authors reported superior results (80% at 10-year follow-up) when the graft was positioned in the subchondral area.

Complications with this procedure include femoral neck fracture, subtrochanteric fracture, graft failure, and donor site morbidity. One study recently reported an incidence of heterotopic ossification of 32% after implantation of vascularized fibular grafts. Despite this relatively high incidence of heterotopic ossification, the authors reported no associated complications or functional deficits in these patients. In light of these data, the vascularized fibular graft is best used for patients with small to medium lesions with precollapse or early collapse disease. Late-stage disease with acetabular changes is a contraindication for this modality.

Nonvascularized Bone Grafting

The rationale for using nonvascularized bone grafting to treat osteonecrosis is to replace necrotic bone with healthy, viable bone or graft substance. Although there are several variations of this procedure, most are straightforward and vary primarily concerning the entry point for graft insertion (core tract, femoral neck, femoral cartilage, and femoral head-neck junction). The technique of bone grafting the femoral head was first described in the 1960s; a strut graft (harvested from ilium, fibula, or tibia) was inserted into the femoral head through an 8- to 10-mm core tract created in the femoral neck from the lateral cortex of the proximal femur. Using this technique, success rates as high as 90% were reported. Similar results were reported in later studies at short-term follow-up. However, this technique is not commonly used today because long-term follow-up of these patients showed failure rates of up to 71% at 14-year follow-up.

Another point of entry, through a trapdoor in the articular cartilage, was first described in 1966, but detailed results using this technique were first reported in 1983. Using cancellous bone as a graft substance, good to excellent results were reported in 8 of 9 hips (90%) at a mean follow-up of 3 years (range, 1 to 9 years). Another study reported clinical success in 20 of 24 hips (83%) with stage III disease using a combination of cortical struts and cancellous bone along with this technique.

The use of a window in the femoral neck as an entry point was first described in 1983. This procedure was combined with an osteotomy and cancellous bone was used as a grafting substance. Clinical results using this technique were reported in 1989. Using autogenous cortical iliac strut grafts, excellent or good results were achieved in 23 of 38 hips (61%) at a mean follow-up of 9 years (range, 2 to 15 years). This technique was further modified by placement of the cortical window at the head-neck junction (the so-called light bulb procedure). Using autogenous iliac crest, the authors reported clinical success in 13 of 15 hips at a mean follow-up of 12 years (range, 10 to 15 years). Another study recently reported clinical success in 18 of 21 hips (86%) at a mean 4-year follow-up using demineralized bone matrix enriched allograft through a window created at the head-neck junction (Figure 4). The development of other ancillary growth factors and cytokines for grafting may increase the popularity and success of this technique in the future.

These procedures are recommended for the treatment of patients with precollapse osteonecrosis or head depression less than 2 mm. Other patients, such as those in whom core decompression has failed, are potential candidates if the femoral head cartilage is intact. It is, therefore, imperative that the cartilage be thoroughly inspected intraoperatively for any irregularities that would preclude the application of one of these techniques. These nonvascularized techniques offer a straightforward, head-preserving procedure that can be easily converted to a total hip replacement if necessary.

Osteotomy

Several types of osteotomies are used in the treatment of osteonecrosis. The most common techniques involve planar (varus and valgus) and multiplanar (transtrochanteric/rotational) methods. In this procedure, the necrotic segment of the femoral head is moved from a weight-bearing position in the acetabulum to a position in which it will bear less weight.

These procedures have been found to have the best results in patients younger than 45 years, those with early postcollapse osteonecrosis with no acetabular involvement, those with small to medium lesions, and those who have not used long-term corticosteroids.

The technique of transtrochanteric osteotomy involves rotating the necrotic segment within the acetabulum to a position where it does not bear weight. Authors of a 1980 study used double osteotomy with a maximum 180° of rotation and were the first to report the results of rotational osteotomies, with the best results found in patients with small lesions. Another study reported successful outcome in 229 of 295 hips (78%) at a mean follow-up of 11 years (range, 3 to 16 years). Although authors in Japan subsequently reported similar results, these results have not been duplicated in the United

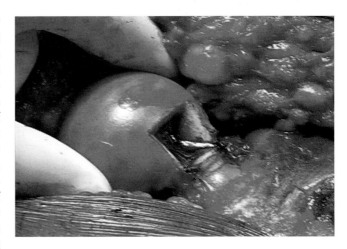

Figure 4 Intraoperative photograph of the cortical window created at the head-neck junction. (Reproduced from Lieberman JR, Berry DJ: *Advanced Reconstruction: Hip.* Rosemont, IL, American Academy of Orthopaedic Surgeons, 2005.)

States. In a series at the Mayo Clinic, for example, only a 17% success rate at 5-year follow-up was reported.

Varus and valgus osteotomies are less technically demanding and have been used more commonly in the United States. Although results vary, several authors have reported success rates of 65% or greater with varus and valgus osteotomies at 5- to 15-year follow-up. One study evaluated outcomes in 37 corrective osteotomies for the treatment of stage II and III osteonecrosis and reported a 76% success rate at a mean follow-up of 11.5 years. In this series, osteotomies were most successful in treating patients with lesions with a combined necrotic angle less than 200° (87%). These findings are similar to those of another study in which osteotomies resulted in better outcomes for patients with smaller lesions. Overall, the use of osteotomies has recently decreased in the United States, perhaps because deforming the proximal femur makes subsequent total hip arthroplasty more difficult to perform.

Joint Arthroplasty Procedures

Limited Femoral Resurfacing

Resurfacing the femoral head is similar in concept to its use in knees for knee replacements in that the diseased cartilage is removed surgically and replaced by a prosthetic joint. Limited resurfacing refers to prosthetic placement on the femoral side only, which then articulates with native acetabular cartilage. Total resurfacing refers to prosthetic replacement of both the femoral and acetabular sides of the joint.

Limited femoral resurfacing can be used in symptomatic patients with medium to large lesions, a collapsed femoral head, and minimal or no acetabular involvement. The potential advantages of limited femoral resurfacing over total hip arthroplasty include lower dislocation rates, bone stock preservation, and easy conversion to total hip arthroplasty if necessary.

The principles of resurfacing arthroplasty of the hip have evolved from the original designs in the 1940s and 1950s. Early designs used glass and other biomaterials but had poor mid- to long-term results. Several recent studies have reported higher success rates using newer designs.

Limited resurfacing is best used in patients with pre-collapse osteonecrosis and pristine native acetabular cartilage. One study found that patients treated with limited resurfacing when symptoms were present for less than 6 months had better outcomes than patients with symptoms for longer periods. These findings may be the result of less macroscopic degeneration of the acetabulum in patients who are treated earlier. Limited resurfacing may also be advantageous in this younger patient population because it allows more activity than a total hip replacement. One study compared the outcomes of limited resurfacing to total hip arthroplasty in patients with osteonecrosis and found that a higher percentage of patients who underwent limited resurfacing maintained high activity levels (60%) compared with the total arthroplasty group (27%) at a mean follow-up of 7 years. Results can generally be expected to yield up to a 90% success rate at 7-year follow-up, although some patients (20%) may have persistent groin pain.

Total Hip Resurfacing

Total hip resurfacing is a treatment option for patients with late-stage osteonecrosis and acetabular involvement. Metal-on-metal designs were first introduced in the mid 1960s, but were abandoned because of high failure rates. With improved technology and extensive experience in Europe, metal-on-metal resurfacing has experienced renewed interest in the United States over the past 5 years. Total hip resurfacing may provide a better treatment alternative to the young patient population because the large femoral head mimics the biomechanics of the native joint. Additionally, young patients might not experience the groin pain that can occur after undergoing hemiresurfacing. However, these devices are still under investigation in the United States, and data regarding long-term outcomes are necessary before it can be determined whether this is a viable option for the treatment of young patients with osteonecrosis.

Total Hip Arthroplasty

Total hip arthroplasty is currently the procedure of choice for patients with late-stage disease in whom bone preserving procedures are not possible. However, historical results for hip replacement in this population have been poor. One study reviewed 55 patients with a mean follow-up of 9.8 years (range, 5 to 14 years) and reported a revision rate of 21%, and several studies have reported equivalent or higher failure rates in this patient population. The likely reason for these poor results is multifactorial. One study showed that necrosis ex-

Table 2	Treatment Algorithm	
Stage	**Treatment**
I (asymptomatic)	Observation
	Pharmacologic therapy, core decompression (controversial)
I (symptomatic)	Core decompression
	Bone grafting (vascularized or nonvascularized)
	Osteotomy
II	Core decompression (small or medium lesions)
	Bone grafting (medium to large lesions)
	Osteotomy
	Limited resurfacing (large lesions)
III	Bone grafting (early collapse)
	Limited femoral resurfacing
IV	Standard total hip arthroplasty
	Total joint resurfacing

tends into the lesser trochanteric eminence causing intramedullary sclerotic changes. These histologic changes, along with a young, active population, may account for the high failure rates for total hip arthroplasty.

Newer designs with improved wear coefficients may improve the longevity of hip replacements in patients with osteonecrosis. One study recently reported a 93.4% success rate at a mean 11.2-year follow-up (range, 10 to 15 years). Another study reported similar results, with a 4% revision rate at a mean follow-up of 4.6 years (range, 2 to 10 years). Although these results are not as good as those for the overall population, they represent a marked improvement over historical results, and will likely improve in the future. Currently, however, it is recommended that hip replacement should be a last resort procedure in patients with late-stage disease.

Treatment Algorithm

For patients with early stage asymptomatic osteonecrosis of the hip, surveillance with serial radiographs every 6 months or until symptoms arise allows adequate time for early intervention should the disease progress or symptoms occur. In asymptomatic patients with no femoral head collapse, there has been debate over whether these patients should be treated either with protected weight bearing or pharmacologic therapy. Although one study reported a 50% likelihood of these hips to collapse, these results have varied with several reports showing less likelihood of disease progression. Therefore, treatment of asymptomatic disease is not recommended. For patients with symptomatic small or medium lesions and no evidence of collapse or pending collapse (crescent sign), a core decompression is appropriate. For patients with medium and large lesions and no femoral head collapse, a bone grafting procedure, osteotomy, hemiresurfacing, or a combination of bone grafting and osteotomy may be appropriate. If there is femoral head cartilage damage without acetabular damage, hemiresurfacing can be used. If there is acetabular damage, total hip replacement (resurfacing or standard) is appropriate (Table 2).

Summary

Osteonecrosis is a disorder that accounts for approximately 10% of the hip replacements performed in the United States. Surgeons should make every attempt to save the femoral head in these patients. Early diagnosis is key and requires an awareness of associated risk factors in symptomatic patients. Various treatment methods exist to save the femoral head, and most of these methods are more successful in early stages of the disease. In patients who need total hip replacements, the results of present-generation prostheses are better than those reported in previous older studies.

Annotated Bibliography

Pathophysiology, Pathology, and Associated Risk Factors

Jones LC, Mont MA, Le TB, et al: Procoagulants and osteonecrosis. *J Rheumatol* 2003;30:783-791.

The authors report an 82% incidence of at least one coagulopathy in patients with osteonecrosis.

Steinberg ME, Mont MA: *Chapman's Orthopedic Surgery*, ed 3. Philadelphia, PA, JB Lippincott, 2001.

This is a comprehensive review of osteonecrosis of the hip and a useful treatment algorithm is provided.

Nonsurgical Treatment

Agarwala S, Jain D, Joshi VR, Sule A: Efficacy of alendronate, a bisphosphonate, in the treatment of AVN of the hip: A prospective open-label study. *Rheumatology (Oxford)* 2005;44(3):352-359.

In this study, the authors show an overall reduction in pain, improvement in function, and disease regression in patients treated who were treated with alendronate 10 mg/day (70 mg/week) along with 500 to 1,000 mg of daily calcium and vitamin D supplements.

Cheng EY, Thongtrangan I, Saleh KJ: Spontaneous resolution of osteonecrosis of the femoral head. *J Bone Joint Surg Am* 2004;86:2594-2599.

The authors report spontaneous resolution of osteonecrosis of the femoral head in 3 of 13 asymptomatic hips.

Surgical Treatment

Beaule PE, Schmalzried TP, Campbell PA, Dorey F, Amstutz HC: Duration of symptoms and outcome of hemiresurfacing for osteonecrosis of the hip. *Clin Orthop Relat Res* 2001;385:104-117.

The authors report an overall survivorship of 79%, 59%, and 45% at 5-, 10-, and 15-year follow-up, respectively.

Calder JD, Pearse MF, Revell PA: The extent of osteocyte death in the proximal femur of patients with osteonecrosis of the femoral head. *J Bone Joint Surg Br* 2001;83:419-422.

The authors implicate osteocyte death as a contributing factor to early failure of total hip arthroplasty in this patient population.

Dailiana ZH, Gunneson EE, Urbaniak JR: Heterotopic ossification after treatment of femoral head osteonecrosis with free vascularized fibular graft. *J Arthroplasty* 2003;18:83-88.

The authors of this study reported a 32% incidence of heterotopic ossification following free vascularized fibular grafting.

Hartley WT, McAuley JP, Culpepper WJ, Engh CA Jr, Engh CA Sr: Osteonecrosis of the femoral head treated with cementless total hip arthroplasty. *J Bone Joint Surg Am* 2000;82:1408-1413.

The authors concluded that cementless total hip arthroplasty is a reasonable treatment option for advanced osteonecrosis of the hip.

Kim SY, Kim DH, Park IH, et al: Multiple drilling compared with core decompression for the treatment of osteonecrosis of the femoral head, in *ARCO Meeting Program, 2003*. Baltimore, MD, Association Research Circulation Osseous, 2003.

This represents the first report of the use of multiple small drilling as a technique for core decompression.

Mont MA, Etienne G, Ragland PS: Outcome of nonvascularized bone grafting for osteonecrosis of the femoral head. *Clin Orthop* 2003;417:84-92.

The authors report an 86% success rate in patients who underwent nonvascularized bone grafting for osteonecrosis of the hip.

Mont MA, Ragland PS, Etienne G: Core decompression of the femoral head for osteonecrosis using percutaneous multiple small-diameter drilling. *Clin Orthop Relat Res* 2004;429:131-137.

The authors report an 80% success rate in treatment of symptomatic stage I disease using this novel minimally invasive technique.

Mont MA, Rajadhyaksha AD, Hungerford DS: Outcomes of limited femoral resurfacing arthroplasty compared with total hip arthroplasty for osteonecrosis of the femoral head. *J Arthroplasty* 2001;16(8 suppl 1):134-139.

At a 7-year mean follow-up for resurfacing and an 8-year mean follow-up for total hip arthroplasty, the authors showed a survival rate of 90% and 93% for hemiresurfacing and THA, respectively.

Phemister DB: Treatment of the necrotic head of the femur in adults: Dallas Burton Phemister (1882-1951). *Clin Orthop Relat Res* 2000;381:4-8.

This is a historical review of the treatment strategy for this disease.

Xenakis TA, Gelalis J, Koukoubis TA, et al: Cementless hip arthroplasty in the treatment of patients with femoral head necrosis. *Clin Orthop Relat Res* 2001;386:93-99.

The authors report a 93% survivorship at mean follow-up of 11.2 years.

Classic Bibliography

Amstutz HC, Dorey F, O'Carroll PF: THARIES resurfacing arthroplasty: Evolution and long-term results. *Clin Orthop Relat Res* 1986;213:92-114.

Boettcher WG, Bonfiglio M, Smith K: Non-traumatic necrosis of the femoral head: Part II. Experiences in treatment. *J Bone Joint Surg Am* 1970;52:322-329.

Dean MT, Cabanela ME: Transtrochanteric anterior rotational osteotomy for avascular necrosis of the femoral head: Long-term results. *J Bone Joint Surg Br* 1993;75:597-601.

Ganz R, Buchler U: Overview of attempts to revitalize the dead head in aseptic necrosis of the femoral head: Osteotomy and revascularization, in *The Hip: Proceedings of the Eleventh Open Scientific Meeting of the Hip Society*. St. Louis, MO, Mosby, 1983, p 296.

Garino JP, Steinberg: Total hip arthroplasty in patients with avascular necrosis of the femoral head: A 2- to 10-year follow-up. *Clin Orthop Relat Res* 1997;334:108-115.

Glueck CJ, Glueck HI, Welch M, et al: Familial idiopathic osteonecrosis mediated by familial hypofibrinolysis with high levels of plasminogen activator inhibitor. *Thromb Haemost* 1994;71:195-198.

Hungerford DS: Bone marrow pressure, venography, and core decompression in ischemic necrosis of the femoral head, in *The Hip: Proceedings of the Seventh Open Scientific Meeting of the Hip Society*. St. Louis, MO, Mosby, 1979, p 218.

Itoman M, Yamamoto M: Pathogenesis and treatment of idiopathic aseptic necrosis of the femoral head. *Clin Immunol* 1989;21:713-725.

Judet R, Judet J, Launois B, Gubler JP: Trial of experimental revascularization of the femoral head. *Rev Chir Orthop Reparatrice Appar Mot* 1966;52:277-303.

Lavernia CJ, Sierra RJ, Grieco FR: Osteonecrosis of the femoral head. *J Am Acad Orthop Surg* 1999;7:250-261.

Merle D'Aubigne R, Postel M, Mazabraud A, Massias P, Gueguen J, France P: Idiopathic necrosis of the femoral head in adults. *J Bone Joint Surg Br* 1965;47:612-633.

Meyers MH, Jones RE, Bucholz RW, Wenger DR: Fresh autogenous grafts and osteochondral allografts for treatment of segmental collapse in osteonecrosis of the hip. *Clin Orthop Relat Res* 1983;174:107-112.

Mont MA, Carbone JJ, Fairbank AC: Core decompression versus nonoperative management for osteonecrosis of the hip. *Clin Orthop Relat Res* 1996;324:169-178.

Mont MA, Einhorn TA, Sponseller PD, Hungerford DS: The trapdoor procedure using autogenous cortical and cancellous bone grafts for osteonecrosis of the femoral head. *J Bone Joint Surg Br* 1998;80:56-62.

Mont MA, Fairbank AC, Krackow KA, Hungerford DS: Corrective osteotomy for osteonecrosis of the femoral head. *J Bone Joint Surg Am* 1996;78:1032-1038.

Rosenwasser MP, Garino JP, Kiernan HA, Michelsen CB: Long-term follow-up of thorough debridement and cancellous bone grafting of the femoral head for avascular necrosis. *Clin Orthop* 1994;306:17-27.

Sugioka Y, Hotokebuchi T, Tsutsui H: Transtrochanteric anterior rotational osteotomy for idiopathic and steroid-induced necrosis of the femoral head: Indications and long-term results. *Clin Orthop* 1992;277:111-120.

Urbaniak JR, Coogan PG, Gunneson EB, Nunley JA: Treatment of osteonecrosis of the femoral head with free vascularized fibular grafting: A long-term follow-up study of one hundred and three hips. *J Bone Joint Surg Am* 1995;77:681-694.

Wagner H, Zeiler G: Idiopathic avascular necrosis of the femoral head: Results of intertrochanteric osteotomy and resurfacing. *Orthopade* 1980;9:290-310.

Chapter 45

Osteolysis

Andrew Grose, MD

Steven B. Zelicof, MD, PhD

Introduction

More than 40 years after Charnley's revolutionary studies in the treatment of degenerative hip disease, osteolysis remains the greatest obstacle to excellent long-term function of total hip arthroplasty. The etiology is clearly multifactorial, involving implant design, bearing surfaces, and patient factors. It is therefore crucial that physicians treating patients with osteolysis have a thorough understanding of the basic science, radiographic evaluation, and general management of osteolysis in patients who have undergone total hip arthroplasty. The term osteolysis is often used interchangeably with the term aseptic loosening. Although osteolysis and aseptic loosening have been used to describe radiographically distinct lesions, it is clear that in both the fundamental process is identical.

What Causes Osteolysis?

Total hip arthroplasty necessarily violates a previously isolated and immune-privileged area. During this violation, two essential events on the path to osteolysis occur: (1) foreign bodies with manmade bearing surfaces are implanted, and (2) the joint space is expanded and redefined in terms of new boundaries to pseudosynovial fluid flow. The new boundaries to this fluid may not be limited to the outer surface of the bone—implants that are not well fixed to the bone allow fluid to migrate along the length of the prosthesis-bone (or cement-bone) interface. The limitations on fluid flow that occur after total hip arthroplasty have been conceptualized as the effective joint space. In some instances, the fluid pressure within the effective joint space may be high. In rat models, increased fluid pressure alone has been shown to cause dramatic osteolysis. Although increased intracapsular pressure has been documented in some patients with osteolytic hips, the contribution of this fluid pressure to osteolysis remains unclear. It is clear, however, that particulate debris from the implants is spread throughout the effective joint space. It is also well documented that the implants used in total hip arthroplasty create particulate debris.

Particulate debris can be produced secondary to either corrosion or wear. Although implant corrosion does occur in physiologic solutions, it does not seem to play a significant role in aseptic loosening. Most particles are from wear of the bearing surfaces, and by far the most numerous of these are submicron polyethylene particles. Up to 500,000 submicron-sized particles per step can be generated from a standard cobalt-chromium femoral head articulating with a polyethylene liner. In addition to polyethylene (or in place of it and in alternate bearing surface replacements), wear debris can consist of polymethylmethacrylate, metals, and ceramics. As it has become clearer that the host's response to wear particles is the primary force behind osteolysis, the disease has been conceptualized as a disease of access—access of the particles to the implant-bone interface and access of the immune system to the particulate debris. Research has subsequently focused on three major areas: (1) the generation of wear debris, (2) the cellular biology of bone resorption, and (3) limiting the effective joint space.

The Biology of Bone Resorption

Early investigations into the membrane surrounding loose implants showed it consisted of many fibroblasts and macrophages, and produced large amounts of inflammatory mediators (prostaglandin E_2, interleukin-1, interleukin-6, tumor necrosis factor-α [TNF-α], and others). It has been postulated that the local macrophage response to debris led to activation of an inflammatory cascade. Polymethylmethacrylate, polyethylene, and titanium have all been shown to stimulate macrophages to produce these cytokines. Particle size, composition, and dose all influence the macrophage response. High doses of particles in the 0.5 to 5.0 μm range induce a maximal response. Larger particles provoke more of a foreign body response, and small particles (< 0.45 μm) do not appear to stimulate cells well. Although polyethylene, titanium, cobalt-chromium, and polymethylmethacrylate have all been shown to produce an abundant macrophage response in vitro, the consensus is that ultra-high

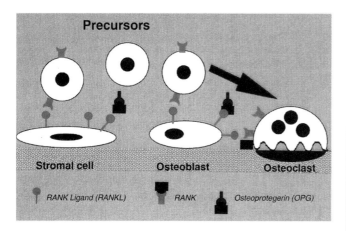

Figure 1 Schematic representation of how, in normal bone physiology, formation and resorption are linked via the receptor activator for nuclear factor kappa B ligand (RANKL)–receptor activator for nuclear factor kappa B (RANK) activation system. RANKL exists as a surface ligand on osteoblasts and stromal cells. It has two known natural receptors: osteoprotegerin and RANK. RANK is a surface receptor existing on macrophage/monocyte cells and osteoclasts.(Reproduced with permission from Clohisy D: Cellular mechanisms of osteolysis. *J Bone Joint Surg Am* 2003;85(suppl 1):4-6.)

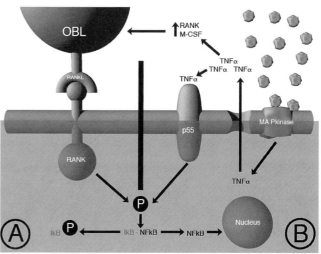

Figure 2 Schematic representation of several mechanisms operating on the monocyte/macrophage lineage to stimulate osteoclastogenesis. Each of these pathways ultimately leads to a freeing of NFκB for migration into the nucleus and regulation of DNA transcription. The shaded area represents the monocyte/macrophage cell. In normal osteoclastogenesis, binding of RANK to RANKL activates a cytosolic phosphorylation (P) cascade. NFκB is a cytosolic transcription factor that has a high affinity relationship with its natural inhibitor, inhibitor of kappa B (IκB). Upon phosphorylation of IκB, IκB-NFκB dissociate, and NFκB moves to the nucleus to regulate transcription. OBL = osteoblast (**A**). Particulate-debris and cell-surface interaction with wear particles activates a mitogen-activated protein kinase (MAPkinase), thereby upregulating TNF-α production. TNF-α upregulates RANKL and monocyte colony stimulating factor (M-CSF) production, thereby driving the RANK-RANKL system. TNF-α also binds to the p55 receptor, leading to intracellular kinase activity and the activation of NFκB pathway independent of RANK (**B**).

molecular weight polyethylene (UHMWPE) is the main culprit in provoking clinically significant osteolysis. (A recent study using a murine model of osteolysis has shown the in vivo response to be significantly greater to UHMWPE when compared with titanium.) It is now clear that although macrophages respond to these particles via both phagocytosis and surface receptor interactions, phagocytosis is not necessary for osteolysis to occur. The end result of macrophage activation is osteoclastogenesis, resulting in a net loss of bone.

Over the past decade, researchers in basic cellular biology have elucidated the normal signaling pathways leading to osteoclastogenesis (Figure 1). Receptor activator for nuclear factor kappa B ligand (RANKL)–receptor activator for nuclear factor kappa B (RANK) and monocyte colony stimulating factor are essential factors in normal osteoclastogenesis. It is also clear that a transcription factor, nuclear factor kappa B (NFκB) is the final common pathway for conversion of the monocyte/macrophage precursor to the osteoclast (Figure 2, *A*). It has recently been shown that new osteoclasts are derived from the circulating monocyte/macrophage pool exposed to the wear debris. Particulate debris is able to activate NFκB independent of the RANKL-RANK system (Figure 2, *B*). Blockade of NFκB activation at several levels has been shown to prevent particle-induced osteolysis. Finally, it has been shown that titanium particulates act to inhibit osteoblast function, possibly further accentuating the effect of osteoclasts in periprosthetic bone. Several studies are underway to actively explore methods of medically altering the molecular biology associated with osteoclastogenesis and bone resorption.

Limiting the Generation of Wear Debris

Although many of the details of the generation of wear particles are beyond the scope of this chapter, any discussion of osteolysis must include an examination of the effects of wear debris and the efforts to eliminate it. Efforts to eliminate wear have focused on improvements in UHMWPE, alternate bearing surfaces, and other component issues. Because most total hip arthroplasties use cobalt-chromium–polyethylene articulations, the overwhelming source of wear debris remains polyethylene. The wear rate of polyethylene, whether calculated as linear or volumetric loss, correlates with the development of osteolysis. Increasing linear wear rates as low as 0.1 mm/yr quadruples the likelihood of osteolysis. A similarly increased risk of osteolysis was found with increases in volumetric wear; each 40 cubic-mm/yr increase led to a threefold increase in osteolysis. Because linear wear rates of less than 0.1 mm/yr have consistently demonstrated low rates of osteolysis, it has been hypothesized that wear lower than 0.05 mm/yr is an acceptable rate, that is, below a proposed osteolysis threshold. This, however, remains a topic of debate.

Several factors are known to affect conventional polyethylene's ability to resist wear, including internal destabilization of the polyethylene, thickness, and internal cross-linking of polyethylene chains. Sterilization by irradiation of polyethylene in air produces free radicals that oxidize the polyethylene chains, leading to early internal instability in the polyethylene component. Prolonged shelf life of the polyethylene before insertion can also lead to oxidation, creating a similar effect. Conventional polyethylene thickness of less than 6 mm has been shown to increase both the rate of wear and osteolysis. It is important to remember that the manufacturer's labeling of the liner thickness refers to the central area, not the periphery. The periphery of the liner is typically thinner, and importantly, it is the periphery of the liner that bears most of the stress. Paradoxically, the same irradiation that produces potentially harmful oxidation can also strengthen UHMWPE. Highly cross-linked polyethylene has been shown in a hip simulator model to dramatically decrease the rate of polyethylene wear, even when articulating with a 32-mm head. Although implant manufacturers may use gamma irradiation to stimulate oxidation and controlled cross-linking, terminal sterilization is accomplished through one of several alternate processes (such as ethylene oxide).

Component issues not specifically related to the bearing surface, such as malalignment of the implant and socket modularity, have also clearly been associated with alteration of wear rates. Increased cup abduction angle has been shown to focus stresses on the outer rim of the cup and lead to early wear, especially in modular systems. Finite element analysis predicts significantly higher peak contact stresses for cups placed in excess of 45° of abduction. Hip simulator experiments confirmed wear rates of 21.7 mg/million cycles for cups placed at 55° compared with 17.2 mg/million cycles at an abduction angle of 45°. Failure to restore femoral offset may also contribute to an increased wear rate. Although it is known that decreasing offset increases the joint reactive force, the clinical demonstration of this as a factor in wear rates has been confounded. Nevertheless, it should be assumed that restoration of offset has a protective effect on the bearing surface. Regarding the effect of socket modularity on wear rates, a direct comparison of modular and nonmodular acetabular fixation showed a dramatically increased rate of osteolysis in modular components (2% versus 22%). In general, modularity causes decreased polyethylene thickness and potentially decreases conformity between the backing and the liner.

Alternate bearing surfaces continue to show promise in increasing the longevity of hip arthroplasty. Low wear rates have been shown recently for ceramic-on-polyethylene bearing implants. Long-term survivorship was excellent even when substandard techniques were used, including 32-mm heads articulating with noncrosslinked polyethylene, inferior stem design, and first-generation cement techniques. Survivorship probabilities were in the range of 80% at 20 years.

Using hard surfaces such as ceramics also theoretically improves the benefits of highly cross-linked polyethylene. The ability of cross-linked UHMWPE to resist wear is inversely proportional to the surface roughness of the articulating head. Cobalt-chromium heads undergo oxidation and abrasion in vivo, leading to increased roughness. Ceramics are relatively resistant to those types of degradation. A report of the 10-year follow-up of a small group of patients who had received alumina-on-cross-linked UHMWPE bearings showed no significant osteolysis. The mean linear wear rate was demonstrated to be 0.02 mm/yr after a 2-year period of bedding-in. Ceramics also demonstrate excellent wear characteristics when used as hard-on-hard bearings. Alumina-on-alumina hip arthroplasty results after 18.5 years of follow-up failed to show any significant linear wear rate in the implanted surfaces. The patients also had minimal amounts of osteolysis. Of the cups requiring revision, only 3 of 19 required any bone graft, and 7 required upsizing to a cup size that was 4 mm larger. Most failures were secondary to acute debonding of the ceramic cup from the cement. It is hoped that design improvements have eliminated the technical reasons for failure in this model.

Zirconium has a long history of use in total hip arthroplasty as outlined in a recent article. Hip simulator models have shown excellent wear characteristics when comparing oxidized zirconium with cobalt-chromium heads, especially when articulating with cross-linked polyethylene. It remains to be seen, however, whether these promising results will yield comparable clinical success.

Metal-on-metal bearings have shown promising results in the short term. A report of 70 prostheses placed in the early 1990s and followed-up for a mean of 5.2 years demonstrated no progressive radiolucencies. Only a single cup was revised for mechanical failure, and two others for recurrent dislocations. None of the femora were revised. Concerns remain, however, regarding the long-term effects of systemic metallosis. Serum cobalt levels have been shown to remain at a constantly elevated state up to 5 years after metal-on-metal hip implantation. The significance of this occurrence is currently unknown. Because of the lack of data on long-term effects, it seems especially prudent not to use these devices in women of child-bearing age and patients with renal failure (serum cobalt is excreted via the kidney).

Additional risk factors have been identified for osteolysis. Long-term follow-up of patients who have undergone total hip arthroplasty has consistently demonstrated young age, male sex, and higher activity levels as significant risk factors (men have been shown to have more than 2½ times the risk of women for osteolysis). Other implant components that increase the risk for osteolysis, such as Hylamer liners, titanium femoral heads, and use of 32-mm femoral heads on noncross-linked polyethylene are no longer used. Nevertheless, clinicians should be aware of their use in the past and take their track record into

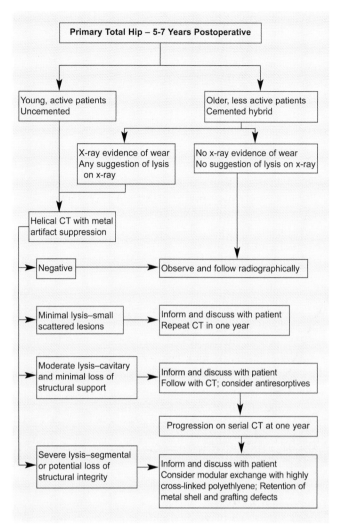

Figure 3 Algorithm for monitoring pelvic osteolysis in patients who have undergone primary total hip replacement surgery. (Reproduced with permission from Stulberg SD, Wixson RL, Adams AD, Hendrix RW, Bernfield JB: Monitoring pelvic osteolysis following total hip replacement surgery: An algorithm for surveillance. *J Bone Joint Surg Am* 2002;84(suppl 2):116-122.)

account when treating a patient with any of these components.

Responding to Osteolysis

As with any potential adverse effect of medical treatment, the management of osteolysis is two-pronged: serial evaluations should be conducted to provide early detection and assessment, and the complication itself should be treated.

Radiographic Surveillance After Total Hip Arthroplasty

Plain radiography has long been known to underestimate the degree of osteolysis. It is now clear that osteolysis may be radiographically as well as clinically silent. Studies using CT to evaluate high-risk patients have documented extensive osteolysis that is not visible using plain radiography. Even combining oblique radiographs

with standard AP pelvis and femoral radiographs only results in a 74% chance that an experienced senior orthopedist will accurately identify a pelvic lesion. Serial examinations are recommended, especially during the first 5 to 7 years of follow-up, to assess patients for both ingrowth and development of lesions and/or loosening. CT has been recommended in young, active patients within the 5- to 7-year period to identify clinically and radiographically silent lesions early. An algorithm was recently devised specifically for assessing pelvic osteolysis (Figure 3). Patients with a high linear wear rate should be considered high risk regardless of age or use pattern and followed appropriately.

Describing and Classifying Osteolysis

It is important to remember that not all osteolysis looks alike. Cementless prostheses that cause osteolysis result in a more expansive and often focal type of lesion. The location and development of that lesion can vary greatly, depending on the implant's ability to limit the effective joint space. In many patients, large bone lesions may be present without compromising the stability of the implant. With cemented implants, however, an interface membrane occurs between the polymethylmethacrylate and bone, causing slow and progressive linear bone loss. This proceeds in a centrifugal direction from the joint, ultimately leading to prosthesis loosening, even when bone loss does not appear to be severe. Implant loosening can be assumed when circumferential radiolucency, migration of the implant, or cracking of the cement mantle is visible.

One difficult issue facing the clinician is when to intervene. Suggested indications include symptomatic lesions, expansive osteolysis involving the posterosuperior acetabular column or > 50% of the cup, an enlarging defect (especially if a high linear wear rate is calculated), and imminent wear-through of the polyethylene liner. Computer-assisted assessment of polyethylene wear has been described, but most clinicians are unlikely to have access to such sophisticated tools. A simple clinical assessment method has been described using only templates of the acetabular prosthesis. The templates must be obtained from the manufacturer, but they have been shown to allow easy and accurate assessment of the remaining polyethylene.

Older classification systems of bone loss (Gruen's model for femora and DeLee and Charnley's model for acetabuli) are primarily descriptive. The American Academy of Orthopaedic Surgeons developed a classification system that further describes the type of lesion (for example, as segmental or cavitary). Simple and elegant classification systems for the femur and acetabulum have also recently been described and have proved beneficial in formulating treatment plans. A review of the specifics of revision hip arthroplasty is beyond the

Table 1 | Classification and Treatment Algorithm for Managing Femoral Bone Loss

Class	Lesion	Recommendation
Type I	Minimal cancellous bone loss	Cemented (provided neocortex removed) or cementless fixation
Type II	Extensive metaphyseal loss, but with intact cortex	Proximal or distal fixation revision implant
Type IIIA	Nonsupportive metaphysis, with > 4 cm of diaphysis preserved for distal fixation	Distal fixation with extensively coated implant
Type IIIB	Nonsupportive metaphysis, with < 4 cm diaphysis preserved	Modular, cementless, tapered stem with flutes for rotational control
Type IV	Nonsupportive isthmus with extensive canal widening	Options include: impaction grafting, allograft-prosthesis composite (younger patients), and proximal femoral replacement (elderly patients)

(Adapted with permission from Valle CJ, Paprosky WG: Classification and an algorithmic approach to the reconstruction of femoral deficiency in revision total hip arthroplasty. J Bone Joint Surg Am 2003;85-A(suppl 4):1-6.

Table 2 | Classification and Treatment Algorithm for Managing Femoral Bone Loss

Class	Lesion	Recommendation
Type I	No significant deficiency	Cemented (if neocortex removed) or cementless fixation
Type II	Contained (cavitary) loss of bone	Proximal and/or distal fixation implant, impaction grafting
Type III	Noncircumferential segmental deficiency	Strut allografting
Type IV	Uncontained bone loss < 5cm; diaphysis intact	Calcar replacing implants
Type V	Uncontained bone loss > 5cm into diaphyseal	Structural allograft or tumor prosthesis

(Reproduced from Gross AE, Blackley H, Wong P, Saleh K, Woodgate I: The role of allografts in revision arthroplasty of the hip. Instr Course Lect 2002;51:103-113.)

scope of this chapter; this topic is discussed in chapter 41. Focus instead is given to recently described classification systems and treatment recommendations.

Treatment

Femoral Deficiency

A classification system and algorithm for the treatment of femoral bone loss has been described and refined and is presented in Table 1. This algorithm is based on the remaining femoral bone's ability to support distal cementless fixation. It is important to remember that the amount of bone loss is only accurately determined after removal of the previous prosthesis, regardless of the classification system used. The authors who described this classification system and algorithm reported frequent use of an extended trochanteric osteotomy during revision surgery. They reported excellent results: 90% or more of the patients with type I, II, or IIIA femoral bone loss who underwent revision using this algorithm showed osseointegration after 8 years. Patients with type IIIB or IV femoral bone loss are challenging to treat. For this patient population, good results have been reported using a combined allograft-prosthesis construct, with 77% of patients in a recent series reported as having successful outcomes.

Pelvic Osteolysis

Pelvic osteolysis presents another set of treatment variables. As stated previously, cemented prostheses tend to loosen before expansive bony destruction occurs. Cementless cups, however, are able to remain well fixed despite large expansile lesions. A classification and treatment algorithm for these lesions is presented in Table 2.

The specific problem of expansile osteolysis in cementless cups has been extensively studied. These implants will often remain stable despite florid osteolysis, and removing the cup can add significant morbidity to the revision procedure. Because there is no acetabular counterpart to the extended trochanteric osteotomy, some studies have reported on the retention of well-fixed, cementless sockets. In these patients, the liner is exchanged and débridement and bone grafting of osteolytic foci is performed as access permits. Specific conditions must be met for socket retention: (1) the components must be in good alignment, (2) the locking mechanism for a new liner must be intact, (3) the metal shell must not be damaged, (4) the new polyethylene must be of adequate thickness, (5) the implant to be retained must have a good track record, and (6) the implant must be modular. Some additional steps must be undertaken to decrease the wear rate that might include any of the following: upgrading to highly cross-linked polyethylene, downsizing the femoral head, or converting the femoral head to a ceramic surface. Good results for short- to medium-term follow-up have been reported using these guidelines. A 50% decrease in wear rate has been shown, along with resolution of many lesions and cessation of progression. One recent article described the attempted salvage of failed locking mechanisms in modular liners that are well fixed and reported reasonable success with the double socket technique (cementing a liner into the cementless cup).

In revision hip surgery, it is important to keep first principles in mind, and remember that any classification system is attempting to answer several basic questions: (1) Which implants, if any, are stable? Are they also well aligned? (2) What type of graft support will the bony defects require? (3) Is there pelvic discontinuity? (4) What is the best surgical approach for the necessary procedure (including contingency plans)? (5) What tools will be necessary to safely extract and insert the components?

Future Medical Therapy

Along with the steady advancement toward the elimination of wear debris, the search for a medical management of osteolysis continues. Bisphosphonates have recently been shown to significantly decrease production of TNF-α in vitro, most likely by causing macrophage apoptosis. Unfortunately, oral doses of bisphosphonates have not been useful in preventing or treating osteolytic lesions. Other studies have shown that a single topical application of a bisphosphonate solution in a rat model dramatically inhibited osteolysis. Gene therapy has shown mixed results. An attempt at using an adenoviral vector to transfect cells and produce a soluble TNF-α antagonist demonstrated a strong inflammatory response to the vector itself, which the soluble TNF antagonist was not able to overcome. Another study reported producing osteoprotegerin by transfected cells and thereby decreased debris-mediated osteolysis to control levels. Additionally, erythromycin was shown to inhibit osteoclast development, absolute osteoclast numbers, and activation of the NFκB system in a titanium debris model. The local delivery of this type of agent to at-risk patients deserves further exploration.

Summary

Osteolysis remains the essential complication associated with total hip arthroplasty. Continued work on the understanding and manipulation of the molecular biology of osteolysis may result in adjunctive and even prophylactic medical therapy of osteolysis. Advancements in the design and production of bearing surfaces may limit the production of particulate debris to levels more easily tolerated by the host. Methods of both primary and revision fixation continue to be improved.

Annotated Bibliography

What Causes Osteolysis?

Clarke IC, Manaka M, Green DD, et al: Current status of Zirconia used in total hip implants. *J Bone Joint Surg Am* 2003;85-A(suppl 4):73-84.

The authors discuss the production methods, clinical performance, and retrieval studies of zirconium bearings to date. The article includes a review of all published studies to date on the clinical data surrounding zirconium implants.

Clohisy JC, Hirayama T, Frazier E, Han S-K, Abu-Amer Y: NF-kB signaling blockade abolishes implant particle-induced osteoclastogenesis. *J Orthop Res* 2004;22:13-20.

The authors of this study report that blockade of the inhibitory kappa B–NFκB dissociation using three different methods effectively prevented polymethylmethacrylate particle-induced osteoclastogenesis.

Dorr LD, Wan Z, Longjohn DB, Dubois B, Murken R: Total hip arthroplasty with use of the Metasul metal-on-metal articulation. *J Bone Joint Surg Am* 2000;82(6):789-798.

In this study, 56 of 70 patients were followed for an average of 5.2 years (range, 4 to 6.8 years). Only one acetabulum was revised for osteolysis. Two other acetabuli were revised because of recurrent dislocation. No femora were revised. No evidence of progressive radiolucencies was observed, nor was any focal osteolysis.

Hamadouche M, Boutin P, Daussange J, Bolander ME, Sedel L: Alumina-on-alumina total hip arthroplasty: A minimum 18.5-year follow-up study. *J Bone Joint Surg Am* 2002;84-A(1):69-77.

The authors of this study performed 118 consecutive total hip arthroplasties in 106 patients over a 2-year period. Twenty-five patients required revision of one or both components; all cemented cup revisions (19 of the 25 necessary revisions) were secondary to acute debonding of the cement-alumina interface, resulting in cup tilt and an unstable component. Linear wear rate was less than 0.025 mm/yr. Variables significant for revision were the abduction angle greater than 45° and cup diameter less than 48 mm.

Hermida JC, Bergula A, Chen P, Colwell CW Jr, D'Lima DD: Comparison of the wear rates of twenty-eight and thirty-two millimeter femoral heads on cross-linked polyethylene acetabular cups in a wear simulator. *J Bone Joint Surg Am* 2003;85-A(12):2325-2331.

Highly cross-linked polyethylene liners were tested in a hip simulator and showed a decrease in wear per million cycles from 16.92 to 2.57 for 32-mm femoral heads and 14.97 to 1.51 in 28-mm femoral heads.

O'Connor DT, Choi MG, Kwon SY, Sung K-LP: New insight into the mechanism of hip prosthesis loosening: Effect of titanium debris size on osteoblast function. *J Orthop Res* 2004;22:229-236.

Rat osteoblasts were shown to demonstrate morphologic changes (thickening of actin fibers) and decreased proliferation in response to titanium particles in the size range of 1.5 to 4 μm.

Orishimo KF, Claus AM, Sychterz CJ, Engh CA: Relationship between polyethylene wear and osteolysis in hips with a second-generation porous-coated cementless cup after seven years of follow-up. *J Bone Joint Surg Am* 2003;85-A(6):1095-1099.

The authors of this study assessed 56 hips to quantify the increased risk associated with increasing linear and volumetric wear rates.

Patil S, Bergula A, Chen PC, Colwell CW Jr, D'Lima DD: Polyethylene wear and acetabular component orientation. *J Bone Joint Surg Am* 2003;85-A(suppl 4):56-63.

In this study, finite element analysis predicted increased peak stresses with increasing cup abduction angle and decreased peak stresses with increasing cup anteversion. Hip simulator wear rates correlated with the difference in predicted peak stresses. Additionally, clinical review of 56 consecutive patients demonstrated a 40% increase in mean linear wear associated with abduction angles greater than 45°.

Sabokbar A, Kudo O, Athanasou NA: Two distinct cellular mechanisms of osteoclast formation and bone resorption in periprosthetic osteolysis. *J Orthop Res* 2003;21:73-80.

Osteoprotegerin and RANK:Fc failed to inhibit TNF-α stimulation of osteoclastogenesis. This suggests that TNF-α and RANK are linked to separate pathways leading to osteolysis.

Teitelbaum SL: Bone resorption by osteoclasts. *Science* 2000;289:1504-1508.

The authors provide a concise review of the knowledge to date regarding osteoclast development, function, and regulation.

Urban JA, Garvin KL, Boese CK, et al: Ceramic-on-polyethylene bearing surfaces in total hip arthroplasty: Seventeen to twenty-one-year results. *J Bone Joint Surg Am* 2001;83-A(11):1688-1694.

In this study, a single surgeon performed ceramic-on-polyethylene total hip arthroplasties in 64 patients using first-generation techniques and a 32-mm femoral head. The average linear wear rate was 0.034 mm/yr. The average volumetric wear was 28.012 mm/yr. The probability of retention of the prosthesis was 95%, 95%, 89%, and 79% at 5, 10, 15, and 20 years, respectively.

von Knoch M, Jewison DE, Sibonga JD, et al: The effectiveness of polyethylene versus titanium particles in inducing osteolysis in vivo. *J Orthop Res* 2004;22:237-243.

A murine model was used to compare the osteolytic response to titanium and UHMWPE particles. Significantly higher bony resorption and osteoclastic response was shown ($P = 0.0165$ and 0.0059, respectively) for the UHMWPE particles. Particle size ranged from 1 to 5 μm.

Wright TM, Goodman SB (eds): *Implant Wear in Total Joint Replacement*. Rosemont, IL, American Academy of Orthopaedic Surgeons, 2000.

The authors provide a review of the multifactorial nature of implant wear and its impact on implant survival.

Young AM, Sychterz CJ, Hopper RH, Engh CA: Effect of acetabular modularity on polyethylene wear and osteolysis in total hip arthroplasty. *J Bone Joint Surg Am* 2002;84-A:58-63.

In this retrospective review of 41 patients with or without acetabular modularity, the authors identified an increased (but not statistically significant) wear rate. A statistically significantly decreased rate of osteolysis (2% versus 22%) was identified for the patients with nonmodular components.

Responding to Osteolysis

Beaule PE, Ebramzadeh E, LeDuff M, Prasad R, Amstutz HC: Cementing a liner into a stable cementless acetabular shell: The double-socket technique. *J Bone Joint Surg Am* 2004;86-A:929-934.

Short-term results were reported for revisions of well-fixed, modular acetabular shells with failed locking mechanisms. The authors found that polyethylene or metal liners were cementing into existing shells. The average follow-up was 5.1 years for 32 patients, among which 6 revisions were performed. Twenty-two percent of hips dislocated, and the 5-year survival rate was estimated at 78%.

Claus AM, Engh CA Jr, Sychterz CJ, Xenos JS, Orishimo KF, Engh CA Sr: Radiographic definition of pelvic osteolysis following total hip arthroplasty. *J Bone Joint Surg Am* 2003;85-A:1519-1526.

The authors conducted this study to determine the sensitivity and specificity of plain radiography in identifying pelvic osteolysis in patients who have undergone total hip arthroplasty. Studies done by an experienced orthopaedist achieved 73.6% sensitivity, even when four radiographic views were offered. The sensitivity for a single radiographic view was 47.2%. The overall specificity was 93%.

Gross AE, Blackley H, Wong P, Saleh K, Woodgate I: The role of allografts in revision arthroplasty of the hip. *Instr Course Lect* 2002;51:103-113.

This article discusses the authors' classification systems for both acetabular and femoral bone loss. Treatment algorithms describing the use of allografts on both sides of the hip as well as outcomes are also discussed.

Maloney WJ, Paprosky W, Engh CA, Rubash H: Surgical treatment of pelvic osteolysis. *Clin Orthop* 2001;393:78-84.

In this study, 68 consecutive instances of pelvic osteolysis were treated based on an algorithm for assessing acetabular salvageability. All patients had liner exchange. All patients with type 1 osteolytic lesions underwent curettage and bone grafting. In those with type 2 lesions, the entire cup was revised, with bone grafting of defects. Approximately one third of the patients with each type of osteolytic lesion showed resolution of osteolysis within a mean of 3.5 years, whereas the other two thirds all showed a decrease in the size of the lesions.

Pollock D, Sychterz CJ, Engh CA: A clinically practical method of manually assessing polyethylene liner thickness. *J Bone Joint Surg Am* 2001;83-A:1803-1809.

The authors of this study used templates obtained from the manufacturer to evaluate femoral head penetration. Comparison of this new method to those of Livermore and Dorr showed it to be significantly more accurate.

Puri L, Wixson RL, Stern SH, Kohli J, Hendrix RW, Stulberg SD: Use of helical computed tomography for the assessment of acetabular osteolysis after total hip arthroplasty. *J Bone Joint Surg Am* 2002;84-A:609-614.

Helical CT with metal-artifact minimization software aided the evaluation of osteolytic lesions in 16 pelves. Patients were chosen for evaluation because of increased risk factors for osteolysis (based on age, activity level, and size). Of the 16 patients included in the study, 13 had significantly more osteolysis on CT than plain radiography, and one of these patients underwent revision based on the CT findings.

Stulberg SD, Wixson RL, Adams AD, Hendrix RW, Bernfield JB: Monitoring pelvic osteolysis following total hip replacement surgery: an algorithm for surveillance. *J Bone Joint Surg Am* 2002;84-A(suppl 2):116-122.

The authors provide an update of previous work using helical CT to evaluate high-risk patients for osteolysis. They found that 48% of patients had osteolysis that was not clinically evident. Half of these patients had no visible evidence of osteolysis on plain radiographs either. Thirty-six percent of these patients had cavitary osteolysis, and 11% had segmental osteolysis. The authors recommended the use of a baseline CT scan at 7 to 10 years postoperatively for the detection of occult osteolysis.

Valle CJ, Paprosky WG: Classification and an algorithmic approach to the reconstruction of femoral deficiency in revision total hip arthroplasty. *J Bone Joint Surg Am* 2003;85-A(suppl 4):1-6.

The authors reported on 71 consecutive femoral revisions that were reviewed at a minimum of 8 years after surgery. Engh's classification system was used to assess stability. They found that 96% of the femoral components were bone ingrown or had fibrous stable fixation.

Future Medical Therapy

Astrand J, Aspenberg P: Topical, single dose bisphosphonate treatment reduces resorption in a rat model for prosthetic loosening. *J Orthop Res* 2004;22:244-249.

The authors of this study found that a one-time topical dose of an alendronate solution significantly decreased bone resorption in a fluid-pressure model of osteolysis in rats.

Classic Bibliography

D'Antonio JA: Periprosthetic bone loss of the acetabulum: Classification and management. *Orthop Clin North Am* 1992;23:279-290.

DeLee JG, Charnley J: Radiological demarcation of cemented sockets in total hip replacement. *Clin Orthop* 1976;121:20-32.

Engh CA, Massin P, Suthers KE: Roentgenographic assessment of the biologic fixation of porous-surfaced femoral components. *Clin Orthop* 1990;257:107-128.

Gruen TA, McNeice GM, Amstutz HC: "Modes of failure" of cemented stem-type femoral components: A radiographic analysis of loosening. *Clin Orthop* 1979;141:17-27.

McKellop HA, Campbell P, Sang-Hyun P, et al: The origin of submicron polyethylene wear debris in total hip arthroplasty. *Clin Orthop* 1995;311:3-20.

Merkel KD, Erdmann JM, McHugh KP, Abu-Amer Y, Ross FP, Teitelbaum SL: Tumor necrosis factor-alpha mediates orthopedic implant osteolysis. *Am J Pathol* 1999;154(1):203-210.

Schmalzried TP, Jasty M, Harris WH: Periprosthetic bone loss in total hip arthroplasty: Polyethylene wear debris and the concept of the effective joint space. *J Bone Joint Surg Am* 1992;74(6):849-863.

Schmalzried TP, Kwon LM, Jasty M, et al: The mechanism of loosening of cemented acetabular components in total hip arthroplasty. *Clin Orthop* 1992;274:60-78.

Shanbhag AS, Jacobs JJ, Black J, Galante JO, Glant TT: Macrophage/particle interactions: Effect of size, composition and surface area. *J Biomed Mater Res* 1994;28:81-90.

Tanzer M, Maloney WJ, Jasty M, Harris WH: The progression of femoral cortical osteolysis in association with total hip arthroplasty without cement. *J Bone Joint Surg Am* 1992;74(3):404-410.

Wroblewski BM, Siney PD, Fleming PA: Low-friction arthroplasty of the hip using alumina ceramic and crosslinked polyethylene: A ten-year follow-up report. *J Bone Joint Surg Br* 1999;81(1):54-55.

Zicat B, Engh CA, Gokcen E: Patterns of osteolysis around total hip components inserted with and without cement. *J Bone Joint Surg Am* 1995;77(3):432-439.

Index